CLERKSHIP
GUIDE

CLERKSHIP GUIDES

Your Essential Guide to Clinical Clerkships

All you need to succeed:

- Practice Cases
- Frequently Asked Questions
- Key Points
- Practice Exam

Other Titles in the *Clerkship Guides* Series

Adams:
Surgical Subspecialties Clerkship Guide

Manley:
Psychiatry Clerkship Guide

Paauw, Burkholder, and Migeon:
Internal Medicine Clerkship Guide

Woodhead:
Pediatric Clerkship Guide

Woodland:
Obstetrics and Gynecology Clerkship Guide

SURGERY CLERKSHIP GUIDE

Gregg A. Adams, MD

Clinical Instructor
Stanford University
  School of Medicine
Stanford, California
Director, Surgical
  Education
Santa Clara Valley
  Medical Center
San Jose, California

Adella M. Garland, MD

Director, Minimally
  Invasive Surgery
Santa Clara Valley
  Medical Center
San Jose, California

Clayton H. Shatney, MD

Clinical Associate Professor
Stanford University
  School of Medicine
Stanford, California
Staff Surgeon
Santa Clara Valley
  Medical Center
San Jose, California

John P. Sherck, MD

Clinical Professor of
  Surgery
Stanford University
  School of Medicine
Stanford, California
Director, Trauma and
  Critical Care
Santa Clara Valley
  Medical Center
San Jose, California

Sherry M. Wren, MD

Associate Professor of
  Surgery
Stanford University
  School of Medicine
Stanford, California
Chief, General Surgery
Palo Alto Veterans Hospital
Palo Alto, California

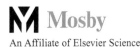 Mosby

An Affiliate of Elsevier Science

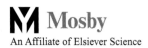
Mosby
An Affiliate of Elsiever Science

11830 Westline Industrial Drive
St. Louis, Missouri 63146

SURGERY CLERKSHIP GUIDE ISBN 0–323–01857–2
Copyright © 2003, Mosby, Inc. All Rights Reserved

Notice

Surgery is an ever-changing field. Standard safety precautions must be followed, but as new research and clinical experience broaden our knowledge, changes in treatment and drug therapy may become necessary or appropriate. Readers are advised to check the most current product information provided by the manufacturer of each drug to be administered to verify the recommended dose, the method and duration of administration, and contraindications. It is the responsibility of the treating physician, relying on experience and knowledge of the patient, to determine dosages and the best treatment for each individual patient. Neither the Publisher nor the editor assumes any liability for any injury and/or damage to persons or property arising from this publication.

The Publisher

Library of Congress Cataloging-in-Publication Data
Surgery clerkship guide / [edited by] Gregg A. Adams ... [et al.].–1st ed.
　　　p.; cm
　　ISBN 0-323-01857-2
　　　1. Surgery–Examinations, questions, etc. 2. Clinical clerkship–Examinations, questions, etc. I. Adams, Gregg A.
　　[DNLM: 1. Clinical Clerkship–Case Report. 2. Surgical Procedures, Operative–Case Report. WO 500 S961003 2004]
RD37.2.S965 2004
617′.0071′55 –dc21　　　　　　　　　　　　　　　　　　2003056136

Acquisitions Editor: William Schmitt
Project Manager: Amy Norwitz
Book Designer: Gene Harris
Developmental Editor: Kevin Kochanski

KI/QWF

Printed in the United States of America.

Last digit is the print number: 9 8 7 6 5 4 3 2 1

This book
is dedicated
to students
of all ages.

Contributors

Gregg A. Adams, MD
Clinical Instructor
Stanford University School of Medicine
Stanford, California
Director, Surgical Education
Santa Clara Valley Medical Center
San Jose, California

Maria D. Allo, MD
Chair, Department of Surgery
Santa Clara Valley Medical Center
San Jose, California

Kristi M. Almo, MD
Clinical Fellow, Minimally Invasive Surgery
Cedars-Sinai Medical Center
Los Angeles, California

Juan A. Asensio-Gonzalez, MD
Unit Chief, Trauma Surgery Service "A"
Division of Trauma Surgery and Surgical Critical Care
Department of Surgery
Associate Professor
University of Southern California Keck School of Medicine
Senior Attending Surgeon
LAC/USC Medical Center
Los Angeles, California

Mirza K. Baig, MD
Department of Colorectal Surgery
Cleveland Clinic Florida
Weston, Florida

Nicole Baril, MD
Staff Physician
Kaiser Hospital
Corona, California

William Bergman, MD
Clinical Associate Professor of Neurosurgery
Stanford University School of Medicine
Director of Neurotrauma
Santa Clara Valley Medical Center
San Jose, California

Thomas V. Berne, MD
Professor of Surgery
University of Southern California School of Medicine
Chief of Surgery
LAC/USC Medical Center
Los Angeles, California

Peter D. Cahill, MD
Clinical Instructor
Stanford University School of Medicine
Stanford, California
Staff Surgeon
Santa Clara Valley Medical Center
San Jose, California

Bipan Chand, MD
Endoscopic Fellow
Cleveland Clinic Foundation
Department of General Surgery
Cleveland, Ohio

Michael Coady, MD
Fellow, Cardiothoracic Surgery
Stanford University School of Medicine
Stanford, California

Gaston Cornu-Labat, MD
Fellow, Hepatobiliary and Pancreatic Surgery
Virginia Mason Medical Center
Seattle, Washington

Alvaro D. Davila, MD
Clinical Assistant Professor of Medicine
Stanford University School of Medicine
Stanford, California
Associate Chief of Gastroenterology
Santa Clara Valley Medical Center
San Jose, California

Raquel E. Davila, MD
Clinical Instructor of Medicine
Division of Gastroenterology
Oregon Health Sciences University
Portland, Oregon

Eric J. Dozois, MD
Department of Surgery
Division of Colon and Rectal Surgery
Mayo Clinic
Rochester, Minnesota

Quan-Yang Duh, MD
Professor of Surgery
University of California, San Francisco,
    School of Medicine
San Francisco, California

Timothy C. Fabian, MD
Professor and Chairman, Department of Surgery
University of Tennessee Health Science Center
Memphis, Tennessee

Victor W. Fazio, MD
Chairman, Department of Colorectal Surgery
The Cleveland Clinic Foundation
Cleveland, Ohio

David V. Feliciano, MD
Professor of Surgery
Emory University School of Medicine
Chief of Surgery
Grady Memorial Hospital
Atlanta, Georgia

Adella M. Garland, MD
Director, Minimally Invasive Surgery
Santa Clara Valley Medical Center
San Jose, California

Stanley M. Goldberg, MD
Adjunct Professor of Surgery
Division of Colorectal Surgery
University of Minnesota
Minneapolis, Minnesota

James E. Goodnight, MD, PhD
Pearl Stamps Stewart Chair and Professor,
 Department of Surgery
University of California, Davis
Davis, California

Ralph S. Greco, MD
Chief, Division of General Surgery
Stanford University School of Medicine
Stanford, California

Steven S. Guest, MD
Clinical Associate Professor of Medicine
Stanford University School of Medicine
Stanford, California
Associate Director, Division of Nephrology
Santa Clara Valley Medical Center
San Jose, California

E. John Harris, Jr., MD
Associate Professor of Surgery
Department of Vascular Surgery
Stanford University School of Medicine
Stanford, California

Kyle Harrison, MD
Resident, Department of Anesthesia
Stanford University School of Medicine
Stanford, California

Marion C. W. Henry, MD
Resident, General Surgery
Stanford University School of Medicine
Stanford, California

David N. Herndon, MD
Professor of Surgery
University of Texas Medical Branch
Chief of Staff
Distinguished Chair in Burn Surgery
Shriners Burn Hospital for Children
Galveston, Texas

Steven K. Howard, MD
Staff Physician
VA Palo Alto Health Care System
Associate Professor of Anesthesia
Stanford University School of Medicine
Stanford, California

David K. Imagawa, MD, PhD
Associate Professor of Surgery and Pathology
Section Chief, Hepatobiliary and Pancreas Surgery
Department of Surgery
University of California, Irvine, Medical Center
Orange, California

Jeff L. Johnson, MD
Assistant Professor of Surgery
University of Colorado Health Science Center
Assistant Director SICU, Denver Health
Denver Health Medical Center
Denver, Colorado

James Kraatz. MD
Adjunct Faculty
University of Minnesota School of Medicine
Burn Unit, Hennepin County Medical Center
Minneapolis, Minnesota

Richard Lafayette, MD
Associate Professor
Associate Chief of Nephrology
Division of Nephrology
Stanford University School of Medicine
Stanford, California

George Lai, MD
Fellow, Division of Nephrology
Stanford University School of Medicine
Stanford, California

John T. Langell, MD, PhD
Resident, General Surgery
Department of Surgery
Stanford University School of Medicine
Stanford, California

Rebecca Legg, MD
Fellow, Critical Care Medicine
Department of Anesthesiology
Stanford University School of Medicine
Stanford, California

H. Peter Lorenz, MD
Associate Professor
Division of Plastic Surgery and Reconstructive Surgery
Stanford University School of Medicine
Stanford, California

Melinda Maggard, MD
Clinical Instructor
Department of Surgery
University of California, Los Angeles,
    Medical School
Los Angeles, California

Louis J. Magnotti, MD
Trauma Fellow
Presley Regional Trauma Center
University of Tennessee
Memphis, Tennessee

Trigg McClellan, MD
Premier Orthopaedics
Summit Care Center
Hermitage, Tennessee

Doug N. Miniati, MD
Chief Resident, General Surgery
Department of Surgery
Stanford University School of Medicine
Stanford, California

Ernest E. Moore, MD
Professor and Vice Chairman
Department of Surgery
University of Colorado Health Science Center
Chief, Department of Surgery
Denver Health Medical Center
Denver, Colorado

Thelinh Nguyen, MD
Division of Vascular Surgery
Barnes Hospital Plaza
St. Louis, Missouri

David D. Oakes, MD
Professor of Surgery
Stanford University School of Medicine
Stanford, California
Staff Surgeon
Santa Clara Valley Medical Center
San Jose, California

Cornelius Olcott IV, MD
Professor of Surgery
Department of Vascular Surgery
Stanford University School of Medicine
Stanford, California

John T. Owings, MD
Assistant Professor
Department of Surgery
University of California, Davis, School of Medicine
Sacramento, California

Jimmy Pak, MD
Vascular Surgery Research Fellow
Department of Surgery
Stanford University School of Medicine
Stanford, California

Edward H. Phillips, MD
Director, Center for Minimally Invasive Surgery
Chairholder, Storz-Berci Chair in Minimally Invasive Surgery
Cedars-Sinai Medical Center
Los Angeles, California

Feza H. Remzi, MD
Staff Surgeon
Department of Colorectal Surgery
The Cleveland Clinic Foundation
Cleveland, Ohio

Alexander S. Rosemurgy II, MD
Professor of Surgery and Medicine
Director, Surgical Digestive Disorders
Director, Division of General Surgery
The Vivian Clark Reeves/Joy McCann Culverhouse
   Endowed Chair for Digestive Disorders and Pancreatic Cancer
University of South Florida
Tampa General Hospital
Tampa, Florida

Bassem Safadi, MD
Assistant Professor of Surgery
Stanford University School of Medicine
Staff Surgeon
Surgical Service
Palo Alto Veterans Hospital
Palo Alto, California

Robert G. Sawyer, MD
Associate Professor of Surgery
Co-Director, Surgical Trauma Intensive Care Unit
University of Virginia School of Medicine
Charlottesville, Virginia

William P. Schecter, MD
Professor of Clinical Surgery
University of California, San Francisco, School of Medicine
Chief of Surgery
San Francisco General Hospital
San Francisco, California

Stephen A. Schendel, MD, DDS
Professor of Plastic Surgery
Department of Surgery
Stanford University School of Medicine
Stanford, California

Paul Schmit, MD
Department of Surgery
University of California, Los Angeles, Medical School
Los Angeles, California

Adam Seiver, MD, PhD, MBA
Clinical Assistant Professor
Stanford University School of Medicine
Stanford, California

John P. Sherck, MD
Clinical Professor of Surgery
Stanford University School of Medicine
Stanford, California
Director, Trauma and Critical Care
Santa Clara Valley Medical Center
San Jose, California

Ming-Sing Si, MD
Resident, Department of Surgery
University of California, Irvine, Medical Center
Orange, California

Gregorio A. Sicard, MD
Professor of Surgery
Division of Vascular Surgery
Barnes Hospital
St. Louis, Missouri

Howard Silberman, MD
Professor of Surgery
University of Southern California, Los Angeles, School of Medicine
Los Angeles, California

Tej M. Singh, MD
Clinical Faculty
Stanford University School of Medicine
Chief, Division of Vascular Surgery
Director of Endovascular Surgery
Santa Clara Valley Medical Center
San Jose, California

Allan Siperstein, MD
Head, Section of Endocrine Surgery
Department of General Surgery
The Cleveland Clinic Foundation
Cleveland, Ohio

Contributors

Payam Tabrizi, MD
Director, Orthopedic Trauma
Department of Orthopedics
Santa Clara Valley Medical Center
San Jose, California

Jesse E. Thompson, Jr., MD
Professor of Surgery
University of California, Los Angeles, School of Medicine
Chairman, Department of Surgery
Olive View/UCLA Medical Center
Sylmar, California

Areti Tillou, MD
Assistant Unit Chief, Trauma Surgery Service "A"
Division of Trauma Surgery
Surgical Critical Care
Department of Surgery
LAC/USC Medical Center
Department of Surgery
Los Angeles, California

L. William Traverso, MD
Clinical Professor of Surgery
University of Washington School of Medicine
Attending Surgeon
Virginia Mason Medical Center
Seattle, Washington

Caesar Ursic, MD
Assistant Professor of Surgery
University of California, San Francisco, East Bay, School of
    Medicine
Trauma Director, Highland General Hospital
Alameda County Medical Center
Oakland, California

Stephen B. Vogel, MD
Professor of Surgery
University of Florida, JHM Health Center
Gainesville, Florida

Steven D. Wexner, MD
Chairman and Residency Program Director
Department of Colorectal Surgery
Chief of Staff
Cleveland Clinic Florida—Weston
Weston, Florida

James E. Wiedeman, MD
Associate Professor of Surgery
Uniformed Services University of the Health Sciences
Staff Surgeon
Mather VA Medical Center
Sacramento, California

Sherry M. Wren, MD
Associate Professor of Surgery
Stanford University School of Medicine
Stanford, California
Chief, General Surgery
Palo Alto Veterans Hospital
Palo Alto, California

Christopher K. Zarins, MD
Professor and Chief, Department of Vascular Surgery
Stanford University School of Medicine
Stanford, California

Preface

Surgery is an enormous subject. Moreover, surgery clerkships provoke an unwarranted amount of anxiety. To effectively study surgery (and relieve your anxiety) you'll need an organized approach to a wide variety of surgical problems. In addition, you'll need a set of skills that includes gathering data and organizing and communicating information to help care for surgical patients. The *Surgery Clerkship Guide* will supply all these needs.

This book is designed to guide you safely through your clerkship and provide a brief reference. It is not intended to be an exhaustive description of the field of surgery. The text is organized into three sections covering basic skills, common presenting complaints or findings, and common surgical problems. Each section gives a straightforward description of surgical problems and an approach to the patient's work-up. A discussion of each problem includes tips for preoperative and postoperative care. *Key Points* in each chapter will help you focus your learning. *Cases* will help put your knowledge to clinical use. *Learning objectives* accompany the answers to each practice case to reinforce important information and generate discussion. At the end of the text is a *multiple-choice exam* to help demonstrate your mastery of the material and prepare you for your clinical exams.

Be prepared for any surgical situation. The *Surgery Clerkship Guide* is a valuable resource for medical students on a surgical clerkship or for students at any level who want to take better care of surgical patients.

Gregg A. Adams, MD

Acknowledgments

The editors and authors would like to thank the staff at Elsevier for their care and attentiveness. We would especially like to thank William Schmitt, Kevin Kochanski, and Amy Norwitz for their thoroughness and patience. Their commitment is apparent throughout this book.

Contents

Section 3 Patients Presenting with a Known Surgical Condition

1

Introduction to the Surgery Clerkship

1

Secrets to Becoming a Successful Surgery Clerk

Welcome to your surgery clerkship. Spending time on a surgical service may seem daunting. Surgery is an enormous topic, and you will be expected to work long hours, taking care of sick patients with unfamiliar problems. Surgery is in fact too big a subject to expect to learn well in one lifetime, let alone in the limited time given to a student. But don't panic. Most of the surgical problems you encounter will become straightforward enough with a little organization. What follows are some helpful hints to approaching surgical patients and their diseases.

DAY-TO-DAY INPATIENT RESPONSIBILITIES

Care of surgical patients is not that different from the care of other patients in the hospital. The differences that do exist relate to the fact that the patients often need or are recovering from an operation. This means that special attention must be paid to wounds, drains, and some specific postoperative rituals designed to minimize postoperative complications.

Where do I fit in on a surgical team?

You will be expected to become an integral member of the surgical team. Assume that you are the patient's primary caregiver and approach each decision with that responsibility. Make sure that you run each decision and any questions you have by the intern or resident who is following the patient with you.

How do I gather information?

Gather your data each morning before the morning work rounds with the team ("prerounds"). Allow yourself 10 to 15 minutes per patient, and leave yourself some extra time for unexpected issues.

The information will come from a variety of sources. Interview the patients if they are conversant, and address their concerns and wishes. Look at the bedside chart that contains the vital signs and intake/output data. Useful information is also found in the main chart if on-call teams or consulting services have left notes. Look at the medication sheet to see if there have been any unexpected changes in the patients' medications. Don't forget to touch base with the nurses or other bedside caregivers to see if they have any new data or concerns. Keep track of the number of days since the last operation and how many days antibiotic therapy has been ordered.

During the day you may be asked to contact various laboratory or radiology departments. Be courteous and identify yourself as a medical student. If you are gathering important information such as culture results or study findings, be sure to get the name of the individual with whom you are speaking.

What information is important?

For new admissions, all information is required. Your history and physical examination (H&P) reports should be complete. Be sure to put the date and time on each. For morning rounds, report any changes in your patient that have taken place overnight, including the patient's vital signs, the fluid intake and output (including the volume and quality of drain output and the volume of urine output recorded in both the last 24 hours and the last hour), and a brief physical examination (including the status of the wound and dressings). There will be specific H&P points to focus on depending on the patient's disease or prior operation.

How do I present information?

Ask your chief resident in what order he or she would like the information presented, or watch a senior resident present and organize your presentations accordingly. Each chief will like to hear the stream of data in a slightly different order or will find one type of information more important than another. Always ask if you have questions, and invite criticism of your presentations.

What are other clues about presentations?

If there is more than one organ system involved in the acute care of the patient, organize the presentation by organ system. Again, ask your chief resident how he or she would like the information to flow.

Be sure to have an assessment and plan in mind. You may not always be right, but it gives you a chance to practice the art of patient care and teaches the importance of anticipation.

How do I approach the operating room?

It is hard to be a medical student. You get very little respect, and you may often feel like you know nothing. Nowhere else in the hospital is that feeling of insignificance more apparent than in the operating room (OR), where everything you do has pitfalls.

Listen carefully to the scrub nurses and the circulating nurses. They will tell you where to stand, what to touch, what *not* to touch, and when to talk.

On arrival to the OR, introduce yourself. Write your name and glove size on the board and ask if there is anything that you can do to help prepare the room or the patient. Remember that the operation really begins long before the first incision, with positioning, prepping, and draping of the patient.

You will be expected to scrub in on all cases unless you are expressly told not to. Review the procedure beforehand, and be prepared to answer questions about the operation. Anatomy is a favorite topic—bone up.

Don't take it personally if your request to look is refused or if the question you were asking is deferred during an operation. Parts of every procedure will require intense concentration. Rarely, unexpected events happen and must be addressed urgently. Ask your question again when the situation is controlled.

DAY-TO-DAY OUTPATIENT RESPONSIBILITIES

How do I approach an outpatient clinic visit?

The clinic is often the first place you will meet a patient, and attendance there is helpful to see how a patient with a surgical problem presents. Be sure to get there on time.

Familiarize yourself with the patient by taking a *brief* look at the chart: postop? new complaint? Go in. Introduce yourself as a medical student. Then perform a problem-directed H&P. This is a short, 5-minute approach, not the hour-long full H&P. If you don't know what to look for, do the best you can, then ask your intern or resident.

Present to the attending surgeon or the chief or senior resident. He or she will fill in the gaps in your presentation with questions, which must be followed up. When you present, have an assessment and plan in mind.

All chart notes will need to be signed by the person who supervised you.

GENERAL PRINCIPLES

Ask questions

One of the biggest mistakes you can make is not asking questions.

Your education is ultimately your responsibility. Make sure you get your money's worth. You may feel like a nuisance at first, but you'll be so much more appreciated once you know what to do. On arrival to a new rotation, ask what's expected of you, how you can be most helpful, and how you'll be evaluated. Ask where the bathroom is, ask when and if you can eat or sleep, and find out about the call rotation. Ask questions of students, interns, residents, and attendings. Don't forget the nurses, social workers, physical therapists, and consultants.

No question is too basic if you don't know the answer. If the time is not appropriate to ask, then write the questions down and look up the answers later.

Your teachers can't guess what you don't know, nor do they expect you to know anything about surgery, so you can direct their teaching. They may answer right away, or they may ask you to look something up and share the information. They may ignore you, but ask anyway.

Certainly ask for help if someone asks you to do something that you've never done before. If you need assistance with a procedure or a consent form, don't hesitate to get help. It is not a sign of weakness—it is a sign of intelligence.

If you especially want to do something, ask. If you'd like to learn procedures or how to operate, let the residents know. The only way to get to do something is to be present and to ask.

Communicate

Communication is another underutilized skill. The dissemination of information is of paramount importance in the smooth running of the team.

Communication begins by *listening* to everyone and by paying attention during rounds and conferences. Useful information is all around you. Then *ask questions* to clarify the information. If you don't understand something, ask. If the time doesn't allow an answer, arrange a more appropriate time to learn. Then *communicate*. Communicate with everyone. You'll find that the therapists and social workers often have key information for the care of the patients. And one third of your education will come from the nursing staff. Listen carefully to them. Respect their experience.

Part of learning the language of medicine is to learn effective communication. Learn how to give an efficient case presentation. Learn to write a clear and concise "SOAP" note. Every chief is different, and you should find out in advance how each one likes presentations and notes done. Don't filter information until you are experienced enough to do so. A resident's saying "vital signs are stable" is different than a student's saying so. You will need to prove that you know what you're talking about. For example, until you know the difference between febrile and afebrile, report the actual temperature.

Always end a presentation with an assessment and a plan. It needn't be right, but you will be expected to have thought about the information that you have just rattled off.

If you notice something happening with one of your patients that you don't understand or didn't expect, tell someone, *especially if it worries you.* It is better to ask someone about normal findings than not to share the worrisome signs that may endanger the patient. ("Is it all right for Ms. Smith to be coughing up blood?")

Get frequent updates on your performance. Find out if you are meeting expectations, what your weaknesses and strengths are, and how you can improve. If you don't find out what the expectations are, how can you possibly exceed them?

Be honest. It is far better to say "I don't know" than to fabricate.

Be respectful

Being respectful applies to everyone, from student to attending surgeon. Be respectful of the patients' privacy, their pain, their bad moods. Respect the wishes of the patients and their families.

Your patient's disease and condition are *confidential information.* Your ability to share in his or her care is a privilege. Be respectful of patients and families, and never identify a patient's name in a public place.

You will interact with other services while on the surgical service. You will be exposed to all forms of bias, prejudice, and occasional bickering. Please be courteous and kind to your colleagues. They have different skill sets than you, and they occasionally will ask you to help them. Likewise, you will need them at some time. These are your future referral sources and middle-of-the-night contacts. Foster good relationships with them—you never know when they might turn up on the credentials committee of the hospital at which you'd like to practice.

Respect diversity. You will see many things in the care of surgical patients. Some you may have never seen before, and some you may not agree with. Divorce yourself from your emotions while you are taking care of patients. They need your help, not your moral judgments.

Be prepared

Find out in advance what is expected of you. Ask your predecessors about the chief resident and attendings. If you are to care for a patient with a disease you know nothing about, learn the basics as quickly as you can. You can fill in the blanks when you have more time.

Time is short, so develop timesaving tools. Find out how the residents or other medical students gather and store their data. What are the shortcuts they take? Not every tool works for everyone, so find what works for you and then stick with it. Residents use many different tools: some have grid cards, others use spiral notebooks. There is no "right" way, as long as the expected information is available when it is needed. Never throw away a patient card, because patients often come back.

Try to stay organized, keep lists, and complete the tasks asked of you. If your workload is overwhelming, let someone know. It may be altered to make your learning more efficient. You won't learn anything by writing 50 notes a day and not having time to read about the diseases you are writing about.

Read about the operations you will help with. Why are they being done? What is the relevant anatomy? What are the possible complications? If you don't know where to read about the operations, ask.

Anticipate

This skill comes with experience.

Taking care of patients is filled with pitfalls and misadventures. If you know the pathophysiology of the diseases and the possible complications of the procedures, you'll be able to know what to watch for. Visualize the complications before they happen, so when a subtle symptom shows up, you'll be prepared to act. Figure out your game plan before bad things happen. Imagine one of your sicker patients having a postoperative complication. What if Mr. X has a myocardial infarction or a pulmonary embolism? Do you know where the crash cart is? Who would you call? When was the last time you looked at your ACLS (advanced cardiac life support) protocols?

Be realistic

Know how long things take. If the rate-limiting step to discharging a patient is the prescriptions, write them first, or better yet, the day before.

Don't assume that the task will get done just because you wrote the order. For example, pay attention to how many of your patients are actually wearing sequential compression devices (SCDs) with the machine functioning while you are on morning rounds. It will be staggering how few. And you will find that it is nearly impossible to keep a nasogastric tube working without constant flushing and fiddling. Trust only the data that you gather yourself. Don't assume.

Keep yourself safe

Keep yourself safe in a physical sense. Use universal precautions by wearing gloves and eye protection when handling dressings or wounds. Learn to handle sharp instruments in a safe manner.

Also keep yourself safe in a psychological sense. Get an adequate amount of sleep when you need it, and stay active in your favorite hobbies and activities, including exercise and personal relationships. Don't believe that the patients do well or poorly due to your action or inaction. The patients have diseases, and diseases are often debilitating or fatal. We, as physicians, have only limited power to affect the outcome. You will be learning to help treat and palliate many diseases, but, for many of the ill, a cure will be elusive.

Every chief is different

Surgery is still a hierarchy. The chief is the top of the totem pole. How that individual deals with that power will vary.

Each chief has specific likes and dislikes. Ask about the patterns that will please him or her. Specifics may include the following:

How does she like presentations?
How long does he leave dressings on after an operation?
What is her definition of fever or abnormal vital signs?
Is he a micromanager or macromanager?

Gather your clues from residents or students who have worked under that chief before. Or ask the chief. Don't be shy—the days of the unapproachable surgical chief resident are long gone. Many remember what it was like to be a student.

Keep in mind that the chief is under an enormous amount of stress. Try not to add to it.

General notes

Remember to be assertive. Do not assume that residents will call you for the OR or to a meeting. You must be in their "back pocket" for much of the rotation so they won't forget about you.

What you get out of your surgical rotation is directly proportional to what you put into it. If you have a special desire to work with patients in the intensive care unit or to do procedures, let the residents know. If you faint at the sight of blood, that, too, is useful information. Surgery is not for every one, and the work is hard. But the rotation should be fun, educational, and fulfilling. You will be able to see the human body in a way that is completely unique. You should leave the rotation with some understanding of what surgeons do and when it is appropriate to call for one.

2

The Surgical Patient

The care of a surgical patient can be divided into three phases: preoperative evaluation, the operating room (OR), and postoperative care. Your workload on a surgery clerkship can be tremendous, and efficiency and organization are essential to providing excellent care. Diagnostic work-ups of specific diseases are discussed with the corresponding chapters of the book; however, there are some things that must be done in the case of all patients to care for them surgically.

PREOPERATIVE PHASE

PREOPERATIVE ASSESSMENT

What is needed at a preoperative clinic appointment?

A history and physical examination (H&P) must be done for each patient who is to undergo surgery. This should include a history of the current illness as well as a directed review of systems that aids in the evaluation of operative risk. Most hospitals have a form for the preoperative H&P with prompts including questions about bleeding tendencies, respiratory disorders, and cardiac history. It is important to include previous operations because they may affect the planned surgical procedures. Current medications (with doses) as well as medication allergies should be documented clearly. Make sure at the preoperative visit that special preparations (i.e., bowel preparation, preoperative laboratory or radiologic studies, type and cross match for banked or donor-designated blood units) are taken care of. Review all studies that have been done during the work-up of the surgical problem. Refer to the attending's note that documents the surgical problem and the decision to operate, because it may indicate special considerations or preoperative studies specific to the surgeon or the planned procedure. A thorough physical examination with special attention to the cardiorespiratory system should be done. In all cases you *must* communicate to the supervising resident or attending surgeon any findings from the history or physical examination that may affect the planned surgery. You should make an effort to participate in the operation and postoperative care of any patients that you examine in the preoperative clinic to maximize the learning experience.

Which preoperative tests should I order?

Fewer preoperative lab tests are being ordered for patients than in the past. For minor procedures requiring only a local anesthetic, no routine preoperative lab studies are needed in healthy patients. In the case of a planned general anesthetic, usually a complete blood count (CBC) and urinalysis are adequate. For major operations a chemistry panel that includes the major electrolytes, blood urea nitrogen (BUN), creatinine, and glucose, and coagulation parameters should be done as well. In many centers the charts of patients having surgery are available the afternoon before. You should review all the lab studies that were ordered in the preoperative clinic at that time and communicate any abnormalities appropriately. If the need for blood transfusions is anticipated, a sample of blood should be sent to the blood bank. (Ask about the regulations regarding consent for transfusion in your hospital. Often merely sending a sample of blood to the blood bank requires that you inform the patient of the risks, benefits, and alternatives to transfusion.) Patients undergoing a general anesthetic for a major procedure who are 45 years of age or older should have a documented normal chest radiograph within 6 months of the procedure, and those older than 60 years of age should have an electrocardiogram (ECG) also.

Which patients require cardiac clearance?

The clinical criteria for assessing risks for cardiac complications after surgery are summarized in Table 2–1. If any of the criteria are identified in the preoperative H&P, the patient should have clearance by the primary care physician or by a cardiologist before scheduling elective surgery. If the cardiac risk is prohibitive or therapeutic measures can be taken to improve the cardiac risk, elective procedures should be canceled or delayed. In cases where the surgery is urgent or emergent, the cardiac risks should be discussed with the patient and the family when possible, and a cardiologist should be involved for perioperative management to minimize risk.

How should anticoagulant medications be managed with surgery?

Older patients are increasingly using "blood thinning" medications (warfarin [Coumadin], clopidogrel [Plavix], aspirin) on a daily basis to reduce the risk of stroke and myocardial infarction.

TABLE 2-1

Preoperative Risk Factors Associated with Postoperative Cardiac Complications

Jugular venous distention or S_3 gallop
Myocardial infarction in the previous 6 months
Premature atrial contractions or rhythm other than sinus on electrocardiogram
3–5 premature ventricular contractions per minute
Age > 70 years
Significant aortic valvular stenosis
Poor general medical condition
    Pao_2 < 60 mm Hg; $Paco_2$ > 50 mm Hg
    K^+ < 3.0 mEq/L; HCO_3 < 20 mEq/L
    Blood urea nitrogen > 50 mg/100 mL; creatinine > 3.0 mg/100 mL
    Elevated transaminase
    Signs of chronic liver disease
    Patient bedridden from noncardiac causes

Modified from Goldman L, Caldera DI, Nussbaum SR, et al: Multifactorial index of cardiac risk in noncardiac surgical procedures. N Engl J Med 297:845, 1977.

Discontinuation of these medications preoperatively reduces the risk of bleeding complications perioperatively, although there is controversy regarding the bleeding risk associated with aspirin use. Appropriate perioperative management of patients on long-term anticoagulation (warfarin) requires that you know the reason for the treatment and the thrombotic risks associated with discontinuation of therapy. For most patients, discontinuation of their therapy in the perioperative period to allow the International Normalized Ratio (INR) to come to 1.2 to 1.3, with reconstitution of therapeutic ranges in 2 to 3 days, is safe. Patients with known major thrombotic complications in the past associated with discontinuation of therapy should be admitted and treated with intravenous (IV) heparin in the perioperative period. Table 2–2 summarizes the most commonly used anticoagulants and their properties.

Should I obtain consent for surgery?

In most institutions medical students are not allowed to obtain consent. Informed consent for surgery has two components. The first is the printed form that is signed and witnessed that includes the type of surgery to be done; the name of the person to be performing the procedure; and the name of the person who explained the risks, benefits, and alternatives to the procedure. Although this document is imperative to allow the patient to enter the operating suite on the day of surgery, it is not a document that holds up in court. The second component is a face-to-face dis-

TABLE 2-2

Commonly Used Anticoagulants and Their Properties

Anticoagulation Medication	Laboratory Values	Mechanism	Time for Preoperative Discontinuation	Reversal Agent (Onset)
Aspirin	↑ bleeding time	Antiplatelet agent	7–10 d	Platelet infusion (immediate)
Clopidogrel (Plavix)	↑ bleeding time	Inhibits ADP platelet aggregation	5 d	Platelet infusion (immediate)
Warfarin (Coumadin)	↑ PT/INR	Inhibits vitamin K–dependent clotting factors	1–3 d	Vitamin K (6–24 hr) FFP (immediate)
Therapeutic heparin	↑PTT	Inhibits multiple clotting factors	2–4 hr	FFP (immediate) Protamine (immediate)
Enoxaparin (Lovenox)	↔ PTT, PT/INR	Inhibits multiple clotting factors	Safe for perioperative	NA
SC heparin	↔ PTT, PT/INR	Inhibits multiple clotting factors	Safe for perioperative	NA

ADP, adenosine diphosphate; FFP, fresh frozen plasma; INR, International Normalized Ratio; NA, not available; PT, prothrombin time; PTT, partial thromboplastin time; SC, subcutaneous.

cussion between the patient (or the person who has legal rights to make medical decisions for the patient) and the surgeon performing the procedure. The chart documentation of this discussion is the legal evidence of "informed consent." Details of the procedure, risks, benefits, and alternatives are explained fully, and all questions are answered to the satisfaction of the patient or the legal decision maker. At the preoperative visit the paperwork portion of the consent is completed; however, the full discussion of the procedure should have already taken place. Nonetheless, additional questions often have come up in the interim between the clinic appointment and the preoperative appointment. In more complex types of surgery you may not be able to field the questions asked. Do not go beyond your knowledge! Call your supervising resident or the attending for the patient if there are questions you cannot answer.

Which patients should receive prophylactic antibiotics?

Postoperative infection is a continuing source of morbidity in the surgical patient. There is also a growing recognition of the deleterious effect of the overuse of antibiotics in the increasing prevalence of pathogenic bacteria with multiple antibiotic resistance. The prudent use of prophylactic antibiotics is warranted in certain surgical situations, as summarized in Table 2–3. The best effect on postoperative wound infection occurs if the antibiotics are used just before an operation and throughout the immediate postoperative period.

Which patients need a bowel prep?

Bowel preparation is used in any case when there is an expectation of resection or reanastomosis of colon. Thus, in planned resections, colostomy takedown, and total proctocolectomies, a full prep that includes both mechanical and antibiotic prep is used. Traditionally a liquid formulation of polyethylene glycol (PEG) is administered the day before surgery to reduce the fecal content within the bowel. Sodium phosphate preparations that are given as a smaller volume are better tolerated by patients with the same effect in reduction of fecal matter and may be a better alternative for older patients who are unlikely to be able to complete a full 4-gallon PEG prep. This is accompanied by the administration of erythromycin base and neomycin in three separate doses orally on the afternoon and evening before surgery (typically 3 PM, 7 PM, and 11 PM) for microbial clearance of the large intestine. You should also consider bowel preparation for aortic aneurysm repair, ventral incisional hernia repairs, or any re-operative abdominal procedure because of the risk of enterotomy.

TABLE 2–3
Operative Situations Warranting the Use of Prophylactic Antibiotics

Small or large bowel resections
Suspected acute appendicitis
Head and neck with opening of
    Oropharynx
    Esophagus
    Trachea
Biliary surgery for
    Acute cholecystitis
    Cholangitis
    Biliary disease in patients >70 years of age
Vascular procedures involving prosthetic grafts
Operations implanting high-risk prosthetics
    Hip replacement
    Knee replacement
    Open reduction internal fixation for traumatic bony extremity injuries
    Mesh hernia repairs

OPERATIVE PHASE

CARE OF THE PATIENT IN THE OR

How should I prepare for the OR?

Check the OR schedule the evening before a scheduled operating day for your surgical team. This way you will be able to read about the case and the disease process in advance and will have an opportunity to ask questions if something is not clear from the reading. Knowledge of the pertinent anatomy and a strategy for operation can be found in any number of surgical atlases. Although you may not understand the nuances of the more advanced procedures, you will certainly learn more during the case if you have some rudimentary knowledge. You should also read through the patient's chart so that you know the symptoms and preoperative radiographic studies that are pertinent. For some cases it is helpful to have the radiographs hung on a light box in the room so that they can be used for reference during the procedure. The more knowledge and interest you exhibit in a case, the more likely you are to be allowed to participate and the more excited you will make your residents and attending staff to teach you.

What precautions should I take to protect myself from potential infectious fluids in the OR?

Universal precautions should be used at all times in the OR. Universal precautions should be in effect before the procedure, when you may start IV lines or help with intubation or positioning; during the operative procedure; and after the procedure as the patient is moved from the OR table to a bed or gurney. Airway or bleeding issues can occur during transport to or from the OR, so you should have gloves available. Protective eyewear or shields are required in the OR by the Occupational Safety and Health Administration.

Each member of the surgical team needs to be acutely aware of sharps and use clear, concise communication. Careful handling of sharps can minimize needle or knife sticks in the OR. This is particularly important in the trauma situation. It is for your own protection that you take the time to review the chart so that you know about documented infectious agents present in any given patient. You should assume that all patients are potential infection risks and take appropriate measures.

Which patients should receive prophylaxis against deep vein thrombosis (DVT)?

Immobilization of surgical patients increases the risk of their forming clots in the veins of the lower extremities, leading to an increased risk of fatal pulmonary embolus (PE). The morbidity associated with deep vein thrombosis (DVT) and PE as well as the morbidity associated with the treatment (systemic anticoagulation) has led to extensive research aimed at preventive measures. Most clots begin to form on the operating table; therefore, preventive measures should begin as soon as the patient is placed on the operating table. Any patient undergoing major surgery is at risk for DVT. Patients undergoing major surgery; those with pelvic fractures, femur fractures, or spinal cord injuries; those undergoing elective knee or hip surgery; or trauma patients should have prophylaxis with support garments and intermittent pneumatic compression devices, with low-dose subcutaneous heparin, or with both. Treatment of documented DVT or PE consists of immediate treatment with heparin with therapeutic partial thromboplastin time (PTT) levels between 60 and 80 maintained until effective warfarin treatment is instituted.

What is in a preoperative note?

This is a brief note usually written in the OR just prior to surgery that states the preoperative diagnosis and indication for surgery. You should document that the risks and benefits and alternatives to the procedure have been discussed with the patient and that he or she understands and wishes to proceed with the planned procedure. This is separate from the consent form and is meant to document the discussions that have taken place with the patient in preparation for the procedure. In cases where the patient is not able to give informed consent (i.e., the patient is a minor child or a conserved patient), document with which person the preoperative discussion took place and the relationship that allows that person to be an appropriate decision maker for the patient (i.e., parent of a minor child, relative, or other designated decision maker for a demented person). In some cases the procedure is emergent and must take place before contact can be made with family. You must state the dire need for the procedure as a life-saving procedure to justify proceeding without formal consent. Check with your resident about the procedure for emergency consent in your hospital.

What is in an operative note?

The operative note should contain all the information needed for someone who did not attend the procedure to understand the events and extent of operation. It should be immediately placed in the patient's chart in the recovery room because the dictated reports may not appear in the chart for several days, and this information may become critical if the patient becomes unstable in the postoperative period. A skeleton of a brief operative note is the following:

Brief Operative Note
Date of procedure:
Preoperative diagnosis:
Postoperative diagnosis:
Procedure:
Surgeon:
Assistants:
Anesthesia:
Findings:
Specimens:
Intraoperative fluids:
    Estimated blood loss:
    Urine output:
    Crystalloid (lactated Ringer's, normal saline):
    Colloid (albumin, packed red blood cells, fresh frozen
        plasma, platelets, etc.):
Drains and tubes:
    Foley catheter, central lines, drains, feeding gastrostomies,
        stoma, etc.

If you dictate a case (rare at the student level, common at the intern/resident level), do it as soon as possible so that the details are fresh in your mind. Initially you may find that having an atlas to refer to while doing your dictation keeps the chronology of the case straight, but be sure that you are dictating the case accurately as you remember it. If you feel uncomfortable dictating a case, ask your attending or senior resident to dictate. The accuracy of the report is much more important than saving face.

POSTOPERATIVE PHASE

POSTOPERATIVE CARE

What is a postoperative check?

The immediate postoperative period constitutes the highest risk for complications resulting from the procedure itself or from the anesthetic. The stress of surgery may cause fluid shifts that will adversely affect the cardiovascular and pulmonary systems. Problems with surgical hemostasis may manifest, and the patient may well be in the midst of physiologic derangements related to the underlying disease. A member of the surgical team should check the patient within the first 6 hours after leaving the OR if the procedure was significant enough to warrant admission postoperatively. The date and time of the examination should be documented in the chart along with the pertinent findings. The note should include documentation of vital signs, inspection of the wound dressing, adequacy of the cardiorespiratory status, pain medications, and urine output. The results of any postoperative lab studies (i.e., CBC or chest radiograph) should be documented. If the patient is found to be unstable for any reason, document the maneuvers that will be instituted to correct abnormalities and immediately notify the senior members of the team and the attending physician.

How do I present a postoperative patient on rounds?

You should present patients comprehensively and succinctly. Surgical chiefs will vary in the amount of information and the format that they prefer for presentations. Ask them early in your rotation, and comply with the format that they are comfortable with.

Most postoperative ward presentations begin with the name and age of the patient followed by what procedure the patients had and what postoperative day they are at (e.g., Mr. Jones is a 50-year-old gentleman who is postoperative day 5 after an open cholecystectomy). This information sets the stage for the rest of the presentation as the patient's progress toward recovery is mentally compared to norms for patients with this magnitude of surgery. If a patient is "off the normal trajectory" toward recovery, it will often prompt diagnostic studies or directed physical examination to detect any potential complications of surgery.

Objective findings such as the vital signs, input and output over the previous 24 hours, and pertinent laboratory values need to be reported, and trends should be noted. Know the status of bowel function and diet, particularly in patients who have undergone abdominal surgery.

You should examine all drains and describe the character of the fluid output as well as the volume, noting if the fluid is bilious, feculent, serosanguineous, or clear or if the character has changed. Ensure that the drain is well secured to the skin. The surgical site should be examined every day. Dressings are usually removed 2 to 3 days after surgery or sooner if the dressing is soaked with fluid or soiled. Excess fluid or soiling may indicate a problem with the surgical wound. Open wounds require dressing changes to débride nonviable tissue and reduce bacterial contamination, and they should be evaluated every day.

PAIN MANAGEMENT IN THE POSTOPERATIVE PATIENT

Pain management presents a particular challenge in the surgical patient. As opposed to medical specialties, in which pain is largely secondary to the underlying disease process, surgery carries with it an obligatory amount of pain. Failure to adequately control postoperative pain can lead to physiologic derangements including tachycardia, impaired respiration, and increases in blood pressure and myocardial oxygen consumption that can increase the risks of poor outcome or complications in the perioperative period.

What are the options for systemic pain relief?

The most common medications used for postoperative pain relief are opioids. These medications can be administered orally, intravenously, or intramuscularly.

The oral opiates are usually formulated in combination with acetaminophen or, less commonly, a nonsteroidal anti-inflammatory medication, and care should be taken to administer a dosing schedule that will avoid overdose and toxicity of the additional component.

Patients who are NPO after an abdominal procedure need to have pain medications delivered parenterally until they are tolerating a diet. The IV route of administration has a faster onset of action than oral or intramuscular medications but a shorter duration of effect that must be taken into account when determining dosing schedules. Patients may have natural or acquired resistance to opioids; therefore, the medication should start at what is considered a safe dose for the size of the patient, then titrated to effect. Every patient is different.

The advent of patient-controlled analgesia (PCA) has helped tremendously in the management of postoperative pain because it avoids the peaks and troughs of opiate effect. The machine is set for delivery of a basal hourly rate, a demand dose that can be delivered by the patient with a lockout period, and maximal hourly doses set to avoid medication overdose. Complications increase with the use of a basal rate to maintain a constant background rate of opiate in the blood, but nonetheless this can be safe when monitored properly and can be helpful particularly in the first 24 hours after a major operation.

Which patients should be considered for regional/epidural analgesia?

Local anesthetics in combination with long-acting opioids can be delivered directly to the epidural space and act synergistically to provide regional analgesia. It reduces the use of and complications of systemic opioids and is particularly helpful in cases of multiple rib fractures, flail chest, and thoracotomy in reducing intensive care unit (ICU) stays and time on mechanical ventilation, reducing the incidence of pulmonary complications. As with PCA, there is a slightly higher risk of pruritus than with the same medications given by IV bolus. The most common side effect of epidural analgesia is hypotension due to the sympathetic block that sometimes accompanies the analgesic effect. Some patients can also develop respiratory insufficiency; thus, the patient should be monitored closely, particularly at the institution of epidural analgesia. A patient must have adequate coagulation parameters and functional platelets to be a candidate for epidural analgesia. Select patients with rib fractures are good candidates for direct intrapleural or intercostal nerve blocks, with the block extending one level above and one level below the rib fractures to attain similar results to an epidural.

How do I manage patients with intractable pain or pain from terminal cancer?

The management of patients with intractable pain requires a comprehensive approach that can often be addressed better in specialized pain centers, which are fortunately becoming more and more common. There are a number of oral opiates as well as transdermal patches that work well for intractable pain. It is preferable to use pain medications that patients can take at home so that they are not confined to a hospital.

It is important to recognize the role anxiety plays in the perception of pain, particularly when it is unrelenting or in conjunction with emotional issues related to the underlying disease process. A sympathetic and clear communication is required so that the patient understands that you are trying to help at multiple levels rather than passing off the symptoms as "psychosomatic" when prescribing an anxiolytic as part of a comprehensive pain plan. Physicians are somewhat unskilled in dealing with end-of-life issues in a patient with pain secondary to terminal disease, although these issues may be quite important to the patient. In this regard specially trained hospice care practitioners can be a great resource for the patient and physician. Many states are now requiring that pain management be part of the medical curriculum and are requiring practicing physicians to take continuing medical education courses in pain management as well.

ANTIBIOTICS IN THE POSTSURGICAL PATIENT

How should antibiotics be managed in the postoperative period?

Antibiotic dosages, antibacterial spectrums, and pharmacokinetics are available in the form of pocket summaries or as software for a personal digital assistant organizer; therefore, these issues are not covered in this text. The use of antibiotics should be reserved for documented infections in the postoperative patient. The temptation is great to "cover" a potential infection in a patient who is not recovering at the rate that would be expected or who has an unexplained fever or leukocytosis. However, nosocomial infections and multiple-resistant organisms are an increasing source of morbidity and mortality and excess expense to the medical system in this country. Coverage should not be unnecessarily broad, because the end result may be to alter the resident flora of the patient and allow the overgrowth of pathogenic bacteria.

APPROACH TO THE CRITICALLY ILL PATIENT

How does the presentation of an ICU patient differ from that of a ward patient?

Because ICU patients often have complex physiologic derangements, they are best presented by systems to maintain organization. As with the ward patient, the basic introduction stating the patient's problem or the procedure done and the number of days that he or she has been under treatment sets the stage for the rest of the presentation. You then proceed with a presentation organized by systems, such that the huge amount of clinical data that are collected and recorded on any given ICU patient in a 24-hour period can be distilled into a comprehensive indication of how the patient is progressing. The note should be written in systems as well so that anyone reading the chart can easily gauge the patient's clinical situation. The following is an outline of an ICU note and presentation for a surgical patient:

ICU Note—Surgical Service
Date and time:
Postop (hospital) day:
    Number of postoperative days
Neurologic:
    Level of function and alertness, Glasgow Coma Scale score
    Sedative and narcotic medications
Cardiovascular:
    Includes heart rate and blood pressure trends
    Special values such as cardiac output and central venous
        pressure where appropriate
    Cardiovascular medications, including pressor drips
    Pertinent findings such as ECG changes or laboratory
        indications of myocardial infarction
Pulmonary:
    Mechanical ventilator settings
    Blood gas information, oxygen saturation
    Chest radiograph findings
Gastrointestinal/gynecologic:
    Input and output
    Laboratory findings such as electrolytes, BUN, creatinine,
        glucose, liver function tests
    Nutritional status: parameters/mode of feeding
Heme/ID (infectious disease):
    Maximal temperature and fever trends

Antibiotic therapy: number of days on therapy
Laboratory values such as CBC, prothrombin time (PT), PTT
Anticoagulation therapy
Assessment/Plan:
Assessment of whether the patient is stable, unstable,
improving, worsening
Mention any planned studies or changes in therapy
Results of consults from other services

When should I discuss code status with a patient or family?

These types of discussions are best done when patients are not in crisis because this gives them the opportunity to think through their wishes. Family members will often need to take over the decision-making process when a patient is critically ill, and this is difficult if these issues have never been discussed. Many patients now have advance directives clearly stating their wishes in a medical crisis. When these issues have not been discussed or when there is disagreement within the family, social services or multidisciplinary ethics committees may be necessary. You should be realistic about the patient's prognosis even if it is poor so that the family can make informed choices about the level of care.

Patients Presenting with a Specific Sign or Symptom

3

Abdominal Mass

The key to evaluation of the abdominal mass is to make a certain diagnosis. Abdominal masses of malignant, infectious, or inflammatory etiologies require rapid treatment, and a definitive diagnosis is needed.

What is an abdominal mass?

An *abdominal mass* may be defined as any conglomeration or mass of tissue, or fluid within a tissue, not ascribable to normal anatomic structures and found within the confines of the anatomic abdomen. It is helpful also to classify masses as superficial within the abdominal wall or deep within the body.

▶ ETIOLOGY

What are the common causes of an abdominal mass?

The most common causes of abdominal masses in the United States are lipoma, hernia, cyst, abscess, appendiceal and diverticular abscesses, colon cancer, and lymphadenopathy. Abdominal masses include a wide variety of pathologic processes, including benign and malignant neoplasia, congenital and acquired lesions (omphalocele, hernia, abdominal aortic aneurysm), inflammatory processes (cyst, Crohn's disease, pancreatic pseudocyst), and infectious disease (appendicitis, diverticulitis with abscess or phlegmon), as well as variants of normal anatomic structures (distended stomach, bowel, or bladder). Description of these entities (e.g., hernia, appendicitis) and their diagnosis and management are also discussed in other chapters.

Common abdominal masses are listed anatomically in Table 3–1 and shown in Figure 3–1.

▶ EVALUATION

When asked to evaluate a patient with an abdominal mass, your goal is to make a definitive diagnosis. With few exceptions in which benignity may be nearly guaranteed (e.g., lipoma), abdominal masses must be worked up until an accurate (usually histopathologic) diagnosis is made.

TABLE 3–1

Common Superficial Masses (Any Quadrant)

Lipoma
Cyst
Abscess
Skin cancer (basal, squamous, melanoma)
Lymph node
Hematoma
Fibroma
Sarcoma
Desmoid tumor
Diastasis recti
Hernia

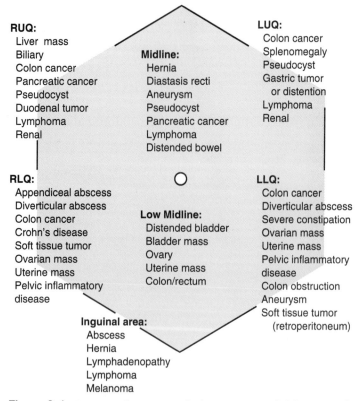

RUQ:
Liver mass
Biliary
Colon cancer
Pancreatic cancer
Pseudocyst
Duodenal tumor
Lymphoma
Renal

Midline:
Hernia
Diastasis recti
Aneurysm
Pseudocyst
Pancreatic cancer
Lymphoma
Distended bowel

LUQ:
Colon cancer
Splenomegaly
Pseudocyst
Gastric tumor
  or distention
Lymphoma
Renal

RLQ:
Appendiceal abscess
Diverticular abscess
Colon cancer
Crohn's disease
Soft tissue tumor
Ovarian mass
Uterine mass
Pelvic inflammatory
disease

Low Midline:
Distended bladder
Bladder mass
Ovary
Uterine mass
Colon/rectum

LLQ:
Colon cancer
Diverticular abscess
Severe constipation
Ovarian mass
Uterine mass
Pelvic inflammatory
disease
Colon obstruction
Aneurysm
Soft tissue tumor
  (retroperitoneum)

Inguinal area:
Abscess
Hernia
Lymphadenopathy
Lymphoma
Melanoma

Figure 3–1. Common deep masses by location. LLQ, left lower quadrant; LUQ, left upper quadrant; RLQ, right lower quadrant; RUQ, right upper quadrant.

What historical points are important?

A thorough history is essential and should include past medical history as well as a description of development of the mass and any associated illnesses. Have there been any previous similar findings? Is there a prior history of malignant, inflammatory, or infectious disease? Was there an injury (hernia, hematoma)? Precise definition of the growth and appearance of the lesion is critical. Is the mass slow growing or was its appearance sudden (aneurysm, pseudocyst, herniation)? Are there any associated signs or symptoms such as abdominal or back pain, fever, nausea, vomiting, jaundice, diarrhea, or weight loss? Is the mass always present or does it come and go (hernia)? The remainder of the history must include prior illnesses, operations, family history, social history, medications, and allergies, and in women, a menstrual, obstetric, and gynecologic history.

What are the steps in physical examination?

Examination of the patient begins with observation. Pay special attention to facial expression, attitude in bed, body habitus, respiratory pattern and rate, pulse, temperature, and mucous membranes. Systemic illness associated with an abdominal mass (e.g., perforated colon with abscess, acute pancreatitis with pseudocyst or abscess, or an abdominal aortic aneurysm) requires more immediate investigation, diagnosis, and management.

Although special attention is paid to the abdominal mass, the remainder of the exam must be complete, especially with respect to the heart, lungs, skin, lymph nodes, and mental status.

Inspect the abdomen and the mass. Is there pulsation, rubor, visible peristalsis, cyanosis, or necrosis or ulceration of the skin? Auscultate over the mass and the abdomen. Is there a bruit or are there bowel sounds within the mass? Is there a silent abdomen (peritoneal irritation)? Palpate gently. Are there peritoneal signs, palpable pulsations, or peristalsis, fluctuance, tenderness, or solidity to the mass? At this point it is critical to define whether the mass appears to be within the abdominal wall or within the true abdominal cavity (or retroperitoneum). Having years of experience in examining abdomens is of great benefit in creating differential diagnoses, but starting out, it is important to keep an open mind and have an organized approach to examination. After attempting to define whether the mass is superficial (abdominal wall) or deeper, try to ascertain whether the mass is fixed to surrounding structures. Gently rock the mass back and forth and try (again, gently) to get your fingers around it. Truly fixed masses tend to be malignant or represent serious inflammatory or infectious processes (colon cancer, perforated Crohn's disease, tuberculoma). A mass that can be reduced back into the abdominal cavity is a hernia until proven otherwise.

Evaluate the adjacent lymph node basins and complete your examination, including a rectal examination in men and both pelvic and rectal examinations in women.

What lab tests are appropriate?

Lab tests are tailored to the individual patient. A 25-year-old man with a reducible umbilical hernia does not need lab tests for diagnosis or prior to repair. A 75-year-old hypertensive smoker with acute abdominal pain and a pulsatile abdominal mass will require a complete blood count, electrolytes, type and cross match, coagulation profile, electrocardiogram, and probably a chest radiograph. In all cases of abdominal masses, the indication for laboratory tests depends on the clinical suspicion and general status of the patient.

What radiographic studies are helpful?

Once again, testing depends on the differential diagnosis and clinical suspicion. Superficial and probably benign masses (hernia, lipoma, cyst, abscesses of the skin or abdominal wall) require no imaging. Suspicion of abdominal malignancy or major infection (appendiceal, colonic, or pancreatic abscess) should lead to abdominopelvic computed tomographic (CT) scanning, usually with oral, rectal, and IV contrast (if not contraindicated). Abdominal ultrasound is helpful at delineating fluid-filled masses and is especially useful in slender patients. Ultrasound is less useful as body size increases and depends on the skill of the operator. Magnetic resonance imaging may be of benefit in diagnosis and characterization of unusual abdominal or retroperitoneal masses and seems particularly helpful in detailing retroperitoneal tumor planes of invasion and in characterizing large complex liver lesions. In most cases CT scanning will suffice.

What other diagnostic tests may be useful?

Prior to beginning more invasive diagnostic interventions, every attempt should be made to determine whether a mass is vascular in origin (aneurysm, pseudoaneurysm, hemangioma) and whether it is a hernia containing the bowel. Also, be mindful that a distended bladder or impacted bowel in obtunded, compromised, or very elderly patients may be misinterpreted as a pathologic lesion.

After these caveats are addressed, the initial test of choice is most often a fine-needle aspiration (FNA) biopsy. This safe and usually not very painful procedure often makes the diagnosis. FNA may be performed with or without radiologic guidance, as each case requires. In some cases even an FNA may be contraindicated due to the potential risk of seeding the needle tract with tumor cells (as in cases of gallbladder carcinoma and hepatoma). Each case should be individualized.

If FNA results are not diagnostic, open incision or excisional biopsy should be performed. Some tumors require histopathologic evaluation of the architecture between cells and require a larger sample than FNA can afford. In these cases (soft tissue tumors, lymphomas), a large core or Tru-Cut needle biopsy is indicated. Whether the mass is incised, excised, or drained and how these procedures are done are determined for each individual patient and clinical scenario, as addressed in other chapters. As stated in the beginning of this chapter, all abdominal masses must be diagnosed so that appropriate treatment plans may be implemented.

▶ TREATMENT

Treatment of abdominal masses varies tremendously depending on the diagnosis. Small, asymptomatic, benign lesions (lipoma, benign nodes, cyst) may be simply observed without surgical intervention. Larger or symptomatic lesions need removal. Abscesses require open or radiographically guided drainage and treatment of the underlying cause. Treatment of other inflammatory and infectious processes must be individualized. Benign and malignant tumors are treated according to established protocols (resection, chemotherapy, radiation therapy). In most cases, hernias are repaired.

K E Y   P O I N T S

- ▶ All abdominal masses need to be diagnosed.

- ▶ There are a wide variety of causes of abdominal masses, and the evaluation is tailored to the suspected cause and to the individual patient.

- ▶ A thorough history and physical examination are the key to accurate diagnosis. Laboratory, radiographic, and other diagnostic tests are indicated only by the suspected etiology.

CASE 3–1. A 44-year-old housewife presents with mild upper abdominal pain and has a large slightly tender "mass" in her left upper quadrant. Three years earlier, she had a 2.5-mm-deep (Clark's level 3) melanoma removed from her left arm and a negative sentinel node biopsy.

continued

CASE 3-1. *continued*

> A. What historical points are important?
> B. What would you look for on physical exam?
> C. What lab tests and imaging studies (if any) would you order?
> D. How would you confirm the diagnosis?

CASE 3-2. A 22-year-old weight lifter is working out at the gym and suddenly develops severe right-sided abdominal pain. By the time he gets to the emergency department, he describes the pain as "8 out of 10." He has difficulty moving, and he has a tender, nonreducible abdominal mass just to the right of the umbilicus. He has direct tenderness and rebound tenderness. He is not nauseated and reports both recent bowel movements and flatus.

> A. What are the key historical points?
> B. What are the keys to his physical examination?
> C. What is your differential diagnosis?
> D. What lab tests or imaging studies will you need?
> E. While taking your medical history, he reports taking warfarin for the past 5 years as treatment for a familial hypercoagulable state. How does this alter your work-up and treatment plans?

4

Abdominal Pain/Distention

What can cause abdominal distention?

In general terms, the abdomen can become distended with air, fluid, or solid tissue. This distention can be generalized throughout the abdomen or localized to one specific region. Most patients with acute, generalized abdominal distention and pain have gaseous distention of the gastrointestinal tract from either ileus or mechanical bowel obstruction. Fluid (blood, succus, ascites, bile, and so forth) can also cause generalized abdominal distention in certain circumstances. This fluid can accumulate either within the lumen of the gastrointestinal tract or within the peritoneal cavity. Finally, localized abdominal distention is seen with solid organ enlargement or neoplastic processes. Progressive disease can lead to more generalized distention, making physical examination problematic (Table 4–1).

What causes abdominal distention in children?

In neonates, intestinal obstruction due to imperforate anus, Hirschsprung's disease (aganglionosis of distal colon), meconium ileus, bowel atresia, and midgut volvulus are common causes of abdominal distention. Necrotizing enterocolitis with resultant ileus or perforation can also lead to distention. In older children, intussusception, Meckel's diverticulum, and midgut volvulus are common etiologies for bowel obstruction, whereas appendicitis is the leading surgical cause of ileus. Children also frequently present with ileus secondary to remote infections. Tumors (Wilms' tumor, neuroblastoma) or hepatosplenomegaly may also result in prominent abdominal distention in children.

What are common causes of small bowel obstruction?

Approximately 85% of all small bowel obstructions are secondary to adhesions, hernias, or neoplasms. In the United States, adhesions from previous surgery (e.g., appendectomy, colon resection, hysterectomy, trauma laparotomy) are the most common cause of small

TABLE 4–1

Causes of Abdominal Distention

Generalized
Bowel obstruction
   Mechanical small bowel obstruction
      Adhesions
      Hernias
      Neoplasms
      Volvulus
      Foreign bodies (gallstones, worms, bezoars)
      Strictures (Crohn's disease, radiation, postoperative)
      Intussusception
   Mechanical large bowel obstruction
      Neoplasms
      Diverticulitis
      Volvulus
      Strictures (inflammatory bowel disease, radiation, ischemic, anastomotic)
      Intussusception
      Fecal impaction
      Foreign bodies
Ileus
   Intra-abdominal causes
      Peritonitis
      Inflammatory focus (appendix, gallbladder, colon, pancreas)
      Intestinal ischemia
   Extra-abdominal causes
      Myocardial infarction
      Pneumonia
      Congestive heart failure
      Head, thoracic, spinal trauma, burns
      Metabolic abnormalities
      Medications
Ogilvie's syndrome (colonic pseudo-obstruction)
Ascites
Hemoperitoneum

Localized
Uterine/ovarian enlargement
Intra-abdominal mass
Organomegaly
Gastric outlet obstruction

bowel obstruction. Worldwide, incarcerated hernias are a more frequent cause. Common small bowel malignancies include adenocarcinoma, carcinoid, sarcoma, and lymphoma. Other less common etiologies of small bowel obstruction include strictures from various causes (Crohn's disease, radiation enteritis, anastomotic sites), intraluminal foreign bodies, intussusception, and volvulus.

What are common causes of large bowel obstruction?

Large bowel adenocarcinoma is by far the most common cause of mechanical large bowel obstruction. It most commonly obstructs the narrow left colon; however, it can be located throughout the length of the large bowel. Diverticulitis complicated by a stricture can also lead to obstruction and may be difficult to differentiate from colon cancer. Other less common causes include sigmoid or cecal volvulus, other strictures, intussusception, fecal impaction, or foreign bodies.

What are intra-abdominal and extra-abdominal causes of ileus?

Ileus, or intestinal paralysis, is most commonly seen after abdominal operations but can be associated with a variety of surgical and medical conditions. Typically, the small bowel, stomach, and colon (in that order) regain peristaltic activity as a postoperative ileus resolves. Peritonitis from a variety of causes can also lead to ileus. Focal inflammatory processes such as appendicitis, cholecystitis, and diverticulitis can result in gaseous abdominal distention. Intestinal ischemia must also be considered. A variety of etiologies outside the abdominal cavity should also be considered in the patient with ileus. Conditions such as myocardial infarction, pneumonia, and congestive heart failure can lead to ileus. Similarly, patients with head, thoracic, or spinal trauma or with burns greater than 25% of body surface area can develop ileus following their injury. Finally, medications and a variety of metabolic derangements must be considered.

What is Ogilvie's syndrome and how do you manage it?

This is acute colonic pseudo-obstruction that most typically occurs in hospitalized patients in the postoperative period (orthopedic, neurosurgery, cardiac surgery), in conjunction with nonabdominal trauma (spine, head), or with a variety of medical conditions (e.g., pneumonia, myocardial infarction). These patients develop massive dilation of the colon, particularly the cecum, with variable noncolicky abdominal pain and failure to pass flatus. Examination reveals a distended and quiet abdomen. Localized tenderness is usually absent unless perforation has occurred. It is essential to exclude a mechanical cause of the colonic distention with sigmoidoscopy and/or a water-soluble contrast enema.

Conservative treatment includes nasogastric decompression and possible placement of a rectal tube. Intravenous neostigmine leads to prompt resolution of the distention in most cases. If this fails, colonoscopic decompression may be needed. Note that neostigmine should be used only after an obstructing lesion in the colon is ruled out and with appropriate cardiovascular monitoring. Operative management is indicated for signs of perforation.

What are some gynecologic causes for abdominal distention?

Ovarian tumors, both benign and malignant, can present with lower abdominal distention in nearly 50% of cases. Pseudomyxoma peritonei is a condition arising from an ovarian mucinous cystadenoma or mucocele of the appendix. It is a locally infiltrating tumor composed of multiple cysts filled with thick mucin and can lead to abdominal distention. Meigs' syndrome is ascites and hydrothorax due to ovarian fibromas. Adhesions from previous gynecologic surgery are a common cause of subsequent small bowel obstruction and abdominal distention.

In what circumstances will fluid accumulate in the peritoneal cavity and cause abdominal distention?

Blood can accumulate in the peritoneal cavity (hemoperitoneum) for a variety of reasons, including blunt abdominal trauma, ruptured ectopic pregnancy, or ruptured aneurysm, or in any patient who has undergone laparotomy. Blood itself does not irritate the peritoneum, but as it clots, peritoneal signs and ileus will develop. Be aware that the abdomen can accommodate most of the patient's blood volume with a change in girth of only 4 to 5 cm. On the other hand, ascites develops more chronically and can lead to massive distention. Physical examination findings include a dull percussion note and a fluid wave. Ascites can be from generalized processes such as chronic renal failure, right-sided heart failure, or malnutrition. More commonly it is related to intra-abdominal factors that cause formation of peritoneal fluid at a more rapid rate than resorption. Chronic liver disease (cirrhosis) is the most common etiology; however, pancreatic ascites, chylous ascites, malignancy, and peritonitis (perforated viscus, bile, tuberculosis) must be considered.

What medications can lead to ileus and abdominal distention?

The most common class of medication that causes ileus is narcotics. Morphine or meperidine given intravenously, by patient-controlled analgesia, or even via epidural catheters can result in prolonged ileus. This becomes an added problem when superimposed on postoperative ileus, peritonitis, or mechanical obstruction. Chemotherapeutic agents are also common causes of painful distention. A variety of other drugs can cause ileus, and it is therefore essential to carefully review the patient's medication regimen. Some of the other less common ones include anticholinergics, phenothiazines, calcium channel blockers, clozapine, tricyclic antidepressants, alpha agonists, and catecholamines.

What are some metabolic causes of ileus?

A variety of metabolic derangements can lead to progressive abdominal distention and pain due to the resultant ileus. Electrolyte abnormalities, particularly hypokalemia, hyponatremia, and hypomagnesemia, can lead to intestinal paralysis. Severe sepsis, even from extra-abdominal sources, can similarly affect the bowel. Other systemic derangements such as hypothyroidism, hypoparathyroidism, and uremia must also be considered. Finally, unusual conditions such as lead poisoning and porphyria can present with abdominal distention.

What causes localized abdominal distention?

Some types of intestinal obstruction such as sigmoid volvulus, closed loop small bowel obstruction, or gastric outlet obstruction may lead to localized rather than generalized distention of the abdomen. Solid organ enlargement (uterus, liver, spleen, kidney), intra-abdominal masses (mesenteric cysts, omental cysts), and ovarian or other neoplasms are other possibilities when the distention appears more localized on physical examination.

▶ **EVALUATION**

What are questions that you should ask a patient with abdominal distention?

The duration of the distention and whether it has been continuous or intermittent are important. Associated symptoms such as pain (persistent or intermittent), nausea and vomiting, and change in bowel habits, particularly obstipation, should be sought. If one is dealing with intestinal obstruction, these associated symptoms may help determine the location or nature of the obstruction. Cramping pain associated with distention but no vomiting (or late vomiting) suggests colonic obstruction. Rectal bleeding, weight loss, anemia, and recent changes in bowel habits are commonly associated with colonic obstruction. Cramps associated with concurrent bilious emesis suggest small intestinal obstruction. Vomiting of food without bile suggests gastric outlet obstruction. Diarrhea may also be seen with partial intestinal obstruction. Chronic diarrhea and weight loss usually accompany Crohn's disease. Fevers, chills, persistent pain, and distention may suggest inflammatory conditions causing ileus or the possibility of intestinal vascular compromise. These latter patients usually have associated weight loss, other manifestations of peripheral vascular disease, and pain out of proportion to the tenderness on the physical examination. You should also ask about prior abdominal operations, gastrointestinal diseases, hernias, malignancies, and abdominal radiation.

How do you examine a patient who presents with abdominal distention?

Prior to direct examination, first observe the patient's mannerisms. The patient who is grimacing and having difficulty finding a comfortable position likely has colicky pain associated with intestinal obstruction. Those appearing malnourished and apprehensive may have a chronic process such as a malignancy or intestinal ischemia. Tachycardia or orthostatic hypotension may suggest severe dehydration from a chronic process or acute hemorrhage. Fever may point to an inflammatory condition in the abdomen. Carefully inspect the abdomen for surgical scars, hernias, venous patterns, or asymmetry. Look for generalized versus localized distention. Auscultate for high-pitched bowel sounds with rushes, suggestive of bowel obstruction, versus absence or decrease in bowel sounds, suggesting ileus. Listen for bruits, indicating vascular lesions of the aorta or mesentery. Percussion aids in localizing abnormal areas of dullness or tympany as well as in eliciting early signs of peritoneal irritation. Be aware that in advanced cases of bowel obstruction, the loops of bowel may fill with fluid and give a dull percussion note. Check for a fluid wave if ascites is suspected. Finally, palpate the abdomen, assessing for organomegaly or abdominal masses. Rectal and pelvic examinations should also be performed to identify distal colonic obstruction, pelvic masses, or hematochezia.

What studies should you order when a patient presents with abdominal pain and distention?

A complete blood count should be performed to look for signs of infection or blood loss. Coagulation studies may be helpful in patients on anticoagulants or with known liver disease. Electrolytes along with blood urea nitrogen and creatinine may provide an assessment as to the degree of dehydration or possible causes of ileus. An acute abdominal series or three-way (upright chest radiograph and flat and upright kidneys, ureter, bladder [KUB]) can help rule out a perforated viscus (free air) and better characterize bowel obstruction.

The KUB may help distinguish between ileus and mechanical obstruction and better define the level of the obstruction to the small or large bowel (Table 4–2). In paralytic ileus, gaseous distention occurs rather uniformly in the stomach, small bowel, and colon. Air-fluid levels can be present, but they usually form "adynamic loops" having air-fluid levels at the same level in a short segment (inverted "U"s). In small bowel obstruction, distended loops can be distinguished by their characteristic valvulae conniventes, which occupy the entire transverse diameter of the bowel. Also, they are located more centrally in the abdomen with dynamic loops showing air-fluid levels at different levels in the same short segment (inverted "J"s). In mechanical large bowel obstruction, colonic haustral markings

TABLE 4–2

KUB Findings in Patients with Gaseous Abdominal Distention

Ileus	Small Bowel Obstruction	Large Bowel Obstruction
Gas in stomach, small bowel, and colon (mild to moderate entire transverse diameter dilation)	Distended small bowel; note that gas pattern forms lines that cross a portion of transverse diameter of bowel (valvulae conniventes)	Distended large bowel; note that gas pattern forms lines that cross only transverse diameter of bowel (haustra)
Variable gas pattern	No colon gas	± Small bowel gas (depends on ileocecal valve competency)
Bowel loops throughout abdomen	Centrally located bowel loops	Peripherally located bowel loops
Air-fluid levels	Air-fluid levels	Air-fluid levels
Inverted U	Inverted J	Inverted J

KUB, kidneys, ureter, bladder.

occupy only a portion of the transverse diameter of the bowel, and the loops are more peripherally located. Associated small bowel distention may or may not be seen, depending on the competency of the ileocecal valve. Be aware, however, that the KUB can appear normal in bowel obstruction.

When the diagnosis remains in doubt, CT scan is used to better characterize the bowel obstruction and also to evaluate for intra-abdominal masses.

TREATMENT

Which patients need admission to the hospital? Which patients need immediate surgery?

Some patients with abdominal distention and minimal associated symptoms can be scheduled for an outpatient work-up. These are patients with suspected solid organ enlargement, masses, or ascites. On the other hand, patients with more acute generalized distention that is associated with pain should be admitted to the hospital. Abdominal catastrophes such as perforated ulcers or leaking aneurysms are usually obvious and require immediate surgery. Other less dramatic inflammatory processes producing ileus, such as appendicitis and cholecystitis, also require timely surgical intervention. Others such as pancreatitis and diverticulitis are initially treated in the hospital with nonoperative means.

The group of patients for whom it is the most difficult to decide on the need for immediate operative therapy is those with bowel obstruction. If a complete, closed loop, or strangulated obstruction is suspected, prompt operation is indicated. On the other hand, chronic recurrent small bowel obstruction from adhesive disease can usually be managed nonoperatively. Large bowel obstruction usually indicates a need for surgical therapy.

How are patients with bowel obstruction initially treated?

Many causes of bowel obstruction may resolve spontaneously. In the initial treatment it is important to recognize that fluid can build up in the intestine proximal to the obstruction and poses an aspiration and perforation risk.

Initial treatment includes bowel rest, intravenous hydration, and nasogastric suction. Resolution of the obstruction will be evident by passage of gas or stool from the colon. If no resolution occurs following 24 to 48 hours of conservative treatment, further evaluation is warranted, such as CT scan or small bowel follow-through radiographs. Peritoneal signs on exam warrant surgical exploration.

K E Y   P O I N T S

▶ Abdominal distention and pain usually mean ileus or mechanical bowel obstruction.

▶ Character of bowel sounds and KUB help differentiate ileus from obstruction.

▶ CT is an extremely useful tool.

CASE 4–1. A 75-year-old man with a known history of diverticulosis presents with abdominal distention and generalized abdominal pain. His past surgical history is significant for an appendectomy when he was young. He has a low-grade fever and a tympanitic, diffusely distended abdomen.

A. Why is his abdomen distended?

B. How would you narrow the diagnosis?

CASE 4–2.

A 45-year-old woman presents to your clinic with a 5-day history of a steady increase in lower abdominal pain associated with lower abdominal distention and occasional diarrhea. Her past surgical history is significant for a total abdominal hysterectomy and cholecystectomy. She is afebrile and the abdomen is dull to percussion. Bowel sounds are decreased.

A. Can the patient have a bowel obstruction with these signs and symptoms?

B. What other etiologies for distention come to mind?

C. What diagnostic tests would have the greatest yield in this case?

5

Acute Abdomen

There may be no greater opportunity to alleviate human suffering and to save lives than in the proper evaluation and treatment of acute abdominal conditions.

▶ ETIOLOGY

What is an acute abdomen?

The acute abdomen is a medical condition whose hallmarks are the onset of persistent abdominal pain (>6 hours) and tenderness. Other characteristic symptoms and signs are often present (e.g., nausea, vomiting, fever, tachycardia), as may be abnormal laboratory and radiographic findings. Early accurate diagnosis and treatment are mandatory because morbidity and mortality are directly proportional to delay. Almost one half of patients presenting to the emergency department with acute abdominal pain require definitive surgical or procedural intervention.

What is the pathophysiology?

Regardless of cause, abdominal pain results from stimulation of either visceral (autonomic) or somatic peritoneal neural pathways. Disease processes (e.g., appendicitis) often initially cause a dull, poorly localized pain (periumbilical) transmitted via bilateral autonomic nerve pathways to the segmental spinal cord center. These nerves innervate smooth muscle in the walls of tubes (intestine, bile ducts, ureters) and are stimulated by stretching, distention, or contraction against resistance. Pain is sensed as a poorly localized ache in certain locations (stomach-epigastrium, appendix-periumbilical region, colon-hypogastrium). Progression of disease results in inflammation of the serosa or the parietal peritoneum with direct stimulation of somatic sensory nerves. Pain is severe and localized unless perforation occurs, in which case the somatic pain is diffuse and generalized.

What are the common causes of the acute abdomen?

The most common causes of acute abdominal pain in order of frequency in the United States are listed in Table 5–1. Abdominal pain may present as diffuse pain or may be localized in a specific place. It is helpful to consider common disease entities by dividing the abdomen into quadrants, as shown in Figure 5–1A; the causes of diffuse abdominal pain are shown in Figure 5–1B.

▶ EVALUATION

Patients with acute abdominal pain mandate immediate surgical evaluation (i.e., see them now!). If possible, narcotics should be held until examination is completed. Early diagnosis and treatment are critical.

What historical points are important?

A thorough history is essential and includes a past medical history as well as a description of the present illness and any associated

TABLE 5–1

Common Causes of Acute Abdominal Pain

Nonspecific abdominal pain (e.g. constipation, food reaction)
Gastroenteritis
Gynecologic disorders
   Mittelschmerz
   Ovarian cyst
   Pelvic inflammatory disease
   Endometriosis
   Other
Acute appendicitis
Biliary
   Gallstones
   Cholecystitis
   Common duct stones
   Cholangitis
Bowel obstruction
Urologic disorders
   Stone disease
   Cystitis
   Pyelonephritis
Enterocolitis
   Inflammatory bowel disease
   Pseudomembranous
   Infectious
   Ischemic
Other
   Pancreatitis
   Hepatitis
   Pneumonitis
   Myocardial ischemia

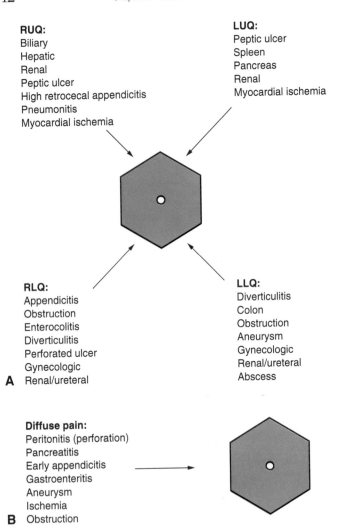

RUQ:
Biliary
Hepatic
Renal
Peptic ulcer
High retrocecal appendicitis
Pneumonitis
Myocardial ischemia

LUQ:
Peptic ulcer
Spleen
Pancreas
Renal
Myocardial ischemia

RLQ:
Appendicitis
Obstruction
Enterocolitis
Diverticulitis
Perforated ulcer
Gynecologic
A Renal/ureteral

LLQ:
Diverticulitis
Colon
Obstruction
Aneurysm
Gynecologic
Renal/ureteral
Abscess

Diffuse pain:
Peritonitis (perforation)
Pancreatitis
Early appendicitis
Gastroenteritis
Aneurysm
Ischemia
B Obstruction

Figure 5–1. *A,* Causes of acute abdominal pain by quadrant. *B,* Causes of diffuse abdominal pain. LLQ, left lower quadrant; LUQ, left upper quadrant; RLQ, right lower quadrant; RUQ, right upper quadrant.

illnesses. Have there been any previous similar episodes? Are there associated illnesses or symptoms? Precise definition of the patient's pain is most important with regard to onset, character, location, duration, and any aggravating or alleviating factors.

The onset of pain may be gradual (appendicitis, bowel obstruction) or acute and catastrophic (perforated viscus). The character of the pain may be mild or severe, constant (appendicitis, diverticulitis, pancreatitis), or intermittent (biliary colic, bowel obstruction, kidney stone). The pain of colic is severe and intermittent, resulting from obstruction of tubes and subsequent contraction of smooth muscles. Patients with colic move about, trying to get comfortable. The location of pain is helpful (as depicted in Figure 5–1A), as is a pattern of migratory pain, seen classically in cases of appendicitis. The duration of pain aids not only in diagnosis but also in assessment of the patient's overall condition; severe pain, nausea, and vomiting lasting 48 hours create a high risk of hypovolemia and electrolyte imbalances and may be associated with significant septic complications. Factors aggravating or alleviating pain should be elicited. Pain that is aggravated by moving, coughing, or deep breathing indicates severe inflammation of the peritoneum (peritonitis).

The remainder of the history must include a description of associated symptoms, prior illnesses, operations, medications, family history, and in women, a menstrual history.

What are the steps to physical examination?

Examination of the patient begins on your arrival with specific attention to facial expression, attitude in bed, body habitus, respiratory pattern and rate, pulse, temperature, and mucous membranes. A motionless, pale, diaphoretic patient with shallow, grunting respirations secondary to diffuse peritonitis (e.g., perforated viscus) is in need of immediate operative intervention.

Although special attention is paid to the abdomen, the remainder of the physical examination must be complete with respect to heart, lungs, skin, and mental status. If possible, narcotics should be held until after the abdominal exam.

Inspection is first. Is there a mass, lump, distention, or visible peristalsis, or are there signs of inflammation?

Palpation of the abdomen must be gentle and start from a point distant from the area of maximal pain and tenderness. Rebound tenderness is best elicited by gentle percussion and palpation or by having the patient cough, laugh, or elevate the legs by tensing the abdomen. These maneuvers reveal peritoneal irritation. Palpation of one side of the abdomen referring pain to the opposite side represents localized peritonitis, as seen with appendicitis (Rovsing's sign), or diverticulitis. Is the abdomen soft or rigid? Is the muscular guarding causing rigidity involuntary or voluntary? Does the patient have pain on rectal or pelvic examination or with thigh extension (psoas sign) or rotation (obturator sign)?

Careful, gentle auscultation is performed. Complete absence of bowel sounds is ominous, often representing diffuse peritonitis as seen with contamination from perforation and overwhelming sepsis. In fact, the presence of normal bowel sounds may reassure one that diffuse peritonitis is not present. Hyperactive or intermittent sounds are detected with obstruction or gastroenteritis. Listen for bruits from a vascular source.

What laboratory studies are appropriate?

Laboratory examination may be extremely helpful. At the least, all patients should submit specimens for a complete blood count, urinalysis, and amylase, and in women of childbearing age, a pregnancy test. Upper abdominal complaints may require a liver panel and lipase level. Electrolytes, blood urea nitrogen, and creatinine reveal volume and metabolic derangements. A coagulation profile may be indicated if considering operative intervention in a patient at risk for coagulopathy (liver disease, warfarin history).

What radiographic studies are helpful?

A chest radiograph should be obtained in all but the most obvious cases and is essential in patients without an obvious diagnosis. Two- or three-view abdominal radiographs may be helpful in those without obvious diagnosis and may reveal fecaliths (appendicitis), stones (biliary or renal), air-fluid levels (obstruction), ground-glass appearance (ascites), or a mass. The use of abdominal computed tomographic (CT) scans, ultrasound, arteriograms, and air-contrast examinations may be indicated and in some cases diagnostic.

In what circumstances is special care warranted?

Accurate diagnosis of abdominal conditions is exceedingly difficult, and therefore abdominal conditions are associated with higher morbidity and mortality rates in certain patient groups. Extensive prior experience in evaluation of these patients is beneficial.

Beware of the acute abdomen in patients at the extremes of life (i.e., infants, the elderly). Communication may be limited by age, debility, dementia, and confusion. Comorbid conditions are frequently present. Patients may be uncooperative.

The immunocompromised patient is difficult to evaluate and at high risk from delayed or inaccurate diagnosis. Most commonly, patients present with a history of steroid consumption. Signs and symptoms (e.g., fever, pain, tenderness) may be masked completely. These patients may not present until late in the course of illness. Patients with human immunodeficiency virus–related states and those receiving chemotherapy are equally challenging and at risk.

Patients with neurologic disorders (paraplegia, quadriplegia) do not sense pain. Systemic signs and symptoms may be the only clues to acute abdominal processes. Liberal use of CT scanning of the abdomen is helpful.

Postoperative patients represent another high-risk group. This includes patients recovering from any major procedure (cardiac, thoracic, general surgical). These patients are taking large doses of narcotics or epidural agents and have varying levels of consciousness. Be wary of the acute onset of abdominal pain in any postoperative patient. This may represent acute cholecystitis, pancreatitis, hemorrhage, or a technical complication of surgery such as iatrogenic bowel perforation (e.g., after a laparoscopic procedure). Early diagnosis and treatment may be life saving.

▶ TREATMENT

Treatment depends on early accurate diagnosis. When an operative condition is identified, surgery should not be delayed. Patients who experienced an intra-abdominal catastrophe (e.g., perforated ulcer or colon) should be taken to operation after resuscitation is initiated. The source of patient instability and systemic collapse is inflammation due to abdominal sepsis, and stability is not obtained until the focus is removed or alleviated. For noncatastrophic cases, when a surgical condition is diagnosed, operation should be performed as soon as possible. Appendectomies and laparotomies for bowel obstruction should not be "scheduled for tomorrow." Morbidity and mortality are minimized by prompt surgical correction. Diagnose early, treat early.

The surgeon will sometimes operate without a diagnosis. Systemic signs associated with abdominal pain, tenderness, rebound, guarding, and rigidity constitute the true "acute surgical abdomen" and mandate immediate exploration even without a preoperative diagnosis. Occasionally in such a case, findings are negative, but the risk of delaying operation far outweighs the risk of the rare negative laparotomy.

K E Y   P O I N T S

▶ The evaluation of abdominal pain begins with a thorough history and physical examination.

▶ Laboratory and radiographic studies are necessary only as clinically indicated.

▶ Special care must be taken when evaluating patients whose comorbidities alter their ability to communicate or sense pain.

▶ Although therapy depends on the etiology, sometimes it is necessary to intervene before reaching a diagnosis.

CASE 5-1. A 45-year-old stockbroker presents to the emergency department with severe abdominal pain. Yesterday, he had a vague ache in his epigastrium with some radiation to his mid back. The pain intensified overnight and then became unbearable. Now the pain is both in his epigastrium and his right lower quadrant. His pulse rate is 120 beats/min, his respiratory rate is 24 breaths/min, he is afebrile, and his blood pressure is 195/82 mm Hg.

    A. What is the differential diagnosis of this pain?
    B. What is the importance of the change in his pain location?
    C. What studies are appropriate?
    D. What therapeutic maneuvers can be done while the diagnosis
       is being made?

CASE 5-2. A 67-year-old woman with a 10-year history of diabetes mellitus presents with a 3-day history of diffuse severe abdominal pain. Her temperature is 38°C and her blood sugar is 568 mg/dL. She is tachypneic, and blood gas analysis shows evidence of metabolic acidosis.

    A. What is the likely diagnosis?
    B. Does this patient need an operation?
    C. What steps are necessary to prepare this patient for the
       operating room?

CASE 5-3. A 59-year-old man with a history of hypertension presents with a 60-minute history of "tearing" abdominal pain that radiates to his back. He has a palpable, pulsatile mass in his abdomen. His pulse rate is 120 beats/min and his blood pressure is 90/40 mm Hg.

    A. What is the likely diagnosis?
    B. What studies are appropriate?
    C. What is the appropriate treatment?

6

Breast Mass

One of the most common referrals to the surgeon's office is for evaluation of a breast mass. The mass is either self-discovered or found on physical exam by a primary physician or gynecologist. Breast cancer is the most common cancer diagnosed in women in the United States and is second only to lung cancer as cause of death from cancer in women annually. Because of this, the appearance of a breast mass can cause considerable anxiety for a patient. More than 500,000 surgical (open) breast biopsies are done each year in the United States, with more than three quarters of those biopsies resulting in benign pathology.

▶ ETIOLOGY

What are the common causes of benign breast masses?

Many of the masses that a surgeon is asked to evaluate are benign. These include simple breast cysts, fibroadenomas, fibrocystic changes, cystosarcoma phylloides, or inframammary lymph nodes. In addition, fat necrosis from breast trauma may present as a mass. Breast abscess can also present as an isolated mass. If the abscess cavity is deep in the breast parenchyma, the skin erythema may be subtle or absent in early lesions.

What are the common causes of malignant breast masses?

Malignant masses of the breast are divided into those derived from breast epithelium, or ducts, and those derived from breast stroma, or lobules. Malignant lesions are further divided into those that are invasive and those that are in situ. In situ lesions exhibit malignant cells that have not yet crossed the basement membrane. The presence of these "precancers" in a biopsy specimen indicates a higher risk of invasive cancer in the future. These patients need to be monitored closely. Some patients have malignancies of other origins in the breast, such as breast lymphoma, or metastases from other primary tumors, such as melanoma. Rarely, neoplasms elsewhere may present with metastatic nodules to the breast.

What are the causes of a painful breast mass?

Many patients are under the misconception that breast cancers in the early stages are painful; therefore, painful lesions of the breast are a cause of great concern in female patients. Painful mass as a presenting symptom of a breast cancer occurs in only 11% of patients. Fibroadenomas, fibrocystic changes, or simple cysts often present with cyclical pain or swelling that is bothersome to the patient. Other causes of painful breast mass include breast abscess or fat necrosis from breast trauma. In evaluating painful breast masses, a history of fluctuation in size of the mass or symptoms due to the mass may be helpful, because cyclical fluctuations are more commonly associated with benign causes of breast masses. Decisions on further evaluation should be made based on the other clinical features of the mass rather than the history of pain.

What is the difference between fibrocystic changes and fibroadenoma?

Symptomatic fibrocystic changes are present in 30% to 50% of women during their reproductive life. Histologically, such changes consist of fibrosis, cysts, and a variable amount of ductal hyperplasia. Fibrocystic changes do not confer an increased cancer risk; however, they do make the breasts somewhat more difficult to examine. The usual pattern of fibrocystic breast disease is diffuse, rubbery, dense texture of the breasts with no real predominant mass. The term *fibroadenoma* refers to a predominant mass that is identified in the breast, usually in a woman who has some amount of fibrocystic changes. The mass is usually mobile with smooth borders. Ultrasound is helpful in distinguishing between a solid fibroadenoma and a cyst caused by fibrocystic breast disease.

▶ EVALUATION

What are the pertinent questions for evaluating a breast mass?

The patient should be asked how and when the breast mass was discovered. If the patient is aware of the mass, you should ask if the mass has changed in size since it was first discovered. Ask if the mass becomes painful or if there are changes in the size of the lesion with menstruation. Ask if there is any history of trauma to the breast, although many women can sustain trauma to the breast without being aware of it. There are questions specific to breast cancer that will help you stratify the risk of malignancy in a patient. These are listed in Table 6–1. Although the presence of any of the historical risk factors should increase the index of suspicion for a potential malignancy, their absence does not exclude the possibil-

---

TABLE 6-1

Pertinent History for Patients with Breast Masses

Family history of breast cancer (premenopausal breast: ↑↑ cancer risk)
Previous breast biopsies demonstrating cancer, in situ cancer, or hyperplasia with atypia
Prior or current abnormal mammographic findings (microcalcifications or spiculated lesions)
Intake of estrogens
Current age (premenopausal or postmenopausal)
Age at menarche (early menarche: ↑ risk)
Age at first pregnancy (late pregnancy: ↑ risk)
Breast-feeding > 6 months: ↓ risk
Prior history of endometrial or ovarian cancer

---

ity that the mass is malignant. Women with the lowest risk factors, who are younger than 45 years of age (premenopausal), and who have negative mammograms and a self-discovered breast mass account for three fourths of patients who have delayed diagnosis of breast cancer.

How do I examine the breast?

The clinical breast exam can be an intimidating examination for medical students early in their training. Comfort with the exam comes with time. Male practitioners may want a chaperone for the exam both for the patient's ease and for medicolegal protection. The first part of the exam consists of examining both breasts to assess symmetry. All efforts should be made to preserve modesty for the patient, but you must see both breasts together at some point in the exam or you may miss subtle differences from side to side. Note any skin changes or dimples or nipple retraction, both with the patient's hands on the hips and with the hands above the head. The patient then lies down with the arm on the side of the exam above the head to distribute the breast tissue evenly on the chest wall. The exam should be systematic such that the entire breast is examined, including the tail of Spence, which extends toward the ipsilateral axilla. The axilla itself is also examined. The clinical breast exam is pictured in Figure 6-1. Lastly, the nipple-areola complex is examined to rule out nipple discharge. Take the opportunity to educate the patient about monthly breast self-examinations as you go through your exam. A surprising percentage of patients are uncomfortable asking about how to do a self-examination.

How do I describe a mass in the chart?

To compare physical findings from one clinic visit to the next, and to correlate physical findings with abnormalities identified on diagnostic radiograph (mammogram, ultrasound, or magnetic resonance [MR] imaging), there should be some uniformity to the manner in

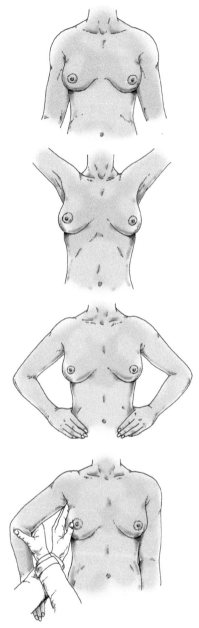

Figure 6-1. Positions for proper breast examination. (Redrawn from Greenfield LJ, Mulholland MW, Oldham KT, Zelenock GB [eds]: Surgery: Scientific Principles and Practices. Philadelphia, JB Lippincott, 1993, p 1241.)

which breast lesions are described. Many surgical breast clinics have forms that include a drawing of the breast so that you can record your findings in a picture. This should be accompanied by a narrative description that includes which breast (left or right) is affected, the approximate size of the lesion, and the character of the lesion (mobile vs. fixed, smooth distinct borders vs. irregular) and its location in relation to the nipple-areola complex. The location should include the quadrant of the breast or the location described as if the breast were the face of a clock with the nipple at the center (e.g., "mass at 7 o'clock, 3 cm from the nipple").

What features distinguish a benign from a malignant breast mass?

When you are evaluating a breast lump in the clinic, it is important to collect the information from the history, the physical exam, and the radiographic features to stratify the risk of the lump's being malignant. The features on physical exam associated with increased risk for malignancy are summarized in Table 6–2. Increasingly, ultrasound is being used in the clinic by surgeons as an adjunct to physical exam, so the distinguishing sonographic features are included as well. Most masses have some benign *and* some worrisome features, and for this reason the majority of masses are sampled for histologic confirmation once they are identified.

TABLE 6–2

Ultrasonographic and Physical Exam Features of Benign Versus Malignant Masses

Low-Risk (Benign-Appearing) Breast Masses	Moderate- to High-Risk (Malignant-Appearing) Breast Masses

Physical exam
  Smooth borders
  Mobile mass
	Physical exam
	  Irregular mass
	  Skin changes: peau d'orange, dimpling
	  Nipple retraction
	  Bloody or brown nipple discharge
	  Axillary masses

Ultrasound
  Smooth, distinct borders
  Hypoechoic (fluid-filled) cyst without
    internal echoes
  Width > depth on sonographic measurements
  No disruption of normal breast architecture
    on sonogram
	Ultrasound
	  Irregular borders
	  Complex internal echoes
	  Intralesional calcifications with shadowing
	  Depth ≥ width on sonographic
	    measurements

Can I evaluate a breast mass without a screening mammogram?

Mammograms are extremely helpful as a part of a comprehensive breast health screening program for women older than 40 years of age. Many younger women have breast tissue that is too dense for mammogram, and the evaluation of masses in this age group is often done without a mammogram. In most cases, scheduling a screening mammogram to fully evaluate the remainder of the breast as well as the contralateral breast can be done without delaying the diagnostic work-up of the palpable mass. Mammography is not perfect and can fail to detect from 10% to 25% of invasive cancers; therefore, palpable masses of the breast need to be evaluated in spite of a negative mammogram.

How do I evaluate the patient with a mass and an abnormality on mammogram?

Carefully review the mammogram before examining the patient by both reading the report and looking at the films. Then carefully compare the findings of your exam with the mammographic findings. If the palpable mass clearly corresponds with the palpable abnormality, a diagnostic work-up of the mass begins with a fine-needle aspiration (FNA) of the palpable mass followed by either excisional biopsy or definitive cancer treatment if the FNA is positive for cancer. If no mass is palpable near the mammographic abnormality, a mammographically placed wire should guide the open surgical biopsy of the lesion. If a palpable mass is present but is not clearly associated with the site of the mammographic abnormality, treat the two lesions as separate entities and work them up in parallel: FNA for the palpable lesion and needle-localized biopsy for the mammographic abnormality.

▶ TREATMENT

What type of biopsy is appropriate for the initial evaluation of the palpable mass?

A flow sheet for the approach to the evaluation of a palpable breast mass appears in Figure 6–2. The definitive treatment of specific types of breast lesions after they are diagnosed is discussed in Chapter 26.

What type of incision should be made for an incisional biopsy?

The options for incisions of the breast for biopsy are shown in Figure 6–3. The location of the incision should be related to the location of

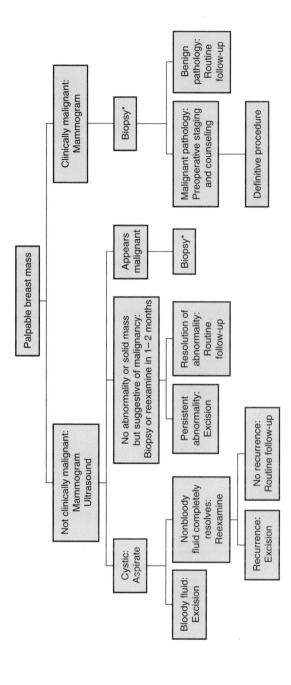

*Biopsy may be fine-needle aspiration (FNA) or excisional. If cytology appears benign or nondiagnostic and mass persists, the lesion should be excised.

Figure 6–2. Algorithm for evaluation of a palpable breast mass.

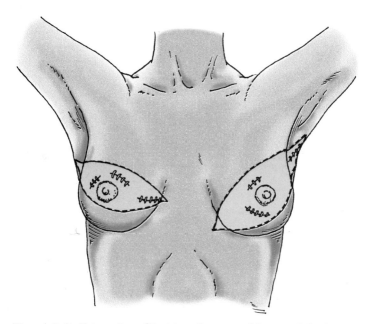

Figure 6–3. Orientation of incisions for surgical biopsy of the breast, shown in relation to potential mastectomy incisions *(shaded areas)*. (Redrawn from Greenfield LJ, Mulholland MW, Oldham KT, Zelenock GB [eds]: Surgery: Scientific Principles and Practices. Philadelphia, JB Lippincott, 1993, p 1246.)

the lesion, with care taken not to have the incision make definitive surgical treatment difficult should the lesion turn out to be malignant. Circumareolar incisions are reserved for infra-areolar lesions. Incisional biopsies can be done under either local or general anesthesia.

K E Y   P O I N T S

▶ Painless breast mass is the most common presentation of breast cancer. Nonetheless, most open biopsies done in the United States are for benign lesions.

▶ Breast masses should be evaluated in a multimodal manner, including clinical breast exam, history for risk stratification, mammography, and, when appropriate, ultrasound or other diagnostic tools such MR imaging.

▶ There is a great deal of overlap in the features of benign and malignant lesions; therefore, tissue confirmation is needed for any persistent breast mass.

▶ Many breast biopsies are done for benign disease; therefore, attention to cosmesis is an important consideration.

CASE 6–1. A 48-year-old woman is sent for evaluation of a breast mass discovered on routine physical examination by her primary care physician. She had presented to her primary physician with a history of new onset of vertigo and multiple falls. On physical examination, she is noted to have a 3×4-cm mass in the upper outer quadrant of the left breast with ill-defined borders and mild skin changes over the mass when she is examined upright. She had not noted the mass but admits that she is not consistent in performing breast self-examinations.

A. What other history would you like to take?
B. How would you manage her mass initially?

She returns 2 weeks after a core needle biopsy of the mass that is consistent with fat necrosis. She has complete resolution of the skin changes, with the mass now half the size on physical exam. The mammogram is negative except for a rounded lesion consistent with fibroadenoma in the contralateral breast that had not changed in the previous three screening mammograms.

C. What was the probable etiology of the mass felt on initial exam?
D. How would your management change if the mass had not resolved partially on her return visit?
E. What would you recommend for the rounded lesion in the opposite breast noted on mammogram?

CASE 6–2. A 20-year-old woman presents with a painful mass in the right breast. The size has nearly doubled since she first noted it 2 months earlier. She has a maternal aunt who died of breast cancer in her 40s. She has a 9-month-old child whom she breast-fed for 7 months. She has never had a breast biopsy or mass in the past. On physical examination she has a 2 × 2-cm firm mass in the left upper outer quadrant at 10 o'clock, 3 cm from the nipple. It is not fixed to the chest wall, and there are no overlying skin changes. The mass has somewhat indistinct borders.

   A. What radiographic tools could you use to evaluate her mass further?

   B. Does the fact that the lesion is painful change your diagnostic work-up?

7

Change in Bowel Habits

What is normal bowel function?

Normal bowel function is a relative term defined as the usual function the patient has experienced over a period of good health. The characteristics of defecation, including the timing, consistency, and frequency, have an established pattern that is normal for that patient. Normal consistency of stool is variable and can range from hard to loose. Similarly, the frequency can span from one stool every 3 days to three stools per day. Diet also plays an important function in defining normal bowel function. The important point is to focus on the patient's usual stool characteristics when the patient felt well or healthy.

How are changes in bowel habits manifest?

The onset of changes in bowel habits is usually gradual. The length of time during which the patient has been aware of a change is often underestimated. Abrupt changes in bowel habits usually represent acute processes such as infectious or inflammatory conditions.

Straining at stool is a frequent complaint grouped under the heading of constipation. A feeling of incomplete emptying of the rectum is also reported in this subgroup. Both complaints focus on rectal outlet pathology. A "recent change in bowel habits" can be a complaint or symptom in patients with colorectal cancer.

▶ EVALUATION

What are important features in evaluating a patient with change in bowel habits?

A thorough history and physical examination are the key to making a diagnosis and identifying patients who may benefit from further evaluation. *Fiber* and *fluid* intake are factors to determine bowel habits: even if dietary fiber is high, poor water intake will cause hard stool.

Medication can affect bowel habits, usually by slowing stool transit, particularly in the elderly population. Supplemental dietary calcium intake can slow transit, as do calcium channel blockers and antidepressants. Unfortunately, all of these compounds are frequently used by the elderly population.

Decreased physical activity is another bowel factor, also common in older patients.

Aging causes progressive diminution of mobility, but trauma can acutely create similar problems.

What are the two common modes of presentation?

1. Diarrhea is usually synonymous with increased stool frequency or increased water or mucus in the stool. It can be broadly classified as acute or chronic and as infectious or noninfectious. A dietary and travel history can be helpful in determining an infectious etiology for a new onset of diarrhea; common causes are summarized in Table 7–1.
2. Constipation is defined as a decrease in stool frequency coupled with an increase in stool hardness. Patients often experience extreme difficulty in defecation and a feeling of incomplete evacuation. Common causes of constipation are summarized in Table 7–2.

How do I investigate a patient with diarrhea?

Because acute diarrheal attacks are often due to infectious agents, cultures should be taken for ova and parasites. Sigmoidoscopy should be performed to diagnose inflammatory, infectious, ischemic, or pseudomembranous colitis. Stools should be checked for *Clostridium difficile* toxin. The patient should be investigated for various benign causes of diarrhea such as lactose intolerance, antibiotics, magnesium-containing antacids, and postoperative conditions such as follows gastrectomy. Biopsy of the colonic mucosa will confirm the diagnosis of microscopic colitis, which is

---

TABLE 7–1

Causes of Infectious Diarrhea

1. Enterotoxigenic bacteria: stimulate the bowel to increase the secretions in lumen (*Staphylococcus aureus*, *Vibrio cholerae*, *Clostridium perfringens*, *Clostridium botulinum*)
2. Invasive organisms: invade the bowel wall and cause ulcerations (*Shigella*, *Campylobacter*, *Yersinia enterocolitica*, *Helicobacter pylori*) or cause an inflammatory response in the bowel mucosa without ulcer formation (*Salmonella*)
3. Parasitic infections: *Giardia lamblia*, *Entamoeba histolytica*, and various worm infections
4. *Cryptosporidium* and cytomegalovirus: commonly cause chronic diarrhea in AIDS and immunocompromised patients

TABLE 7–2	

Diarrhea Chronicity
Acute   Often indicates an organic disease state (e.g., mechanical bowel obstruction, adynamic ileus from trauma or peritoneal irritation)   *Chronic*   Neurologic problem (e.g., irritable bowel syndrome, Hirschsprung's disease)   Electrolyte disorder (hyperglycemia, hypercalcemia)   Psychological disorder

now recognized as a definite entity and an important cause of diarrhea, particularly in elderly women.

Patients with persistent or chronic diarrhea need stool cultures and visualization of the mucosa with sigmoidoscopy. Biopsy, both for histology and for culture and sensitivity, is reasonably reliable to rule out viral causes of microscopic colitis. Less than 10% of mucus-secreting villous tumors cause diarrhea; however, both benign and malignant tumors can present with loose stool and increased stool frequency.

Any patient with severe or longstanding symptoms of diarrhea should be tested and treated for dehydration and electrolyte abnormalities.

Which constipated patient needs further evaluation?

If there is no suspicion of neoplasia, the evaluation and treatment of constipation can be pursued without further studies.

Recent onset of constipation, bloody stools, pain, fever, anemia, and weight loss are suggestive of neoplasia, and further investigations are necessary in these patients. Colonoscopy with bowel preparation is the investigation of choice; however, flexible sigmoidoscopy with barium enema may be an acceptable alternative.

If an organic cause of constipation is suspected, sigmoidoscopy and serum chemistries should be performed.

▶ TREATMENT

How do I treat a patient with change in bowel habits?

Treatment mainly depends on the cause of the change in bowel habits. Based on the assessment of fluid status in the initial evaluation of the patient with diarrhea, intravenous fluid resuscitation may be needed. Antibiotics are useful in cases of invasive bacterial or cytotoxic infectious diarrhea, whereas antispasmodics should be used with caution and should be avoided in patients with fever or bloody diarrhea. Obviously, other treatments depend on the specific cause identified.

Constipated patients with no organic cause may benefit from a high-fiber diet. If the patient fails a trial of conservative treatment, further investigations such as sigmoidoscopy, colonoscopy, or barium enema should be performed to direct treatment toward a specific cause. In patients with cancer and selected patients with functional causes, surgery may be indicated.

K E Y   P O I N T S

▶ A complete history and thorough physical examination are necessary to evaluate changes in stool habits.

▶ Laboratory investigation is necessary only in selected cases.

▶ Change in bowel habit is the key symptom in colorectal cancer.

▶ Presence of other symptoms such as rectal bleeding, abdominal pain, anemia, and signs of abdominal mass increases the suspicion of cancer.

CASE 7–1.   A 54-year-old man presents complaining of a gradually decreasing caliber of his stools and constipation during the last 6 months. He has no significant past medical history. He has continued to work as a grocery store manager but states that he feels really tired by the end of the day.

    A. What is the probable diagnosis, based on his complaints?
    B. What history is important to obtain?
    C. What initial studies are important to obtain at the first office visit?
    D. What follow-up should be arranged?

8

Free Intraperitoneal Air

The surgeon is generally called to evaluate a patient with free intraperitoneal air identified by radiographs. These films are generally obtained to evaluate a patient presenting to the emergency department or on the hospital ward with abdominal pain.

▶ ETIOLOGY

What is free intraperitoneal air?

Free intraperitoneal air refers to the presence of extraluminal air within the peritoneal cavity, that is, air outside of the gastrointestinal tract. Free intraperitoneal air must be distinguished from retroperitoneal air (usually presenting along the border of the psoas muscle), intraluminal air-fluid levels in the gastrointestinal tract, air in the portal vein, and air located in loculated intra-abdominal abscess cavities. Retroperitoneal air can be caused by a posterior perforation of the duodenum (usually due to blunt trauma) or retroperitoneal perforation of the rectum or colon. Occasionally a patient with extensive subcutaneous emphysema has air in the soft tissues overlying the abdominal wall, which can confuse the inexperienced clinician.

What is the etiology of free intraperitoneal air?

The most common cause of intraperitoneal air is a recent laparotomy or laparoscopy. Free intraperitoneal air may be present on a radiograph up to several days following abdominal surgery. The great concern when free intraperitoneal air is identified is the possibility of a perforation in the gastrointestinal tract. The hole can be present anywhere from the gastroesophageal junction to the rectum.

Occasionally, a patient receiving positive-pressure ventilation or a patient with a major tracheobronchial airway injury can present with pneumomediastinum. The air in the mediastinum under pressure can dissect down from the mediastinum into the peritoneal cavity.

▶ **EVALUATION**

What radiographic views should be ordered if I suspect free intraperitoneal air?

An upright posteroanterior chest radiograph is the best way to demonstrate free intraperitoneal air. The air is most easily seen when it accumulates between the right hemidiaphragm and the liver, accounting for the idiomatic expression "free air under the diaphragm" (Fig. 8–1). Some patients are too ill to tolerate the upright position prior to the chest radiograph. If this is the case, the patient may be placed in the left lateral decubitus position for several minutes (the right side of the abdomen is elevated). This position allows the free intraperitoneal air to rise to the right lateral abdominal wall (Fig. 8–2).

Some inexperienced clinicians order a flat plate of the abdomen and an upright abdominal radiograph to search for free intraperitoneal air. These views (particularly the upright abdominal radiograph) may demonstrate the free intraperitoneal air if the diaphragm is seen. However, the real role of these two radiographic views in the evaluation of a patient with an acute abdomen is the demonstration of multiple intraluminal air-fluid

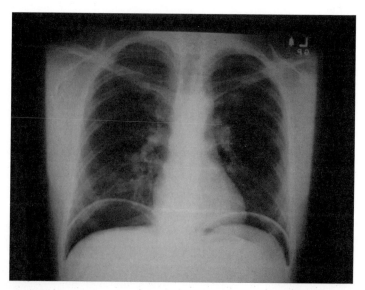

Figure 8–1. Radiograph depicting extraluminal gas as "free air under the diaphragm."

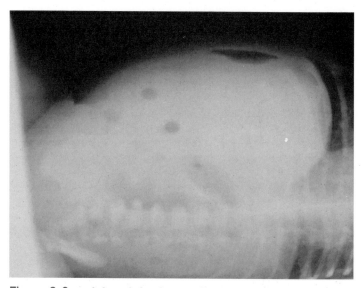

Figure 8–2. Left lateral decubitus radiograph depicting extraluminal gas.

levels characteristic of a bowel obstruction. An astute radiologist can recognize very subtle signs on the flat plate and upright abdomen that suggest free intraperitoneal air. However, as a general rule, an upright chest radiograph should always be ordered in addition to a flat plate and upright abdominal radiograph if hollow viscus perforation is suspected.

The abdominal computed tomographic (CT) scan is playing an increasingly important role in the evaluation of patients with acute abdominal pain. Many clinicians omit routine abdominal radiographs and proceed directly to the abdominal CT scan. The abdominal CT scan is an excellent test to identify both free intraperitoneal and retroperitoneal air (Fig. 8–3). This examination also gives important information regarding free intraperitoneal fluid, loculated intra-abdominal fluid collections, or bowel wall thickening, as well as the state of solid organs such as the liver, spleen, pancreas, and kidneys.

What is the clinical significance of free intraperitoneal air?

The identification of free intraperitoneal air is a critical clinical finding because almost all patients who present with abdominal pain

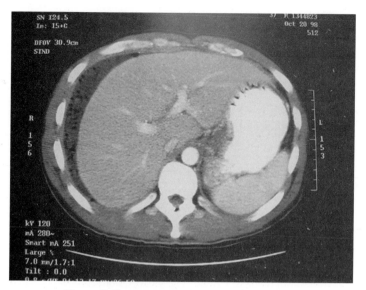

Figure 8–3. CT scan depicting extraluminal gas.

and who have "free air under the diaphragm" require surgical intervention. In other words, the finding of free intraperitoneal air helps distinguish those patients who require an operation from those who can be managed nonoperatively.

Do all patients with free intraperitoneal air need an operation?

"Surgeons operate on patients, not x-rays." This aphorism is a basic principle that must be internalized by the aspiring surgeon to avoid serious error. The approach to the patient with acute abdominal pain is guided by a careful history and physical examination. The direction and tempo of the work-up are also in part determined by the hemodynamic stability of the patient. This subject is covered in detail in Chapter 5.

The presence of free intraperitoneal air in the patient with an acute abdomen is such a dramatic and significant finding that there must be clinical circumstances of real substance to prevent operative evaluation of the patient's abdomen.

A recent laparotomy or laparoscopy within the past several days can result in residual free intraperitoneal air without morbid significance. Without the history of recent laparotomy or significant mediastinal emphysema, the most likely diagnosis is a hollow viscus perforation.

▶ TREATMENT

What are the treatment options in a patient with free intraperitoneal air?

As previously implied, clinically stable patients with free intraperitoneal air due to recent surgery or pneumomediastinum do not require surgical intervention.

The treatment rendered to patients with perforation of a hollow viscus depends on the site of perforation and, in some instances, the duration of the symptoms and the overall medical status of the patient. The perforation may be located in the intra-abdominal esophagus, the stomach, the intraperitoneal duodenum, the small intestine, the intraperitoneal colon, or the intraperitoneal rectum. Perforations of the retroperitoneal duodenum (Fig. 8–4), colon, or rectum (Fig. 8–5) lead to retroperitoneal air that can be distinguished from intraperitoneal air on the abdominal CT scan.

Perforations of the intra-abdominal esophagus are not common and occur for the most part as a complication of endoscopy. Small perforations in clinically stable patients are managed with observation and antibiotic therapy. Otherwise, surgical intervention is necessary. The classic noniatrogenic esophageal perforation, Boerhaave's syndrome, occurs in the left side of the chest after a bout of vomiting (often associated with excessive alcohol intake or

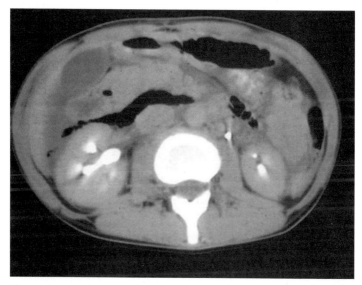

Figure 8–4. CT scan depicting the extraluminal gas pattern resulting from a perforation of the retroperitoneal duodenum.

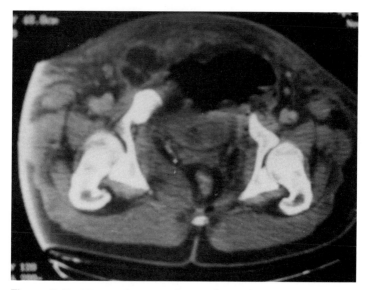

Figure 8–5. CT scan depicting the extraluminal gas pattern resulting from a perforation of the rectum.

gluttony). The patient presents with chest pain and mediastinal emphysema and usually has a left pleural effusion, fever, and leukocytosis. The diagnosis is confirmed by a water-soluble contrast swallow demonstrating contrast extravasation into the left chest. As with clinically significant endoscopic perforation, emergency left thoracotomy, esophageal repair, and drainage are essential to save the patient.

The stomach may perforate as a result of benign ulcer disease, malignancy, or trauma. Trauma is an extremely unusual cause of gastric perforation owing to the thickness of the stomach wall. When a gastric ulcer perforates, the possibility of a malignant ulcer should be entertained. Gastric cancers typically have heaped-up edges but can sometimes be difficult to distinguish from benign ulcer disease. A frozen section can often make the diagnosis at the time of surgery. However, the correct diagnosis of a gastric cancer sometimes may not be made until completion of a careful examination of multiple slides of formalin-fixed tissue several days after surgery. At a minimum, perforated gastric ulcers should be excised and the defect closed. Many times, a formal gastrectomy is indicated. The factors governing these operative decisions are beyond the scope of this chapter.

Peptic ulcer disease typically occurs in the first and second (intraperitoneal) portions of the duodenum. Peptic ulcers can also occur in the prepyloric region of the stomach. "Anterior duodenal ulcers perforate, causing peritonitis, and posterior duodenal ulcers penetrate (into the gastroduodenal artery), causing gastrointestinal hemorrhage." This surgical aphorism describes the usual behavior of duodenal ulcers, causing complications requiring surgical care. On rare occasions, a large circumferential ulcer can perforate and penetrate at the same time, causing both peritonitis and gastrointestinal hemorrhage. Perforated duodenal ulcers are treated by plication rather than excision. Occasionally a patient with a perforated duodenal ulcer presents as clinically stable with mild abdominal pain, free intraperitoneal air, but no definite signs of peritonitis. These ulcer perforations may be already sealed by the omentum or by the liver. In unusual circumstances, these patients may be treated by nasogastric suction, antibiotics, and close observation. This treatment decision should be made only by an experienced surgeon. Almost all patients with a perforated duodenal ulcer require surgery.

The most common cause of small bowel perforation is trauma. Penetrating trauma is the most common type. However, small bowel perforation due to blunt trauma is a relatively frequent occurrence and should be ruled out in all patients who present with abdominal pain after blunt abdominal trauma. Other disease processes such as a closed-loop small bowel obstruction, ischemia, inflammatory bowel disease, small bowel lymphoma, Meckel's diverticulum, foreign bodies, cytomegalovirus infection, and typhoid fever can cause small bowel perforation.

Colon and rectal perforations can occur as a result of large bowel obstruction, ischemia, diverticulitis, colitis, and foreign body perforation. The treatment includes laparotomy, resection of the affected portion of bowel, or closure of the perforation with primary anastomosis. The decision to create a colostomy versus primary reanastomosis depends on the site of perforation, the extent of peritoneal contamination, and the general health of the patient.

K E Y P O I N T S

▶ In the patient who has not had recent surgery, free intraperitoneal air is almost always due to bowel perforation.

▶ The hole in the gastrointestinal tract can be anywhere from the gastroesophageal junction to the rectum.

▶ Free intraperitoneal air is best diagnosed by CT scan or an upright chest radiograph.

▶ Most patients with free intraperitoneal air require surgical intervention.

CASE 8–1. A 35-year-old man presents to the emergency department at 4 AM complaining of sudden onset of upper abdominal pain since 9 PM. He took some aspirin and went to bed. However, the pain has been unrelenting and he could not sleep. On exam, the patient has a normal blood pressure, but he is tachycardic and diaphoretic. He is in obvious distress due to pain. His abdomen is boardlike, with decreased bowel sounds and generalized tenderness. His abdominal musculature is tense on deep palpation, and he complains of pain on sudden release of your hand.

A. What is your initial general diagnosis?
B. What laboratory and radiographic studies should be ordered?
C. What is your most likely course of action?

9

GI Bleeding

The source and rate of gastrointestinal (GI) bleeding determine patient presentation, symptoms, signs, and treatment. Bleeding can be massive or occult. The site of bleeding can be in the upper GI tract, defined as originating above the ligament of Treitz (the duodenojejunal junction), or in the lower GI tract, below the ligament of Treitz.

IMPORTANT TERMS

Hematemesis—vomiting of blood
This implies large-volume upper GI hemorrhage, as might be seen with a bleeding peptic ulcer, a Mallory-Weiss tear at the gastroesophageal junction, or bleeding gastroesophageal varices. Emesis that has the appearance of "coffee grounds" denotes blood that has been in contact with gastric acid long enough to cause breakdown of hemoglobin.

Hematochezia—passage of blood per rectum
This term implies that a significant volume of fresh blood is being passed from the rectum. The blood loss is significant, fast, and ongoing (red bowel movements, possibly with clots). Hematochezia usually implies lower GI blood loss but can also be a consequence of large-volume upper GI bleeding.

Melena—dark, tarry bowel movements
This term implies slower blood loss than hematochezia or may represent past blood loss. The most frequent source of melena is the lower GI tract, but it can also be due to significant blood loss originating from a more proximal GI source.

Occult GI hemorrhage—blood loss determined by testing normal-looking stools for blood
This is a common cause of anemia. Sites of blood loss can be upper GI or lower GI and may involve cancer, ulcer disease, arteriovenous malformations, or more uncommon problems such as hemobilia (blood loss into the biliary tree).

▶ ETIOLOGY

The evaluation of patients with GI bleeding depends on presentation, age, history, and physical examination.

The manner in which the blood is passed is helpful in determining the source and thereby the diagnostic and therapeutic plan for a patient. For a patient who presents with hematemesis, it is imperative to consider those upper GI sources that may result in rapid blood loss. Table 9–1 provides a list of causes of upper GI bleeding.

For patients who present with melena, hematochezia, or occult GI blood loss, the differential diagnosis would include all those listed in Table 9–1, as well as causes of lower GI blood loss listed in Table 9–2.

What historical points are clues to the origin of the bleeding?

The amount of blood loss is important. Some causes of GI hemorrhage, such as cancer, inflammatory bowel disease, and intussusception, may result in small-volume blood loss. With high-volume blood loss per rectum, consider the causes of hematemesis (see Table 9–1) as well as diverticular disease (usually of the right colon), arteriovenous malformations (usually of the right colon), and ischemic colitis (usually of the sigmoid colon).

Patient age at presentation is important. Older people are more likely to have cancer or diverticular disease. Adolescents are the most likely to have juvenile polyps. Age can guide us in our considerations but is not an absolute. There is no consistent definition of "too young" or "too old."

A detailed history should focus on "who," "what," and "when." Learn about the patient. Is there a history of liver disease, anticoagulation use, nonsteroidal anti-inflammatory drug use, cancer, trauma, and so forth? How did the bleeding become apparent? When did the bleeding present: days ago or hours ago? Has it happened before? Is it ongoing?

TABLE 9–1
Upper GI Tract Causes of Bleeding
Peptic ulcer (duodenal or gastric ulcer) Gastritis Variceal bleeding (esophageal/gastric varices, gastric venous congestion) Mallory-Weiss tear (at the gastroesophageal junction) Arteriovenous malformation, arterial aneurysm Cancer (esophageal, gastric, duodenal)

TABLE 9–2

Lower GI Tract Causes of Bleeding

Diverticular disease of the colon
Arteriovenous malformations of the small bowel/colon
Colorectal cancer
Inflammatory bowel disease
Ischemic colitis
Intussusception
Juvenile polyps
Meckel's diverticulum
Anorectal disease, including hemorrhoids

The physical examination should seek evidence of liver disease, trauma, anorectal disease, and any disorders or diseases that might cause GI bleeding or promote it.

► EVALUATION

What tests should be ordered?

A complete history and physical examination should narrow the differential diagnosis. Then, directed diagnostic tests should be undertaken. The haste with which they are undertaken depends on the patient's condition and the rate of ongoing bleeding. The tests should focus on the patient's status and the site of bleeding.

Send laboratory tests, such as a complete blood count, serum chemistries, and coagulation studies, and have blood typed and cross matched.

Place a nasogastric tube in those patients with notable acute blood loss to evacuate the stomach and to detect intragastric blood.

GI bleeding should lead to consideration of early diagnostic and therapeutic endoscopy. Endoscopy allows determination of the bleeding site and cause of bleeding, as well as possible intervention through injection, banding, or cautery. Angiography can be useful for patients bleeding rapidly from sites beyond the pylorus. If blood loss is occult and the patient is well, GI contrast study can be a valuable diagnostic test.

For rapid bleeding proximal to the ligament of Treitz, endoscopy is usually the approach of choice. However, endoscopy may not be possible or definitive. In that case angiography may be necessary as an alternative to an undirected operative exploration. Note that surgical treatment is often much more extensive if the site of bleeding is not localized preoperatively.

Bleeding scans are helpful in a limited number of patients—those bleeding from places too low or too high to be visualized with endoscopy and those who are bleeding at a rate too low to be seen on angiography. Angiography is thought to be useful with bleeding at 3 mL/min or more. Bleeding scans are helpful at lesser rates, generally thought to be 0.5 to 3 mL/min. Unfortunately, the accuracy of such scans is variable, and it is often hard to define locale.

▶ TREATMENT

How should GI bleeding be treated?

Treatment focuses on the problem behind the bleeding, with attention to improving coagulopathy and overall patient well-being. Resuscitation should begin on patient presentation.

Intravenous access is obtained with large-bore IVs, and fluid resuscitation with crystalloid is started. Administration of blood products is reserved for a documented need (anemia or coagulopathy). Correction of coagulopathy is imperative.

Place a nasogastric tube. Is there blood in the nasogastric tube? The presence of bile without blood implies bleeding beyond the ampulla of Vater.

Begin antacid therapy. Use an H_2 receptor blocker or a proton pump inhibitor for ulcer-related bleeding.

For variceal bleeding, consider the administration of octreotide or vasopressin.

Upper endoscopy is indicated to diagnose and possibly treat upper GI sources of bleeding. Lower tract endoscopy may be useful for diagnosis, but optimal results require a complete bowel preparation.

Balloon tamponade may be used to compress bleeding gastric and esophageal varices temporarily. Remember that patients with portal hypertension and varices are also likely to bleed from peptic ulcers.

Angiography can be used for diagnosis and intervention of lower tract sites of bleeding and is useful when endoscopy has not found the site of hemorrhage.

Bleeding scans are also used in patients with significant acute blood loss who are not amenable to or have failed diagnostic endoscopy and who are bleeding at a rate too slow for diagnostic angiography.

Emergency operative intervention is indicated to correct the cause of uncontrollable hemorrhage. If the bleeding can be stopped by any other means, operative intervention, if indicated, can be undertaken under better, elective circumstances when the procedure will not be encumbered by ongoing bleeding and the resultant coagulopathy or by lack of preoperative optimization, such as a bowel preparation. "Blind" resections for bleeding are condemned but are infrequently indicated as life-saving measures. The specific resection undertaken is based on the best information available at the time.

KEY POINTS

▶ The source and rate of bleeding determine the patient's presentation and treatment.

▶ Upper GI sources of blood loss should also be considered in patients who present with melena or hematochezia.

▶ GI endoscopy should be considered soon after a complete history and physical examination are done.

CASE 9–1. A 60-year-old alcoholic presents with hematemesis.

    A. What are early considerations?
    B. What is the diagnosis?
    C. What is the goal of therapy?

CASE 9–2. A 70-year-old man presents with anemia and Hemoccult-positive stool.

    A. What are the likely diagnoses and the treatment priorities?

10

Hemoptysis

▶ ETIOLOGY

What is hemoptysis?

Hemoptysis is a common problem that accompanies a large spectrum of respiratory and nonrespiratory disorders. *Hemoptysis* is defined as the expectoration of blood or bloody sputum. It may range from blood-tinged sputum to frank blood. It often indicates the presence of a serious or life-threatening underlying disorder. *Massive hemoptysis* is defined as the expectoration of at least 100 to 300 mL of blood within a 6-hour period or more than 600 mL of blood within a 24-hour period. *Exsanguinating hemoptysis* is defined as bleeding at a rate exceeding 150 mL/hr. This is a true emergency, requiring simultaneous treatment and evaluation; mortality rates range from 12% to 50%. Massive hemoptysis is most commonly observed in tuberculosis (TB), bronchiectasis, lung abscess, fungal infections, and bronchogenic carcinoma. Whereas bleeding from the gastrointestinal (GI) tract (hematemesis) causes death by exsanguination, hemoptysis can be fatal owing to lack of effective gas exchange (asphyxiation).

Several factors determine outcome associated with hemoptysis: preexisting pulmonary insufficiency, poor cough effort, age, anticoagulation, rate/volume of blood loss, and mechanism of pulmonary bleeding. It is necessary that the examining clinician approach each case of hemoptysis, regardless of quantity of blood, as though it were a serious underlying disease process.

What are the common causes of hemoptysis?

The causes of hemoptysis are numerous, with more than 100 identified in the literature (Table 10–1). Infection is the most common cause worldwide. In the United States, the most common cause of hemoptysis in adult patients is bronchitis. Neoplasia is the second most common cause, with bronchogenic carcinoma the most common diagnosis. Hemoptysis is so common in bronchogenic carcinoma that it should be regarded as the most common etiology in patients between 40 and 60 years of age, especially in smokers. The differential diagnosis of hemoptysis is narrower in children, in whom hemoptysis is a relatively uncommon complaint (Table 10–2).

TABLE 10–1

Causes of Hemoptysis

Infectious
Bronchitis
Bronchiectasis
Tuberculosis
Pneumonia
Lung abscess
Fungal infection
Parasitic infection

Cardiac
Left ventricular failure
Mitral stenosis
Pulmonary hypertension
Bacterial endocarditis
Pulmonary embolism
Arteriovenous malformation
Tracheobronchovascular fistula

Trauma
Blunt
Penetrating
Inhalation injury
Iatrogenic

Miscellaneous
Foreign body
Broncholithiasis
Endometriosis
Freebase cocaine use
Vitamin C deficiency
Radiation therapy

Munchausen syndrome
Idiopathic

Neoplastic
Bronchogenic carcinoma
Primary lung tumor
Bronchial adenoma
Lymphoma
Leukemia
Metastatic lung cancer
Carcinoma of contiguous cardiovascular
    structures

Immunologic
Goodpasture's syndrome
Amyloidosis
Collagen vascular disorders
Pulmonary hemosiderosis
Wegener's granulomatosis
Systemic lupus erythematosus

Congenital
Cystic fibrosis
Kartagener's syndrome
Bronchial cyst

Hematologic
Coagulopathy
Thrombocytopenia
Disseminated intravascular coagulation
Anticoagulation medication
Thrombolytic therapy

In children, the most common causes include pneumonia, foreign bodies, and tracheobronchitis.

What are the principal sources of bleeding into the lung in patients with hemoptysis?

Bleeding into the lungs is from one of four primary sources.

1. *Bronchial arteries:* The bronchial arteries are the source of most episodes of massive hemoptysis because, unlike the pulmonary arteries, the blood is under systemic pressure. The bronchial arteries supply the conducting airways, the vasa vasorum of the large pulmonary arteries, and the pleura. These vessels arise from the aorta directly or from intercostal arteries. In up to 5% of patients, the anterior spinal artery may derive from the bronchial artery, creating a risk for paraplegia if these

TABLE 10–2

Causes of Hemoptysis in Children

Cause	Incidence (%)
Pneumonia	20
Foreign body	15
Tracheobronchitis	15
Unknown	15
Cystic fibrosis	8
Trauma	5
Neoplasm	5
Arteriovenous malformation	5
Cardiac disease	3
Hemosiderosis	3
Nasopharyngeal bleeding	3
Tuberculosis	3

Data from Torn LWC, Weisman RA, Handler SD: Hemoptysis in children. Ann Otol Rhinol Laryngol 89:420, 1980.

arteries are embolized as part of treatment. These arteries proliferate and become tortuous in inflammatory states. The bronchial arteries are the source of bleeding in most chronic parenchymal lung infections, such as lung abscesses and TB. They are also the source in bronchogenic carcinoma, endobronchial metastasis, and broncholithiasis.

2. *Pulmonary arteries:* The pulmonary arteries are rarely associated with major bleeding. Arteriovenous malformations may be supplied with blood from the pulmonary arteries. Bleeding in patients with a pulmonary embolism arises from the pulmonary artery. It is the source of bleeding in iatrogenic catheter-related hemoptysis from a Swan-Ganz catheter.

3. *Pulmonary veins:* The pulmonary veins are associated with bleeding in cases of trauma or inflammatory states.

4. *Systemic fistulas:* Systemic fistulas are very rare causes of bleeding.

▶ EVALUATION

What are the steps in the initial evaluation of hemoptysis?

The first step is to confirm the origin of the bleeding. Is the bleeding from the respiratory tract or the GI tract (hematemesis)? An attempt should also be made to quantify the amount of blood loss. A thorough history should be obtained. Benign conditions are usually responsible when hemoptysis has been occurring for many years (chronic bronchitis, cystic fibrosis). Obtain the patient's medical records. This may contain clues (i.e., if the patient has a history of TB) or uncover forgotten procedures (a bronchoscopy in the past). Assess the risk factors for lung cancer, especially in patients older than 40 years of age.

What key questions should I ask a patient with hemoptysis?

- Description of symptoms: Ask about fevers, recent infections, trauma, and heart disease
- Past hemoptysis history: Is the hemoptysis new? How long has the patient been symptomatic?
- Recent chest trauma
- History of unilateral or bilateral leg swelling
- Underlying cardiopulmonary disease
- History of upper airway, sinus, or upper GI problems
- Previous history of hemoptysis
- Recent infectious symptoms
- Use of tobacco: How long has the patient smoked?
- Recent travel: Remember that recent travel to foreign countries may expose patients to TB and parasitic infections
- Work environment: Obtain information regarding occupational and environmental exposures (asbestos, arsenic, nickel, beryllium, iron oxides)
- Medications: Review use of anticoagulants and salicylates
- History of drug use (cocaine)
- Family history of hemoptysis

How do I distinguish hemoptysis from hematemesis?

It is important to distinguish hemoptysis from hematemesis. Hemoptysis, which results from bleeding from the tracheobronchial tree, is associated more often with a cough and respiratory symptoms. It often is alkaline, is bright red with clots, and often has the frothiness of expectorate. One can identify pulmonary macrophages in the expectorate.

Hematemesis, which results from bleeding from the upper GI tract, is associated often with esophagogastric symptoms, alcohol use, hepatic disease, and vomiting. It is frequently brown or "coffee ground" in color, acidic in pH, and without frothiness. There are no pulmonary macrophages in the expectorate, and often food particles are present.

What are the key features to note on physical examination?

On examination, it is important to note whether the patient is febrile. High-grade fevers may be suggestive of an infectious process.

Examine the mouth, gums, and pharynx. Foul-smelling breath may suggest a lung abscess or pneumonia. Palpate the neck to assess for lymphadenopathy, indicating malignancy or infection. Carefully examine the chest. Bruises may suggest trauma. Wheezing is heard in patient with bronchogenic carcinoma or foreign body. Patients with pneumonia may have tactile fremitus or dullness to percussion. Carefully listen to the heart for mitral stenosis murmur. Examine the abdomen for enlargement for the spleen or liver. Splenomegaly may be secondary to TB, congestive heart failure, or lymphoma. Clubbing of the fingers may be secondary to lung cancer, infective endocarditis, or chronic obstructive pulmonary disease. The presence of ecchymosis and petechiae may suggest a hematologic disorder or coagulopathy.

What diagnostic tests are important to obtain in these patients?

The most important initial diagnostic test is a chest radiograph. A good-quality chest radiograph may suggest TB, pneumonia, lung abscess, pulmonary infarction, or cancer. All patients should be placed on a pulse oximeter to assess oxygenation; an arterial blood gas is useful if there is evidence of desaturation. A complete blood count, platelet count, prothrombin time, and partial thromboplastin time are recommended for all patients. A blood sample for type and cross match should be obtained in all patients who have had significant blood loss or who are unstable. In general, computed tomographic scan should be considered the initial study (after chest radiograph) in patients not actively bleeding. Bronchoscopy should be considered for those who are actively bleeding. When bronchoscopy fails to localize the bleeding site, selective arteriography may be used to assess the bleeding site.

▶ TREATMENT

How do I stabilize patients with massive hemoptysis?

The patient must be rapidly assessed and managed. The initial focus should be on stabilization. The following factors are the most important in the initial evaluation: oxygenation, gas exchange, hemodynamic state, airway patency, and ability to clear blood. In the treatment of hemoptysis, patient evaluation and management must occur simultaneously. If the bleeding is significant or there is already evidence of airway compromise, the patient should be immediately intubated. An orotracheal route is preferred. A cardiac monitor and pulse oximeter should be placed. If the patient does not need early intubation, cough suppression is usually advocated. Two large-bore intravenous lines should be placed and blood sent for routine lab studies and type and cross match. Bronchoscopy allows for assessment of the airway and bleeding. It also allows for the passage of vasoconstrictor drugs, cold saline lavage, and laser photocoagulation. Aspirin or other nonsteroidal anti-inflammatory drugs should be discontinued. Coagulopathy status should be corrected.

How does one adequately ventilate patients with massive hemoptysis?

If the location of the bleeding is known, the patient should be placed with the involved lung in the dependent lateral decubitus position to prevent blood from spilling over into the noninvolved lung. Airway control is paramount. Isolation of the bleeding lung can be achieved by intubation with either a single- or double-lumen endotracheal tube (ETT). For right-sided bleeding, the single-lumen cuffed ETT can be advanced into the left main stem bronchus under bronchoscopic guidance to allow unilateral lung ventilation while spillage from the right lung to the left is blocked. For left-sided bleeding, the ETT is placed in the trachea while a Fogarty catheter is placed in the left main stem bronchus to avoid spillage into the right lung. Placement of the ETT into the right main stem bronchus is easier to perform; however, it is usually avoided because it occludes the take-off of the right upper lobe bronchus, thereby losing gas exchange from the right upper lobe as well as the entire left lung.

For patients who have multiple sites of bleeding or bilateral disease, how can I control ongoing bleeding?

Bronchial–pulmonary artery embolization is a useful treatment option for patients with massive hemoptysis. It is used for patients who have multiple sites of bleeding or bilateral disease, for nonsurgical patients, or as a temporizing measure for patients who are awaiting surgery.

In patients with massive hemoptysis, how can I identify the site of bleeding?

The bleeding site can often be quickly visualized by flexible bronchoscopy once the patient is intubated. Bronchoscopy can be performed through the ETT, though it is often limited by the size of the flexible scope. Rigid bronchoscopy, on the other hand, is able to effectively remove large clots but must be performed in the operating room.

Angiographic evaluation and embolization of bleeding vessels are also useful.

When should surgery be considered?

Surgery is indicated for patients who have been unresponsive to other measures and who have massive unilateral hemoptysis and adequate pulmonary reserve. Because embolization has been so successful, surgery is now being considered more as an elective treatment for selected individuals rather than as emergent therapy.

K E Y   P O I N T S

▶ Hemoptysis ranges from blood-tinged sputum to exsanguinating hemorrhage.

▶ Massive hemoptysis is a medical emergency.

▶ The most common causes of hemoptysis are bronchitis and cancer.

CASE 10-1. A 68-year-old man with a 50 pack-year smoking history presents to the emergency department with massive hemoptysis. He is intubated for airway control and stabilized. His chest radiograph demonstrates a 2.5 × 2 cm spiculated mass in his left upper lobe.

    A. What vessel is the most likely source of the bleeding?

    B. On bronchoscopic examination, he is found to have multiple sites of ongoing bleeding. What is the most effective way of controlling the bleeding?

    C. What are the most common causes of hemoptysis in the United States?

11

Inguinal/Scrotal Swelling

What conditions result in swelling in the inguinal area?

The most common condition resulting in inguinal swelling is a groin hernia. Inguinal hernias bulge above the inguinal ligament (a line between the symphysis pubis and the anterior superior iliac crest), and femoral hernias bulge below it. An indirect inguinal hernia is due to a persistence of the processus vaginalis and can bulge into the scrotum. A direct inguinal hernia is due to a weakness in the floor of the inguinal canal and normally remains in the groin. The precise differentiation between a direct and indirect inguinal hernia cannot usually be made on physical examination and is not important in planning therapy. Enlarged lymph nodes can also cause groin swelling and simulate a hernia, particularly if matted and fixed in the deep location (Table 11–1).

How do I differentiate lymphadenitis from an incarcerated inguinal hernia?

This may be a difficult matter, especially if the chronicity of the swelling is uncertain. Both situations present with tender, irreducible groin masses. Frequently, diligent attempts at reduction of the mass are successful, confirming the diagnosis of hernia. Fevers may accompany lymphadenitis, but be cautious not to miss a strangulated hernia, which can also cause fever. Signs of bowel obstruction suggest a hernia. Ultrasound may suggest an enlarged node rather than a hernia; however, if the diagnosis is uncertain, urgent surgical exploration of the mass is the safest approach.

Can a gonad be present in the groin?

In males, an undescended testicle presents as an inguinal swelling. Most often it has been documented in early life that the testicle is not in the scrotum. Acute pain can be related to torsion of this undescended testicle. In young females, it is not uncommon to palpate an ovary in an indirect hernia sac.

TABLE 11-1
Causes of Inguinal and Scrotal Swelling
Inguinal Adenopathy Hernia/hydrocele Undescended testicle *Scrotal* Testicular torsion Torsion of appendix testis Epididymitis Mumps orchitis Varicocele Spermatocele Testicular tumor Idiopathic scrotal edema Hernia/hydrocele

What other conditions can result in swelling in the scrotum?

Testicular torsion, torsion of the appendix testis, epididymitis, orchitis, and trauma result in painful swelling in the scrotum. Varicoceles, spermatoceles, hydroceles, and testicular tumors typically do not cause pain.

How do I differentiate a hydrocele from an indirect inguinal hernia in a young child?

Young children may present with a sudden swelling in the groin or scrotum that is quite alarming to the parents. Owing to the short distance between the internal inguinal ring and the scrotum, both a hydrocele and an indirect inguinal hernia may cause a rather diffuse, elongated swelling from the groin to the scrotum. The first step is to patiently attempt to reduce the mass through the internal inguinal ring with steady, direct pressure. Complete reduction of the mass confirms that it is an inguinal hernia. If the mass cannot be reduced, you must differentiate between an incarcerated inguinal hernia and a communicating hydrocele. If the child has no evidence of pain or tenderness with the mass and has manifested no gastrointestinal symptoms, it is unlikely to be an incarcerated hernia. In addition, a hydrocele may transilluminate when a bright light source is placed against it. On physical examination, press the spermatic cord against the pubis and decide whether it is thickened. A distinct elongated thickening is felt in the case of a hernia, whereas no mass is felt above the upper extent of a hydrocele.

How do I differentiate testicular torsion from epididymitis?

Both conditions can lead to a diffusely swollen and tender scrotum, making differentiation difficult. Epididymitis rarely occurs in males younger than 20 years of age. Its onset is more insidious and may be associated with fever, chills, and dysuria. Prehn's sign involves lifting the scrotum up off the examining table and supporting it. The pain is alleviated in patients with epididymitis, whereas the pain is worsened in patients with testicular torsion. The lie of the testicle in torsion may be more horizontal than the normal vertical position, and the epididymis may be palpated anteriorly. The "blue dot" sign, transilluminating the scrotum and looking for a blue mass at the upper pole of the testicle, is suggestive of torsion of the appendix testis.

▶ EVALUATION

What historical factors are important when evaluating inguinal/scrotal swelling?

Ask whether the swelling has been noted previously and whether it is constant or intermittent. Typically, patients with hernias will have noted a reducible bulge at some time. Hernias may be associated with straining during coughing, urination, or bowel movements. Therefore, ask about a history of smoking, asthma, chronic obstructive pulmonary disease, urinary hesitancy, or constipation. Any history of trauma should be noted. Be careful, however, in ascribing the swelling to injury. Frequently, the traumatic event calls attention to a preexisting yet undiscovered condition, such as a testicular tumor. History of fever, recent sexually transmitted diseases, or lower extremity skin infections may point to an infectious cause. Fever, chills, night sweats, and weight loss suggest lymphoma. Sudden testicular pain and swelling in an adolescent is torsion until proven otherwise.

How do I examine a patient with a suspected inguinal hernia?

First, have the patient stand in front of you while you sit on a stool. Have the patient show you where he or she noticed a bulge if one is not evident. Carefully observe the groin for any bulges with the patient in the relaxed state, while performing a Valsalva maneuver and while coughing. Direct palpation of the skin of the groin may help confirm a bulge during Valsalva. In male patients, invaginate the scrotal skin with your index finger and run it up into the inguinal canal. Have him cough, and feel for bulging tissue against your finger. Next, have the patient lie supine on the examining table and repeat these maneuvers.

What additional studies may be helpful in the evaluation?

Most inguinal and scrotal swellings can be diagnosed by careful physical examination. If an infectious cause is suspected, a complete blood count and urinalysis should be ordered. If a testicular neoplasm is suspected, tumor markers (beta human chorionic gonadotropin, alpha fetoprotein) should be sent. To help diagnose an incarcerated hernia, a plain abdominal film may show an obstructed bowel gas pattern or bowel gas outside the abdomen. Be aware, however, that a Richter's hernia (in which only a portion of the bowel wall is involved in the incarceration) can still strangulate and not cause bowel obstruction. Ultrasound may be useful to characterize an ill-defined inguinal mass in an obese patient. For suspected testicular torsion, prompt Doppler ultrasonography may aid in the diagnosis.

▶ TREATMENT

Which inguinal and scrotal swellings require prompt operation?

Both incarcerated inguinal hernia and testicular torsion need surgical correction without delay. Attempts at reduction to convert an incarcerated to a reducible inguinal hernia are warranted, particularly in children, assuming there are no signs of strangulation such as skin redness, fever, or other systemic symptoms. Failure to reduce the hernia mandates immediate operation to prevent the sequelae of strangulation. For testicular torsion, an operation should be performed within 4 hours from the beginning of symptoms.

When is a scrotal incision used and when is an inguinal incision used?

When a patient with inguinal or scrotal swelling is taken to the operating room, it is essential to make the correct incision. If one suspects an inguinal or femoral hernia or communicating hydrocele, an inguinal incision is made as for an elective inguinal hernia repair. If one suspects a testicular neoplasm, a similar groin incision is made, delivering the testicle into the field for inspection. It is a major error to incise the scrotal skin in the presence of a testicular cancer, as the scrotal skin draws into pelvic rather than inguinal lymphatics.

If you are dealing with torsion of a testicle or an appendix testis, a scrotal incision is appropriate. Also, when dealing with noncommunicating hydroceles in adults, a scrotal incision also is best.

K E Y   P O I N T S

▶ The history and physical examination usually lead to an accurate diagnosis.

▶ Don't delay treatment of an incarcerated hernia or testicular torsion.

CASE 11-1. A 2-year-old boy is brought to the emergency department with a swelling in the right groin and scrotum that the mother noticed earlier in the day. The child has remained active without fever, vomiting, or complaints of pain in the groin. The mother states that she has noticed some intermittent swelling in the right scrotal region in the past. Examination reveals an elongated mass extending from the groin to the scrotum that is nontender.

   A. List two conditions in your differential diagnosis. How would you distinguish between the two on physical examination?
   B. If the mass reduces on your examination, what is your plan? How about if the mass cannot be reduced?

CASE 11-2. A 21-year-old man comes to you regarding acute scrotal pain that began the previous evening. The patient relates a history of mild trauma to the region 2 days earlier while riding his bicycle. The scrotum is now diffusely swollen, thickened, and tender. He states that he is having some trouble urinating and has some generalized malaise.

   A. What is in the differential for this patient?
   B. List other physical exam findings or additional tests that may help you better define the diagnosis.
   C. What would prompt you to take this patient to surgery?

CASE 11–3. A 56-year-old man sees you regarding an intermittent bulge he has noticed in his left groin. He gets a nagging, dull ache in the area after being on his feet for prolonged periods.

A. Describe a systematic approach to the physical examination of this region. If a reducible groin hernia is detected, list three predisposing factors that you should question the patient about. Why is this important?

B. Can you differentiate among an indirect inguinal hernia, a direct inguinal hernia, or a femoral hernia on your physical examination?

12

Jaundice

What is jaundice?

Jaundice occurs when the breakdown products of heme metabolism (bile pigments) accumulate in excess quantities in tissues throughout the body. *Hyperbilirubinemia* is another term often used to describe this condition. Jaundice becomes apparent when the serum bilirubin is greater than 3 mg/dL.

Where does bilirubin come from?

Nearly 80% of the daily production of bilirubin comes from the catabolism of hemoglobin in decaying red blood cells as they circulate through the reticuloendothelial compartments. The remainder is from the degradation of myoglobin, hepatic heme, and hemoproteins, including the cytochromes.

What are the essential steps of bilirubin metabolism?

Heme is catalyzed by the microsomal enzyme heme oxygenase to produce a green pigment called *biliverdin*. Biliverdin is then reduced by biliverdin reductase to bilirubin IX-α, which is the unconjugated form of bilirubin. These enzymes are present in high concentrations within cells of the reticuloendothelial system, monocytes, macrophages, and hepatocytes.

Unconjugated bilirubin circulates in plasma bound to albumin until it reaches the liver.

The bilirubin-albumin complex then diffuses through the sinusoidal pores to the plasma membrane, where it dissociates. Unconjugated bilirubin then freely enters the hepatocytes, where it is conjugated with glucuronic acid. This conjugation process markedly increases its water solubility, allowing for excretion across the canalicular membrane into bile. Colonic bacteria partially degrade conjugated bilirubin into urobilinogen, which in part gives stool its characteristic color.

What forms of bilirubin are measurable in serum?

The van den Bergh reaction is the most widely used method to quantitate both the total serum bilirubin concentration and the direct-reacting fraction composed of conjugated forms of bilirubin. The indirect-reacting fraction (unconjugated bilirubin) is simply the numeric difference between the total serum bilirubin and the conjugated bilirubin concentrations.

What is the classification of jaundice?

There are two types of jaundice: unconjugated hyperbilirubinemia and conjugated hyperbilirubinemia. Unconjugated hyperbilirubinemia may result from increased bilirubin production or from impaired hepatic bilirubin uptake and storage. Overproduction of bilirubin occurs with hemolysis (e.g., erythrocyte abnormality, hemolytic anemias, hypersplenism, infarction), ineffective erythropoiesis (thalassemias), or hematoma breakdown. Posthepatitis hyperbilirubinemia, neonatal jaundice, drug reactions, Gilbert's syndrome, and Crigler-Najjar syndromes are associated with decreased hepatic bilirubin uptake.

Conjugated hyperbilirubinemia is divided into intrahepatic or extrahepatic causes. Intrahepatic disorders include cholestatic syndromes (e.g., Rotor's syndrome, Dubin-Johnson syndrome, primary biliary cirrhosis), hepatocellular dysfunction of any cause (e.g., viral hepatitis, hepatic cirrhosis, drugs, toxins, postoperative jaundice, sepsis, malignancies, infiltrative disorders), and metabolic disorders (e.g., cholestasis of pregnancy, benign recurrent intrahepatic cholestasis). Extrahepatic etiologies include biliary tract diseases (e.g., choledocholithiasis, tumor, cysts, strictures) or pancreatic pathology (e.g., pancreatitis, neoplasms, cysts).

▶ EVALUATION

How do patients with unconjugated hyperbilirubinemia present?

These patients typically have a mild form of jaundice. There is no bilirubin in the urine, and the stool and urine color are normal. Splenomegaly is found in most patients with jaundice due to hemolytic disorders. Sickle cell crisis with infarction or acute hemolysis is associated with severe bone pain, fatigue, malaise, or abdominal pain.

Jaundice in neonates is a common presentation of unconjugated hyperbilirubinemia. In most cases its cause is multifactorial and is transient, with peak bilirubin levels achieved within 5 days.

Another common condition is Gilbert's syndrome, which is seen in 5% to 10% of the population. The total serum bilirubin is typically between 1.0 and 5.0 mg/dL and is predominantly unconjugated. The condition is asymptomatic and has an excellent prognosis. Periods of stress or fasting intensify the hyperbilirubinemia.

How do patients with conjugated hyperbilirubinemia present?

The cholestatic syndromes are characterized by the presence of hyperbilirubinemia plus pruritus, malaise, and acholic stools. These patients can also be asymptomatic.

Patients with hepatocellular dysfunction or cirrhosis may present with combinations of signs and symptoms, depending on the severity and chronicity of the illness. Symptoms are often nonspecific and may include fatigue, malaise, anorexia, insomnia, confusion, fever, amenorrhea, easy bruisability, and right upper quadrant pain. Physical examination may reveal ascites, tender hepatomegaly, spider angiomata, painful gynecomastia, palmar erythema, asterixis, and fetor hepaticus.

Do patients with biliary obstruction present differently?

No. Right upper quadrant pain, dark urine, and acholic stools can occur along with jaundice. A history of unintentional weight loss is suggestive of malignancy. The triad of jaundice, fevers or chills, and right upper quadrant pain suggests ascending cholangitis. Positive fecal occult blood tests or silver-colored stools may be seen with ampullary tumors. Physical signs may also include ascites, a palpable gallbladder (Courvoisier's sign), hepatomegaly, and cachexia.

A thorough history and physical examination provide critical clues in the evaluation of the patient with jaundice. Additional testing is indicated to arrive at the proper diagnosis.

What laboratory tests are helpful?

Serum alanine aminotransferase (ALT) and aspartate aminotransferase (AST) levels are critical in the early evaluation of the jaundiced patient. These enzymes are generally elevated with hepatocellular damage such as that caused by viral hepatitis. ALT is a more specific indicator of liver injury than is AST. An elevated alkaline phosphatase level suggests biliary obstruction, cholestasis, or infiltrative liver disease (e.g., granulomas, malignancy, amyloidosis). Alkaline phosphatase may be derived not only from hepatic sources but also from intestine, bone, and placenta. A concomitant rise of gamma-glutamyltransferase (GGT) or 5'-nucleotidase levels is indicative of a hepatic origin for alkaline phosphatase. The prothrombin time is a useful indicator of overall hepatic production of key proteins and clotting factors. An elevated prothrombin time may indicate profound liver dysfunction.

What radiographic studies are useful?

Ultrasonography (US) and computed tomography (CT) are highly sensitive for the demonstration of biliary dilation. US is often the initial study for the evaluation of extrahepatic biliary obstruction. It can detect gallstones with a sensitivity of nearly 95%.

CT offers little advantage over US for the detection of biliary dilation. However, CT has the ability to trace the course of bile ducts, detect patterns of ductal dilation, and visualize with accuracy small parenchymal masses as well as adjacent structures (vascular, intestinal, and pancreatic).

Magnetic resonance imaging is the most accurate tool for the detection of hepatic hemangiomas, adenomas, and focal nodular hyperplasia. Increasingly, magnetic resonance cholangiopancreatography is being used as a noninvasive modality to detect pancreaticobiliary strictures, stones, anomalies, and tumors.

Percutaneous transhepatic cholangiography is performed by interventional radiologists. A fine needle is introduced into the liver parenchyma and advanced into a peripheral bile duct. A cholangiogram is obtained and provides precise visualization of the biliary tree. This modality also allows for biliary drainage and stenting. Currently, its use is limited to evaluation of complex biliary lesions or for failed endoscopic interventions.

Is there a role for endoscopic evaluation?

Endoscopic retrograde cholangiopancreatography (ERCP) allows for direct visualization of ampullary lesions, pancreatic ductal diseases, and biliary tract abnormalities. It is the most precise of all tests for detecting the cause, extent, and location of extrahepatic obstruction. Furthermore, ERCP offers the advantage of therapeutic intervention such as papillotomy, stone extraction, tissue sampling, and biliary stenting. Complications of ERCP include pancreatitis, cholangitis, perforation, and bleeding. Endoscopic US, where available, is extremely sensitive for the detection of biliary stones and for staging of pancreatic neoplasms.

When is a liver biopsy indicated?

Liver biopsy is the only test capable of confirming the diagnosis of specific liver diseases and for determining the histologic severity and prognosis of many forms of hepatocellular dysfunction.

▶ TREATMENT

This section is devoted to the management of obstructive jaundice.

The ultimate goal in the management of obstructive jaundice is establishing biliary drainage. Surgical, endoscopic, and percutaneous modalities are the available means of achieving this goal. A multi-disciplinary approach that successfully incorporates these techniques is by far the best treatment strategy. Adjunctive medical therapy may include the use of antibiotics for infection, narcotics for pain relief, and antihistamines for relief of pruritus.

What surgical options are available?

The surgical management of choledocholithiasis may include choledochotomy (common bile duct exploration) with stone extraction, choledochoduodenostomy, or other biliary enteric bypass procedure. Benign bile duct strictures are best managed surgically with either choledochojejunostomy or Roux-en-Y hepaticojejunostomy. The Whipple procedure remains as the only possible curative treatment of obstructing pancreatic neoplasms. Surgery provides the only means of cure for resectable bile duct cancers.

What do percutaneous drainage techniques accomplish?

This modality allows for tissue sampling, biliary drain placement, stone extraction, balloon dilation of strictures, and placement of biliary endoprostheses. These prostheses are extremely helpful for the palliation of unresectable proximal bile duct tumors. Complications of this procedure include bleeding, hemobilia, and infection.

What endoscopic options are available?

Endoscopic sphincterotomy and stone extraction, with or without stent placement, is the procedure of choice for common bile duct stones, cholangitis, and acute biliary pancreatitis.

ERCP plays an important role in the management of malignant unresectable strictures, benign strictures, and papillary stenosis.

K E Y   P O I N T S

▶ Jaundice occurs when the serum bilirubin level exceeds 3 mg/dL.

▶ A knowledge of bilirubin metabolism is critical for understanding the various causes of jaundice.

▶ Jaundice is divided into two types: unconjugated hyperbilirubinemia and conjugated hyperbilirubinemia.

▶ History, physical examination, and appropriate use of laboratory, histologic, radiologic, and endoscopic tests are essential for accurate diagnosis.

▶ A multidisciplinary approach, including surgical, percutaneous, and endoscopic techniques, is critical for optimal management of obstructive jaundice.

CASE 12–1. A 65-year-old man presents to the emergency department with a 3-month history of intermittent epigastric pain, nausea, vomiting, and anorexia. He also reports the onset of jaundice and clay-colored stools about 2 weeks earlier. He has noted some weight loss of about 10 pounds. The physical examination is notable for a temperature of 101°F, heart rate of 110 beats/min, jaundice, and mild epigastric tenderness.

A. What further history should you elicit?
B. What tests should be obtained?
C. How should this patient be managed?

13

Leg Pain, Ulceration, and Swelling

What are common causes of leg pain?

Leg pain has multiple etiologies, including trauma, muscle cramps, electrolyte deficiencies (e.g., hypokalemia and hypocalcemia), osteoarthritis, infection (cellulitis), compression of the neurospinal canal, deep tumors and masses, deep venous thrombosis, compartment syndrome, acute ischemia, and peripheral vascular disease.

What causes intermittent claudication and rest pain?

Intermittent claudication is pain or fatigue in the muscles of the lower extremity that is caused by walking and relieved by rest. The usual etiology is peripheral vascular disease that results in poor arterial inflow to the exercising muscles, but spinal cord compression or nerve root injury (neurogenic claudication) may also be the cause. The pain increases in severity with walking, and eventually the patient stops. The pain is described as "cramps" in the leg muscles, and it improves after a short period of inactivity. Claudication most commonly occurs in the calf muscles, but iliac artery narrowing may result in gluteal or thigh pain on activity.

Rest pain is a grave symptom caused by ischemic neuritis. It is usually a severe burning pain confined to the foot. It may be localized to the vicinity of an ischemic ulcer or pregangrenous toe. It is aggravated by extremity elevation and improves with placing the foot in the dependent position, for example, when standing or hanging the leg over the side of the bed.

What are the common causes of lower extremity ulcers?

Lower extremity ulcers can be caused by trauma or infection. More common are those caused by arterial disease, venous insufficiency, or neurotrophic factors (Table 13–1).

TABLE 13-1

Differential Diagnosis of Common Leg Ulcers

Type	Usual Location	Pain	Bleeding with Manipula-tion	Lesion Character-istics	Associated Findings
Ischemia	Distally, on dorsum of foot or toes	Severe, particularly at night, relieved by dependency	Little or none	Irregular edge, poor granulation tissue	Trophic changes of chronic ischemia, absent pulses
Stasis	Lower third of leg ("gaiter" area)	Mild, relieved by elevation	Venous ooze	Shallow, irregular shape, granulating base, rounded edges	Stasis dermatitis
Neuro-trophy	Under calluses or pressure points (e.g., plantar aspect of 1st or 5th metatar-sophalangeal joint)	None	May be brisk	Punched out, with deep sinus	Demonstrable neuropathy

From Rutherford RB (ed): Vascular Surgery, 4th ed. Philadelphia, WB Saunders, 1995, p 9.

What are the possible etiologies of lower extremity swelling?

As depicted in Table 13–2, there are many causes of lower extremity swelling, ranging from medical to surgical. These include venous, lymphatic, cardiac, and lipid factors.

What is dependent rubor?

In advanced atherosclerotic disease, the skin of the foot may display a characteristic ruborous cyanosis on dependency. It is caused by a combination of poor inflow, stagnant blood in the capillary network, vasodilation, and high oxygen extraction. This results in dark capillary blood that manifests in the common finding of a purple foot.

TABLE 13-2

Differential Diagnosis of Chronic Leg Swelling

Clinical Feature	Venous	Lymphatic	Cardiac Orthostatic	"Lipedema"
Consistency of swelling	Brawny	Spongy	Pitting	Noncompressible (fat)
Relief by elevation	Complete	Mild	Complete	Minimal
Distribution of swelling	Maximal in ankles and legs, feet spared	Diffuse, greatest distally	Diffuse, greatest distally	Maximal in ankles and legs, feet spared
Associated skin changes	Atrophic and pigmented, subcutaneous fibrosis	Hypertrophied, lichenified skin	Shiny, mild pigmentation, no trophic changes	None
Pain	Heavy ache, tight or bursting	None or heavy ache	Little or none	Dull ache, cutaneous sensitivity
Bilaterality	Occasionally, but usually unequal	Occasionally, but usually unequal	Always, but may be unequal	Always

From Rutherford RB (ed): Vascular Surgery, 4th ed. Philadelphia, WB Saunders, 1995, p 8.

▶ **EVALUATION**

What are risk factors for peripheral occlusive disease?

Risk factors include tobacco use, hypertension, elevated cholesterol level, diabetes, sedentary lifestyle, obesity, and family history of peripheral or cardiac disease.

What physical characteristics help distinguish ulcer etiologies?

Ulcers caused by arterial disease are usually painful, do not bleed, and are on the lateral aspect of the lower extremity. Ulcers caused by venous insufficiency are usually on the medial aspect of the lower leg, bleed easily, are pain free, and are associated with edema and skin discoloration.

What is the work-up for intermittent claudication?

Start with a good history and physical exam. After understanding the patient's complaints and appreciating the risk factors, perform a thorough physical exam of the lower extremities. After palpating the pulses and listening for femoral bruits, closely examine both lower extremities, looking for ulcers, hair loss, brittle toenails, or other lesions. Once this is complete, calculation of the ankle brachial index is required for each extremity (see Chapter 36). If neurogenic claudication is suspected, magnetic resonance (MR) imaging of the spine is indicated to evaluate for spinal cord compression.

What imaging will help in the work-up of peripheral occlusive disease?

After the history and physical exam are completed, duplex ultrasound, lower extremity arteriograms, or MR angiograms with reconstructions may assist in diagnosing areas of poor arterial inflow and help in planning treatment strategies.

What is the work-up for venous insufficiency?

After a thorough history and physical, a duplex ultrasound may be performed to rule out deep vein thrombosis and document sites of valvular incompetence.

▶ TREATMENT

The treatment of arterial insufficiency is discussed in Chapter 36.

Venous insufficiency resulting in swelling and ulceration is treated with leg elevation and compression stockings. If deep venous thrombosis is present, systemic anticoagulation is necessary. If sites of venous valvular incompetence can be identified, selective ligation of perforating vessels may be performed.

K E Y   P O I N T S

▶ Thorough and pertinent history and physical exam are important in evaluating lower extremity complaints.

▶ A broad medical and surgical differential diagnosis must be considered.

▶ Work-up for intermittent claudication is based on specific history, physical findings, and initially noninvasive approaches.

▶ Vascular ulcers of the lower extremity may have arterial or venous etiologies.

CASE 13-1. An 82-year-old woman with a history of hypertension and diabetes mellitus presents to your clinic with complaints of left calf pain when walking two blocks. The pain subsides after she rests 5 minutes. She denies any other medical problems.

A. What other pertinent history is needed?
B. What is your differential diagnosis?
C. What tests would be appropriate?
D. How would you initiate treatment?

14

Lymphadenopathy

What are the causes of lymphadenopathy?

The causes of lymphadenopathy are protean, as listed in Table 14–1. General categories include (1) infection (bacterial, viral, parasitic, spirochetal, chlamydial, mycobacterial, or fungal); (2) malignancy (intrinsic to the node or metastatic); (3) drug reactions (phenytoin, serum sickness); and (4) miscellaneous conditions (sarcoidosis, lupus). Of lymph nodes that are eventually biopsied, approximately 40% are abnormal but without specific diagnosis on histologic examination or culture. Three conditions account for the majority of the remaining 60%: metastatic malignancy (25%), intrinsic malignancy (i.e., lymphoma) (20%), and tuberculosis (10%). Generalized lymphadenopathy is caused by systemic disease, whereas local or regional adenopathy may represent either local (rubella, infection, tumor) or systemic (HIV, tuberculosis) disease.

When is lymphadenopathy pathologic?

Although lymph nodes usually are too small to appreciate on exam, palpable nodes are not always pathologic. Small "shotty" nodes less than 1 cm in size are common in the neck and groin and if the patient is otherwise well are of no concern. Conversely, palpable nodes in a patient with associated constitutional signs and symptoms of fever, weight loss, night sweats, or fatigue need evaluation. A lymph node larger than 1.5 cm that is not resolving over a few weeks should be investigated. Any lymph node greater than 3 cm should be considered highly suspicious of malignancy. Reactive, tender nodes appear quickly in response to an infection and then slowly regress over 6 weeks. Sometimes these reactive nodes will not disappear completely but remain small and palpable, but the important thing is that they did regress. Most patients younger than 30 years of age have benign lymph nodes, whereas lymphadenopathy in a patient older than 50 years is usually due to a malignancy.

TABLE 14–1

Diseases Associated with Generalized Lymphadenopathy

Benign reactive hyperplasia
Infections
Viral diseases
    Infectious mononucleosis (Epstein-Barr virus)
    Varicella zoster
    Cytomegalovirus
    Rubeola, rubella
    Hepatitis B
    HIV, including AIDS
Bacterial
    Streptococci, staphylococci, *Salmonella, Brucella*, tularemia, *Listeria, Pasteurella pestis,*
      Haemophilus ducreyi, cat-scratch fever, syphilis, leprosy
Fungal/protozoal/mycobacterial
    Histoplasmosis, toxoplasmosis, coccidioidomycosis
    Chlamydia
    Mycobacterium
    Filariasis
Collagen vascular disorders
    Rheumatoid arthritis, systemic lupus erythematosus, Sjögren's syndrome
Endocrine disorders
    Hyperthyroidism, hypoadrenocorticism, hypopituitarism
Hypersensitivity states
    Serum sickness, drug reaction (phenytoin, hydralazine, allopurinol)
Miscellaneous
    Dermatomyositis, Kawasaki's disease (mucocutaneous lymph node syndrome)
    Amyloidosis, sarcoidosis
    Lipid storage diseases (Gaucher's disease, Niemann-Pick disease)
    Histiocytosis
Neoplasia
    Hodgkin's disease
    Non-Hodgkin's lymphoma
    Acute and chronic leukemias
    Angioimmunoblastic lymphadenopathy

What history is important to obtain?

Key factors are (1) patient age; (2) size, shape, and consistency of the nodes; (3) location of adenopathy; and (4) duration and rate of change. Important components of the history include whether the patient is immunocompromised, has symptoms of acute viral syndromes, and has constitutional signs and symptoms such as weight loss, night sweats, or fatigue. Patients with lymphoma may have an altered tolerance to alcohol or may report itching after showering. Patients with a history of tobacco or alcohol use are more likely to have malignancy. Environmental factors such as recent travel or exposure to animals or geographic locations conducive to histoplasmosis, Q fever, and so forth should be sought. Does the patient have another acute or chronic illness or any new drug ingestion? Signs and symptoms such as chest tightness, dysphagia, shortness of breath, and facial swelling suggest mediastinal disease. Abdominal fullness, early satiety, or pains radiating to the back or shoulders indicate intraperitoneal etiology. Unilateral leg swelling after deep venous thrombosis has been excluded should prompt a pelvic computed tomographic (CT) scan to exclude regional lymphadenopathy causing extrinsic compression.

How does HIV positivity relate to lymphadenopathy?

Human immunodeficiency virus (HIV) is associated with lymphadenopathy as an initial manifestation following seroconversion or in the latter stages of HIV as a persistent generalized lymphadenopathy. HIV-positive patients with CD4 counts greater than 200/µL may have generalized lymphadenopathy that persists; these nodes are usually smaller than 1.5 cm. Any node larger than 1.5 cm or an asymmetry of distribution should prompt investigation. When the CD4 count is between 200 and 500/µL there is an increased rate of Hodgkin's and non-Hodgkin's lymphoma, Kaposi's sarcoma, and tuberculosis. When the CD4 count is less than 100/µL, consider *Mycobacterium avium* complex or fungal or suppurative infection as the underlying etiology.

What is the differential diagnosis of lymphadenopathy?

Conditions mimicking lymphadenopathy include lipomas, rheumatoid nodules, sebaceous cysts, ganglion cysts, thyroglossal duct, or branchial cleft cysts. Enlarged parotid or submandibular glands may feel nodular. Cutaneous clues to the differential diagnosis include a rash on the palms or soles in secondary syphilis, erythema nodosum in tuberculosis or sarcoid, and a malar rash in lupus. Mononucleosis may show pharyngeal exudate. Splenomegaly may accompany mononucleosis, leukemia, or lymphoma. Hyperthyroidism may show tremor, whereas lupus or rheumatoid arthritis may have associated synovitis.

What are Virchow's, Irish's, and Sister Mary Joseph's nodes?

Virchow's node is a left supraclavicular lymph node that is usually due to a gastrointestinal, renal, testicular, or ovarian malignancy. A right supraclavicular node may be due to a pulmonary, mediastinal, or esophageal tumor. *Irish's node* is a left axillary node due to gastric cancer. *Sister Mary Joseph's node* is paraumbilical adenopathy due to an intra-abdominal malignancy.

What can cause axillary adenopathy?

Although the most common cause of axillary lymphadenopathy is an ipsilateral injury or infection in the arm or hand, unilateral adenopathy raises the specter of breast cancer, so a thorough breast exam and mammogram should be part of the evaluation. Remember that male breast cancer accounts for 1% of cases; thus, always examine the male breast as well.

What can cause hilar lymphadenopathy?

Bilateral hilar adenopathy may be due to benign infectious causes such as coccidioidomycosis, tuberculosis, or histoplasmosis. Skin testing or antigen titers (drawn before skin testing is done) may help in the differential diagnosis. Sarcoidosis may cause hilar adenopathy and should be considered in a patient with joint pain, erythema nodosum, or uveitis. Malignancy such as bronchogenic carcinoma or lymphoma should be suspected in a patient with a mediastinal mass, pleural effusion, or pulmonary mass associated with either bilateral or unilateral adenopathy.

What can cause inguinal lymphadenopathy?

Chronic, small "shotty" nodes are common in the inguinal region due to either subclinical or low-grade infections in the lower extremities or perineum. Genital ulceration followed by the appearance of either unilateral or bilateral inguinal adenopathy should raise the suspicion of venereal disease as the cause. The differential diagnosis includes syphilis, herpes, chancroid, lymphogranuloma venereum, and granuloma inguinale. A careful social history and examination can elucidate these as the etiology. Inguinal metastasis from rectal, vaginal, penile, and cervical cancer stress the importance of a complete physical examination, including digital rectal exam and a bimanual pelvic exam. Melanoma metastasis is also a cause, and a thorough examination for discolored lesions should be done.

What can cause cervical lymphadenopathy?

The neck is the most common location for lymphadenopathy. Many benign etiologies account for bilateral cervical adenopathy associated with fever and fatigue, including infectious mononucleosis, pharyngitis, primary HIV infection, cytomegalovirus, herpes simplex virus, and secondary syphilis. Inflamed cervical nodes are usually due to staphylococcal or streptococcal infection. Treatment is with antibiotics, and if the node is frankly fluctuant, incision and drainage will be necessary. Tuberculosis adenitis (scrofula) typically presents as a slowly enlarging, mildly symptomatic node of several weeks' to months' duration that may or may not be fluctuant. The diagnosis should be suspected in a patient with a history of tuberculosis, a positive purified protein derivative (PPD), or an abnormal-appearing chest radiograph. When the diagnosis is suspected and there is no evidence of disease elsewhere to provide the diagnosis, node excision is done and the patient is started on antitubercular drugs until the final culture results are available.

A hard submandibular or anterior cervical node, especially in the elderly, often represents a metastasis from a head and neck malignancy. Lung, breast, and thyroid cancer may also metastasize to anterior cervical nodes. Fine-needle biopsy confirms the diagnosis, and then the primary tumor should be sought with a thorough head and neck exam, including triple endoscopy, to evaluate the nasal, bronchial, and esophageal passages.

▶ EVALUATION

What are the key points on physical examination?

Careful palpation should be performed of the occiput, periauricular area, the entire neck, supraclavicular fossa, axillae, abdomen, and groin and epitrochlear spaces. On physical exam, five points should be elucidated: size, location, consistency, inflammation, and fixation.

Infections are the most common cause of lymphadenopathy and are suggested by clinical symptoms and signs such as fever, rash, or local abscess. Hard nodes may be due to malignancy or fibrosis from prior inflammation. Lymphoma and leukemia usually produce firm, rubbery nodes. Pyogenic infection produces tender, fluctuant nodes, although these may also result from advanced tuberculosis or necrotic tumors. Fixation to other nodes or to the deep fascia or dermis suggests neoplasm. Look for associated erythema or streaking or for associated wounds. Pay attention to old incisions—the patient may not remember having had a "mole" removed that in fact was a melanoma.

What radiographic studies are important?

CT scanning can detect nodes as small as 0.5 cm. Pedal lymphangiography delineates the size and characteristics of pelvic and low retroperitoneal nodes. It has largely been supplanted by CT scans but may be useful in the case of a patient with lymphoma and an equivocal CT scan. The drawbacks of pedal lymphangiography are that it is invasive, potentially morbid, and contraindicated in patients with pulmonary disease or a dye allergy.

Gallium scanning may be helpful. Neoplastic lymphoid tissue and also some solid tumors such as melanoma take up gallium. Enlarged lymph nodes that take up the gallium are likely to be neoplastic, but enlarged nodes that do not take up gallium are not necessarily benign because many tumors do not avidly bind the gallium.

Because there is a significant false-positive and false-negative rate with gallium scans, they should be viewed as an adjunct measure once the diagnosis is found, not as a first-step study.

Which laboratory studies are helpful?

Extensive testing is rarely indicated. If on initial history and physical exam no clear underlying cause is elucidated, a complete blood count (CBC) with differential, erythrocyte sedimentation rate, and chest radiograph will help narrow the differential diagnosis. Atypical lymphocytes on CBC may point toward mononucleosis, toxoplasmosis, or a viral infection. Monospot can be sent, although it may be negative in 10% of patients with mononucleosis. If tuberculosis is considered on chest radiograph, a PPD should be placed; if sarcoid is suspected, an angiotensin-converting enzyme (ACE) level may be checked. Coccidioidomycosis, cytomegalovirus, histoplasmosis, and toxoplasmosis serology can be checked if the differential points that way. Patients with HIV risk factors should have testing, and those with marked inguinal adenopathy should be checked for sexually transmitted diseases.

When is a biopsy helpful?

As a general rule, the larger the node and the older the patient, the more likely that a neoplasm is present. Do not delay when cancer is suspected. If the node is small and the clinical suspicion and physical exam suggest a viral infection, watchful waiting for 2 to 4 weeks may be undertaken, but the patient must be reexamined to confirm stability or regression. If the node enlarges or does not resolve, biopsy is indicated. Lymph nodes greater than 2 to 3 cm in diameter, particularly when multiple, have a high risk of malignancy in any age group in any location and should be evaluated promptly.

What are the biopsy options?

There are two types of biopsy: needle and excisional. In general, fine-needle aspiration (FNA) is a quick and easy way to make a preliminary diagnosis of malignancy. It has minimal morbidity and can be done at the time of the initial visit. The main requirements are an experienced cytopathologist and communication between the clinician and pathologist. If the patient has generalized lymphadenopathy, try to avoid the inguinal nodes for biopsy, because these are the most likely to be falsely enlarged from subclinical infection. Neck nodes provide a specific diagnosis 70% of the time, axillary nodes 50%, and inguinal 40%; thus, go for the neck node first. As many as 85% of attempts yield a diagnosis.

If the FNA yields malignancy, the next step is localization of the primary and appropriate intervention. If the FNA reveals suspicion for lymphoma, an excisional biopsy will be needed for architectural diagnosis. If the FNA is nondiagnostic, excisional biopsy should be done. Thoracic or abdominal nodes may be approached for FNA with CT or ultrasound guidance, although often an open biopsy is required.

For head and neck malignancies, a needle biopsy is preferred as the initial step to prevent contamination of the tissue planes for subsequent definitive treatment.

For an excisional biopsy, at least 1 g of tissue should be obtained. Preferably, the node should be sent fresh to pathology, but if that is not possible it should be sent in saline as opposed to formalin so that marker studies, immunocytochemistry, and cultures can be done.

K E Y P O I N T S

▶ Features that would suggest further evaluation of a node by biopsy include size larger than 1.5 cm, age older than 50 years, history of tobacco or alcohol use, or other constitutional symptoms.

▶ A complete history and physical exam narrow the differential diagnosis. When the diagnosis is uncertain and the suspicion of malignancy is low, a period of observation for 2 to 4 weeks can be undertaken, but the patient must be reexamined.

▶ Extensive laboratory studies are not needed.

CASE 14–1. A 20-year-old woman comes for evaluation of a neck lump of 2 days' duration. She is well now but reports that last week she had the "flu." She has no significant past medical history. On exam the only finding is a slightly tender, mobile 2-cm mass anterior to the right sternocleidomastoid muscle.

A. What is your differential diagnosis? List five possibilities.
B. What tests should you order?
C. A week later the lab results are all normal and the patient returns. What is your plan?

CASE 14–2. A 60-year-old man comes for his annual physical. He smokes 2 packs per day and used to drink heavily but reports he has "cut down." He feels well. On exam he has a 1.5-cm firm, fixed mass in the left anterior neck.

  A. What is your differential diagnosis?
  B. What tests do you order? If a biopsy is done, should you do an FNA or excisional biopsy?

15

Mental Status Changes

What are the categories of causes of mental status changes?

Causes are categorized into CNS diseases, medications, medication withdrawal, metabolic derangement, organ failure, and global infection or serious illness (Table 15–1).

What is the significance of mental status change in the surgical patient?

Cognitive function is the most complex of all physiologic processes and is therefore easily affected by minimal derangements in any of the body's organ system functions. Changes in mental status are quite common in the postoperative patient, who is affected by anesthesia, pain, changes in medications, critical illness, and hospitalization. Causes of mental status changes are varied, from a benign exacerbation of chronic dementia to an immediately life-threatening epidural hematoma. Management requires the immediate exclusion or treatment of the life-threatening problems and long-term diagnosis and prevention of the recurrent ones.

What are the usual terms used to characterize levels of consciousness?

Confusion is a state characterized by a disturbance of global attention and inability to maintain a coherent stream of thought. *Lethargy* denotes a state of sluggishness or sleepiness from which the patient is easily awakened. *Stupor* is a state from which the patient can be aroused only by vigorous stimuli. *Coma* is the state in which the patient appears asleep and cannot be aroused. Because of many definitions of terms for level of consciousness, an objective assessment such as the Glasgow Coma Scale is most valuable (see Chapter 35).

TABLE 15-1

Causes of Mental Status Changes

Central Nervous System
Infection (e.g., meningitis, abscess)
Vascular (cerebrovascular accident, transient ischemic attack, vasculitis)
Trauma
Tumor
Primary dementia
Encephalopathies
Seizures

Medications
Narcotics, sedatives, hypnotics, anesthetics
Antidepressants, anticonvulsants
Anti-inflammatory (steroidal and nonsteroidal)
Others

Medication Withdrawal
Alcohol
Sedatives

Metabolic Derangements
Abnormalities of glucose, sodium, calcium, acid-base
Endocrinopathies

Organ Failures
Renal, hepatic, respiratory, circulatory, multiple

Global Infections or Serious Illnesses

▶ **EVALUATION**

How do you differentiate between delirium and dementia?

Delirium is a global transient impairment of cognition characterized by clouded sensorium, agitation, confusion, and misinterpretation of the environment (hallucinations, illusions, and delusions). Other clinical features may include disorientation, anxiety, combativeness, paranoia, irritability, hyperexcitability, altered motor behavior, incoherent speech, insomnia, decreased level of consciousness, inappropriate behavior, and disinhibition. Delirium is a common disorder, reported in 10% to 15% of surgical patients. It is potentially reversible and may be recurrent.

Dementia is an irreversible state of loss of memory, cognitive function, and recognition.

Causes of primary dementia include Alzheimer's disease, multi-infarct dementia, and Parkinson's disease. Dementia is usually chronic but may have acute exacerbations, as in "sun-downer's syndrome"—a confusional state recurring in the evening, especially in hospitalized and postoperative patients with dementia. Both delirium and dementia may be causes of confusion.

What immediate steps must be taken when encountering a patient in an acute confusional state or other acute change in mental status?

First, as in all emergencies, airway, breathing, and circulation (ABCs) must be evaluated and abnormalities corrected. Hypoxia, hypoglycemia, and septic shock are sometimes overlooked causes of mental status changes and should be clearly excluded prior to giving sedative medications. A brief assessment of neurologic status should be noted.

Second, steps must be taken to ensure that the patient is not at risk to others or self. Judicious application of restraints and sedation may be required even to prevent the confused patient from discontinuing tubes, drains, and catheters critical to medical care.

Third, the cause of the mental status change should be carefully evaluated and treated.

What should be the focus of history in a patient with acute mental status change?

Confused or agitated patients may not be able to provide an adequate history but should be queried for information they can provide. The medical record may reveal a previous baseline mental status examination, a medical condition that may be the cause, or medications that may have been omitted or given in excess as a source of mental status change.

What should be the focus of the physical examination of a patient with acute mental status change?

In addition to documenting a complete neurologic exam, the physical exam should look for pinpoint pupils (suggestive of narcotic use), unequal pupils (suggestive of mass lesion), papilledema (suggestive of increased intracranial pressure [ICP]), and nuchal rigidity (suggestive of meningitis). There should also be a search for evidence of head trauma (bruising, periorbital or periauricular ecchymosis, or hemotympanum).

What are the elements of a complete mental status examination?

A thorough mental status examination should document the following:

1. Level of consciousness: awake and alert, lethargic, stuporous, comatose, or AVPU (*a*lert, responds to *v*ocal stimuli, responds to *p*ain, *u*nresponsive)
2. General appearance: behavior and physical condition (e.g., neat, unkempt)
3. Mood: depressed, restless, agitated, labile
4. Form of thought: information flow clear, loose associations, flights of ideas, perseverations
5. Content of thought: delusions or concrete ideations
6. Perceptions (interpretation of environment): illusions or hallucinations
7. Orientation: person, place, time
8. Registration: ability to learn and repeat new information
9. Recall of recent events
10. Long-term memory
11. Language
12. Judgment

What laboratory tests should be ordered to help determine the cause of acute mental status changes?

Serum glucose should be immediately determined, but glucose may be given before waiting for results. An electrolyte panel will demonstrate abnormalities of serum calcium, magnesium, and sodium. Renal failure may be excluded as a source by a normal blood urea nitrogen (BUN). An elevated serum ammonia level may point toward hepatic failure as a source. When indicated, blood or urine should be sent for drug screen. Blood gas analysis will exclude hypoxia. Depressed thyroid function tests may point toward hypothyroidism.

Patients who have lateralizing signs on neurologic exam require emergency head computed tomography (CT), transfer to an intensive care unit to maintain ABCs, and contact with a neurosurgeon. Also, if no medical or metabolic source is found, consideration should still be given to CT of the head to exclude mass lesions. If meningitis is suspected by the presence of fever or nuchal rigidity, a lumbar puncture (LP) is indicated. In a patient with increased ICP, however, an LP may precipitate brain stem herniation, so elevated ICP must be excluded by physical exam and head CT prior to performing the LP.

What are the clinical findings associated with acute alcohol withdrawal?

Alcohol withdrawal commonly occurs 24 to 48 hours after the last drink and is a potentially fatal complication. Signs and symptoms include change in mental status; autonomic hyperactivity (sweating, tachycardia); nausea and vomiting; coarse, rapid hand tremors;

delirium tremens with vivid hallucinations; seizures; and Korsakoff's psychosis or Wernicke's encephalopathy.

What are some causes of mental status change that may be a major threat to life and thus must be evaluated and treated emergently?

Patients with acute change in mental status require emergent treatment. Immediately treat hypoglycemia, alcohol withdrawal, hypoxia, medication overdose, sepsis, central nervous system (CNS) infection, and CNS mass lesions including tumor or epidural or subdural fluid collections that may lead to brain stem herniation. Most concerning are lateralizing signs and mental status changes after trauma or neurosurgery or in a patient at risk for sepsis.

▶ TREATMENT

What actions should be taken if medication overdose is determined to be a possible source?

For drug overdose (OD), when possible, give a reversal. If a narcotic is suspected, give naloxone HCl (Narcan) 2 mg IV. If this is effective, remember that the naloxone half-life is short and check the patient later to confirm that another dose is not needed. For possible benzodiazepine OD, give flumazenil (Romazicon), remembering that administration is associated with a risk of seizure. Current flumazenil dosage recommendations are 0.2 mg over 30 seconds, then 0.3 over 30 seconds, repeat to 3 mg. For questions or for other drugs, consult poison control.

How is acute alcohol withdrawal treated?

After airway and breathing are ensured, circulation should be supported by aggressive fluid and electrolyte replacement. Some sedation is always required, and very large doses are often needed, beginning with either chlordiazepoxide HCl (Librium) or diazepam (Valium).

To prevent encephalopathy, intravenous vitamins should be given, including multivitamins, thiamine 100 mg, and folate 1 mg ("banana bag"). Also in the treatment regimen may be magnesium sulfate, antiepileptics, and haloperidol lactate (Haldol). Glucose should always be given to exclude and treat hypoglycemia in the patient with altered mental status; however, it may precipitate Wernicke's encephalopathy if thiamine is not also administered.

K E Y   P O I N T S

▶ Acute mental status changes may be the first sign of severe systemic abnormalities, such as hypoxia, hypoglycemia, or sepsis.

▶ Acute mental status changes may represent a medical or surgical emergency. After ensuring ABCs, the causes should rapidly be determined and treated.

▶ Acute confusional state is common in the surgical patient. Dementia should not be assumed as the cause, because the cause may be a large variety of disease states, some critical.

▶ Delirium from alcohol withdrawal commonly presents 24 to 48 hours after cessation of drinking and may be immediately life-threatening due to the severe perturbations of metabolic and mental states.

CASE 15–1. A 65-year-old man has just returned from the recovery room, having undergone a partial foot amputation for gangrene. Past medical history is negative except for the presence of untreated hypertension and insulin-dependent diabetes. The ward nurse calls you requesting nasal oxygen because the patient is still very sleepy and not breathing deeply, and the oximeter alarm keeps going off, bothering the other patients.

A. Outline your course of action.

CASE 15–2. A 44-year-old homeless man is admitted to the surgical service for IV antibiotic treatment of neglected cellulitis on the left leg. The admission history and physical exam do not mention social habits and note the neurologic exam to be "normal." On morning rounds of hospital day 2, he states he is feeling better, then asks why the bus is taking so long to arrive. He is also flicking at his bed sheets and, when asked, responds that he sees large roaches crawling on his bed. Examination reveals that he is slightly warm with a pulse of 110 beats/min and a normal blood pressure.

A. What is the most likely cause of his confusion?
B. Outline a plan for care.

16

Nausea and Vomiting

▶ ETIOLOGY

Although surgeons are asked to evaluate both outpatients and inpatients with nausea and vomiting, the differential diagnoses are not the same.

What are the most common causes of nausea and vomiting in outpatients?

In the outpatient setting, causes of nausea and vomiting are most commonly nonsurgical (Table 16–1). Nonspecific infectious illnesses predominate. Most common are viral syndromes either systemic or localized to the gastrointestinal (GI) tract. Bacterial or parasitic infections of the GI tract can also occur. Gastric and intestinal irritation may result from direct toxins (e.g., ethanol or products of microbial infection), specific food intolerance, over-the-counter medications (e.g., aspirin or other nonsteroidal anti-inflammatory agents), or prescription medications (e.g., antibiotics or narcotics). Crohn's disease and, less commonly, ulcerative colitis may present with nausea. Many of these conditions can be diagnosed following a thorough history of the present illness.

Medical conditions not directly related to GI physiology may also present with nausea and vomiting. These include myocardial infarction or ischemia, pregnancy, endocrine disorders (e.g., diabetic ketoacidosis, gastroparesis, or adrenal insufficiency), renal failure associated with uremia, and lesions of the central nervous system (e.g., tumors, meningitis, migraine headache, hydrocephalus, and labyrinthitis). Psychogenic causes of nausea include stress, intense emotional responses, anorexia nervosa, and bulimia.

Conditions that potentially need aggressive intervention are more germane to the surgeon. Early in the work-up, specific evaluation for the possibility of mechanical bowel obstruction should be undertaken. Obstruction may occur at any level of the GI tract, from the esophagus to the anus. The small bowel is most commonly involved in Western countries, with obstruction most often due to postoperative adhesions. Incarcerated hernias are also quite common causes of small bowel obstruction. Pancreatitis and the serious sequelae of pancreatitis, including pseudocyst formation,

TABLE 16–1
Common Causes of Nausea and Vomiting in the Outpatient

Infectious or Inflammatory Etiologies
Viral, bacterial, or parasitic gastroenteritis
Systemic viral illness
Serious nonviral systemic infections
Inflammatory bowel disease

Toxic Conditions
Food intolerance
Alcohol ingestion
Other known toxin
Nonsteroidal anti-inflammatory agents
Other medications

Systemic Conditions
Myocardial ischemia
Pregnancy
Diabetes mellitus
Renal failure with uremia
Central nervous system conditions
Psychogenic causes

Mechanical and Other Gastrointestinal Conditions
Bowel obstruction
Pancreatitis/pancreatic lesions
Biliary tract disease/obstruction
Intra-abdominal abscess/peritonitis
Massive gastrointestinal bleeding

hemorrhage, abscess formation, and necrosis, are also frequently seen as causes of nausea and vomiting. Other acute abdominal conditions such as spontaneous bacterial peritonitis, perforated or inflamed diverticula, or abdominal trauma can also lead to nausea and vomiting. Finally, nausea and vomiting associated with marked hematemesis may represent bleeding esophageal varices, bleeding gastric or duodenal ulcer, Mallory-Weiss tear, or any of a number of other conditions that require early endoscopic and occasionally operative treatment.

What is the significance of bilious vomiting?

Bile in the vomitus indicates reflux of duodenal contents into the stomach. In adults, this is common and may be nonspecific. However, if a bowel obstruction is present, bilious vomiting indicates that the site of obstruction is distal to the second portion of the duodenum. Bilious vomiting in infants may signify malrotation or midgut volvulus and requires emergency evaluation and treatment.

What is the significance of vomiting undigested food or vomiting shortly after eating?

If intestinal obstruction is suspected, a careful history can help diagnose the level of pathology. Esophageal pathology, including tumors, strictures, and motility abnormalities (e.g., achalasia), may present with dysphagia (difficulty swallowing), odynophagia (pain associated with swallowing), or vomiting. If vomiting is a predominant symptom, it will occur soon after eating and include nondigested food. These symptoms may also be found with gastric obstruction, but the time between food ingestion and the vomiting of partially digested stomach contents may be variable due to the reservoir capacity of the stomach. More generalized intra-abdominal pathology, such as peritonitis or pancreatitis, can present with extreme food intolerance, leading to vomiting immediately after eating.

What causes feculent vomiting?

Feculent vomiting refers to a stool-like odor of the vomitus. Truly feculent vomiting is rare. When it occurs, it suggests mechanical obstruction of the GI tract in the distal small bowel or the colon. This condition suggests a more long-standing process that has developed over hours to days, allowing time for the majority of the proximal GI tract to dilate and expand prior to the onset of vomiting.

What is the importance of constipation and obstipation associated with nausea and vomiting?

Constipation is the failure of passage of stool, whereas *obstipation* is the absence of passage of flatus. Either sign may be associated with nausea or vomiting and may suggest a mechanical obstruction or paralytic ileus. Failure of normal GI function requires a different evaluation process than conditions associated with the ongoing passage of stool or gas.

What are the most common causes of nausea and vomiting in a postoperative patient?

The differential diagnosis of nausea and vomiting in postoperative patients differs from those patients who are outpatients or those without a history of abdominal procedures (Table 16–2).

In the immediate postoperative period, many patients suffer from nausea as an aftereffect of general anesthesia. However, the most common cause of postoperative nausea and vomiting is paralytic ileus. If severe, this condition may take days to weeks to resolve.

Of more concern is an early bowel obstruction, which may be due to adhesions, internal herniation, or occlusion of an anastomosis or stoma. Differentiation of mechanical obstruction from a paralytic

TABLE 16–2

Common Causes of Nausea and Vomiting in the Postoperative Patient

Medication (narcotics, antibiotics, anesthetic agents, chemotherapy)
Paralytic ileus
Early mechanical bowel obstruction
Stricture or edema of anastomotic site or stoma
Pancreatitis
Intra-abdominal infection
Anastomotic leak or bowel perforation

ileus can be difficult and may require contrast studies. Often, observation is sufficient if a reasonable amount of time is allowed for the spontaneous resolution of a postoperative ileus.

Generalized abdominal tenderness or frank peritonitis associated with nausea or vomiting may signify the presence of an intra-abdominal abscess or anastomotic leak and should be evaluated promptly. Pancreatitis in the postoperative period can occur and may require a high level of suspicion to diagnose. Finally, many medications used in postoperative patients may cause nausea or vomiting (see later).

What drugs are most commonly associated with nausea in hospitalized patients?

Many medications have been associated with some incidence of nausea or vomiting. The most common offenders are narcotics, antibiotics (particularly those given orally), and chemotherapeutic agents (less commonly used in surgical patients). Changing the class of antibiotic or type of narcotic agent may sometimes alleviate symptoms. Related conditions may include antibiotic-associated enteritis (including *Clostridium difficile*–associated colitis) and diarrhea, either of which may present with nausea or food intolerance. Treatment of *C. difficile* colitis may include cessation of antibiotics, if possible, and administration of either metronidazole or oral vancomycin.

▶ **EVALUATION**

What are the pertinent aspects of the history of present illness in a patient with nausea and vomiting?

Nausea and vomiting are present in a large number of conditions; therefore, the correct diagnosis of the etiology requires a carefully obtained history. The duration and severity of symptoms must be ascertained. Recent ingestion of new medications or foods is an important clue, as is review of recent alcohol intake. An infectious etiology is suggested by a history of exposure to other family members or contacts with similar complaints. Associated symptoms of diarrhea, myalgia, fever, or chills also give important information. Questions about changes in bowel habits are important to thoroughly evaluate the possibility of bowel obstruction. The nature of the vomited material or the presence of blood or undigested food, for example, will help narrow the differential diagnosis. Other questions to help assess possible specific etiologies include the presence or absence of headache or chest pain, as well as the date of the last menses in women.

What are the important aspects of the past medical and surgical histories?

Patients should be questioned about medication use as well as a history of those illnesses that may be associated with nausea and vomiting. These may include cardiac disease, migraine headache, diabetes mellitus, peptic ulcer disease, inflammatory bowel disease, and cholelithiasis. The past surgical history is critical for surgeons, because the presence of unequivocal bowel obstruction in a patient who has never had an intra-abdominal operation is an indication for urgent surgical exploration. The specific incision used for prior procedures is also important because some, such as a Pfannenstiel or a right lower quadrant appendectomy incision, are associated with a lower incidence of obstruction. Clearly, the exact nature of prior operations is also important, because prior bowel resection and anastomosis or procedures for malignancy might suggest an etiology for mechanical obstruction at the operative site.

What are the significant findings on physical examination?

Although a good overall physical examination is necessary, a careful examination of the abdomen is clearly of greatest importance. This assessment should begin with observation to assess for discomfort or distention, then auscultation to assess the presence and characteristics of bowel sounds. High-pitched or tinkling bowel sounds are indicative of obstruction. Palpation with close attention to distention and points of tenderness is informative, because the degree and level of distention or pain may be related to the location of the obstruction. The site of tenderness may also localize an inflammatory process. Percussion to assess tympany is an excellent means to help differentiate pathology secondary to gaseous bowel distention and ascites from other conditions not associated with paralytic ileus or obstruction. Of specific importance is a detailed search for abdominal, incisional, or inguinal hernias as well as a rectal examination to rule out low rectal lesions and the presence of blood in the stool.

Which laboratory tests are important?

Routine laboratory tests (Table 16–3) are most useful to assess the degree of dehydration and metabolic derangement associated with vomiting. The most common electrolyte abnormality associated with prolonged vomiting is hypochloremic metabolic alkalosis. Other findings may include an elevated hematocrit or hypokalemia. Other tests may be helpful but nonspecific (e.g., an elevated white blood cell count in the setting of inflammation) and should be reserved to confirm a suspected diagnosis. After a differential diagnosis is suggested by the history and physical examination, appropriate tests may be performed to rule out specific conditions. These may include an amylase or lipase determination to rule out pancreatitis, troponin or creatine kinase levels to rule out myocardial ischemia, liver function tests to rule out hepatic or biliary pathology, beta human chorionic gonadotropin to rule out pregnancy, or urinalysis to rule out urinary tract infection or nephrolithiasis.

TABLE 16–3
Common Tests Used to Evaluate Patients with Nausea and Vomiting
Laboratory Tests, Nonspecific Serum chemistries, metabolic panels Complete blood count
Laboratory Tests, When Indicated Troponin, creatine kinase-MB Amylase, lipase Beta human chorionic gonadotropin Drug screens Liver function tests, hepatitis serologies Stool culture
Radiology Three-way of the abdomen (upright and supine abdominal films and chest radiograph) CT scan of the abdomen/pelvis Biliary ultrasound or scintigraphy Upper gastrointestinal contrast study Contrast enema
Other Studies Esophagogastroduodenoscopy Endoscopic retrograde cholangiopancreatography Gastric emptying studies Mesenteric angiography or MRI

What radiologic examinations are frequently obtained in evaluating nausea and vomiting?

Not all patients who present acutely with nausea and vomiting require radiographic studies. These tests should be ordered with specific findings in mind (see Table 16–3). Most commonly, plain films of the abdomen are obtained, including an upright and supine view of the abdomen and an upright chest radiograph (collectively called a "three-way" study of the abdomen). These studies may reveal any of several pertinent findings, including air-fluid levels indicating bowel obstruction, free intraperitoneal air indicating bowel perforation, or evidence of localized ileus associated with focal inflammatory process. Computed tomography (CT) should be reserved for situations with a high likelihood of establishing a definitive diagnosis, such as a focal lesion or pancreatitis. CT is also highly sensitive in detecting small amounts of intraperitoneal air.

For more chronic cases of nausea or vomiting, studies may include contrast studies of the esophagus, stomach, or intestine; nuclear imaging studies of the swallowing apparatus, biliary excretion, or gastric emptying; ultrasound to evaluate the biliary tree or pelvic anatomy; or angiography and magnetic resonance imaging to evaluate the adequacy of blood flow or bile flow to the bowel.

What other tests are sometimes used to diagnose the cause of nausea or vomiting?

Esophagogastroduodenoscopy (EGD) is used acutely for the diagnosis and treatment of hematemesis, as well as electively for more chronic symptoms. Less frequently, endoscopic retrograde cholangiopancreatography or colonoscopy is used in a more extensive evaluation. When a differential diagnosis is narrowed by history and physical examination and supported by laboratory and radiographic studies, other specific tests may be indicated. These may range from electrocardiogram to specialized stool serologies to lumbar puncture to perhaps even exploratory laparoscopy or laparotomy.

What are important complicating sequelae of prolonged nausea and vomiting?

Vomiting may lead to several fluid and electrolyte disorders. Chief among these are dehydration, a diagnosis that frequently can be made on physical examination (dry mucous membranes, skin tenting, tachycardia) and confirmed by laboratory tests (elevated hematocrit, elevated blood urea nitrogen (BUN)-to-creatinine ratio). Prolonged vomiting may lead to hypokalemia and mild metabolic alkalosis, associated with a paradoxical aciduria as hydrogen ions are excreted in exchange for the resorption of potassium in the kidneys. Aggressive replacement of potassium and fluid is necessary in these patients. If nausea and vomiting are even more chronic, weight loss and malnutrition will also result. It is also possible to detect acid erosion of the enamel of the teeth with frequent vomiting.

▶ **TREATMENT**

How are nausea and vomiting treated?

The initial treatment of nausea and vomiting includes identification and correction of the underlying cause. Life-threatening causes, such as bowel obstruction, should be treated urgently. Infectious etiologies should be sought and appropriate antibiotics administered.

Once appropriate steps have been taken to correct underlying causes, the actual symptoms of nausea and vomiting may be addressed. Commonly used antiemetic medications are listed in Table 16–4.

Prolonged symptoms of vomiting may result in dehydration and electrolyte abnormalities, which must be corrected.

TABLE 16–4

Common Antiemetic Agents

Drug Name	Drug Type	Dose
Promethazine hydrochloride (Phenergan)	Phenothiazine	25-50 mg PO, PR every 4-6 hr 25 mg IM every 4-6 hr 12.5 mg IV every 4-6 hr Peds: 0.5-1.0 mg/kg/dose PO, PR, or IM
Prochlorperazine maleate (Compazine)	Phenothiazine	5-10 mg PO, PR 3 or 4 times per day 5 mg IV over 2-3 min Peds: 0.13 mg/kg/dose
Trimethobenzamide hydrochloride (Tigan)	Related central agent	250 mg PO 3 times per day 200 mg PR, IM every 6-8 hr Peds: 100 mg/dose if patient is >30 lb
Metoclopramide monohydrochloride monohydrate (Reglan)	Dopamine antagonist	10 mg PO, IM, IV 1 hr before meals and at bedtime
Cisapride (Propulsid)	Prokinetic agent	10-20 mg PO before meals and at bedtime
Ondansetron hydrochloride (Zofran)	Serotonin 5-HT$_3$ blocker	8 mg PO, IV 3 times per day IV form may be given in a single 32-mg dose every day if desired

PO, orally; PR, rectally; IM, intramuscularly; IV, intravenously; Peds, pediatric.
From Adams GA, Bresnick SD: On Call Surgery, 2nd ed. Philadelphia, WB Saunders, 2001.

K E Y   P O I N T S

▶ A careful history is important to narrow a large differential diagnosis.

▶ Physical examination can help rapidly determine the likelihood of the need for urgent surgical intervention.

▶ A specific set of conditions are associated with nausea and vomiting in the postoperative patient.

▶ Complete bowel obstruction in a patient with no prior history of abdominal surgery or infection is an indication for urgent surgical exploration.

▶ The majority of laboratory, radiographic, and invasive studies are performed only with a specific diagnosis in mind.

▶ Administration of antiemetic medication follows only after careful evaluation of the patient and correction of underlying causes.

CASE 16–1. A 56-year-old man presents to the emergency department with a 3-day history of nausea and vomiting. He has no significant past medical history. He has never had an operation. On physical examination, he has a distended, tympanitic abdomen and no evidence of hernias. On plain films of the abdomen, he has signs of a small bowel obstruction and he has a normal chest radiograph. A CT scan shows dilation of the small bowel to the level of the mid or distal ileum.

    A. What is the most relevant aspect of this patient's past medical and surgical histories?

    B. Based on his physical examination and radiologic studies, what is your differential diagnosis?

    C. What should your first major therapeutic intervention be?

CASE 16–2.

A 36-year-old man presents with nausea and vomiting of 2 days' duration. His abdomen is distended and tympanitic. He has a long midline abdominal scar from a prior splenectomy following a motor vehicle accident. His routine laboratory test results are all within normal limits. Plain films of his abdomen reveal signs of an early or partial small bowel obstruction.

A. What is the significance of the man's prior operation?
B. Should this man have his abdomen explored?

17

Neck Mass

What are the common causes of neck masses?

Neck masses generally fall into three categories: congenital, inflammatory, and neoplastic. The majority of neck masses in children fall under the first two categories, whereas the incidence of neoplasia increases with age.

What are the common congenital neck masses, and how do they present?

Congenital lesions account for 55% of neck masses in children. The clues to the diagnosis are the location, the appearance, and a history that is present for months or years. The most common congenital neck masses include the following:

1. Thyroglossal duct cyst, which is related embryologically to the descent of the thyroid primordium from the foramen cecum to where the thyroid is located and therefore can be present anywhere along this tract. It usually presents as a 2- to 4-cm mass in the midline below the hyoid bone and elevates with tongue protrusion. It commonly presents after an upper respiratory tract infection in children. However, it can present at any age, with 35% of cases presenting after 40 years of age.
2. Branchial cleft cysts, which are the abnormal development of the branchial clefts that can result in fistulas, sinus tracts, or cysts. Branchial cleft cysts present as neck masses often developing in childhood or early adulthood after an upper respiratory tract infection. Second branchial cleft cysts are the most common type and present as neck masses below the angle of the mandible and anterior to the sternocleidomastoid.
3. Lymphangiomas or cystic hygromas, which are soft, fleshy masses that transilluminate.
4. Hemangiomas, which are very common in infants and children. They can present as superficial lesions or can be deep, presenting as subcutaneous masses. Most involute as the child grows.

5. Dermoid cysts and teratomas, which occur as midline masses, but unlike thyroglossal duct cysts, they do not move with tongue elevation.
6. Others, including those such as thymic cyst, bronchogenic cyst, and laryngocele.

What are common inflammatory neck masses?

Inflammatory masses in the neck can be lymph nodes, abscesses, or masses arising from the thyroid and salivary glands.

1. Lymphadenopathy: reactive lymphadenopathy can result from a focus of an infection in the head and neck. Common examples include acute bacterial infections such as pharyngitis, tonsillitis, tooth abscess, or otitis. Other common infections include toxoplasmosis, infectious mononucleosis, cat-scratch disease, primary human immunodeficiency virus (HIV) infection, brucellosis, cytomegalovirus, and tuberculosis.
2. Abscesses: subcutaneous abscesses can arise from cutaneous lesions such as a furuncle or an infected keratinous cyst. Thyroglossal duct and branchial cleft cysts can get infected and can present as abscesses. Parapharyngeal and peritonsillar abscesses can cause unilateral neck swelling, mimicking a neck mass.
3. Inflammatory conditions involving the thyroid gland include Graves' disease, acute thyroiditis, or subacute thyroiditis. Salivary glands can develop infections such as parotitis in mumps, acute suppurative parotitis, parotid abscess, and recurrent acute sialoadenitis.

What are common neoplastic neck masses?

Common tumors presenting as neck masses include metastatic disease, lymphomas, thyroid tumors, and tumors of the salivary glands. Benign soft tissue tumors such as lipomas are fairly common, whereas sarcomas are rare.

The lymphatic drainage of the neck is rich, and any malignancy involving the scalp, face, and aerodigestive tract can present in the neck as a metastatic lymph node. In addition, some of the deep cervical and supraclavicular lymph nodes may become involved in the spread of cancers from the abdomen and thorax.

Tumors of the thyroid gland include benign neoplasms such as adenomas, which may or may not be functional. Most malignant tumors of the thyroid are well-differentiated neoplasms such as papillary and follicular carcinoma. Other less common thyroid cancers include medullary, undifferentiated, and metastatic carcinomas and lymphomas.

Neoplasms of the salivary glands constitute about 5% of all head and neck tumors, and about 70% of those are tumors of the parotid gland. Whereas most tumors of the parotid are benign, 60% of submandibular gland tumors are malignant. Common benign parotid tumors include pleomorphic adenomas, Warthin's tumor, adenoma, and oncocytoma.

▶ EVALUATION

What is this neck mass?

The work-up of a neck mass depends on the initial impression. The key is to narrow the differential diagnosis based on the history and physical examination (H&P). In addition to obtaining information on the characteristics of the mass as well as systemic symptoms, it is important to inquire about the history of smoking, alcohol intake, tuberculosis exposure, trauma, travel, occupation, environmental exposure, and sexual behavior.

The evaluation is often made easier by determining the nature of the lesion based on the exam (i.e., is this a lymph node, thyroid mass, parotid mass?) and by placing the neck mass in one of the categories listed earlier. This, of course, would only serve as a guide because some masses won't fit any of these classifications, such as multinodular goiter, acquired laryngocele, and traumatic carotid pseudoaneurysms.

Congenital lesions tend to occur in childhood and early adulthood and have characteristic features and location. Most are diagnosed clinically without further tests.

This feels like an inflammatory cervical lymph node. What should I do next?

If you suspect that the lymph node is inflammatory or reactive based on the H&P, the effort should focus on determining the primary cause. Primary sources of infection such as dental abscess, tonsillitis, skin infection, or ear infection should be checked for. If a primary bacterial infection is suspected to be the cause, a trial of antibiotics is indicated. A complete blood count is often a helpful test to begin with. Other tests that may be helpful in select cases include tuberculin skin test, *Toxoplasma* titers, Monospot, *Brucella* titers, and HIV testing. Imaging is usually not necessary. If a lymph node that is thought to be inflammatory continues to grow past 2 to 4 weeks despite appropriate treatment, a fine-needle aspiration (FNA) should be performed.

This lymph node is suspicious for cancer. What should I do next?

FNA confirms the diagnosis with a high degree of accuracy, especially for squamous cell carcinomas, adenocarcinomas, and metastatic thyroid cancers. Further imaging with computed tomographic (CT) scan or magnetic resonance imaging is helpful in the work-up and staging if a malignancy is suspected.

For metastatic squamous cell carcinomas, a complete head and neck examination, including panendoscopy of the upper aerodigestive tract, is mandatory. Patients who are at risk include those with a long-standing history of cigarette smoking and alcohol intake. Suspicious areas as well as the base of the tongue and nasopharynx should be biopsied. For metastatic disease, physical examination, panendoscopy, and CT scan will detect the primary tumor in about two thirds of patients. Some authors recommend tonsillectomy if no primary tumor is identified.

Open biopsy of a suspected metastatic lymph node is contraindicated. Some studies have shown this to be detrimental and associated with a higher risk of local recurrence. FNA can be diagnostic in most cases of lymphoma, but an open biopsy may be needed to establish the type.

This feels like a thyroid mass. What should I do next?

When evaluating a patient with a thyroid mass, the following should be taken into consideration:

- The duration as well as rate of growth
- Symptoms indicating inflammation, local invasion, or compression, such as pain, hoarseness, stridor, and dysphagia
- Symptoms of hypothyroidism or hyperthyroidism
- Age, sex, family history, and location that the patient was born or has spent a significant portion of his or her life; this is particularly important in areas where goiter is endemic or where widespread radiation exposure has occurred such as in Chernobyl or Hiroshima
- History of low-dose radiation in infancy or childhood, which is associated with an increased risk of thyroid cancer

The physical examination should determine the size and firmness of the mass and whether it is fixed or mobile. It is important to determine whether it is a solitary nodule or part of multinodular thyroid goiter or diffuse swelling. The presence of cervical adenopathy is usually a sign of a metastatic disease. Manifestations of hypothyroidism or hyperthyroidism as well as extrathyroidal manifestations of Graves' disease should be checked.

The H&P, in most cases, guides the clinician in the direction of the diagnosis. FNA has become the mainstay in establishing the diagnosis of thyroid nodules. FNA diagnoses simple thyroid cysts if the mass completely disappears on aspiration of clear fluid. FNA is usually not indicated in patients with stable multinodular goiter or clinically evident Graves' disease or thyroiditis.

It is critical to have a skilled cytologist interpret the aspiration. FNA cytology results are reported as benign, malignant, indeterminate, or suspicious. It is difficult to distinguish follicular carcinoma from adenoma by FNA, and the report usually is read as follicular

neoplasm, indeterminate, or suspicious for malignancy. An unsatisfactory or inadequate sample is recorded in 10% to 20% of aspi-
rates. FNA can be repeated if the sample is unsatisfactory or
inadequate. If the diagnosis is not established, surgical excision is
recommended.

Other diagnostic tests are of value, including ultrasound, which
can determine the size and number of the lesions and whether they
are cystic or solid. It is also useful in the follow-up of nodules if no
operation is planned. Radionuclide scanning is now used less frequently, largely replaced by FNA. Nodules are described as hot or
cold based on the uptake of iodine. Whereas hot nodules rarely turn
out to be malignant, 20% of cold nodules do. CT scanning is of limited value and is rarely used in the work-up of thyroid nodules.

This feels like a salivary gland mass. What should I do next?

The three pairs of major salivary glands are the parotid, submandibular, and sublingual glands. It is important to determine if
the enlargement is related to an infection such as mumps or parotitis or to a tumor. FNA has become the mainstay in establishing the
diagnosis of salivary gland tumors. Chronic enlargement of the
parotid gland can sometimes be seen in patients with conditions
such as diabetes, gout, sarcoidosis, and malnutrition.

▶ TREATMENT

How are neck masses treated?

Treatment of a neck mass depends on the etiology. The first step of
appropriate therapy is an accurate diagnosis. In general, congenital masses are approached with surgical resection only if they
become symptomatic. Treatment of inflammatory neck masses
entails discovery and correction of the underlying cause. Treatment
of neoplastic masses is specific to the tumor type and may include
surgical resection, external beam radiation, and/or chemotherapy.

K E Y   P O I N T S

▶ The differential diagnosis of a neck mass is extensive.
   The key to evaluating a neck mass is obtaining a careful
   and thorough H&P. This would lead to the diagnosis in
   most patients and would guide further cost-effective
   tests.

continued

▶ A complete head and neck examination, including panendoscopy, is essential in the work-up of metastatic cervical lymphadenopathy.

▶ FNA is a simple, effective, and highly accurate method that can be used as an adjunct for establishing the diagnosis for most neck masses.

▶ Suspected reactive lymphadenopathy that does not resolve after 2 to 4 weeks despite appropriate treatment should be worked up further with an FNA.

CASE 17–1. A 65-year-old man, with a 60 pack-year history of smoking, presents with a progressively enlarging left-sided neck "lump" of 2 months' duration. He also reports mild dysphagia for solid foods for the past 3 weeks. Physical examination reveals a 3-cm hard lymph node anterior to the left sternocleidomastoid.

A. How would you begin the evaluation?
B. What is the most likely diagnosis?
C. Would you recommend a cervical lymph node biopsy?

CASE 17–2. A 45-year-old man presents with a progressively enlarging neck "lump" of 3 months' duration. The patient does not have pain, hoarseness, or dysphagia and is clinically euthyroid. Examination reveals a 2-cm firm mass in the left thyroid lobe and is otherwise unremarkable.

A. How would you start the evaluation?
B. Do you think an FNA is indicated?
C. What would be the next step if the FNA is reported as inadequate?

18

Nipple Discharge

Nipple discharge is a frequent reason for referral to a general or breast surgeon. The majority of patients referred for nipple discharge have a benign underlying cause. However, breast cancers are thought to originate in the lining of the milk duct, and certainly this is not a symptom to be ignored. The proper evaluation of women with this presenting symptom helps sort out those patients who need surgical excision to rule out malignancy.

▶ ETIOLOGY

What are the benign causes of nipple discharge?

The most common benign breast processes that can cause nipple discharge are ductal papilloma, duct ectasia, or fibrocystic changes. Other causes that are not directly related to the breast are pituitary adenomas (prolactin producing) and medications that may affect serum prolactin hormonal levels (Table 18–1). Women who are postpartum may produce small amounts of expressible liquid for prolonged periods after cessation of breast-feeding, particularly with continued nipple stimulation.

What are the malignant causes of nipple discharge?

The possibility of an underlying breast cancer associated with nipple discharge is the major reason for referral of these patients to a breast or general surgeon. Most breast carcinomas originate from the ducts and have the potential to cause nipple discharge. Both invasive ductal carcinoma and ductal carcinoma in situ (DCIS) can cause discharge that is usually bloody. About 9% of patients with cancer have nipple discharge as the presenting symptom; however, even so, the most common underlying etiology of bloody nipple discharge is still benign.

▶ EVALUATION

How do I evaluate nipple discharge in the clinic?

The pertinent history should include patient age, menopausal state, history for breast cancer risk stratification, and medications taken

TABLE 18-1

Medications Associated with a Presentation of
Nipple Discharge

Medication	Common Usage
Phenothiazines	Neuroleptic Psychotic disorders
Metoclopramide	Antiemetic—nausea, cancer Upper GI promotility agent—GERD, diabetic gastroparesis
Reserpine	Antihypertensive Essential hypertension, CAD
Butyrophenones (i.e., haloperidol [Haldol])	Major tranquilizer Behavioral modification, psychotic disorders
Verapamil	Ca^{2+} channel blocker Hypertension, rhythm disturbances, CAD
Tricyclic antidepressant	Restores norepinephrine and serotonin levels Depression, neuritic pain
Cimetidine	Histamine receptor antagonist PUD, GERD, gastritis
Estrogens	Hormone replacement therapy Birth control

CAD, coronary artery disease; GI, gastrointestinal; GERD, gastroesophageal reflux disease; PUD, peptic ulcer disease.

presently or in the recent past (including but not limited to hormone replacement or birth control). The characteristics of the discharge are an essential part of the history. Benign nipple discharge is usually nonspontaneous (requiring breast or nipple manipulation), bilateral, emanating from multiple ducts, and nonbloody. The characteristics that increase the index of suspicion for malignant causes of nipple discharge are unilateral discharge, spontaneous discharge (staining of the bra, shirt, or bedclothes), or frankly bloody discharge. The relative risk of a malignant etiology is higher in a postmenopausal woman who has new onset of unilateral nipple discharge. Most of the women in this age group should have a diagnostic work-up (biopsy). When examining the breast, you should try to express fluid with manual pressure at the nipple or in the breast. Note whether the discharge is coming from a single duct or multiple ducts and whether manipulation of a particular quadrant of the breast results in the discharge.

What is the color of normal and worrisome nipple discharge?

Normal nipple discharge can have a variety of appearances, such as clear, milky white, yellow tinged, or brown to dark green. Clear or light-colored fluid is usually easily identified as not worrisome, particularly if it is bilateral, but it may prompt a work-up for an underlying hormonal disorder or reaction to medications. Frankly bloody discharge is clearly worrisome; however, not all bloody discharge is red or necessarily obvious. Hemoglobin that has degraded can appear green or brown rather than red, and very dark fluid may or may not have blood in it. The best manner to evaluate the fluid is to test directly for occult blood. Simply express fluid with manual pressure at the nipple or the adjacent breast and apply it to the cards usually used to detect occult blood in stool samples. An applied developer changes color if there is blood present. Those women with blood present should have further work-up (biopsy).

Should I do a smear for cytology on the fluid?

Usually the amount of fluid that is able to be expressed is relatively small and thus the specimen is likely to have dried out and degraded to a degree that will not allow useful information to be gained by this method. If you have a pathologist who will process the specimen immediately in the clinic, it may yield good histology. A woman with bloody discharge who has negative cytology still needs further diagnostic work-up to rule out a malignant cause, and a woman with suspicious cytology can still have benign (papilloma with atypia) or precancerous (DCIS) conditions rather than invasive cancer.

How are ductography and ductal lavage used in the evaluation of nipple discharge?

Ductography and ductal lavage are new diagnostic tools that are being evaluated for their usefulness in both screening populations of women for breast cancer and evaluating patients with nipple discharge. Ductography involves placing a tiny fiberoptic camera into the duct for visual inspection of the duct. As it is a new technology, its availability is limited, as is the number of breast surgeons who are trained in its use. There is an overlap in the appearance of benign and malignant causes of bloody discharge when evaluated by ductography alone, but the sensitivity and specificity of the test are improved with the addition of ductal lavage and cytologic examination of the lavage specimen. Some studies indicate that the use of fluorescent cell sorters can determine the ploidy (amount of DNA per cell) of the cells in the lavage and may help distinguish benign from malignant etiology. This should be tempered with the knowledge that many well-differentiated breast cancers are diploid when examined after complete excision, which may limit the usefulness of flow cytometry. Again, these are new technologies whose use has not been fully evaluated and are mainly available at tertiary breast centers in academic institutions; however, they are promising advances to limit the negative biopsy rate in patients with bloody nipple discharge.

How do I evaluate a patient who had discharge last month but now does not?

When a woman comes in stating that she had discharge for some period but that it has now resolved, you should attempt to express fluid manually. If you are able to do so, test the sample for occult blood. If you are not able to express fluid, you must rely on a meticulous history to decide the relative risk. If the character and color of the fluid are more consistent with a benign cause, you can reassure the patient. If the appearance is more worrisome, you may want to reexamine that patient at a different time in her cycle and try to express fluid again at the follow-up examination. In any case you should educate her on the features associated with malignant causes (discharges that are unilateral, spontaneous, or bloody) and tell her to return for reevaluation if anything changes. There is power in the statement "there is nothing to worry about" when it is said by a health care provider, and it may cause a patient to ignore worrisome changes that develop. If the patient does not seek care and there is a malignancy that becomes apparent in the future in that breast, it can adversely affect the prognosis and is a common source of lawsuits. Patients need to know when to come back for reevaluation, must have easy access to you, and in some sense must have "permission" to come back if anything changes. This should be accompanied by communication with the referring physician, again stating what changes in clinical status would warrant repeat evaluation.

What is the significance of abnormal-appearing skin of a nipple and a history of nipple discharge?

The presence of skin abnormalities associated with blood on the shirt, bra, or bedclothes should be taken seriously. New onset of retraction or inversion of the nipple can indicate the presence of a malignant breast process, even in the absence of nipple discharge. Irritation of the nipple can be a sign of Paget's disease of the breast, a rare form of ductal carcinoma involving the main ducts. It is associated with skin changes at the nipple where the ducts exit. The skin changes around the nipple are often subtle; thus, a meticulous examination of the nipple is essential. The patient usually notes irritation or itching of the nipple and may find dried blood on clothing from an erosion or ulceration of the skin. The diagnosis is made by biopsy of the irritated or ulcerated area, and the prognosis is much better in those women who have a diagnosis established before there is an associated palpable lesion. It is often mistaken for contact dermatitis or breast/skin infection. Any irritation of the nipple needs to have completely resolved before the patient is discharged from care.

Should all women with nipple discharge have a screening mammogram or ultrasound?

Any woman who is older than 40 years of age should have a mammogram to correlate with physical findings. Occasionally there are changes that will revise your index of suspicion for malignancy. The presence of suspicious findings on mammogram may cause you to do an excision that you otherwise may not have done. Ultrasound can be helpful, particularly in the evaluation of a subareolar mass associated with nipple discharge. You may find a simple cyst that is amenable to percutaneous drainage. The reality in breast care is that no diagnostic tool is perfect, particularly when used alone. A complete evaluation requires information from the history, examination, imaging studies, and cytology studies via fine-needle aspiration (FNA) when possible.

▶ TREATMENT

What type of biopsy is appropriate for bloody nipple discharge?

Most biopsies for bloody nipple discharge in the absence of a mass are termed *duct explorations*. The involved duct is identified in the operating room by manual expression. The duct is then cannulated, often with a lacrimal probe, to identify the direction that it takes away from the nipple. There are options for the incisions: either radially following the duct from where it exits the skin or circumareolar with identification of the duct using the probe. Either method is cosmetically acceptable, which is an important consideration, because most of these patients (particularly the younger patients) have a benign cause for the discharge. The involved duct can also be identified intraoperatively by placing a small needle or cannula into the orifice for injection of methylene blue. My preference is for use of the lacrimal probe, because it is less messy and gives a tactile method of identifying the duct.

What type of biopsy is appropriate for bloody nipple discharge in the presence of a mass?

When a mass is present, the biopsy should include the mass. In most women, the involved duct and the mass are near the areola and can be handled through the same circumareolar incision. Nipple discharge with an associated lump is much more likely to yield a diagnosis of carcinoma than is nipple discharge alone, even if bloody. Therefore, patients with a palpable lump should be explored with surgical biopsy rather than observed, even if an FNA of the lesion is negative. Potential sampling error limits the negative predictive value of FNA.

Are duct explorations warranted in all patients with profuse, single-duct discharge?

A large percentage of patients have benign pathology after duct exploration, even with profuse, single-duct bloody discharge. There is continued debate about proper management. Some authors advocate close observation and education for patients who are reliable and compliant. However, breast cancer in any form has a better prognosis if caught at its earliest (nonpalpable) stage. This is the reason that comprehensive breast care includes self-examination, annual mammography (combined with additional imaging techniques as appropriate), and annual physical examination by a physician. Extensive patient awareness of the risks is advocated. Less invasive means of identifying those patients who are more likely to have a malignancy are in development (ductography and ductal lavage). Many oncologists think that eventually biochemical markers will be able to precisely identify those patients that are at true risk for breast cancer. Currently, exploration of a duct with bloody discharge with meticulous attention to cosmesis and good functional result is the acceptable paradigm, because in many patients no malignancy will be identified.

What is the definitive treatment if a malignancy is identified?

If the biopsy does reveal a malignancy, the involvement of the nipple-areola complex makes it impossible to preserve the nipple. This makes breast conservation surgery less attractive, because most patients are unhappy with the cosmetic result if the nipple and central portion of the breast are missing. However, many of these patients are suitable candidates for reconstruction (immediate or delayed) with a skin-sparing mastectomy. In Paget's disease of the breast, about 5% of the patients without a mass have positive lymph nodes, and with a mass present that percentage goes up. As in all cases of breast malignancy, axillary sampling or sentinel node biopsy should accompany the breast resection. These patients should also have the initial staging laboratory studies and chest radiograph.

How does the treatment differ if a man presents with nipple discharge?

Nipple discharge in a man is typically associated with florid gynecomastia. Unilateral gynecomastia, though rare, cannot be differentiated from male breast cancer by palpation alone. FNA can usually identify the mass as gynecomastia, but occasionally there is atypia, which is of concern. Gynecomastia may regress if the underlying cause (e.g., medications, alcoholic liver disease, drug use) is treated. In some cases the mass or discharge is persistent and a subcutaneous mastectomy or liposuction can be done to return the contour to normal. Liposuction should not be considered in any patient who has a predominant mass or atypical cells of any type on FNA because it potentially compromises what may need to be a cancer operation.

K E Y   P O I N T S

▶ Nipple discharge is most commonly benign, more frightening than it is dangerous.

▶ Unilateral, profuse, spontaneous bloody discharge from an isolated duct with the presence of a palpable mass is the highest risk for malignancy. However, all bloody nipple discharge should warrant an exploration to rule out malignancy, unless ductography and ductal lavage are available at your institution.

▶ The surgical management of nipple discharge is evolving, and periodic review of the surgical, oncologic, and radiologic literature is essential to providing a continued excellent standard of care.

CASE 18–1. A 40-year-old woman is sent for
consultation concerning nipple discharge. She states that the discharge is occasionally reddish brown and she noted it since the beginning of the summer. She thinks that it is worse now that she is swimming daily for a master's swim program and has asked that her club decrease the chlorine in the pool. She thinks that her family physician has blown this out of proportion but knew that he would bug her until she agreed to see you.

    A. How would you assess the risk of malignancy in this patient?
    B. You decide that her situation warrants a surgical exploration. What if she initially refuses biopsy?
    C. Her pathology comes back as intraductal papilloma. What is the appropriate follow-up?

CASE 18–2. A 22-year-old college student presents
to your office with new onset of nipple discharge. She had
recently attended a health fair at her college where breast
self-exam was taught and noted the first time she did an exam
that she was able to express yellow fluid from both breasts.
She worried that she has cancer, because her neighbor had
breast cancer with associated discharge.

   A. What history would you want from her?
   B. What would be your first step in treatment? Does she need
      treatment?

19

Postoperative Bleeding

▶ ETIOLOGY

Hemorrhage is a primary concern for the surgeon in the postoperative period. Although bleeding may be self-limited or easily controlled by external pressure, some episodes of bleeding can lead to significant hemodynamic compromise or even death.

What are the categories of postoperative bleeding?

There are two basic types of postoperative hemorrhage: (1) generalized bleeding caused by loss of normal hemostatic defenses and (2) localized bleeding from the surgical site. Differentiation between these two categories of bleeding can be difficult but may lead to significant management differences. One should always keep in mind that both of these two categories of bleeding may be present in a hemorrhaging patient, and both may result in hemodynamic aberrations if the blood loss is great.

Generalized postoperative bleeding is the result of a coagulopathic state. This type of bleeding tends to present as diffuse bleeding from capillary beds that have been disrupted during the surgical procedure. The loss of normal hemostatic mechanisms may be due to a preexistent bleeding tendency. Numerous hematologic disorders can induce a profound coagulopathic state. These include acquired and hereditary disorders affecting the individual factors of the hemostatic cascade, as well as quantitative and qualitative disorders of platelet function. Other common causes of the coagulopathic state include hepatic insufficiency, renal failure, and over-the-counter or prescription medications. A coagulopathic state may also be acquired in the perisurgical period. Common causes include hypothermia, dilutional coagulopathy from excessive crystalloid resuscitation, and consumptive coagulopathy due to large operative blood losses. Additionally, patients undergoing cardiac and some vascular procedures will be anticoagulated with heparin as part of the normal operative course.

Localized postoperative hemorrhage usually occurs from an isolated source at the surgical site. This is generally due to loss of hemostatic control such as a loose tie, suture line disruption, or displaced surgical clip. This type of bleeding may be self-limited or controlled by external pressure, as in the case of superficial wound bleeding. In other instances, it may be necessary to return to the operating room for exploration of the surgical site and ligation of the bleeding vessel or tissue to gain control of hemorrhage.

Although less common, the stress of surgery can provoke localized bleeding from other sources. These include gastrointestinal bleeding from gastric and duodenal ulcers, arteriovenous malformations, gastric and esophageal varices, or inflammatory bowel disease. The astute clinician also inspects for iatrogenic sources of bleeding such as traumatic placement of endotracheal tubes, urinary drainage catheters, central venous lines, and nasogastric tubes.

Can postoperative bleeding be prevented?

Aside from good surgical technique, a thorough preoperative history and physical examination are of paramount importance in identifying medical comorbidities that can predispose the patient to postoperative bleeding. A carefully performed history should inquire about a family or patient history of bleeding disorders, easy bruisability, or excessive bleeding after superficial skin lacerations or dental procedures. One should also determine the patient's risk of liver disease with a focus on alcohol history, exposure to hepatotoxic chemicals, or risk of exposure to viral hepatitis through sexual contacts, previous blood product transfusions, maternal history of viral hepatitis, or intravenous (IV) drug use. The physician should also ask about known history of peptic ulcer disease or history of gastrointestinal or genitourinary bleeding, manifest by hematemesis, hematochezia, melena, hematuria, or menorrhagia. It is also important to inquire about the use of all medications that may increase bleeding risk; these include but are not limited to warfarin, enoxaparin, aspirin and other nonsteroidal anti-inflammatory drugs, adenosine diphosphate inhibitors, or glycoprotein IIb/IIIa inhibitors.

A thorough physical examination should include a careful assessment of the integument for signs of bleeding such as ecchymoses or petechiae. It is also important to inspect for signs of hepatic insufficiency, including spider telangiectases, icteric sclerae, jaundice, ascites, or abdominal varices. A rectal examination with stool occult blood testing is also part of every preoperative physical examination.

The surgeon should use the history and physical examination to guide further preoperative work-up. This can include laboratory studies such as a complete blood count (CBC), prothrombin time (PT), activated partial thromboplastin time (aPTT), bleeding time, fibrinogen level, or liver function tests. If one or more comorbid risk factors for bleeding are identified, adequate intervention must be taken before the patient is admitted to the operating room.

▶ EVALUATION

What are the signs and symptoms of postoperative bleeding?

Some episodes of bleeding can be easily diagnosed, especially when the source of hemorrhage can be visualized. When evaluating a patient for postoperative hemorrhage, the physician must pay careful attention to the physical findings present. In initial stages of bleeding, the volume of blood loss may be small and the patient asymptomatic. As bleeding progresses or with copious bleeding, patients often present with mental status changes such as confusion, lethargy, or obtundation. With hemodynamically significant bleeding, the patient will also develop tachycardia, tachypnea, low urine output, and hypotension. This presentation complex is consistent with a hypovolemic state inducing compensatory physiologic changes and resultant deficiencies in end-organ perfusion. Bear in mind that inadequate postoperative pain control can present as tachycardia, tachypnea, and agitation. Thus, it is important to treat pain adequately and observe parameters such as urine output and blood pressure when evaluating a patient for possible postoperative hemorrhage.

On examination, a patient who has lost a significant blood volume may feel cold and clammy. Capillary refill time will be excessive (i.e., >2 seconds) as compensatory peripheral vasoconstriction occurs in an attempt to divert blood centrally to preserve vital organ perfusion. Expeditiously but carefully perform a head-to-toe assessment of the patient for the source of bleeding. The surgical dressing must be removed and the wound area explored for bleeding or hematomas. If a nasogastric tube is in place, evaluate the effluent for blood indicative of an upper gastrointestinal bleeding source. If intraoperative drains were placed, evaluate the quantity and quality of the drainage for signs of active hemorrhage. The same evaluation should be performed for chest tubes and urinary catheters, if present. If no obvious source of bleeding is present, and a jugular or subclavian central line was placed, listen to the breath sounds and consider a chest radiograph to evaluate possible hemothorax.

What laboratory values are useful?

If bleeding is suspected, ensure that blood is typed, cross matched, and available in the event that transfusion becomes necessary. Laboratory analysis can be helpful in the evaluation. A CBC, PT, aPTT, and disseminated intravascular coagulopathy (DIC) panel should be sent. These laboratory studies allow evaluation of the patient's hematocrit (recognizing that it may not be low initially after an acute bleed), platelet count, and integrity of the intrinsic and extrinsic coagulation cascade.

▶ TREATMENT

How do I manage postoperative bleeding?

While the diagnostic work-up is underway, prompt resuscitation of the patient is of absolute importance. Ensure adequate control of the patient's airway, breathing, and circulation before attending to other areas of concern. Volume resuscitation with crystalloid fluids should be started while the laboratory evaluation is being completed. The patient should have at least two large-bore peripheral IV catheters (≥18 gauge). Adequate fluid resuscitation should ensure return of normal hemodynamics and urine output (>0.5 mL/kg/hr).

Obvious sources of active hemorrhage should be controlled with manual pressure when possible. Hypothermia should be aggressively treated with warming blankets and use of IV infusion warmers. The operative team should be mobilized in preparation for emergent return to the operating room. If the patient is stable, it may be appropriate to await laboratory studies while continuing resuscitative steps. If the patient is unstable, rapid resuscitation and immediate return to the controlled setting of the operating room are essential. Resuscitation may require the use of non–cross-matched blood, if typed and cross matched blood is not yet available.

How do laboratory studies assist in the management of postoperative bleeding?

Laboratory values can be helpful in guiding therapy. The surgeon must assess each laboratory value in the context of the individual patient's postoperative course. A mildly low red blood cell volume in a stable patient can be followed with serial hematocrit determinations to ensure stabilization. A falling hematocrit can indicate the presence of bleeding but may also be secondary to dilution of red blood cells by large quantities of crystalloid fluids. Remember that a patient with an acute bleeding episode, regardless of the amount of blood loss, can exhibit a normal or stable hematocrit if not enough time has passed for fluid equilibration to have occurred. In the event of significant anemia, rapid transfusion of packed red blood cells (PRBCs) must be instituted. For large-volume PRBC resuscitation, a rapid warming infuser should be used to prevent hypothermia with its associated coagulopathic state. Serum calcium levels must be monitored when administering large-volume PRBC transfusions. Citrate, a blood preservative present in PRBCs, binds serum calcium, a necessary electrolyte factor for hemostasis.

A low platelet count can be present secondary to heavy bleeding, DIC, or drug reaction. Although a platelet count of greater than 50,000/μL is usually adequate in a surgical patient, it is prudent to replace platelets to above this value when a patient is hemorrhaging. In patients with qualitative platelet dysfunction, such as in the setting of renal failure, platelet transfusion should be instituted in the actively bleeding patient, despite the absence of thrombocytopenia. Other beneficial therapies in this setting include desmopressin or aminocaproic acid to help correct qualitative platelet dysfunction.

An elevated PT and aPTT indicate a deficiency in the coagulation cascade in a bleeding patient, and a significant elevation in either of these values should be corrected immediately. Fresh frozen plasma (FFP) is a sufficient temporizing intervention in most patients. In stable patients who are suspected of bleeding secondary to a coagulopathic state, administration of FFP may be the only intervention needed. These patients need serial laboratory studies and may need frequent transfusions with FFP throughout their course. This is especially true in patients with liver dysfunction. Vitamin K supplementation may be useful in long-term correction of factor deficiencies. Recall that patients who have received intraoperative heparin initially have elevated aPTT values and may require reversal of anticoagulation with protamine in the face of active bleeding.

Serum fibrinogen concentration is a useful study in hemorrhaging patients. Low levels may be present due to DIC or consumption of clotting factors secondary to heavy bleeding. When hypofibrinogenemia is identified, it should be rapidly corrected to normal levels with cryoprecipitate, because its conversion to fibrin is a crucial step in hemostasis.

K E Y   P O I N T S

▶ Postoperative bleeding may be caused by generalized abnormalities in clotting mechanisms, inadequate surgical hemostasis, or both.

▶ Once postoperative bleeding has been diagnosed, rapid resuscitation, correction of coagulopathy, and operative exploration are the mainstays of treatment in the unstable patient.

▶ Although operative exploration may be avoidable in stable patients, this decision must be made judiciously. When it is determined that a return to the operating room is necessary, this must be done without delay, because the patient's life depends on it.

▶ Bleeding patients can deteriorate rapidly. Through the vigilance, foresight, and expertise of the surgeon responsible for their care, certain disaster can be averted in these patients.

CASE 19–1. You are called to evaluate a 33-year-old woman who underwent a right modified radical mastectomy earlier that day for breast cancer. The nurse reports the patient has lost 650 mL of bloody fluid from her subcutaneous drain over the past 3 hours. On evaluation you find a young women in no apparent distress. She is alert, complaining of mild incisional pain, and is concerned about the blood loss. Her vital signs reveal a heart rate of 84 beats/min, blood pressure of 124/62 mm Hg, respiratory rate of 16 breaths/min, and oxygen saturation of 97% on room air. The subcutaneous drain is connected to bulb suction and the bulb is full of bloody fluid.

A. What should you do to further evaluate this patient?
B. How should you manage this patient?

20

Postoperative Fever

Postoperative fever, the most common finding in surgical patients, is responsible for the bulk of nursing calls to physicians at night. It is estimated that as many as 40% of patients have temperature elevations after major surgery. In most cases the fever resolves and is not problematic. Fever is usually broken down into two categories: (1) low-grade temperatures less than 101.5°F and (2) high-grade temperatures greater than 101.5°F. Fever may be secondary to an infection or surgical complication and therefore patients need to be clinically assessed. Clinical assessment should include checking patient vital signs, pulmonary exam, abdominal exam, inspection of the operative site, and overall assessment of how ill a patient appears.

▶ ETIOLOGY

It is important to understand the potential causes of postoperative fever so that a differential diagnosis can be constructed. The common causes of postoperative fever are represented in Table 20–1. The timing of the fever in relation to the operation is important. The longer the time from operation when patients present with a fever, the more likely it is from an infectious cause.

What causes fever presenting in the first 48 hours postoperatively?

The first 48 hours is the most common time a noninfectious fever presents. The primary cause of these fevers is atelectasis. Frequently, after major operations there are small to large areas of the lung that do not fully re-expand. This inexpansion is caused by a variety of factors, including effects of general anesthesia, diminished lung function secondary to abdominal incisions, pain interfering with deep breathing, supine positioning, and poor mobilization of pulmonary secretions. Streptococcal wound infection is an unusual cause of fever in the immediate postoperative period that must be excluded.

What causes fever presenting postoperative days 3 to 5?

In this period, atelectasis is a less likely reason for the fever. Increasingly, infectious causes of fever must be investigated. The

TABLE 20-1	
Etiology of Postoperative Fever	
Infectious	**Noninfectious**
Pneumonia	Atelectasis
Urinary tract infection	Deep venous thrombosis
Wound infection	Drug fever
Clostridium difficile colitis	Pulmonary embolism
IV line or site infection	Hematoma
Abscess	Transfusion reaction
Peritonitis	Alcohol withdrawal
Bacteremia	Adrenal insufficiency

common causes of fever at this time are pneumonia, urinary tract infections, and intravenous (IV) site infections. Early wound infections may also be present. Prognostic signs associated with a high likelihood of infectious causes are temperatures greater than 101.5°F, elevated white blood cell count (>10,000/μL), and significant comorbid medical conditions.

What causes fever presenting on day 5 or later?

All fevers in this period should be assumed to be secondary to an infection until proven otherwise. This is the period when complications from surgery such as anastomotic leak, abscess formation, and wound infections present. Infections related to catheters or other foreign bodies are also a significant cause of this type of fever. Assessment of the patient must include an understanding of what operation has been performed to anticipate possible related complications.

▶ EVALUATION

All patients should be examined when a postoperative fever is discovered. Pulse and blood pressure need to be assessed to identify patients who are becoming hypotensive and critically ill (evidence of sepsis). A focused physical exam including auscultation of breath sounds, inspection of all IV sites (both central and peripheral), inspection of the incision and surrounding operative area, and an abdominal exam should be performed.

How do I evaluate a patient presenting with fever in the first 48-hour postoperative period?

Evaluation beyond a physical exam is rarely indicated in this group of patients. Specifically, it is not recommended to routinely obtain blood cultures, complete blood count (CBC), urine culture, sputum cultures, or chest radiograph. The yield of this work-up is minimal without some clinical suspicion of a more serious problem besides atelectasis. Physical exam of the wound and IV sites is sufficient to rule them out as a source of infection at this time, unless the patient complains of a specific symptom, such as dysuria or cough.

How do I evaluate a patient presenting with fever on postoperative days 3 to 5?

A focused physical exam should be performed to rule out common etiologies. Careful attention should be paid to the pulmonary exam because pneumonia is common in this group. It is appropriate at this time to consider obtaining a chest radiograph, CBC, urinalysis, urine culture, and possibly blood cultures. Patients who have central IV catheters in place must be considered for line removal and culture of the line tip. It is vital to inspect and palpate surgical wounds to rule out infection.

How do I evaluate a patient presenting with fever on day 5 or later?

Late fevers should be carefully worked up because these often represent a complication or serious problem. A physical exam needs to be performed to evaluate vital signs, lungs, heart, abdomen, surgical site, and catheter sites. Knowledge of the operation performed is vital to this evaluation. Patients who have had intestinal surgery may have disruptions of nascent anastomoses. Further, if the surgical site involved a body cavity (abdomen, pelvis, thorax), a deep abscess may form in that cavity following the operation. Directed lab and radiographic evaluation is indicated. If there is no obvious pulmonary, urinary, or IV catheter site infection, it is reasonable to consider a computed tomographic (CT) scan to look for sources of intra-abdominal infection. Evaluation of the wound is also critical because this is a common time for postoperative wound infections to present. It is also important to note whether the patient has been having diarrhea, which would suggest either an intra-abdominal abscess or *Clostridium difficile* colitis. Deep venous thrombosis is another cause of fever that can be overlooked, and if there is clinical suspicion, venous duplex ultrasonography should be performed.

▶ **TREATMENT**

How are postoperative fevers treated?

Treatment of postoperative fever depends on the etiology.

Atelectasis. The primary treatment of this disorder is patient mobilization, deep breathing, coughing, and use of the incentive spirometer. It is vital to make sure the patient has adequate analgesia to encourage good pulmonary toilet. If there is a concentrated area of atelectasis by physical exam, chest physical therapy may be helpful. No medical intervention is necessary.

Wound Infection. Infected wounds need to be opened to eliminate any undrained fluid collections and to allow access for local wound care. Simple wound infections may be treated with local wound care alone; antibiotics may be added if there is evidence of cellulitis. Routine wound cultures are not usually necessary, unless there is extensive cellulitis. A wound culture in this case may be helpful in directing antibiotic coverage for the cellulitis.

Urinary Tract Infection. The first indication of a urinary tract infection may be symptoms of painful urination. Urinalysis may demonstrate white blood cells, nitrates, or leukocyte esterase. A urine culture should be obtained if there is a positive urinalysis. Antibiotic therapy may be initiated immediately without waiting for the culture results. Culture results are useful for directing specific antibiotic therapy if necessary.

Pneumonia. The clinical presentation of pneumonia is fever, productive cough, and an infiltrate on chest radiograph. Sputum culture and Gram stain are important to guide treatment. Empiric antibiotic should be started to target nosocomial organisms, especially gram-negative ones. See also Chapter 27 for a full discussion of pneumonia.

Intra-abdominal Abscess. Treatment for intra-abdominal abscess is individualized based on the clinical condition of the patient and on the CT scan findings. Most often, if there is a solitary abscess that is amenable to percutaneous catheter drainage, this technique should be performed. Gram stain of the aspirate and broad-spectrum antibiotics against gram-negative and anaerobic organisms are usually started.

IV Catheter Infections. The line should be discontinued and the tip sent for culture. If there is evidence of cellulitis around the site or the patient is very ill, empiric antibiotics should be started. Therapy is usually targeted at gram-positive organisms. Some centers treat infected catheter tips with removal alone, reserving antibiotic therapy for patients with positive blood cultures or other evidence of systemic infection.

K E Y P O I N T S

▶ Postoperative fever in the first 48 hours after surgery is common and most often secondary to atelectasis.

▶ Fevers on postoperative days 3 to 5 are commonly caused by urinary tract infection, pneumonia, line infection, and wound infections.

▶ For fevers on postoperative day 5 and beyond, patients need to be carefully evaluated to rule out an intra-abdominal abscess, deep wound infection, or other surgical complication as the cause of the fever.

CASE 20–1. A 19-year-old man had an appendectomy for perforated appendix earlier in the day. He now has a temperature of 102.5°F.

A. What is your differential diagnosis?
B. What should you do?

21

Shock

▶ ETIOLOGY

What is shock?

Shock is an abnormal physiologic state in which there is inadequate oxygen available to the cells. Lack of oxygen leads to lack of energy, loss of cellular integrity, organ failure, and ultimately death.

What is the relationship between oxygen delivery and shock?

Figure 21–1 is a diagram of the applied physiology of oxygen delivery that is relevant to shock. Let's work backward from right to left through this diagram to understand the pathophysiology of shock.

Shock occurs when there is oxygen debt. Oxygen debt is the difference between oxygen demand (which is the amount of oxygen the cells need to maintain normal function) and oxygen consumption (which is the amount of oxygen the cells are actually using).

Surgery patients often have conditions that increase oxygen demand, such as fever (an increase of 10% per degree Celsius), injury (especially burns), and excessive work of breathing. Surgery patients often need to achieve higher than normal levels of oxygen consumption to match demand and avoid shock.

Oxygen consumption depends on two factors: oxygen delivery and oxygen extraction. Let us start with oxygen delivery. Oxygen delivery is the product of cardiac output (CO) and oxygen content (Cao_2). (The formula is $CO \times Cao_2 \times 10$; the factor of 10 makes the units mL O_2 per minute). Oxygen delivery thus has a cardiac component (CO) and a pulmonary/blood component (Cao_2).

The cardiac component is emphasized in traditional discussions of shock, which focus on perfusion. Let's continue to work backward, tracing the factors that determine cardiac output. Cardiac output is the product of heart rate and stroke volume. Abnormalities in either heart rate or stroke volume (or both, as in severe tachycardia) can produce shock. Stroke volume is the difference between left ventricular end-diastolic volume (preload) and end-systolic volume.

Left ventricular end-diastolic volume is determined by left ventricular filling pressure and by left ventricular compliance. Hypovolemic shock, with decreased filling pressure from decreased intravascular volume, is the most common cause of shock in surgical patients. Decreased left ventricular compliance occurs in ischemic cardiac disease, where the poorly perfused myocardium becomes stiff and requires higher pressures to distend.

Left ventricular end-systolic volume is determined by contractility and afterload. Abnormalities in contractility and afterload occur primarily in cardiogenic shock.

Perfusion, however, is only part of the oxygen delivery story. The pulmonary and blood component of oxygen delivery, Cao_2, is also a key component of oxygen delivery. Cao_2 is the product of arterial oxygen saturation and hemoglobin (Hgb) concentration, with a small component of dissolved oxygen dependent on Pao_2. The formula is

$$(Hgb \times Sao_2 \times 1.34) + (0.003 \times Pao_2)$$

Going deeper, Sao_2 depends on Pao_2, as given by the oxygen-Hgb dissociation curve. Proceeding even further, the Pao_2 is determined by the Pao_2, with shunting and $\dot{V}/\dot{Q}$ abnormality determining the $Pao_2 - Pao_2$ gradient. Finally, Fio_2 is a major factor determining Pao_2, as described by the alveolar gas equation. To summarize, low Hgb, shunting, and $\dot{V}/\dot{Q}$ abnormality all reduce Cao_2, decrease oxygen delivery, and contribute to shock.

Oxygen delivery quantifies how much oxygen is presented to the tissues, but tissues must first extract oxygen for it to be available to the cells. The ability of the tissues to remove oxygen from capillary blood—which Figure 21–1 denotes as the *maximum (Max) extraction*—is primarily determined by vasoregulation, which governs the matching of perfusion with metabolic need. In general, extraction increases in shock states (usually up to a maximal extraction value of about 50%) to compensate for either increased oxygen demand or reduced oxygen delivery. Severe systemic inflammation, however, impairs vasoregulation, reduces the value of maximum extraction, and thereby contributes to shock. This is often the case in the systemic inflammation found with severe infection.

What are the important shock syndromes in surgery?

Four important shock syndromes are hypovolemic shock, cardiogenic shock, obstructive shock, and septic shock. These syndromes result from one or more abnormalities in the oxygen transport mechanism shown in Figure 21–1.

What is the pathophysiology of hypovolemic shock?

Hypovolemic shock starts with a decrease in intravascular volume. This is associated with decreased preload and thus decreased stroke volume. Although heart rate may increase to compensate, cardiac output decreases. Oxygen delivery, which is the product of

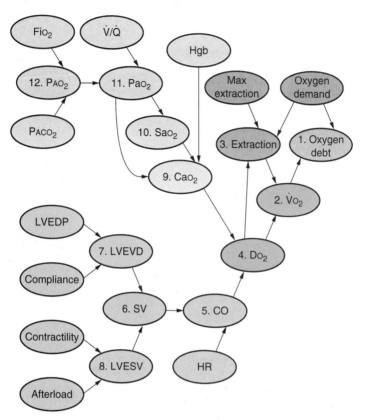

Figure 21–1. Oxygen delivery and the pathophysiology of shock. This is a diagram of the relationships underlying oxygen delivery. Each oval denotes a physiologic variable. Each of these variables depends on other variables, which are found by tracing back the arrows that lead into the oval. For example, oxygen debt is determined by oxygen demand and $\dot{V}o_2$ (oxygen consumption). The diagram shows the qualitative relationships between the key variables. Note that the variables available for manipulation by the clinician are at the periphery of the diagram, with no arrows leading into them, such as LVEDP, Fio_2, and Hgb. The different shades denote different organ systems or separate portions of the shock cascade. Intervention may be made at several different points in the cascade.

The following is a key to the abbreviations, with units, of the terms used in the figure and in the mathematical expressions used in the numbered list on the opposite page.

$\dot{V}o_2$, oxygen consumption, mL/min
Do_2, oxygen delivery, mL/min
CO, cardiac output, L/min
Cao_2, oxygen content of arterial blood, mL/100 mL
HR, heart rate, beats/min
SV, stroke volume, mL
LVEDV, left ventricular end-diastolic volume, mL
LVESV, left ventricular end-systolic volume, mL

Hgb, hemoglobin g/100 mL
SaO_2, saturation of oxygen in arterial blood
P_{50}, value where Hgb is 50% saturated
2,3 DPG, 2,3 diphosphoglycerate, mmol/100 mL
PaO_2, partial pressure of arterial oxygen, mm Hg
PAO_2, partial pressure of alveolar oxygen, mm Hg
$\dot{V}/\dot{Q}$, $\dot{V}/\dot{Q}$ abnormality
FiO_2, fractional inspired oxygen
$PACO_2$, partial pressure of alveolar carbon dioxide, mm Hg
RQ, respiratory quotient
PB, barometric pressure, mm Hg
PH_2O, partial pressure of water, mm Hg

For those who want to dig deeper into the quantitative relationships, the following—where well defined—are the mathematical expressions underlying the relationships. The list numbers correspond to the numbered items in the figure.

1. Oxygen debt = Oxygen demand − $\dot{V}O_2$
   Note: Oxygen debt represents the *accumulation* of this difference over time.
2. $\dot{V}O_2$ = Extraction × DO_2
3. Extraction = *Minimum* [maximum extraction, oxygen demand/DO_2]
   Note: *Minimum* is a function that takes the lesser of the two values. In this case the Extraction is either the Maximum Extraction or the Oxygen Demand/DO_2, whichever is *less*.
4. DO_2 = CO × CaO_2 × 10
5. CO = HR × SV
6. SV = LVEDV − LVESV
7. LVEDV = f(LVEDP, Compliance)
   Note: LVEDV is a complex function of LVEDP and compliance. In general, as LVEDP and compliance increase, LVEDV increases.
8. LVESV = f(Contractility, Afterload)
   Note: LVESV is a complex function of contractility and afterload. In general, as contractility increases and afterload decreases, LVESV decreases. (Remember, a *decreased* LVESV gives an *increased* SV.)
9. CaO_2 = (SaO_2 × Hgb × 1.34) + (PaO_2 × 0.003)
10. SaO_2 = f(PaO_2, P_{50})
    Note: This function is the familiar, sigmoid-shaped oxygen-Hgb dissociation curve. P_{50} is another complex function of temperature, 2,3 DPG, $PaCO_2$, and pH.
11. PaO_2 = f($\dot{V}/\dot{Q}$, PAO_2)
    Note: PaO_2 is a complex function of $\dot{V}/\dot{Q}$ abnormality and PAO_2. In general, as $\dot{V}/\dot{Q}$ decreases and PAO_2 increases, PaO_2 increases.
12. PAO_2 = (FiO_2 × [PB − PH_2O]) − ($PACO_2$/RQ)
    Note: this is the approximate version of the alveolar gas equation, where PB − PH_2O typically is 713, and RQ typically ranges from 0.7 to 1.0.

cardiac output and arterial oxygen content, thus falls. As delivery falls, extraction increases and initially oxygen consumption is maintained. Ultimately maximal extraction is reached, and decreases in delivery bring decreased oxygen consumption. Oxygen consumption falls below oxygen demand and the patient is in shock.

Important clinical situations for hypovolemic shock in surgery patients include bleeding; fluid losses from the gastrointestinal tract; and inflammation-associated fluid losses into the interstitium, both local (e.g., pancreatitis) and generalized (e.g., the systemic inflammatory response syndrome, or SIRS).

What is the pathophysiology of cardiogenic shock?

Cardiogenic shock starts with a decrease in myocardial contractility. Decreased contractility leads to increased end-systolic volume, decreased stroke volume, and decreased cardiac output. Oxygen delivery drops. Extraction increases to compensate, but when maximal extraction is reached, any further drop in delivery leads to a drop in oxygen consumption. When oxygen consumption falls below demand, the patient is in shock. A common setting for cardiogenic shock is myocardial infarction, with death and dysfunction in ischemic myocytes.

What is the pathophysiology of obstructive shock?

In obstructive shock, a blockage or pressure gradient prevents venous return from reaching the left heart. This leads to decreased left-sided preload and pathophysiologic consequences similar to those of hypovolemic shock. The difference is that in obstructive shock, right-sided filling pressures are high (not low, as in hypovolemic shock).

In tamponade, even though filling pressures may appear high, fluid in the pericardial sac reduces the diastolic transmural pressure gradient and thus decreases end-diastolic volumes. Decreased preload leads to decreased stroke volume and decreased cardiac output.

In tension pneumothorax, pleural air under pressure raises intrathoracic pressure and reduces venous return from the periphery. Twisting of the mediastinum may also produce further vascular obstruction. As in tamponade, transmural filling pressures fall, end-diastolic volumes decrease, stroke volume declines, and cardiac output is reduced.

In pulmonary embolism, clot in the pulmonary artery raises afterload on the right heart, which fails. Venous return is blocked in the right heart. Right-sided pressures are high, but left-sided pressures are low, with low left-sided preload and thus decreased cardiac output.

What is the pathophysiology of septic shock?

In septic shock there are multiple defects in oxygen delivery. Septic shock starts with infection triggering a network of inflammatory mediators. These mediators increase oxygen demand. At the same time they impair vasoregulation and extraction. Cardiac output increases. Increased oxygen delivery initially compensates for decreased extraction and thereby maintains oxygen consumption equal to demand.

As the infection progresses, however, the mediators act to reduce oxygen delivery. First, endothelial injury and capillary leak allow fluid to pass out of the vascular space faster than it returns via lymphatics. The patient becomes edematous, and filling pressures fall. With decreased preload, cardiac output falls. Second, mediators act as myocardial depressant factors, impairing cardiac contractility and reducing cardiac output further. Third, edematous lungs develop shunt and V̇/Q̇ abnormality that lead to a fall in Pao_2, decreased Sao_2, and decreased Cao_2. Ultimately the patient faces decreased oxygen delivery and oxygen consumption at the same time that oxygen demand is increased. The result is oxygen debt and shock.

▶ EVALUATION

What are the signs of shock?

Signs of shock on physical exam include cool and clammy skin, tachycardia, decreased peripheral pulses, hypotension, mental status changes, and oliguria. Laboratory signs of shock include metabolic acidosis and elevated serum lactate. Signs of shock from pulmonary arterial catheter measurements include low cardiac output, low oxygen consumption (calculated $\dot{V}o_2 = CO \times (Cao_2 - Cvo_2) \times 10$), and low oxygen delivery ($CO \times Cao_2 \times 10$).

▶ TREATMENT

What is the management of shock?

The management of shock in surgical patients proceeds through the ABCs of resuscitation, as follows:

- ■ Airway (A)
    - ☐ Ensure adequate airway, using jaw-thrust maneuvers, oral or nasal airways, and, if necessary, endotracheal intubation.

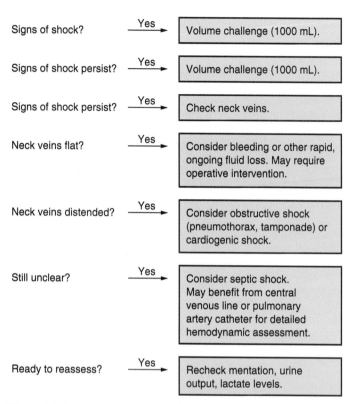

Figure 21–2. Management of circulation in the ABC approach to shock. As noted in the text, shock management follows the ABCs, where airway (A) and breathing (B) management precede the management of circulation (C), presented here. The signs of shock include hypotension, oliguria, and lactic acidosis.

- Breathing (B)
  - ☐ Ensure adequate breathing. This may require mechanical ventilation.
- Circulation (C) (Fig. 21–2)
  1. Rapidly infuse 1000 mL (20 mL/kg) crystalloid solution, such as normal saline. In many cases this is enough to correct the poor perfusion.
  2. If there are still signs of shock, repeat the 1000-mL infusion.
  3. If there is still no improvement, evaluate the neck veins. If the neck veins are distended, consider obstructive shock, such as pneumothorax, tamponade, or pulmonary embolism. If you are unable to evaluate the neck veins, consider placing a central venous catheter.

4. If there is no improvement and the neck veins are flat, consider hemorrhage. If there is history of trauma or recent operative procedure, start packed RBC cell transfusion and consider a procedure for definitive control of bleeding.
5. If there is no improvement after the 2000-mL infusion and the neck veins and central venous pressure measurements are not conclusive, consider placing a pulmonary artery catheter.
6. If the pulmonary artery measurements are consistent with hypovolemia, treat with volume, blood, and definitive control of fluid losses. A patient who is bleeding or who has peritonitis usually requires an operative procedure.
7. If pulmonary artery measurements are consistent with cardiogenic shock, treat with afterload reduction, inotropes (such as dopamine, epinephrine, or dobutamine), or a balloon pump. Echocardiography is useful to evaluate cardiac function. The patient may need definitive therapy for myocardial ischemia.
8. If pulmonary artery measurements are consistent with septic shock, treat with volume, inotropes, and vasopressors (such as vasopressin, norepinephrine, or phenylephrine [Neo-Synephrine]). Search for a source of infection, which may require definitive surgical management. Treat with empirical antibiotics until you identify the organism and sensitivities.

■ Reassess
1. Reassess the response to resuscitation repeatedly. Although blood pressure increases and heart rate decreases serve as useful indicators, the goal should be adequate delivery of oxygen to the tissues. A resuscitated patient will have restoration and maintenance of normal end-organ function as shown by improved mentation, resolution of oliguria (urine output at least 0.5 mL/kg/hr), and correction of lactic acidosis.

K E Y P O I N T S

▶ Shock is oxygen debt.

▶ Oxygen debt results from one or more defects in the oxygen transport mechanism shown in Figure 21–1.

▶ There are four key shock syndromes: hypovolemic, cardiogenic, obstructive, and septic.

▶ Management starts with attention to airway (A) and breathing (B) and proceeds to circulation (C).

continued

▶ The goal of shock treatment is restoration of adequate oxygen delivery and restoration of normal end-organ function.

▶ Most surgical patients with shock are hypovolemic and respond to volume administration.

▶ Treatment of shock requires attention to the underlying problem: stop the bleeding, drain the infection, and relieve the pneumothorax or tamponade.

CASE 21-1. A 25-year-old man crashes his motorcycle. He is brought to the emergency department with a blood pressure of 90/50 mm Hg.

    A. What shock syndrome does this patient most likely have? What is the pathophysiology?
    B. What other signs of shock would you likely find in this patient?
    C. What are your first priorities in managing this patient? The patient does not respond to an infusion of 2000 mL of normal saline. What do you do now?

CASE 21-2. A 56-year-old man is sent home from the emergency department after complaining of abdominal pain. He now returns 10 days later with high fever, severe diffuse abdominal pain, and peritonitis. His blood pressure is 80/50 mm Hg.

    A. What shock syndrome does this patient most likely have? What is the pathophysiology?
    B. What is your approach to managing this patient?

22

Shortness of Breath

▶ ETIOLOGY

Shortness of breath (SOB), or "dyspnea," is a common complaint in the hospitalized patient. This symptom becomes clinically important when it occurs at a level of exertion that is unacceptably low for the patient; given its subjective nature, this can vary dramatically among individuals. SOB can present acutely or paroxysmally, or it can be chronic and a marker for a wide range of conditions and diseases ranging from benign to life-threatening. A rapid and accurate assessment of a patient presenting with SOB is always warranted. The sensation of dyspnea can be caused by anatomic, physiologic, neurologic, mechanical, and psychological factors. If the onset is acute, it is important to establish an etiology quickly so potential life-saving treatment can be started.

What causes dyspnea?

The actual pathophysiologic mechanism that causes dyspnea is poorly understood. The control of respiration is a complex feedback loop involving the brain stem, chemoreceptors, stretch receptors in the lung, and mechanoreceptors in the musculature of the chest wall and diaphragm. Disease processes involving any of these areas can result in the sensation of dyspnea. However, there is no area of the cerebral cortex that, when stimulated, produces dyspnea; conversely, there is no cortical lesion that ablates dyspnea.

How do patients experience dyspnea?

Although some patients describe being uncomfortably aware of their breathing, others experience and describe these subjective sensations in a different way, such as "air can't get all the way down," "I cannot get enough air," or "I feel tightness in the chest."

What is the differential diagnosis for dyspnea?

The differential diagnosis of dyspnea is long and varied (Table 22–1).

TABLE 22–1

Differential Diagnosis for Dyspnea

Abdominal tumor or ascites	Myocardial infarction
Anaphylaxis	Neuromuscular disease
Anemia	Obesity
Arrhythmia	Parenchymal lung disease
Asthma, bronchitis, chronic obstructive pulmonary disease	Pericardial effusion, tamponade
Atelectasis	Pulmonary edema
Chest wall trauma, contusion	Pneumonia
Congestive heart failure	Psychological (anxiety)
Diabetic ketoacidosis ("Kussmaul breathing")	Pneumothorax
Electrolyte abnormalities	Pregnancy
Fever	Pulmonary embolism
Hypoxemia	Pulmonary hypertension
Intracardiac shunt	Rib fractures, splinting secondary to pain
Kyphoscoliosis	Sepsis
Metabolic acidosis	Spinal cord injury
Mucus plug	Upper airway obstruction, aspiration
	Valvular heart disease

▶ **EVALUATION**

What should the initial assessment of a patient with SOB include?

The patient should be quickly examined, starting with the ABCs (airway, breathing, circulation). The patient's airway should be checked for patency. Check the quality and rate of the respiratory effort. Supplemental oxygen by facemask should be applied, and a measure of oxygenation (via pulse oximetry or arterial blood gas) should be obtained. Finally, the rate and quality of the pulse should be checked, and a blood pressure measurement should be obtained. If the patient is in severe distress or becomes hemodynamically unstable, he or she should be transferred to the intensive care unit (ICU) for possible endotracheal intubation and close monitoring.

What is the secondary assessment of the patient with SOB?

Given the varied causes of dyspnea, a quick but thorough history and physical exam should be performed. The history should focus on the circumstances surrounding the onset of symptoms; the relationship to physical activity; the aggravating or precipitating factors; the ameliorating factors; and the presence of related conditions (e.g., smoking, occupational exposures). Vital signs should be reevaluated, followed by a focused physical examination. The patient's position should be noted. Perioral or nail bed cyanosis indicates hypoxia.

Pallor may indicate anemia; diaphoresis may represent fever or increased work of breathing or it can be a symptom of a myocardial infarction or pulmonary embolus. A new rash or hives may be secondary to anaphylaxis or other allergic reaction. Check the patient's mental status and evaluate the pupils for size and reactivity. Check the mouth for foreign bodies and the presence of emesis or blood in the oropharynx, and suction appropriately. Check the neck for jugular vein distention, tracheal deviation, and the presence of suprasternal retractions. Auscultate the heart for the presence of murmurs, rubs, or muffled heart sounds. Palpate the chest for signs of crepitus or rib fractures, and note any asymmetrical movement. Auscultate all lung fields for decreased breath sounds, crackles, or wheezing. Percuss the chest to evaluate signs of consolidation, fluid, or tympany. The abdomen should be palpated for signs of rigidity, and the femoral pulses should also be palpated. The extremities should be examined for clubbing or edema. The calves should be inspected for evidence of deep venous thrombosis.

What are the common physical findings of dyspnea and associated diseases?

Physical findings vary depending on the cause of the dyspnea. An outline of physical findings and associated conditions is presented in Table 22–2.

What diagnostic tests should be performed?

The patient should be continuously monitored while further tests are obtained. A chest radiograph should be ordered immediately to check for pneumothorax, pulmonary edema, focal consolidation (pneumonia), pleural effusion, skeletal abnormality, or cardiomegaly. A 12-lead electrocardiogram helps detect myocardial ischemia or infarction, arrhythmias, or the presence of new right heart strain—an $S_1Q_3T_3$ pattern would be indicative of pulmonary embolus. A complete blood count (to check for anemia) and a panel 7 with magnesium, calcium, and phosphate (to check for electrolyte abnormalities or worsening renal function) should be drawn. An arterial blood gas determination provides useful acid-base information and quantifies the degree of hypoxia and assesses the adequacy of ventilation. In asthmatic patients, bedside spirometry, including forced expiratory volume in 1 second (FEV_1) and forced vital capacity (FVC), can determine peak flows and give useful information (i.e., adequacy of treatment). If the patient is suspected of having a pulmonary embolus, then a $\dot{V}/\dot{Q}$ scan or chest computed tomography (CT) angiography should be obtained. An echocardiogram can provide useful information about contractile and valvular function of the heart. Finally, patients may need a fiberoptic evaluation of the airway to rule out mechanical obstruction.

TABLE 22-2

Physical Findings Associated with Clinical Conditions

Physical Findings	Associated Disease or Condition
Increased respiratory rate	Multiple causes
Diaphoresis	Myocardial infarction, fever, pulmonary embolus, stress
Substernal and costal retractions	Upper airway obstruction
Cyanosis	Hypoxia
Paradoxical abdominal breathing	Chest muscle weakness, airway obstruction
Wheeze	COPD, asthma, CHF
Crackles	Pulmonary edema, pneumonia
Shallow, rapid breathing	Muscle weakness, anxiety
Deep or shallow breathing	CNS insult, diabetic ketoacidosis
Pursed-lip breathing	COPD
Hives and rash	Allergic reaction, anaphylaxis
Stridor	Upper airway obstruction
Unilateral breath sounds	Pneumothorax, pleural effusion
Pink, frothy sputum	Pulmonary edema
Cough and purulent sputum	Pneumonia
Muffled heart sounds	Cardiac tamponade, CHF
Focal neurologic deficits	CNS insult
Obesity	Decreased respiratory reserve
Skin pallor	Anemia
Tracheal deviation, tympany on percussion of chest	Pneumothorax
Skin crepitus	Rib fracture
Clubbing of fingers and toes	Chronic hypoxemia
Cough	Pneumothorax, pneumonia
Jugular venous distention	CHF
Hepatojugular reflex, pedal edema	CHF

CHF, congestive heart failure; CNS, central nervous system; COPD, chronic obstructive pulmonary disease.

▶ **TREATMENT**

What are the common treatments for dyspnea?

The treatment is disease specific, but all patients should receive supplemental oxygen at concentrations to keep SaO_2 greater than 94% while further treatment is being implemented and diagnostic tests are being performed. Patients in impending respiratory failure should be intubated and transferred to the ICU for further work-up and therapy. Patients suspected of having a pulmonary embolus should be anticoagulated first while awaiting further tests. A significant pneumothorax should be treated by placement of a chest tube. Pleural effusions can be percutaneously drained. If a myocardial infarction is diagnosed, patients should receive aspirin and beta-blockers. If the patient is in pulmonary edema, treatment includes diuresis, reverse Trendelenburg positioning, nitrates, and morphine. Patients with pneumonia or sepsis should be started on broad-spectrum antibiotics. Glucose and electrolyte abnormalities should be normalized, and severe anemia should be corrected with blood transfusion. Any significant neurologic change warrants a head CT. Albuterol and ipratropium breathing treatments should be given to the wheezing patient. Anxiety can produce dyspnea, but it should be a diagnosis of exclusion entertained only after all other diseases have been ruled out. The patient's condition should be continuously monitored, and unless there is a prompt resolution of symptoms, patients should be transferred to a monitored bed for close observation.

Why should pulmonary function be optimized preoperatively?

Dyspnea and a low Pao_2 are the two most accurate preoperative predictors of adequacy of postoperative ventilation. Patients with poor pulmonary function preoperatively have improved outcome postoperatively when aggressively treated. Treatment includes bronchodilator drugs, antibiotics, chest physical therapy, and cessation of smoking.

What are the most common causes of dyspnea due to cardiac causes?

The most common causes of cardiogenic SOB are poor left ventricular compliance due to ischemia or hypertrophy and increased circulating blood volume (volume overload, restricted forward blood flow such as in mitral stenosis). The presence of congestive heart failure significantly increases perioperative risk, and optimization likely will improve patient outcome.

K E Y   P O I N T S

▶ Dyspnea can be caused by a wide variety of diseases and conditions.

▶ A careful but expeditious evaluation of any patient with dyspnea is always warranted.

▶ Life-threatening causes of dyspnea should be ruled out before less serious causes are entertained.

▶ Any patient with dyspnea requires supplemental oxygen and close monitoring until appropriate diagnosis and treatment are instituted and the patient's condition improves.

CASE 22–1. A 35-year-old man presents to the emergency department with acute dyspnea. His respiratory rate is 35 breaths/min, and he appears tired and in distress.

A. What are the primary objectives in the immediate treatment of this patient?

B. What is included in the initial management?

C. What would lead you to consider endotracheal intubation of this patient?

23

Urine Output Changes

Urine output is a vital measurement of organ perfusion and may be the first sign of major physiologic derangements. If a patient also has altered vital signs, immediate evaluation and treatment are crucial. But even with normal vital signs, urgent evaluation (within 30 to 60 minutes) and aggressive treatment may prevent the development of shock and renal failure.

Derangements in urine output can include decreased urine output (oliguria, anuria), increased urine output (polyuria), or blood in the urine (hematuria).

DECREASED URINE OUTPUT

▶ ETIOLOGY

What defines oliguria and anuria?

Adequate urine output for an adult is 0.5 to 1 mL/kg/hr. Oliguria in adults is defined as urinary output of less than 400 mL/day. Anuria in adults is defined as urinary output of less than 50 mL/day.

Adequate urine output for children 1 year old and older is 1 mL/kg/hr, and for children younger than 1 year it is 2 mL/kg/hr. Urine output less than 0.5 mL/kg/hr represents anuria.

What is the etiology of oliguria?

The etiology of oliguria is divided into three groups: prerenal causes (kidney perfusion), renal causes, and postrenal causes (obstruction) (Table 23–1).

Prerenal Causes. The most common cause of oliguria in the surgical patient is intravascular fluid deficit. This fluid deficit may result from the surgical illness (anorexia, vomiting, or diarrhea), the operation (intraoperative fluid and blood losses), or the postoperative recovery (third-space losses into the interstitial spaces, postoperative hemorrhage, insensible losses from wounds, or sepsis).

TABLE 23-1

Common Causes of Oliguria

Prerenal	Renal	Postrenal
Volume depletion	Glomerular nephritides	Ureteral obstruction (must
Third spacing	Acute glomerulonephritis	be bilateral)
Hemorrhage	Vasculitis	Retroperitoneal mass
Gastrointestinal losses	Malignant hypertensive nephropathy	Sloughed papillae
Renal losses	Renal thrombosis	Strictures/valves
Poor cardiac output	Tubular interstitial	Stones, clots
Congestive heart failure	Pyelonephritis	Bladder neck obstruction
Tamponade	Hypercalcemia	Prostatic hypertrophy
Myocardial infarction	Multiple myeloma	Tumor
Pulmonary embolus	Acute interstitial	Sphincter spasms
Shock/sepsis	nephritis	Strictures/valves
Hepatorenal syndrome	Acute tubular necrosis	Bladder rupture
	Postischemic injury	Blocked catheter
	Prolonged vasopressor use	
	Nephrotoxic agents	
	Antibiotics	
	Contrast dye	
	Anesthetics	
	Nonsteroidal anti-inflammatory	
	drugs	
	Chemotherapeutic agents	
	Vascular problems	
	Emboli	
	Renal vessel thrombosis	

From Adams G, Bresnick S: On Call Surgery, 2nd ed. Philadelphia, WB Saunders, 2001, p 404.

Renal Causes. Renal causes of oliguria are numerous. The specific cause may be suggested by changes in the urinary sediment. In the critically ill surgical patient, acute renal failure may be caused by a series of renal insults (such as hypotension, sepsis, nephrotoxic agents), and this cause is determined only after prerenal and postrenal causes have been aggressively treated and excluded.

Postrenal Causes. Urinary obstruction soon after operation is often due to urinary retention. This results from a combination of interference with the autonomic system from anesthesia and drugs and loss of bladder tone from overdistention. This cause can be prevented by insertion of a bladder catheter prior to long operative procedures. Benign prostatic hypertrophy is common in older men. Bladder stones and clots are less common causes. Obstruction is even less commonly due to bilateral ureteral obstruction, but this should be considered in patients with recent pelvic surgery and abdominal neoplasms.

▶ EVALUATION

What are the initial steps in the evaluation of low urine output?

Because there is definite urgency in resolving the problem, it's best to immediately and simultaneously proceed with evaluation and treatment.

Clinical assessment of volume status (prerenal causes) should include the history (of vomiting, diarrhea, recent surgery or trauma) and physical exam (for dry skin, flat neck veins, changes in mentation).

Renal failure (renal cause) may be suspected by a history of nephrotoxic medications or other renal insults such as shock. Examination in the patient with obstruction (postrenal causes) may reveal lower abdominal distention and/or a large prostate.

What laboratory studies are helpful in the evaluation of urine output changes?

Serum electrolyte, blood urea nitrogen (BUN), and creatinine determinations are useful tools to assess both the severity of dehydration and general kidney function. A urinalysis and urine electrolytes also give information that may diagnose a renal cause of oliguria. Polyuria may be due to hyperglycemia, so serum and urine glucose levels should be checked if uncontrolled diabetes is suspected.

▶ TREATMENT

What is the optimum approach to the treatment of the patient with oliguria?

The most common cause of diminished urine output is inadequate intravascular volume (prerenal cause), and it is reasonable to begin intravenous (IV) volume resuscitation while other causes are being excluded. A rapid bolus of normal saline (500 or 1000 mL bolus in adults, or 20 mL/kg in children) should be given while an evaluation is in progress. There is no detriment to this bolus, and it may be diagnostic as well as therapeutic if the initial bolus restores adequate urine volume. The role of diuretics in oliguria remains controversial. A number of studies have shown that diuretics confer no long-term benefit in the prevention or treatment of acute renal failure (ARF), and their use may certainly exacerbate hypovolemia. Studies have also shown that dopamine confers no benefit in the prevention of ARF.

Patients with postrenal causes (obstruction) are often the easiest to diagnose and treat, and this cause should be excluded first. This cause should be suspected when the urine output stops suddenly or fluctuates widely.

The treatment for bladder outlet obstruction is to insert a bladder catheter (Foley). If the postvoid residual volume is more than 400 mL, the catheter should be left in place to allow distended bladder muscles a chance to recover. In a patient who already has a catheter, it should be flushed with 20 to 30 mL of sterile saline to confirm patency and possibly dislodge obstructing debris. More than once, an extensive evaluation and treatment of oliguria have been started when the cause was only a plugged Foley catheter. Catheter irrigations should be done with extreme caution soon after bladder or kidney surgery. After the catheter is placed, watch for postobstructive diuresis and replace fluids and electrolytes as needed (begin by replacing urine with D-5 ½ normal saline). Antibiotics should be given prior to any manipulation of an infected urinary tract.

When oliguria is not corrected by initial fluid replacement or by relief of bladder outlet obstruction, further evaluation must be done. An accurate estimate of intravascular volume may require direct measurement of central venous or pulmonary artery pressure (see Chapter 32). Urine should be sent for routine and microscopic analysis. Serum and urine should be sent to the lab for electrolytes and osmolarity, preferably before or more than 12 hours after diuretics are administered, and fractional excretion of sodium (FE_{Na}) should be calculated (see Table 32–6 in Chapter 32). The results of these values may aid in determining cause (Table 23–2).

Antidiuretic hormone is increased in settings of stress, which include operations and trauma. Significant fluid retention is to be expected after major operations. The syndrome of inappropriate antidiuretic hormone is diagnosed (see Table 23–2) by the presence of high urine sodium with low serum sodium and osmolarity and is treated initially by maintaining normal intravascular volume.

Given the possibility of impending renal failure, all nephrotoxic medications (especially aminoglycosides and nonsteroidal anti-inflammatory drugs) should be stopped and doses of other drugs should be adjusted when renal failure develops. Intake of potassium, magnesium, and aluminum should be limited, and levels should be monitored.

INCREASED URINE OUTPUT

▶ ETIOLOGY

What defines polyuria?

Polyuria is defined as urinary output of more than 3000 mL/day.

What are the causes of polyuria?

Causes of high urine output may be grouped into water diuresis (urine osmolarity <250) or solute diuresis (urine osmolarity >250). Water diuresis may be appropriate (in response to polydipsia, excess hypotonic IV fluids, or resorption of edema) or inappropriate (diabetes insipidus). Solute diuresis may be appropriate (after saline loading or relief of urinary obstruction) or inappropriate (hyperglycemia).

> ► **EVALUATION**

How are the specific causes of polyuria diagnosed and treated?

Postoperative Resorption of Third-Space Fluids. The diagnosis of appropriate water diuresis and appropriate solute diuresis is determined by history and examination of fluid intake and output records. Postoperative resorption of third-space fluids (physiologic diuresis) causes increased urine output several days after surgery or trauma and is a reassuring sign of resolution of edema. This does not require treatment other than curtailing excess IV fluids. Rarely, patients with limited cardiac reserve develop symptoms from the hypervolemia (congestive heart failure or atrial fibrillation from atrial distention), and these patients can benefit from further diuresis with low-dose dopamine or furosemide. Postobstructive diuresis usually resolves spontaneously if normovolemia is maintained.

Diabetes Insipidus. Diabetes insipidus (DI) results from the loss of antidiuretic hormone/vasopressin secretion from the pituitary (neurogenic) or from decreased responsiveness to this hormone by the kidney (nephrogenic). Neurogenic DI may follow head trauma, cerebral edema, pituitary tumors, or neurosurgical procedures. DI is diagnosed by comparing urine and plasma electrolytes (see Table 23–2) that show relatively low urine sodium and specific gravity. Patients can sometimes become rapidly dehydrated with massive urine outputs. Treatment is with immediate volume restoration and vasopressin administration.

Uncontrolled Diabetes Mellitus. Uncontrolled diabetes mellitus is a common cause of polyuria. When the serum glucose is higher than 300 mg/dL, the kidney's ability to absorb glucose is overwhelmed and glucosuria results, with resultant polyuria. The hyperglycemia is controlled with insulin.

High-Output Renal Failure. High-output renal failure occurs in patients who have loss of renal concentrating ability and manifest rising serum BUN and creatinine. This is treated the same as other causes of renal failure, in addition to maintenance of normovolemia. Remember that azotemia (renal failure) may present with oliguria but also with normal or increased urine output.

TABLE 23–2

Laboratory Findings in Several Causes of Change in Urine Output

Cause	Blood			Urine			
	Na	**BUN**	**BUN/Cr**	**Output**	**SG**	**Na**	**Fe$_{Na}$**
Prerenal	—	Incr	>10:1	Decr	>1.020	<40	<1%
ATN	—	Incr	>10:1	—	<1.020	>40	2–3%
SIADH	Decr	Decr	>50:1	Decr	Incr	>100	Varies
DI	Incr	Incr	<5:1	Incr	Decr	<10	—

ATN, acute tubular necrosis; BUN, blood urea nitrogen; Cr, creatinine; Decr, decreased; DI, diabetes insipidus; FE$_{Na}$, fractional excretion of sodium; Incr, increased; Na, sodium; SG, serum glucose; SIADH, syndrome of inappropriate antidiuretic hormone.
From Adams G, Bresnick S: On Call Surgery, 2nd ed. Philadelphia, WB Saunders, 2001, p 407.

Excessive Diuretic Use. Excessive diuretic use is diagnosed by history and treated by lowering the dosage.

Salt-Wasting Nephritis. Salt-wasting nephritis demonstrates relatively high urine sodium. Nephritis is caused by a host of medications and often manifests with rash, fever, pyuria, and flank pain. Allergic nephritis caused by penicillin-related drugs, especially methicillin, often arises after 10 days of treatment and demonstrates eosinophils in the urine. Treatment is by removing the toxic agent; some clinicians recommend a short dose of corticosteroids.

Increased Output Following Obstruction. Following resolution of a significant postrenal obstruction, the kidneys respond by increasing output. This can lead to polyuria sufficient to cause hypovolemia. The treatment is rehydration.

HEMATURIA

▶ **ETIOLOGY**

What is hematuria?

Hematuria (blood in the urine) may be gross (seen visually) or determined by dipstick or microscopic analysis. Suspected hematuria should be confirmed by proper microscopic analysis and is defined >1 red blood cell per high-power field (RBC/hpf); after a trauma, defined as >3 RBC/hpf in men and >5 RBC/hpf in women.

What is the differential diagnosis of hematuria?

A presumptive diagnosis of the cause of hematuria may be made from the history and urine exam. Bleeding at initiation of the stream usually comes from the urethra. If the bleeding occurs at the end of the stream, the source is usually the prostate or bladder neck.

▶ EVALUATION

What tests are helpful in differentiating causes of hematuria?

A urinalysis is useful. With casts, dysmorphic RBCs, and protein-uria, consider glomerular disease. With pyuria, dysuria, bacteria, and white blood cell casts, consider urinary tract infection.

Hematuria that doesn't clear with initial treatment must be further evaluated, and renal and bladder tumors must be excluded. A urologist may suggest computed tomographic scan of the kidney and may perform endoscopic examination of the bladder and urethra.

Post-traumatic hematuria (>5 RBC/hpf) is managed differently than other causes (see Chapter 35). Pelvic fractures should raise concern about possible bladder and urethral injuries that are suggested by blood at the urethral meatus, a high-riding prostate on rectal exam, and any perineal hematoma. In these cases, a urethral catheter should not be placed until urethral injury is excluded by a normal retrograde urethrogram.

What entities can be confused with hematuria?

Using only the dipstick test for hematuria may give false-positive results from hemoglobinuria, myoglobinuria, and ascorbic acid administration.

A bright pink color in the drainage tubing is not hematuria and results from a chemical interaction of some antibiotics and the plastic tubing.

A brownish color may be a late sign of myoglobinuria. Begin aggressive IV fluids to ensure a brisk diuresis, look for and remove sources of myoglobin (e.g., with débridement, fasciotomy, or amputation as indicated), and confirm the diagnosis with a check of urine myoglobin and serum creatinine phosphokinase.

Medications such as phenazopyridine (Pyridium) or dietary agents such as beets can also cause discolored urine in the absence of hematuria.

▶ TREATMENT

What is the treatment of hematuria?

The established cause is treated definitively and the urine rechecked for resolution. Treatment may be as simple as a short course of antibiotics for cystitis or as complex as partial nephrectomy for renal tumor.

K E Y   P O I N T S

▶ Urine output is a vital measurement of organ perfusion.

▶ Alterations in urine output may be the first sign of major physiologic derangements.

▶ The onset of oliguria requires immediate simultaneous evaluation and treatment.

▶ The most frequent cause of oliguria in surgical patients is an intravascular fluid deficit.

CASE 23–1. A 29-year-old motorcyclist sustains rib fractures, a liver injury, and severe comminuted right tibia and fibular fractures. He's treated with laparotomy and closed reduction and casting of his leg. At 3 AM the next morning, you receive a call that his urine output has gone from 40 mL/hr to none the last hour. His vital signs are stable.

    A. What are the most likely causes?
    B. After telling the nurse you will see the patient at the 6:00 AM prerounds, what orders should you give prior to returning to sleep?
    C. What immediate actions should be taken?

CASE 23–2.
A 45-year-old man is 4 days following a fall from scaffolding and craniotomy for the resulting subdural hematoma. He remains comatose with normal vital signs. You note that his urine output has been gradually increasing for the past 4 hours from 100 mL/hr to 650 mL/ hr.

A. What is the most likely cause of the polyuria?
B. How is the diagnosis confirmed?
C. How is this disorder treated?

24

Wound Problems

The management of wounds has always been one of the cornerstones in the practice of surgery. Key developments in surgery have directly related to practices that led to a decrease in wound complications. Nevertheless, wound complications continue to constitute around 50% of complications related to surgical procedures.

DESCRIPTION OF WOUNDS

How are wounds described?

Closed. A wound is described as *closed* when the skin is approximated. An example is a surgical incision that is closed with sutures or staples. The wound heals by *primary intention*. Re-epithelialization takes place within 48 hours of injury, and healing is rapid and with minimal wound contracture.

The wound-healing process takes place through well-defined phases. Within minutes the wound is infiltrated with polymorphonuclear cells and the *inflammatory phase* begins. These cells are gradually replaced with macrophages that play an important role in phagocytosis, removal of injured tissue, and recruitment of fibroblasts. In clean wounds with minimal tissue loss, such as a surgical incision, the inflammatory phase takes a few days. The *cellular phase* starts around the third day postinjury when fibroblasts start appearing and new capillaries start forming. A new connective tissue matrix is deposited and the wound edges start to weld. This is followed by the *proliferative phase* when collagen deposition starts about the fourth or fifth day and increases steadily for about 3 weeks. *Scar remodeling* with turnover of collagen continues for months and years later.

Open. *Open* wounds where the skin has not been approximated heal by *secondary intention*. Those wounds are often infected or have tissue necrosis. The healing process involves the build-up of granulation tissue that is made of inflammatory cells, ground substance, fibroblasts, and capillaries. The wound heals by scar formation and wound contraction in a relatively slow process. An example of an open wound is an incision that is opened following development of a wound infection. Wounds are sometimes left open if there is a substantial risk of infection or tissue loss. An example of this would be a patient who was operated on for a perforated colon. The skin would be left open to prevent the chance of a wound infection, by allowing drainage of potentially infectious fluids and access to the wound for débridement.

Occasionally, if an open wound is clean for approximately 5 days after injury, the wound edges can be reapproximated at that time. This process is referred to as *delayed primary closure*.

How are postoperative wounds classified with respect to their infectious risk?

Experimental studies have shown that the risk of wound infection is related to the bacterial count/volume of tissue (risk increases when the bacterial count is $>10^5$/g of tissue). These studies correlate with the clinical observation that the risk of infection increases with the degree of bacterial contamination at the time of operation. Based on that, surgical wounds are classified into four groups, as follows:

1. *Clean wound:* The incision is created under sterile conditions. There is no preexisting infection, and there is no contact with the gastrointestinal (GI), genitourinary (GU), or respiratory tracts. Examples include inguinal hernia repair, knee replacement, and vascular bypass. The risk of wound infection in this group is approximately 1%.
2. *Clean-contaminated wound:* The wound is in contact with the GI, GU, or respiratory tract, but there is no significant spillage or underlying infection. Examples include gastrectomy, laryngectomy, and small bowel resection. The risk of wound infection is approximately 5%.
3. *Contaminated wound:* The wound is in contact with the GI, GU, or respiratory tract with significant spillage or underlying infection. Examples include acute, nonperforated appendicitis and colon resection with spillage. The risk of infection is approximately 15%.
4. *Dirty wound:* The wound is old (4 to 6 hours) or is in contact with gross infection such as fecal peritonitis and perforated viscus. The risk of wound infection is higher than 40%.

WOUND MANAGEMENT: GENERAL GUIDELINES

Regardless of the etiology, the approach to wound management is to facilitate the healing process and to ensure that the conditions for tissue repair are ideal. This includes stopping further tissue injury, controlling any infection, eliminating nonviable tissue, and optimizing blood flow to the affected area.

How are wound infections prevented?

The key to preventing a wound infection is avoiding contamination and minimizing tissue injury during the procedure. Normal skin is colonized with bacteria; therefore, skin prepping to minimize bacterial count is essential. The administration of antibiotics prior to skin incision reduces the risk of wound infection and is especially indicated in clean-contaminated and contaminated cases. In cases where the risk of infection is high, it is prudent to leave the wound open and consider delayed primary closure. Other factors increase the risk of infection and should be taken into account when making that decision. Those include—among others—advanced age, poor nutritional status, diabetes, long operative time, tissue hypoperfusion, radiation, and malignancy.

How are acute wounds handled?

Acute traumatic wounds can present as lacerations, abrasions, or crush injury. Attention should be focused initially on controlling the bleeding, cleansing the wound, clearing foreign objects, and débriding nonviable tissue. Most lacerations can be safely closed primarily once these measures are accomplished. The wound should not be closed if it is old (>6 hours) or contaminated or if there is extensive tissue injury. The wound should be left open to heal by secondary intention or delayed primary closure. Patients should be asked about the status of immunization to tetanus and vaccinated as indicated.

How are chronic wounds handled?

Chronic wounds, such as pressure sores, venous stasis ulcers, and nonhealing irradiated wounds, can pose a challenge. The underlying disease process should be addressed and local tissue perfusion should be optimized. For example, if a patient has a nonhealing foot ulcer and arterial occlusive disease, revascularization would be necessary for the ulcer to heal. Similarly, the general health and nutrition of the patient should be optimized. In some instances poorly healing or nonhealing wounds are treated with excision and coverage with well-vascularized myocutaneous flaps.

IMMEDIATE WOUND PROBLEMS

How are wound infections handled?

A wound infection typically manifests approximately 5 days postoperatively with erythema, induration, pain, and purulent discharge. If a wound infection is suspected, the wound should be opened and the purulence drained. A superficial wound infection involves the skin and subcutaneous tissue, whereas a deep infection may involve the fascia. The administration of intravenous antibiotics is often unnecessary, unless the patient develops systemic manifestations of an infection or cellulitis. The wound is then managed with wet-to-dry dressings changed two or three times daily to facilitate the secondary intention healing and to keep the wound clean.

How are seromas and hematomas treated?

These are fairly common complications of wounds and present with a collection of fluid or blood under the incision. Typical signs of infection are absent. Most fluid collection resorbs spontaneously. Aspiration is indicated if the fluid collection is causing symptoms or is not resolving spontaneously.

What is a wound dehiscence?

A wound dehiscence (typically described in abdominal incisions) indicates that the fascial closure has been disrupted and a defect in the fascial closure has developed, or it may indicate suboptimal surgical technique. It is usually associated with a deep wound infection. The diagnosis is made by visual inspection and by palpation (feeling the defect). Occasionally a dehiscence can develop without signs of a wound infection. The history of copious clear fluid discharge through the incision around the fifth postoperative day is a typical presentation. The treatment is surgical reclosure, with approximation of the fascial defect either primarily or with prosthetic mesh. Occasionally, if there is no associated evisceration or uncontrolled infection, wound dehiscence can be managed nonoperatively with local wound care and by allowing the wound to heal by secondary intention. An incisional hernia develops as a late sequela of dehiscence.

What is an evisceration?

Evisceration occurs when abdominal contents bulge through the fascial dehiscence. Patients with evisceration should be taken immediately to the operating room for abdominal wall closure.

How do necrotizing soft tissue infections differ from simple wound infections?

Necrotizing wound infection is a relatively uncommon complication, but it is ominous and should be recognized immediately. It is a rapidly invasive soft tissue infection that can involve all wound layers, including fascia and muscles. It manifests with pain, fever, rapidly progressive erythema, induration, and skin blisters. The patient usually develops fever and hemodynamic changes such as tachycardia and hypotension. The treatment is surgical débridement of all infected and necrotic tissue as soon as the diagnosis is made. The wound is typically reexamined within 24 to 48 hours and may require further débridement. Most necrotizing soft tissue infections are polymicrobial, but some are caused by single organisms such as beta-hemolytic streptococci or *Clostridium perfringens*. The administration of intravenous antibiotics is an important adjunct to surgical débridement (see Chapter 31).

LONG-TERM WOUND PROBLEMS

How are sinus tracts and fistulas handled?

A fistula (communication between a hollow viscus and the skin) can develop as a wound complication. Examples include enterocutaneous (intestine to skin), pancreaticocutaneous (pancreatic duct to skin), or gastrocutaneous (stomach to skin) fistulas. They commonly present after an abscess has been drained through the wound but the organ secretions, whether they are succus, stool, bile, or pancreatic fluid, continue to drain through the open wound.

A sinus tract is a persistent, nonhealing opening in the wound that connects to a deeper, nonhollow structure. A sinus tract usually connects to a focus of persistent infection such as suture granuloma, infected prosthesis, or osteomyelitis.

What are a hypertrophic scar and a keloid?

A hypertrophic scar is excessive scar deposition that is confined to the wound site. It may regress without intervention but otherwise can be successfully treated with excision and wound closure without tension, often using Z-plasty, flap repair, or skin grafting.

A keloid, on the other hand, is excessive scar formation that extends beyond the wound site. Keloids are more common in blacks than in whites and have a familial predilection. Keloid is a more difficult problem to treat, with very high recurrence following simple excision. The most common method of treating keloids consists of local injection of corticosteroids with excision of the excessive scar, leaving a thin rim of keloid, so as not to expose the underlying subcutaneous tissue.

What is an incisional hernia?

It is estimated that hernias develop in 2% to 10% of abdominal or flank incisions. The risk of incisional hernia formation increases with the development of a wound infection. Other risk factors include age, obesity, malnutrition, chronic obstructive pulmonary disease, and a history of abdominal aortic aneurysm. Incisional hernias can manifest at any time following the operation and present with a bulge through the incision that is usually reducible. Incisional hernias can develop complications, including incarceration, strangulation, and intestinal obstruction. The principles of surgical repair rest on the concept of approximating the fascia without tension. In most cases, the fascial defect is repaired with prosthetic mesh.

K E Y P O I N T S

▶ Wound complications represent 50% of all surgical complications.

▶ Wound complications include infection, seroma, and dehiscence.

▶ Wound infections are treated by opening the incision and packing the wound.

CASE 24–1. A 54-year-old man has a sigmoid cancer and a sigmoid resection is planned for the next day.

A. What steps should be undertaken to minimize the risk of a wound infection?

B. On the sixth postoperative day, purulent drainage is noted at the lowermost aspect of the wound with induration and erythema. What is your diagnosis, and what should be done?

C. At 3 months' follow-up, the wound is healed except for a small opening in the skin that exudes a small amount of pus. What is the likely cause?

CASE 24–2. A 25-year-old man sustains a 7-cm laceration on the dorsal aspect of his forearm from shattered glass. He presents to the emergency department 3 hours later.

A. How should the patient be treated, and how should the wound be handled?

B. If the patient had presented to the emergency department 12 hours following the injury, how would your treatment differ?

Patients Presenting with a Known Surgical Condition

25

Inguinal and Abdominal Wall Hernias

What is a hernia?

A hernia is a defect in the abdominal wall, congenital or acquired, resulting in a protrusion of abdominal contents through the defect. This may result in local discomfort, or the contents may become entrapped (incarcerated) or the blood supply compromised (strangulated), requiring emergency surgery.

What are the types of inguinal hernias?

Inguinal hernias are divided into direct, indirect, and femoral types. Indirect hernias are the most prevalent and represent a persistent processus vaginalis where the hernia sac travels through the internal ring.

Direct hernias are next most common and describe a defect in the floor of the inguinal canal. If large enough, the hernia sac may descend through the external ring. Direct hernias are thought of as wear-and-tear hernias.

Femoral hernias are the least common of inguinal hernias and represent a hernia sac descending below the inguinal ligament, medial to the femoral vein. These are uncommon hernias but are seen more frequently in females than males. Femoral hernias are suspected when a mass is found below the inguinal ligament on the medial aspect of the upper thigh.

What are the types of abdominal wall hernias?

Abdominal wall hernias may include umbilical, epigastric, or incisional types. These are illustrated in Figure 25–1. Umbilical hernias occur at the umbilicus and represent a weakness in the abdominal wall. In children, umbilical hernias are congenital and may spontaneously close by 2 years of age. In adults, umbilical hernias are considered acquired and develop secondary to increased intra-abdominal pressure, as seen in pregnancy or ascites.

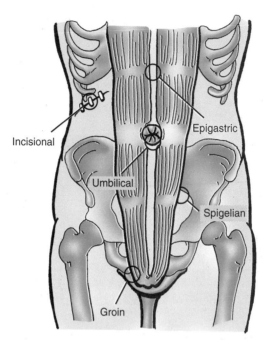

Figure 25–1. Sites of abdominal wall hernias.

Epigastric hernias are located between the umbilicus and xiphoid process in the midline. These hernia sacs protrude through the linea alba of the rectus muscle.

Incisional hernias occur in approximately 2% to 10% of abdominal sites. They result from a breakdown of the fascia secondary to inadequate healing, infection, or excessive strain of the tissue.

▶ EVALUATION

What signs and symptoms are associated with a hernia?

The patient may present with a symptomatic or asymptomatic groin or abdominal mass. Symptoms may include pain. If the hernia is incarcerated, it may present as a bowel obstruction with nausea, vomiting, and abdominal distention. It is important to determine the duration of the mass and if it spontaneously reduces. Incarceration may lead to strangulation if the mass is not reduced immediately. Reduction may be done at the bedside if tolerable to the patient or may require immediate surgical intervention. For most patients with spontaneously reducible hernias, the site may become progressively tender as the day goes on secondary to undue stress at the wall defect. Hernias also tend to get larger over time. Signs of strangulation with ischemia may include fever, tachycardia, and skin changes overlying the hernia sac. These skin changes may include erythema, warmth, or abdominal tenderness and represent a surgical emergency requiring reduction of the hernia and investigation of the contents.

What historical points are important?

Evaluation should also include a history to elicit any causes of increased intra-abdominal pressure. These include any history of urinary, gastrointestinal, or pulmonary obstructive symptoms. If any of these symptoms are present, it is prudent to rule out any underlying colonic, pulmonary, or urologic abnormality.

What is the physical exam for inguinal hernias?

A complete set of vital signs should be obtained, and particular attention should be paid to the presence of a fever and evidence of tachycardia. A complete physical exam should be completed in anticipation of surgical intervention. Attention should then be paid to the hernia site. The area should be visually inspected for the presence of a mass and any overlying skin changes. If the mass is in the inguinal region, it can be mistaken for many other entities, as seen in Table 25–1.

Abdominal examination should include visual inspection to look for abdominal distention or evidence of previous scars. The presence and quality of bowel sounds should be noted to identify a bowel obstruction. The abdominal wall is palpated with the fingers overlying the inguinal region while the patient is asked to cough or strain. This maneuver should reproduce the hernia. A finger can also be placed into the inguinal canal via the scrotum, and again the patient can strain or cough to reproduce the hernia.

TABLE 25–1

Differential Diagnosis for Groin Mass

Hernia
Lymphadenopathy
Lipoma
Hydrocele
Varicocele
Aneurysm or pseudoaneurysm
Sebaceous cyst
Hidradenitis
Epididymitis

What is the physical exam for abdominal wall hernias?

Hernias of the abdominal wall are found using the same technique as for inguinal hernias. If a hernia is not obvious, ask the patient to stand upright and try the same maneuvers. The exam is only complete once the contralateral side is examined to ensure there is not an additional contralateral hernia. Figure 25–1 represents the locations for frequently seen hernias.

What diagnostic tests are necessary?

Imaging studies are not necessary unless there is any question about the diagnosis. On physical exam most other entities can be excluded. Hydroceles can be transilluminated. Lymphadenopathy is not reducible. However, ultrasound and computed tomography can sometimes help when a difficult hernia cannot be found and the patient still has symptoms.

▶ TREATMENT

What are the indications for surgery?

Almost all hernias should be repaired unless surgical risk is prohibitive. Given the low risk of a hernia repair, even patients with multiple comorbidities should be strongly considered for operation because of the increased morbidity and mortality associated with an emergent repair.

What are the key points of inguinal anatomy?

Mastering the inguinal anatomy entails understanding a few general landmarks. First, it is important to distinguish between an inguinal and a femoral hernia. Femoral hernias are found below the inguinal ligament and on the medial aspect of the upper thigh. Inguinal hernias are found lateral to the pubic tubercle and medial to the anterior iliac spine. The preoperative distinction between indirect and direct hernias may be difficult and is of little clinical significance. This distinction is best determined once Hesselbach's triangle is clearly identified. The boundaries of the triangle consist of the rectus muscle medially, the inguinal ligament inferiorly, and the epigastric vessels superiorly. This is illustrated in Figure 25–2. Direct hernias are seen within this triangle, whereas indirect hernias are seen protruding through the internal ring.

Other important structures include the muscles, ligaments, cord structures, and nerves. The posterior wall of the inguinal canal is composed of the transversalis fascia and the aponeurosis of the transversus abdominis muscles. Direct hernias are a result of weakness in the posterior wall. The external oblique fibers reside super-

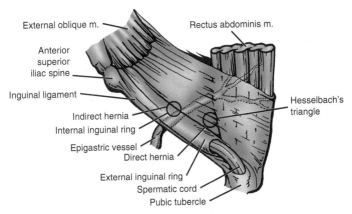

Figure 25–2. Inguinal anatomy.

ficially to the cord and the hernia sac. The internal oblique fibers join the transversalis muscle to form the superior aspect of the inguinal region. The ilioinguinal ligament makes the inferior edge of the inguinal region, which is important to identify when the repair is undertaken. The musculature and ligaments are seen in Figure 25–2.

The cord structures consist of the vas deferens (males), the round ligament (females), the testicular artery and vein (males), the lymphatics, and the autonomic nerves. Careful attention needs to be paid to avoid injury to any of these structures. The nerves of importance include the ilioinguinal, iliohypogastric, and genital branches of the genitofemoral nerve. The ilioinguinal nerve is encountered usually just below the external oblique fibers and adjacent to the cord. Division of any of these nerves may result in sensory deficits in the groin, the base of the penis, or the medial upper thigh or on the side of the scrotum or labia. The floor of the inguinal canal also encompasses the femoral vessels and nerve. This is important when trying to locate a femoral hernia.

How is an open inguinal hernia repair performed?

Open inguinal hernia repairs require dissection of the inguinal anatomy, identification of the type of hernia, and choice of hernia repair. Classically, hernias were repaired with suture and included types such as the eponymous McVay, Bassini, and Shouldice repairs. However, these are falling out of favor owing to the associated postoperative pain and incidence of hernia recurrence. Newer techniques use a prosthetic mesh to provide a tension-free repair that allows for less postoperative pain and faster recovery.

The Shouldice repair is used for both direct and indirect hernias. It uses a multilayer, imbricated repair with running sutures to close the inguinal floor. In this repair the inguinal floor is divided and then sutured to the internal oblique superiorly and to the inguinal ligament inferiorly. The conjoined tendon is then sutured to the inguinal ligament to complete the repair. The Bassini repair is also used for both indirect and direct defects. The repair uses multiple interrupted, nonabsorbable sutures to approximate the conjoined tendon to the shelving edge of the inguinal ligament. The McVay repair can be used for the repair of indirect, direct, and femoral hernias. This repair reapproximates the transversus abdominis to Cooper's ligament, which resides below the inguinal ligament. This closes the empty space medial to the femoral vein and lateral to the pubic tubercle.

What repair techniques use prosthetic mesh?

Open hernia repairs that use prosthetic mesh include the plug-and-patch repair and the Lichtenstein repair. The Lichtenstein technique uses a mesh sheet to create a tension-free repair. It may be used for both direct and indirect hernias. The groin dissection is carried out as described before, and the inguinal floor is reconstructed by securing the mesh to the inguinal ligament inferiorly and to the internal oblique superiorly. A slit is then made in the mesh at the level of the internal ring, and the cord structures are encircled with the mesh. The finished repair is demonstrated in Figure 25–3. It is important not to strangulate the cord structures by making the opening too narrow. The plug-and-patch repair is similar to the Lichtenstein repair, but it also involves the use of a mesh plug, which is placed into the inverted and reduced hernia sac. This repair is completed with laying mesh over the inguinal floor and securing it to the inguinal ligament and the internal oblique with interrupted, nonabsorbable suture.

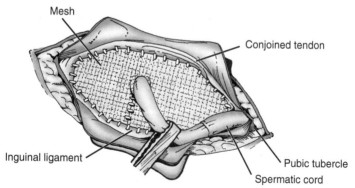

Figure 25–3. Tension-free mesh repair of an inguinal hernia.

How is a laparoscopic inguinal hernia repair performed?

The two most common types of laparoscopic repairs include the transabdominal preperitoneal (TAPP) hernia repair and the totally extraperitoneal (TEP) hernia repair. These repairs have been advocated when a patient has bilateral inguinal hernias or a recurrent inguinal hernia that has failed conventional open repair. Other advantages include less postoperative pain and faster recovery time. The disadvantages of these approaches include the need for general anesthetic, which may not be tolerated by the elderly population, and the risk of inadvertent injury to intra-abdominal structures with the TAPP repair.

Both laparoscopic repairs incorporate prosthetic mesh for the hernia repair. The TAPP repair includes the placement of three trocars in the abdominal cavity with insufflation and the creation of a preperitoneal space. The hernia sac is then reduced and the mesh secured to Cooper's ligament inferiorly and to the undersurface of the rectus superiorly and anteriorly.

The TEP repair incorporates the same repair but does not violate the abdominal cavity. A preperitoneal space is created with the use of a dissecting balloon that is placed posterior to the rectus muscle but anterior to the posterior fascia. The mesh is then secured in a similar fashion to the TAPP repair.

How do the different types of inguinal hernia repairs compare?

Overall comparisons have been made between the different types of open repairs and between the open and laparoscopic techniques. The overall recurrence rates with open hernias that do not use prosthetic mesh vary from series to series, the type of repair, and the surgeon doing the repair. The key element to recurrence appears to be the amount of tension placed on the repair. Therefore, one may conclude that repairs that cause the least amount of tension, such as the Lichtenstein and plug-and-patch techniques, offer the least chance of recurrence. Other complications common to hernia repairs are listed in Table 25–2.

Comparisons between open and laparoscopic techniques have been done in a prospective, randomized fashion and have not demonstrated any disadvantage to the laparoscopic technique except for the necessity of general anesthetic and the initial additional expense of the laparoscopic equipment. However, the initial short-term follow-up has demonstrated similar recurrence rates and the benefit of faster recovery, especially when recurrent or bilateral hernias are approached in the laparoscopic fashion. Complications from the laparoscopic techniques are somewhat different from those from the open procedure. The general anesthetic has its own potential side effects, as does the pneumoperitoneum. TAPP repairs may cause injury to the intra-abdominal contents because the

TABLE 25–2

Complications After Open Hernia Repair

Bleeding
Infection
Seroma formation
Nerve injury or entrapment
Urinary retention
Testicular pain, orchitis, epididymitis

repair requires entry into the abdominal cavity. However, the indications and benefits to open versus laparoscopic repairs remain areas of evaluation in surgical practice.

What types of abdominal wall hernia repairs are there?

The most common abdominal wall hernias include umbilical, epigastric, and incisional hernias. Some of the more uncommon abdominal wall hernias are listed and briefly described in Table 25–3.

Repair of any abdominal wall hernia requires its identification and then a closure of the fascial defect. Most small defects can undergo primary repair if there is no undue tension and the fascial edges can be clearly defined. Larger defects usually require the use of some type of prosthetic mesh and can be done in an open or a laparoscopic fashion.

How is an open abdominal wall hernia repair performed?

In the open repair the patient is placed in the supine position and undergoes general anesthesia. An incision is placed over the hernia sac, and the sac is carefully separated from the surrounding subcutaneous tissue. The fascial edge is then circumferentially exposed in preparation for the repair. The sac may be entered and excised to prevent any injury to the bowel during closure, or it may be reduced and left in place to prevent direct contact of the mesh

TABLE 25–3

Uncommon Abdominal Wall Hernias

Spigelian	Located lateral to the rectus sheath below the level of the umbilicus
Grynfeltt	Occurs in the superior lumbar triangle
Petit's	Occurs in the inferior lumbar triangle
Obturator	Occurs within the obturator canal and may cause compression of the nerve, leading to pain in the region of the hip, knee, or inner thigh

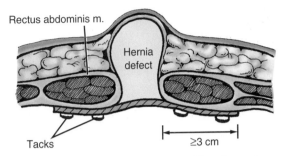

Figure 25–4. Laparoscopic ventral hernia repair.

with the underlying bowel. If mesh is used, nonabsorbable suture is secured to both the fascial edge and the mesh in either a running or interrupted fashion. The subcutaneous tissue and skin are then closed.

How is a laparoscopic abdominal wall hernia repair performed?

This requires a general anesthetic and the placement of three or four trocars through the anterior abdominal wall. Placement of these trocars is crucial and should be done as lateral to the hernia edge as possible. Once the hernia sac is reduced, it need not be excised. It is important to remove all of the abdominal contents prior to the placement of the prosthetic mesh. The repair entails placing the mesh intra-abdominally and then securing the mesh to the peritoneal surface by a tacking or stapling device. The laparoscopic repair allows for the detection and repair of multiple abdominal wall hernias and also places the mesh at a greater distance from the fascial edge, thereby decreasing the chance of recurrence, as seen in Figure 25–4. Laparoscopy also offers less postoperative pain and reduces the incidence of wound infections.

K E Y   P O I N T S

▶ Hernias are defects in fascial planes.

▶ Symptoms arise when underlying tissue pushes through the defect and may result in incarceration or strangulation of the underlying tissues.

▶ All hernias should be surgically repaired if the patient is a surgical candidate.

continued

▶ There are both open and laparoscopic approaches to most types of hernias.

▶ The key to successful repair of an inguinal hernia is tension-free reconstruction of the fascial defect.

CASE 25–1. A 30-year-old man, with no significant past medical history, presents with a tender right groin mass. He states that the mass has been present for approximately 2 months, beginning after he moved some furniture. On examination you find a 2-cm reducible mass in the right groin. He has no abdominal tenderness and no evidence of a left groin mass.

    A. What is the differential diagnosis?
    B. What tests would you order?
    C. What type of repair would you recommend?

CASE 25–2. A 65-year-old man, 10 years status post abdominal aortic aneurysm repair, presents with a 2-day history of abdominal distention, nausea, and vomiting. He is otherwise healthy. On physical exam you note an obese male in mild distress. He is mildly tachycardic and complains of mild abdominal pain. Abdominal examination reveals a healed midline scar, high-pitched bowel sounds, abdominal distention, and mild diffuse tenderness. A mass is felt in the midline just above the umbilicus and has overlying erythema and tenderness.

    A. What is the diagnosis?
    B. What should the next step be?
    C. What is the operative approach?

26

Breast Disease

BENIGN BREAST DISEASE

The evaluation and treatment of breast disease are a prominent component of any surgical practice. There is a tendency to focus on the treatment of cancers of the breast. However, benign conditions of the breast account for most of the breast patients seen in surgical clinics. Understanding the normal physiology of the breast is important to recognizing pathology.

▶ PHYSIOLOGY OF THE FEMALE BREAST

What is the anatomy of the breast?

Breast anatomy consists of anatomic units called *lobules*, each having a series of elongated ductules that coalesce to form a total of 10 to 20 ducts that drain the entire breast. Fibrous connective tissue bands, called *Cooper's ligaments*, run between the lobules from superficial to deep. These ligaments support the contour of the breast. The venous and lymphatic drainage patterns in the breast are primarily to the ipsilateral axilla, although medial lesions can drain into the internal mammary nodes.

What regulates the development of the female breast?

Estrogen, progesterone, and prolactin are the principal hormones involved in the development of the female breast. Estrogen, a fat-soluble hormone, acts in the cell nucleus to induce the production of RNA and eventually estrogen-induced proteins. These include the progesterone receptors.

Breast development results from shifts in hormones and begins at approximately 10 years of age and starts with elevation of the nipple. Nonovulatory fluctuations in hormone levels cause enlargement of the breast and the nipple-areola complex. At approximately 12 to 13 years of age, nonovulatory cyclical changes in hormone levels lead to the onset of menses, and further development of the breast occurs. By age 15 to 16, the nonovulatory cycles are replaced by ovulatory cycles, which cause the breasts to take on an adult appearance. Full maturity of breast tissue does not occur until pregnancy, when there is tremendous ductal, alveolar, and lobular growth due to progesterone, prolactin, and chorionic gonadotropin to prepare the breast for lactation. Three months after cessation of lactation, breast lobules atrophy without the loss of the number of lobules. When a woman reaches menopause, the glandular portions of the breast are replaced by fat.

What is the mammary ridge and what is its significance in humans?

The milk line, or mammary ridge, first appears at 5 weeks' gestation and runs from the base of the lower limb to the base of the upper limb. During normal development, the breast tissue along the mammary ridge recedes, except for the tissue on the thorax. Occasionally breast tissue remains from the rudimentary mammary ridge and results in the appearance of accessory breast tissue. Such tissue, although more common in the axillae, can appear anywhere along the ridge, including in the labia majoris. Young patients often first note the presence of accessory breast tissue with the onset of menses, when the tissue cyclically fluctuates in size and degree of tenderness. Just like the normal breast tissue, accessory breast tissue has a risk of malignant transformation. Masses in accessory breast tissue need to be evaluated using the same criteria that are used in the breast.

What breast changes accompany pregnancy and lactation?

During pregnancy there is tremendous growth of both ducts and lobules to prepare the breast for the production of milk. By the immediate postpartum period, the breasts may have up to tripled in size. The abrupt drop in circulating hormone levels that occurs at delivery, combined with the effects of prolactin, triggers the production and release of colostrum and eventually breast milk. Lactating women are at increased risk of forming abscesses or suppurative mastitis. This is attributed to the propensity for blockage of ducts, combined with areolar skin breakdown as a port of entry for bacteria. Most women with mastitis during breast-feeding respond to antibiotics, warm compresses, and pumping breast milk from the involved breast to avoid engorgement. Occasionally an abscess requires surgical drainage.

Can mastitis and breast abscesses occur in women who are not breast-feeding?

Although lactating women are certainly at more risk for mastitis and breast abscesses, these conditions can occur in women who are not actively breast-feeding. The treatment is the same, with warm compresses and antibiotics and surgical drainage of any abscesses. Often the fluctuance is deep within the breast parenchyma. In these cases, ultrasound is helpful in identifying those patients who require surgical drainage. Rarely, a woman is diagnosed as having a breast abscess and the pathology indicates inflammatory breast cancer. If there is any chance that the lesion could be malignant, a biopsy including the skin is obtained.

What are fibrocystic changes?

Symptomatic fibrocystic changes are present in 30% to 50% of women during their reproductive life. Histologically it consists of fibrosis, cysts, and a variable amount of ductal hyperplasia. Unless some atypia is noted, it does not imply an increased risk for development of cancer. When a woman with fibrocystic changes forms a predominant mass, it is called a *fibroadenoma*. The mass is usually mobile with smooth borders. Like fibrocystic changes, a fibroadenoma tends to fluctuate in size and degree of tenderness with the menstrual cycle.

What is mastodynia?

Mastodynia, or painful breasts, is a common complaint in women with benign breast disease. The pain can be cyclical or constant and be either associated with a predominant mass or diffuse. Only about 11% of malignancies present as a painful mass; however, each mass needs to be evaluated whether or not it is painful. In those women who have cyclical pain without a predominant mass, reassurance that this is a benign condition often suffices. Physical examination, including lung and chest wall exams, can usually discriminate breast pain from chest wall pain. For pleuritic pain or costochondritis, reproducing the pain with palpation of the ribs or with deep inspiration is helpful. Treatment of this type of pain with nonsteroidal anti-inflammatory medications usually leads to resolution of symptoms. For women with cyclical pain attributable to the breast itself, treatment with hormonal agents such as oral contraceptives or danazol or tamoxifen often controls symptoms. Many women do better once they are reassured that there are no worrisome findings on physical examination or mammogram to suggest malignancy. Pain that has progressively become worse or more constant requires investigation with a chest computed tomographic (CT) scan and a mammogram, with biopsy of any mass that is identified, regardless of risk category.

Can benign breast masses be distinguished from malignant masses on the basis of clinical findings?

There are certainly clinical features that can reassure you that the breast lesion is benign. However, because of the overlap in clinical appearance and presentation of benign and malignant breast disease, only a few lesions in select women with the lowest risk category should be evaluated without some manner of tissue confirmation. There are several benign entities that have a great deal of overlap in the radiographic appearance with malignant lesions. Sclerosing adenosis, a variant of fibrocystic changes, is commonly detected on mammogram as clustered microcalcifications without palpable lesion. Histologic findings of sclerosing adenosis include regular appearance of the nuclei and the absence of mitotic figures. Radial scars and fat necrosis may present with spiculated lesions on mammogram and may even have overlying skin changes such as skin dimpling. Lesions with these features should not be observed without at least a needle biopsy. Mammary duct ectasia has a clinical presentation that is identical to an infra-areolar carcinoma, often with dark discharge and nipple retraction.

MALIGNANT BREAST DISEASE

▶ ETIOLOGY

Breast cancer is the second leading cause of cancer deaths in women. It accounts for 44,000 deaths annually in the United States, and 150,000 new cases are diagnosed each year. The female-to-male ratio is 150:1. The most common presentation of breast cancer is the appearance of a new lump discovered either on physical examination by the patient's clinician or by self-exam. For this reason the appearance of a new lump warrants a tissue diagnosis in most cases. Chapter 6 reviews the work-up of a breast mass, as well as the risk factors that increase the relative risk that any given mass will harbor malignancy. Although these criteria are helpful in thinking about the work-up of a mass, many women develop breast cancer without any identifiable risk factor other than simply having a breast.

▶ EVALUATION

How are women screened for breast cancer?

The early identification of breast cancer is critical to improve outcome. Comprehensive breast screening programs to help reduce breast cancer deaths in the United States include the use of mammography starting at 40 years of age, annual breast exams by a physician, and monthly breast self-examination. Other examinations such as ultrasound and magnetic resonance imaging are becoming increasingly important in breast cancer care.

What is the general organization of cancer centers?

Once breast cancer has been diagnosed, the patient is best treated using a multidisciplinary approach that includes access to a general or oncologic surgeon, a plastic surgeon, a medical oncologist, a radiation oncologist, and social services. Such multidisciplinary centers are being established around the country. However, excellent care can be delivered without a dedicated center. The surgeon who initially diagnoses the cancer reviews individual cases at tumor boards that meet regularly in most hospitals with the input of physicians from each of these specialties and provides the proper referrals based on the recommendations of the multidisciplinary board. Breast cancer care is an area of medicine that has been evolving with the help of ongoing research studies. The amount of data in the surgical and medical oncology literature is formidable. Continuing accumulation of data from large multicenter trials is helping us improve the care we deliver to women with breast cancer now as well as in the future.

▶ TREATMENT

Most breast cancers arise from the ductules or from the lobular stroma. Operative and postoperative management are tailored according the stage of disease and the general health of the patient. The ability of the patient to tolerate and benefit from chemotherapeutic regimens or courses of radiation therapy is discussed before final recommendations are made. The spectrum of disease ranges from precancerous or in situ lesions to widely metastatic or locally advanced tumors. For most breast cancers, surgical treatment precedes chemotherapy or radiation therapy. The exceptions are widely metastatic cancers, inflammatory cancers, and, more recently, locally advanced cancers. In some cases the only role of the surgeon is to provide an adequate specimen for measuring histologic markers for prognosis and for planning specific courses of therapy.

How does the management of a precancerous lesion differ from that of a cancerous lesion?

In situ breast cancers, or precancerous lesions, can be of lobular origin, i.e., lobular carcinoma in situ (LCIS); or epithelial- or ductal-origin ductal carcinoma in situ (DCIS). The term *in situ* indicates that the lesion has cellular features of carcinoma but shows no signs of invasion past the basement membrane.

DCIS accounts for 50% of the cancers diagnosed by needle-localized breast biopsy, because it commonly presents with microcalcifications on a mammogram. The significance of these lesions is as markers for risk of concurrent or future incidence of cancer in the ipsilateral side. Previously, the presence of DCIS on a biopsy specimen with any degree of cellular atypia was an indication for mastectomy. Currently, surgeons may attempt wide excision for low-grade, non-comedo-type DCIS as an initial procedure, going on to mastectomy for lesions that are found to have features of multi-focal disease or continued positive surgical margins after attempts at wide excision. Foci of microinvasion where negative margins are achieved are amenable to breast conservative surgical therapy with axillary lymph node sampling, or sentinel node biopsy. Post-operative radiation therapy to the involved breast, following excision with clear margins, decreases the risk of recurrent DCIS, as well as the risk of invasive carcinoma's developing in the future. Nonetheless, these are patients that warrant close follow-up for their lifetime. A treatment algorithm for patients with DCIS is given in Figure 26–1. Patients found to have microinvasion of lymph nodes should be considered for antiestrogen treatment postoperatively.

LCIS, as contrasted with DCIS, is a marker of increased risk for the development of invasive cancer in both the contralateral and ipsilateral breasts. LCIS is most often an incidental finding on breast biopsies done for nearby palpable or mammographically visible lesions. LCIS is rarely palpable, nor does it tend to contain internal calcifications. Patients diagnosed with LCIS on histologic examination have up to 12 times the lifetime risk of developing an invasive breast cancer over the general population. Previous treatment algorithms recommended bilateral mastectomy for incidental LCIS. The cancers that develop in patients who present with LCIS are more often invasive ductal carcinomas rather than invasive lobular carcinoma. Bilateral mastectomies are still the best option for patients with a strong family history of breast cancer or a history of ovarian cancer; however, close follow-up with semi-annual mammograms and physical examination is reasonable. Patient preference also plays a role in the decision-making process. For many women, the fear of developing breast carcinoma is so overwhelming that bilateral mastectomy is their preference. These patients should have a consultation with a plastic surgeon to decide whether reconstruction is desirable and to discuss the timing and types of reconstruction that are appropriate. An algorithm for the treatment of LCIS is presented in Figure 26–2.

What is the initial staging for patients diagnosed with invasive breast cancer?

Further therapy for breast cancer depends on the stage of the tumor. The staging depends on the size of the tumor and the presence of lymph node invasion as set in the guidelines of the American Joint Committee on Cancer using the TNM staging system (Table 26–1). Patients should be staged initially with a careful history and physical examination. If there are any indications of distant metastases, such as focal neurologic abnormalities, headache,

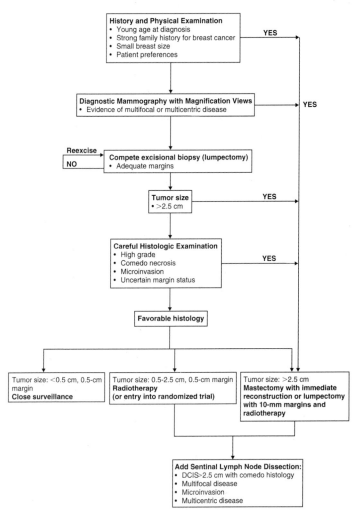

Figure 26–1. Treatment algorithm for patients with ductal carcinoma in situ (DCIS). (From Cameron JL [ed]: Current Surgical Therapy, 7th ed. St. Louis, Mosby, 2001, p 724.)

persistent cough, or bony pain, the patient should be evaluated with CT scan and bone scan. Initial work-up for those without worrisome findings on history and physical examination should include a chest radiograph and screening labs, including complete blood count and liver function tests. Many patients want to know the stage of their cancer as soon as the results of the initial biopsy are available. Careful explanation of how you are going to get the information (further surgery and tests) and assurance that you will help them

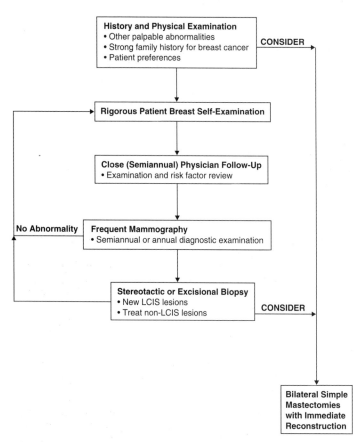

Figure 26–2. Treatment algorithm for patients with biopsy-proven lobular carcinoma in situ (LCIS). (From Cameron JL [ed]: Current Surgical Therapy, 7th ed. St. Louis, Mosby, 2001, p 726.)

access the appropriate input from specialists will put them more at ease. You should also provide information on cancer support groups, because patients often benefit from interaction with other patients who have similar experiences.

How do you decide between mastectomy and breast-conserving therapy?

Previously, mastectomy was the only surgical option for patients diagnosed with breast cancer, but breast-conserving therapy is now becoming more common in modern surgical practice. Multiple studies have shown that treatment with lumpectomy and axillary dissection, combined with postoperative radiation therapy, is equiv-

TABLE 26–1

AJCC TNM Staging System for Breast Cancer

Primary Tumor (T)

TX	Primary tumor cannot be assessed
T0	No evidence of primary tumor
Tis	Carcinoma *in situ*
Tis (DCIS)	Ductal carcinoma *in situ*
Tis (LCIS)	Lobular carcinoma *in situ*
Tis (Paget's)	Paget's disease of the nipple with no tumor
T1	Tumor 2 cm or less in greatest dimension
T1mic	Microinvasion 0.1 cm or less in greatest dimension
T1a	Tumor more than 0.1 cm but not more than 0.5 cm in greatest dimension
T1b	Tumor more than 0.5 cm but not more than 1 cm in greatest dimension
T1c	Tumor more than 1 cm but not more than 2 cm in greatest dimension
T2	Tumor more than 2 cm but not more than 5 cm in greatest dimension
T3	Tumor more than 5 cm in greatest dimension
T4	Tumor of any size with direct extension to (a) chest wall or (b) skin, only as described below
T4a	Extension to chest wall, not including pectoralis muscle
T4b	Edema (including peau d'orange) or ulceration of the skin of the breast, or satellite skin nodules confined to the same breast
T4c	Both T4a and T4b
T4d	Inflammatory carcinoma

Regional Lymph Nodes (N)

NX	Regional lymph nodes cannot be assessed (e.g., previously removed)
N0	No regional lymph node metastasis
N1	Metastasis to movable ipsilateral axillary lymph node(s)
N2	Metastases in ipsilateral axillary lymph nodes fixed or matted, or in clinically apparent ipsilateral internal mammary nodes in the *absence* of clinically evident axillary lymph node metastasis
N2a	Metastasis in ipsilateral axillary lymph nodes fixed to one another (matted) or to other structures
N2b	Metastasis only in clinically apparent ipsilateral internal mammary nodes and in the *absence* of clinically evident axillary lymph node metastasis
N3	Metastasis in ipsilateral infraclavicular lymph node(s) with or without axillary lymph node involvement, or in clinically apparent ipsilateral internal mammary lymph node(s) and in the *presence* of clinically evident axillary lymph node metastasis; or metastasis in ipsilateral supraclavicular lymph node(s) with or without axillary or internal mammary lymph node involvement
N3a	Metastasis in ipsilateral infraclavicular lymph node(s)
N3b	Metastasis in ipsilateral internal mammary lymph node(s) and axillary lymph node(s)
N3c	Metastasis in ipsilateral supraclavicular lymph node(s)

Distant Metastasis (M)

MX	Distant metastasis cannot be assessed
M0	No distant metastasis
M1	Distant metastasis

Stage Grouping

Stage	T	N	M
Stage 0	Tis	N0	M0
Stage I	T1*	N0	M0
Stage IIA	T0	N1	M0
	T1*	N1	M0
	T2	N0	M0
Stage IIB	T2	N1	M0
	T3	N0	M0
Stage IIIA	T0	N2	M0
	T1*	N2	M0
	T2	N2	M0
	T3	N1	M0
	T3	N2	M0
Stage IIIB	T4	N0	M0
	T4	N1	M0
	T4	N2	M0
Stage IIIC	Any T	N3	M0
Stage IV	Any T	Any N	M1

*T1 includes T1mic

alent to modified radical mastectomy in terms of both local and regional control, as well as survival. The patient must be willing and able to comply with postoperative radiation treatments. Table 26–2 summarizes the factors important in selecting patients for breast conservation. Note that at the top of the list is patient preference, because most patients presenting with cancer are appropriate candidates for either method of surgical treatment.

What is the significance of histologic markers for breast cancer?

Histologic markers are used to determine the prognosis in individual cases of breast cancer and to guide therapy. The presence of estrogen and progesterone receptors on breast cancer specimens is a marker of a more well-differentiated tumor and allows the medical oncologist to determine whether hormonal manipulation with tamoxifen will be useful. The presence of the tumor marker Her 2-neu in a given specimen is a poor prognostic indicator, but the strength of the reaction can determine whether monoclonal antibody treatment is indicated. Other histologic markers indicating the aggressive nature of the tumor, such as the S-phase fraction, the presence of mitotic figures, or aneuploidy, are helpful in determining the risk of recurrence (Table 26–3) and in planning the type and length of adjuvant treatment that are indicated.

How does the management of inflammatory carcinoma differ from that of other forms of breast cancer?

Inflammatory breast cancer is a rare neoplasm characterized by an aggressive course and invasion of cancer cells into the lymphatics of the skin. Clinically, there are skin changes and often erythema in a rapidly enlarging breast mass. Skin punch biopsy can make the diagnosis. Metastases tend to occur early and widely. The preferred treatment consists of chemotherapy and radiation; mastectomy is withheld for those rare patients with nonhealing wounds or intractable pain. Many patients have rapid regression and necrosis

---

TABLE 26–2

Criteria for Choosing Breast-Conserving Surgery

Patient preference
Willingness and ability to complete a course of radiation therapy
No prior therapeutic radiation treatment to the ipsilateral breast
Single primary tumor or anatomically confined in situ lesion
Ability to achieve negative surgical margins
Tumor ≤ 4 cm or a breast-to-tumor ratio that allows good cosmesis
Ability to follow patient with mammography
Patient reliability

TABLE 26-3

Histologic Prognostic Indicators in Breast Cancer

Prognostic Factor	Increased Risk of Recurrence	Decreased Risk of Recurrence
Size	T2, T3	T0, T1
Hormone receptors	Negative	Positive
DNA flow cytometry	Aneuploid	Diploid
Histologic grade	High	Low
Tumor labeling index	<3%	>3%
S-phase fraction	>5%	<5%
Lymphatic or vascular invasion	Present	Absent
Cathepsin D	High	Low
Her 2-neu	High	Low or absent
Epidermal growth factor receptor	High	Low

of the tumor once therapy has started. These are challenging patients to treat, and communication with the medical oncologist throughout therapy is critical.

How does pregnancy or lactation affect the work-up of breast mass?

Breast cancer is discovered during pregnancy in 1:3000 pregnancies. The work-up is often delayed, because the changes that are felt in the breast are often attributed to the pregnancy. Once a diagnosis of breast cancer has been established by needle or excisional biopsy, the treatment algorithms are essentially the same, with decisions being made based on the stage and histologic markers of the tumor. If the breast cancer is discovered early in pregnancy and the administration of chemotherapy cannot be safely delayed until after delivery, the pregnancy may need to be terminated. Cancer discovered late in pregnancy can be treated surgically safely, and adjuvant therapy is instituted as soon as possible after delivery. Breast cancers discovered in an actively lactating mother are treated in the same manner as breast cancers in a nonlactating woman. There is a slight increase in wound care complications due to leakage of milk at the incision.

How does breast cancer differ in men?

There are 900 to 1400 new cases of breast cancer in men annually. The disease is theoretically easier to screen for by physical examination because of the lack of significant breast tissue to mask the appearance of a mass. However, male breast cancer is typically discovered at a more advanced stage, most likely due to a lack of understanding that the appearance of a mass could represent a malignancy. Breast-conserving therapy is not really an issue in male breast cancer for two reasons: First, the only recognizable component of an anatomic breast in men is the nipple-areola complex, and thus the asymmetry of complete mastectomy is minimal; second, the masses in male breast cancer are in such proximity to the nipple that negative margins would not be achievable without resection of the nipple-areola complex.

BREAST RECONSTRUCTION

Which patients are candidates for immediate reconstruction after mastectomy?

Ample evidence exists that immediate reconstruction after mastectomy improves the emotional impact of mastectomy for patients;

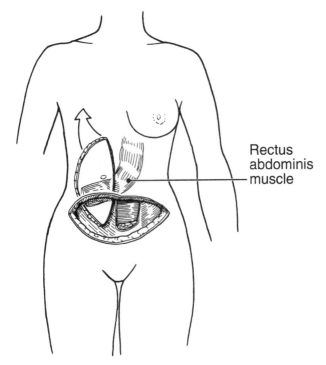

Rectus abdominis muscle

Figure 26–3. Drawing of pedicled transverse rectus abdominis myocutaneous (TRAM) flap. The blood supply for the flap comes from the superior epigastric vessels. The flap is tunneled beneath the upper abdominal skin to reach the chest wall. (From Cameron JL [ed]: Current Surgical Therapy, 7th ed. St. Louis, Mosby, 2001, p 742.)

however, not all patients are candidates for reconstruction. In terms of tumor size and stage, patients who opt for mastectomy with lesions that are stage 0, I, or II should be offered plastic surgery consultation to discuss the possibility of immediate reconstruction. Those patients with locally advanced tumors or those with tumors close to or invading the chest wall should be advised that reconstruction would be best delayed until local control of tumor is ensured. They may still wish to discuss the options for delayed reconstruction before undergoing mastectomy to help with the emotional aspects associated with losing a breast.

The best cosmetic results are achieved with a transverse rectus abdominis myocutaneous (TRAM) flap, and it is the most common autogenous flap, as outlined in Figure 26–3. Patients who are older, who smoke, who are at risk for poor wound healing, or who have had multiple abdominal procedures are not candidates for autogenous tissue reconstruction with a TRAM or latissimus dorsi flap. Flap reconstruction is a much more complex and lengthy operation, so patients who are poor anesthetic risks secondary to underlying medical problems will most likely be rejected for reconstruction. However, these patients may be considered appropriate for immediate reconstruction with an implant or for placement of a tissue expander to prepare the area for a delayed reconstruction. The best practice is to offer referral to any patient who may be a candidate for reconstruction and allow the plastic surgeon to present the options and explain the scope and complexity of the procedures, so that the patient can make an informed decision.

K E Y   P O I N T S

▶ Evaluation of the breast is a prominent part of surgical practice.

▶ The majority of open biopsies reveal benign pathology. Therefore, attention to cosmesis is important.

▶ Comprehensive screening programs that include the use of mammography, breast self-exam, and annual examination by a physician help identify breast cancer at early stages, improving patient outcome.

▶ For most patients with breast cancer, breast-conserving therapy with postoperative radiation is equivalent to mastectomy in terms of outcome.

▶ A multidisciplinary approach to breast cancer care improves patient satisfaction and care.

CASE 26–1.

A 65-year-old Hispanic woman presents with a finding of microcalcifications in the left upper outer quadrant of the breast on screening mammography. She has a history of DCIS of the right breast 5 years earlier and had a wide excision and breast irradiation at that time. She has no family members with breast cancer. She has a 40-pack-year smoking history and currently smokes one-half pack/day. Her medical history is significant for non-insulin-dependent diabetes mellitus and peripheral vascular disease. On physical examination she has a well-healed transverse scar in the upper outer quadrant of the right breast. There is no predominant mass on physical exam.

A. How would you proceed with biopsy?
B. Does her history of DCIS increase the risk that this lesion is cancerous?

She undergoes biopsy and a 0.8-cm invasive ductal carcinoma is found.

C. What are her surgical options for definitive treatment?
D. Would they be different if her prior radiation had been to the same rather than the contralateral breast?

CASE 26–2.

A 58-year-old woman is referred to you for evaluation of a breast mass associated with erythema. She was initially treated with antibiotics with limited improvement, but over the last 3 weeks has a mass that is increasing in size. On physical examination she has extensive skin changes and erythema. The entire breast has a firm, rubbery consistency and is quite tender. She has matted lymphadenopathy in the ipsilateral axilla and has several cervical lymph nodes that are mildly enlarged. She has a chest radiograph that was ordered by her primary care physician, which is normal. Labs are notable for elevated transaminase levels. Except for the obvious breast mass, her physical exam is normal.

A. What is the most likely diagnosis?
B. How would you establish the diagnosis?
C. What additional staging exams would you order?

27

Pulmonology

ASTHMA

Asthma is an obstructive airway disease characterized by airway inflammation; recurrent exacerbations with dyspnea, wheezing, and cough; and pronounced airway responsiveness to stimuli that cause little or no response in nonasthmatic patients (airway hyper-reactivity). Approximately 5% of the U.S. population has this disease. Asthma most frequently develops in childhood but can present in adult life at any age. The disease course is remarkable for its recurrent exacerbations interspersed with symptom-free or mildly symptomatic periods.

▶ ETIOLOGY

Asthma is classified by the stimulus that provokes exacerbations (i.e., exercise-induced, allergen, aspirin-sensitive, occupational, cold-induced, and emotional) and by the severity of symptoms the patient experiences (mild-intermittent, mild-persistent, moderate-persistent, and severe-persistent). These classification schemes help clinicians with the treatment of asthma by identifying the triggering stimuli, the severity of the disease, and the patient's concomitant need for medicinal therapy.

What is the pathophysiology of asthma?

There is a wealth of information on the pathologic abnormalities found in the airways of asthmatic patients but no clear explanation of how these abnormalities surface and lead to clinical asthma. Airway inflammation is always present with cellular infiltrates in airway mucosa, airway edema, and elevated levels of cytokines. Other abnormalities of asthmatic airways include smooth muscle hypertrophy, increased mucus secretion, ciliary dysfunction, and mucus cell proliferation. The end result of all of these abnormalities is the narrowing of airways with increased resistance to airflow resulting in airway obstruction. This process occurs in a patchy distribution throughout the small and large airways of the tracheobronchial tree in mild asthma and in a more diffuse distribution in moderate to severe asthma.

▶ EVALUATION

What symptoms suggest the diagnosis of asthma?

The cardinal symptoms of asthma are chest tightness, shortness of breath, wheezing, and anxiety. There are variants of asthma in which cough, hoarseness, or night-time insomnia are the only symptoms. The severity of asthma and the provoking stimulus predict how often and when a patient with asthma will become symptomatic. Patients with mild asthma often complain of symptoms only at night or with specific exposures to triggers such as dust, pollens, animal dander, or cold temperatures. As the severity of asthma increases, patients can experience symptoms more frequently, with a greater number of inciting stimuli, and without an identifiable trigger.

What findings on physical exam are consistent with asthma?

With symptomatic asthma exacerbations, vital sign abnormalities include tachypnea and tachycardia. When airway obstruction is severe, pulsus paradoxus, an exaggerated fall in blood pressure with inspiration, may be present. Examination of the chest shows hyperinflation with hyper-resonance on percussion and can show accessory muscle use with active retraction of intercostal muscles. Auscultation elicits the cardinal sign of asthma: wheezing. Wheezing tends to be more prominent during exhalation but often can be heard throughout the respiratory cycle. Rhonchi are sometimes present, indicating the accumulation of secretions in the larger airways. Expiration is prolonged in comparison to inspiration. In severe cases of airway obstruction, wheezing may not be present and breath sounds are difficult to auscultate. Cyanosis, when present, signals the presence of respiratory failure.

What laboratory studies should be ordered?

Acute exacerbations are easily identified by exam findings, but most of these findings are poor predictors of the severity of the exacerbation. Arterial blood gas (ABG) analysis and spirometry are the best tools for predicting the severity of an exacerbation. On ABG analysis, respiratory alkalosis with mild hypoxia is typical of mild to moderate exacerbations. As the exacerbation proceeds, a metabolic acidosis appears, which reflects the increased metabolic demands from the work of breathing. As the exacerbation progresses toward respiratory failure, the $Paco_2$ normalizes and a respiratory acidosis adds itself to the acid-base disturbance.

Spirometry can also be used to judge the severity of an exacerbation. Forced expiratory volume in 1 second (FEV_1) and peak expiratory flow rate (PEFR) are depressed in asthma. In emergency situations, PEFR is easy to obtain and can be repeated multiple times to follow the progress of the patient during therapy. Most asthmatic patients know their maximal PEFR and what decrease in PEFR signals danger for them. In those patients without this knowledge, PEFRs less than 50% of predicted are indicative of a severe exacerbation. Additionally, PEFRs that remain depressed or worsen with therapy signal severe exacerbations and the need for closer monitoring and intensification of therapy.

Other laboratory findings that are found in some asthmatic patients include peripheral eosinophilia, increased levels of serum IgE, and positive wheal-and-flare testing for allergies. The sputum in asthma can appear purulent without concomitant infection. Charcot-Leyden crystals (crystallized eosinophil lysophospholipase), Curschmann's spirals (mucus and cells forming bronchiolar casts), and Creola bodies (groups of ciliated epithelial cells) found in the sputum of asthmatic patients change the color and consistency of the sputum, causing the apparent purulence.

What are the radiographic findings in asthma?

Chest radiography in asthma often shows the large lung volumes, flattened diaphragms, and hyperlucency that are typical of the obstructive diseases. These findings are not pathognomonic for asthma. However, chest radiography is useful to find additional causes for an asthmatic patient's symptoms such as pneumonia and the rare complications of pneumothorax or pneumomediastinum.

What are the electrocardiographic findings in asthma?

Sinus tachycardia is the most common finding on electrocardiogram (ECG) in asthma exacerbations. Right bundle branch block, anterior lead ST changes, atrial fibrillation, multifocal atrial tachycardia, and electrical alternans all can be seen during acute exacerbations.

▶ TREATMENT

Treatment of asthma has two goals: to relieve acute obstruction and to reduce the frequency and severity of acute attacks.

What therapies relieve acute airway obstruction?

The first goal is to relieve the acute worsening of airway obstruction during an asthma exacerbation. Removal of the inciting agent, if known, is the first step. Pharmacotherapy is the second step.

Medications used in acute exacerbations include β-agonists, ipratropium, and corticosteroids.

β$_2$-agonists such as albuterol are delivered locally to obstructed airways via metered-dose inhalers (MDIs) or nebulizers. The handheld MDIs are difficult to use and require instruction from health care personnel on their proper use. Patients who cannot master the technique of MDI use can either add an easy-to-use spacer device to the MDI or switch to a nebulizer device for drug delivery. Patients in the midst of an exacerbation may be unable to use an MDI secondary to their respiratory distress. In cases like this, nebulized β$_2$-agonists should be used.

The anticholinergic drug ipratropium has marginal benefits in acute asthma exacerbations. Like the β$_2$-agonists, it is delivered via MDIs or nebulizers. Both the β$_2$-agonists and ipratropium are generally well tolerated, but they can cause dose-limiting tachycardia, and β$_2$-agonists can cause hypokalemia.

Systemic corticosteroids are given to patients with severe exacerbations. Intravenous (IV) boluses of hydrocortisone or methylprednisolone are administered initially, and the patient is transitioned to 40 to 60 mg per day of oral prednisone once clinical improvement allows it. Systemic steroids should be tapered off rapidly within 1 to 2 weeks of starting. Some patients present already on chronic systemic steroids—these patients should also be bolused initially with higher doses of IV corticosteroids and tapered, as their clinical condition permits, back to their usual dose of oral prednisone.

How is chronic asthma controlled?

The second goal of asthma therapy is chronic control of the disease. Medications used for this purpose aim to decrease the number of exacerbations and to minimize any symptoms between exacerbations. These medications include corticosteroids, long-acting β$_2$-agonists, methylxanthines, leukotriene antagonists, and cromolyn.

The long-acting β$_2$-agonist salmeterol is dosed twice daily via MDI. This medication, because of its long half-life, is not suitable for emergency use. However, it does reduce the number of exacerbations, the severity of exacerbations, and the amount of symptoms between exacerbations when used regularly.

Control of airway inflammation with corticosteroids is the mainstay of chronic asthma management. Steroids can be given via MDI, orally, or intravenously. IV administration is reserved for severe exacerbations. The locally administered, inhaled corticosteroid preparations are best for chronic management. They are efficacious in preventing airway inflammation and limiting symptoms with few of the systemic side effects seen with oral or IV corticosteroids. The most common side effect of inhaled steroid medications is oral thrush. Having the patient rinse after every use can easily control this. Other side effects such as cataracts and growth retardation in children are also observed with chronic inhaled steroid use.

The latest and most promising drugs in the asthma armamentarium are the leukotriene inhibitors. These drugs are given in oral preparations, are easily tolerated, and can have considerable efficacy. They have quickly become the second or third choice for patients with asthma symptoms not controlled easily with occasional rescue albuterol MDI use.

The methylxanthines, aminophylline and theophylline, are third- or fourth-line choices for chronic asthma management. Theophylline, the more common of the two, can be administered in once- or twice-daily oral preparations. A narrow therapeutic index and the need for serum drug level monitoring make this drug a less appealing choice for chronic asthma management. Nonetheless, it does offer some patients with refractory asthma symptomatic relief.

Finally, the mast cell membrane stabilizer, cromolyn, can have benefit in chronic asthma. This medication is best suited for those with allergen-triggered asthma. Like salmeterol, this medication needs to be used chronically for it to show its benefits.

What are the surgical considerations in a patient with perioperative asthma?

Like patients with chronic obstructive pulmonary disease (COPD), patients with asthma require extra vigilance on the part of the surgeon. Preoperatively, the surgeon should ascertain the severity of the patient's asthma and what triggers exacerbations. This helps the surgeon manage any postoperative respiratory complaints more effectively. Circumstance permitting, the asthmatic patient should have minimal or no symptoms preoperatively and should be on a stable medication regimen.

The preoperative evaluation by the anesthesiologist should reveal if the patient has had previous intubations for asthma exacerbations, whether the patient has had previous procedures requiring tracheal intubation and what the outcome of those were, what degree of lung dysfunction the patient has, and if any medications (aspirin) or medical compounds (latex) trigger exacerbations. This information allows both the surgical team and the anesthesiologists to be prepared for any bronchospasm that may occur during the case or immediately postoperatively and to help avoid any iatrogenic exacerbations.

Postoperative pulmonary toilet is essential for an uncomplicated recovery. This starts with good pain control to prevent splinting and accumulation of secretions. Bronchodilator therapy followed by encouragement of coughing helps minimize bronchoconstriction and aids the asthmatic patient with secretion clearance. Asthmatic patients, like other patients, should be encouraged to perform incentive spirometry to prevent atelectasis and postoperative pneumonia.

Finally, any postoperative patient who develops symptomatic bronchospasm should be evaluated for a cause such as the interval development of pneumonia or a medication-triggered exacerbation. After a thorough evaluation to detect any inciting cause, the patient can be treated symptomatically with bronchodilators and, if necessary, corticosteroids.

K E Y   P O I N T S

▶ The pathophysiology of asthma leads to airway narrowing, increased resistance to flow, and eventual airway obstruction.

▶ Chest tightness, shortness of breath, and wheezing, coupled with expiratory wheezing on physical exam, are suggestive of asthma.

▶ Mainstays of therapy are β_2-agonist and anticholinergic inhalers and systemic or inhaled steroids.

CASE 27-1. A 26-year-old woman presents to the emergency department with an "asthma attack." She reports 1 day of worsening shortness of breath, wheezing, and cough. On physical exam, she is tachypneic with a respiratory rate of 26 breaths/min and tachycardic with a heart rate of 115 beats/min. She appears moderately distressed and has some accessory muscle use with respiration. Chest auscultation elicits diffuse wheezing without rhonchi. This patient may need further questioning to assess which "triggers" caused this attack. Her evaluation might include a peak flow test. Her treatment may include administration of methylprednisolone or possible intubation.

A. What would be the most reasonable first step?

CASE 27-2. A 69-year-old asthmatic woman comes to you for preoperative evaluation. She wishes to have an elective artificial hip replacement. She states that her arthritic

continued

CASE 27–2. *continued*

hip, not her asthma, limits her activities. She has not had an
asthma exacerbation for more than a year, and she reports
that her PEFR has remained at 450 L/min (85% of predicted)
during that time. Her medications include an albuterol MDI
that she has not used this month and an inhaled steroid
preparation that she uses daily. On physical exam, she
appears well and in no distress. Chest exam is normal, and
auscultation elicits wheezing only on forced expiration.

A. Given the options available for evaluating her pulmonary status
(e.g., recommending no further work-up for asthma, obtaining
preoperative pulmonary function tests [PFTs] or arterial blood
gas sampling [ABGs], recommending preoperative use of
bronchodilators and spirometry, or canceling elective surgery),
what is the most appropriate preoperative recommendation?

CASE 27–3. A 42-year-old woman is referred to
your pulmonary office for preoperative evaluation for an
elective ventral hernia repair. The patient's history is
remarkable for a long history of moderate, persistent asthma.
She has had four or five admissions for asthma and one
intubation in the last 10 years. She recognizes several triggers
of her asthma symptoms, including cold air, cats, and seasonal
pollens. She tells you that the last couple of weeks have been
particularly bad for her asthma as she has had daily
symptoms and has used extra albuterol to control her
symptoms. Other than the albuterol, her medications include
an inhaled steroid preparation and salmeterol. During the
springtime, she also takes an antihistamine medication and a
nasal steroid for her seasonal allergies. Her physical exam is
remarkable for a heart rate of 102 beats/min and for diffuse
wheezing with a prolonged expiratory phase on chest
auscultation. A chest radiograph obtained at the time of her
visit shows hyperinflated lung fields but no infiltrates.

A. What do you recommend to your surgical colleagues and to
the patient?

CHRONIC OBSTRUCTIVE PULMONARY DISEASE

COPD encompasses diseases of airflow obstruction and includes chronic bronchitis and emphysema. This airway obstruction manifests in a reduced maximum expiratory flow and a slow, forced expiration. Most of the airway obstruction is slowly progressive and not reversible. The diagnosis of chronic bronchitis relies on clinical criteria and is defined as the presence of a productive cough for at least 3 months during two consecutive years without other local cause such as bronchiectasis. Emphysema is an anatomic diagnosis and is defined as permanent, abnormal enlargement or destruction of the air spaces distal to the terminal bronchioles. Often a patient can meet the criteria for both diseases, because one disease does not preclude the presence of the other. Patients with COPD can also demonstrate airway hyper-reactivity and inflammation that show an overlap with another obstructive disease of the airways, asthma.

▶ ETIOLOGY

The hallmark symptoms of COPD are cough and breathlessness in a patient with a long smoking history. Although nonsmokers with significant second-hand smoke exposure, α_1-antitrypsin deficiency, or certain environmental exposures can develop COPD, this is the exception, not the rule. Most patients do not present with symptoms before they reach their 50s. Patients with symptoms suggestive of COPD prior to the age of 40 or who do not have a smoking history should have an evaluation for the less prevalent causes of COPD and for diseases that can mimic COPD, such as bronchiectasis and adult-onset asthma.

What is the pathophysiology of COPD?

The course of COPD begins with the narrowing of peripheral airways. The causes of this narrowing are many and include inflammation, enlargement of mucous glands, increased mucus production, squamous metaplasia, and smooth muscle hypertrophy. Loss of septal tethering and, in some patients, bronchoconstriction lead to further airway obstruction. These processes cause distal airway obstruction and loss of elastic lung recoil. As the disease process progresses, expiration becomes difficult and there is less resistance to chest wall expansion. Lung hyperinflation results and the patient has a lessening ability to exhale forcefully or fully. With continued tissue destruction and airway obstruction in the distal airways, alveolar capillary destruction occurs even as air trapping worsens. These areas of ventilation with low or no perfusion are referred to as dead space. The accumulation of dead space is one of the ways ventilation and perfusion in the lung become mismatched. It is defects in ventilation/perfusion ($\dot{V}/\dot{Q}$) matching that causes the hypoxia and hypercarbia seen in advanced COPD.

▶ **EVALUATION**

What are the symptoms of COPD?

The cough found in COPD is chronic and can produce varying amounts of sputum. Sputum production in the absence of an acute chest illness rarely exceeds 60 mL/day. Typically, the cough begins in the morning only but may become constant and be the most overwhelming symptom for the patient, especially when increasing sputum production and purulence suggest an acute exacerbation. COPD exacerbations may or may not be triggered by infections and are characterized by increasing cough, purulent sputum production, wheezing, and shortness of breath. In the late stages of disease or if a new infection is severe, exacerbations can cause respiratory failure with hypoxia and hypercarbia.

The breathlessness found in COPD occurs when airway obstruction is already moderate to severe. This is rare before the age of 40 and typically occurs in the 6th or 7th decade. This dyspnea initially occurs only with exertion but eventually occurs at rest as the disease process worsens.

What are the physical exam findings in COPD?

Exam findings in COPD depend on the severity of the illness and on the body habitus of the patient. Early in the course of COPD the only physical finding may be end-expiratory wheezing with forced expiration. As the disease progresses and lung hyperinflation ensues, the anterior-to-posterior diameter of the chest increases and the diaphragms flatten and move less with breathing. This is reflected in the physical exam with the "barrel chest," decreased breath sounds, and decreased heart sounds that are stereotypical for COPD.

In its end stage, cyanosis, accessory muscle hypertrophy, and signs of right-sided heart failure such as jugular venous distention, hepatomegaly, and peripheral edema may develop. Anorexia and weight loss also are typical of end-stage COPD as the work of breathing leads to increased energy requirements even as the dyspneic patient finds eating more and more difficult. End-stage patients often position themselves to relieve dyspnea. They sit forward with their weight supported on the palms of outstretched arms and breathe through pursed lips.

COPD patients with acute exacerbations show more prominent wheezing and decreases in peak expiratory flow rate. They also may show signs of infection such as fever, persistent cough, and purulent sputum production. The most concerning finding in an acute exacerbation is the altered mental status or obtundation that may herald hypercapnic respiratory failure and the need for emergent intubation.

What are the radiographic findings in COPD?

Although computed tomographic (CT) scanning, especially high-resolution scanning, is most sensitive and specific for detecting the pathologic lesions of COPD, its cost and limited availability make it the second-line test behind chest radiography. Lateral and frontal chest radiographs are useful not only for diagnosis but also to exclude other pathology in symptomatic patients.

Emphysema is an anatomic diagnosis of distal air space destruction and enlargement. On chest radiograph these emphysematous changes can be seen as large lung volumes, flattened diaphragms, enlarged retrosternal air space, lung field hyperlucency, and a narrowed inferior-directed cardiac silhouette. Other signs that may be seen with plain radiography include bullae and the enlarged right cardiac border and the prominent hilar vascularity seen with pulmonary hypertension.

Chronic bronchitis, unlike emphysema, is a clinical diagnosis and as such does not have characteristic radiographic findings. Patients may show bronchial cuffing, which is the thickened opacification of bronchial walls seen in cross section. This is not pathognomonic for chronic bronchitis and can be seen in other disorders. Patients with chronic bronchitis may also demonstrate the radiographic findings found in emphysema. These disorders can occur concurrently in a patient.

Chest radiography is also a helpful tool in patients with acute exacerbations. Review of the chest radiograph in these situations often reveals a source of the worsening symptoms such as a new lung infiltrate, lobar collapse, or pneumothorax.

What are the findings on spirometry and ABG analysis in COPD?

Pulmonary function testing (PFT) is important in the diagnosis of COPD, in monitoring its progression, in gauging the severity of acute exacerbations, and as a preoperative tool to estimate the anticipated risk of surgical morbidity and mortality in patients with COPD. Full PFT includes five components: flow measurements, volume measurements, diffusing capacity of carbon monoxide, flow-volume curves, and ABG analysis. The hallmark of COPD is decreased flow rates and increased lung volumes on PFT measurements. In patients with COPD, the key measurements include forced expiratory volume in 1 second (FEV_1), vital capacity (VC), FEV_1/VC ratio, and the arterial partial pressure of oxygen (PaO_2) and of carbon dioxide ($PaCO_2$) from ABG analysis. FEV_1 measures the amount of air (in liters) that is forcibly exhaled in the first second of exhalation when starting from the end of a maximal inhalation. VC measures the volume of air (in liters) that can be maximally exhaled after a maximal inhalation.

A decrease in FEV_1/VC ratio may be the first sign of mild COPD. As the disease progresses into moderate to severe stages, changes in FEV_1 are the best indicators of disease progression. An FEV_1 of greater than or equal to 70% of predicted based on the patient's age, height, and sex indicates mild disease; an FEV_1 of 50% to 69% of predicted signifies moderate disease; and patients with less than 50% of their predicted FEV_1 have severe disease. This has not only disease-specific prognostic implications but also surgical prognostic implications because patients with moderate and severe COPD have an increased risk of postsurgical morbidity and mortality.

Peak expiratory flow rate (PEFR) and flow-volume curves can also give estimates of the severity of airway obstruction. PEFR is especially useful in evaluating airway obstruction in the hospitalized patient. This measurement can be done at the bedside by untrained personnel and entails the patient's giving a maximal expiratory effort into a small hand-held flow meter. The meter then reads the peak flow velocity of the expired air in milliliters per second. PEFR can be obtained repeatedly over short intervals and can be used to monitor the effectiveness of bronchodilator therapy in the acutely ill patient. It can also evaluate the status of the postoperative patient. PEFRs of less than 200 mL/sec reflect severe airway obstruction, but even more important than the absolute value is the trend of PEFRs over several measurements. Decreasing PEFR over time despite bronchodilator therapy heralds developing respiratory failure.

Flow-volume curves are the domain of trained pulmonologists. However, postoperative patients often require continued mechanical ventilation. Most of today's ventilators display flow-volume curves, flow-time curves, and measurements of airway resistance. All of these give the astute clinician clues to the severity of any given patient's degree of airway obstruction. Patients with active airway obstruction on mechanical ventilation show lower peak flow rates, flattening of the expiratory limb of the curve, and larger lung volumes on flow-volume curves. Flow-time curves in the patient with active airway obstruction show the expiratory part of the curve not returning to its baseline. This indicates that the patient is still exhaling when the next inhalation begins. This airway obstruction leads to the development of air trapping and further increases in peak and mean airway pressures. Concomitant with this is increased difficulty in ventilating the patient and increased risk of barotrauma and hemodynamic compromise.

The final investigation is ABG analysis. In the evaluation of chronic COPD the presence of hypoxia and hypercarbia as reflected in a Pao_2 below 60 and $Paco_2$ above 40 indicates severe disease. In acute exacerbations changes in pH and Pao_2 reflect the ability of the patient to compensate for the acute episode. A normal pH regardless of the level of Pa_{CO_2} reflects a compensated state. Likewise, worsening hypoxia without a change in pH should prompt a search for other pathology such as pneumonia or pulmonary embolus.

▶ **TREATMENT**

What are the treatments for COPD?

Therapy for COPD aims at slowing disease progression, preventing acute exacerbations, relieving symptomatic airway obstruction, and correcting physiologic abnormalities. Smoking cessation is the only intervention shown to slow disease progression. Other preventive measures include administration of pneumococcal and seasonal influenza vaccines and the aggressive treatment of bacterial and viral respiratory illnesses. Despite its usual viral etiology, antibiotics have been shown to improve the outcome of acute bronchitis in patients with COPD and should be prescribed when patients present with the bronchitic symptoms of worsening cough and increased sputum production in the absence of an identifiable infiltrate on chest radiography.

The mainstays of chronic therapy for relief of acute worsening of airway obstruction are β_2-agonists such as albuterol. The anticholinergic drug ipratropium is also an effective bronchodilator and can be given with β_2-agonists. Typically, these drugs are dispensed through MDIs with the help of a spacer device. In acute situations, or when the patient is unable to master the technique involved with MDI use, the drugs can be nebulized. These drugs are typically well tolerated and do decrease the symptoms of wheezing, dyspnea, and cough, but they can cause dose-limiting tachycardia, and β_2-agonists can cause profound hypokalemia.

Other drugs such as theophylline and corticosteroids are controversial in the treatment of COPD. Theophylline can improve morning respiratory symptoms and when administered at bedtime prevents night-time decreases in FEV_1. In advanced cases of COPD, which are complicated by pulmonary hypertension, theophylline can improve ventricular contractility and promote pulmonary vascular dilation. These effects can improve symptoms and exercise capacity. However, theophylline's marginal benefits, its narrow therapeutic index, and the need for monitoring of serum levels of the drug limit its clinical usefulness.

Corticosteroids likewise have limited clinical usefulness. Inhaled steroids have never been shown to be of benefit either as chronic maintenance therapy or as adjuncts in acute exacerbations and are not recommended for use in COPD. Oral and IV corticosteroids can improve FEV_1 marginally, shorten length of hospital stay, and prevent relapse in the short term in patients hospitalized for acute exacerbations. Oral corticosteroids may also benefit a few patients who experience persistent debilitating symptoms despite optimal dosing of β_2-agonists and anticholinergic MDIs. It is not yet known how to predict which patients will show benefit with oral corticosteroids. Given the multiple side effects of chronic steroid use such as weight gain, skin fragility, hyperglycemia, osteoporosis, cataract development, personality change, hypertension, and increased risk for gastrointestinal bleeding, steroids should be continued only in patients with documented improvement in FEV_1 and exercise capacity.

In advanced COPD where patients have hypoxia either with ambulation or during rest, oxygen therapy also improves symptoms and increases exercise capacity. Oxygen therapy should be prescribed in patients with measured PaO_2 of less than 55; with oxygen saturations of less than 89% at any time; with evidence of pulmonary hypertension, cor pulmonale, or mental or psychological impairment attributable to their lung disease; or with polycythemia with hypoxemia.

What are the surgical issues in COPD?

Patients with moderate or severe COPD defined as an FEV_1 of less than 70% predicted or a $PaCO_2$ of greater than 45 at baseline have increased risk for surgical morbidity and mortality. Specifically, these patients have an increased likelihood of developing postoperative pulmonary complications such as atelectasis, pneumonia, and respiratory failure. The amount of increased risk depends on the severity of lung disease and the type of surgery undertaken.

Type of Surgical Procedure. The type of surgical procedure is the first important factor in estimating postoperative risk. Lung resections carry the greatest risk, especially in patients with marginal pulmonary function to start with. In these high-risk procedures, patients with COPD should have preoperative evaluations, starting with spirometry, and an ABG. Those with depressed FEV_1 or with CO_2 retention should have further work-up because these tests are sensitive enough to detect those with increased risk from the procedure but not specific enough to determine who should not have surgery. One way to assess the relative risk of the procedure is to estimate the anticipated loss of lung function with lung resection. Clinicians can estimate the anticipated loss of FEV_1 by obtaining dual lung perfusion scintigraphy. This test reports the amount of perfusion to each lung. With this information, the amount of total lung perfusion that each lung contributes can be deduced. The predicted postoperative FEV_1 will be the product of the preoperative FEV_1 multiplied by the percent of the total lung perfusion that the remaining lung has. Though there is no absolute amount of FEV_1 agreed on by experts, most would say that postoperative predicted FEV_1 should remain above 800 mL to 1 L or it should be greater than 40% of predicted, given the patient's age, height, and sex, for the surgery to be undertaken. Alternatively, recent studies have looked at the value of preoperative measurement of maximal oxygen uptake during exercise (max $\dot{V}O_2$). Max $\dot{V}O_2$ values below 15 mL/kg/min and below 10 mL/kg/min predict higher complication rates and higher postoperative mortality, respectively.

Max $\dot{V}o_2$ testing and predicted postoperative FEV_1 measure two different aspects of lung function and may complement each other for preoperative evaluation. Further studies are needed to evaluate the optimal testing required for preoperative evaluation for lung resection.

Location of Surgical Incision. Another important consideration in estimating postoperative risk of complications is the location of the surgical incision. Thoracic and high abdominal incisions carry the highest risk because they often cause transient diaphragmatic muscle dysfunction and splinting with respiration from the pain of the incision. This can worsen atelectasis and reduce the patient's ability to clear secretions. From this substrate comes perioperative pneumonia and respiratory failure. To prevent these complications, incentive spirometry should be taught to the patient early on and preferably in the preoperative period. It is more difficult for a patient who may be in pain or who may have a depressed sensorium from sedative or narcotic medications to learn how to perform incentive spirometry adequately. Also, when possible, regional blocks should be used for anesthesia instead of, or as an adjunct to, general anesthesia. These techniques avoid endotracheal intubation and the risks associated with general anesthesia and mechanical ventilation. They also can be continued postoperatively when they offer the advantage of good pain control without the deleterious side effects, such as respiratory depression, that are associated with systemically administered narcotics.

More distal incision sites, including lower abdominal incisions, have less risk of perioperative pulmonary complications. However, patients still require a vigilant approach with perioperative incentive spirometry, encouragement of cough, suctioning when appropriate, and an adequate regimen of bronchodilator therapy.

Smoking Cessation. The most important measure for preventing postoperative pulmonary complications in COPD patients undergoing surgery is smoking cessation. When possible, encourage patients to stop smoking at least 8 weeks prior to surgery. For more urgent surgical procedures, have patients stop smoking immediately and prescribe nicotine substitutes throughout their hospitalization to ease the postoperative nicotine withdrawal symptoms.

K E Y   P O I N T S

▶ The pathophysiology of COPD is airflow obstruction from chronic bronchitis, emphysema, and other diseases that cause airway narrowing.

▶ The mainstays of evaluation are PFT and ABGs.

▶ Moderate to severe COPD can significantly increase morbidity and mortality in surgical patients.

CASE 27-4. A 65-year-old man returns to your clinic for follow-up 4 weeks after discharge from a hospitalization for a COPD exacerbation. The patient has finished a tapering course of steroids and a 2-week course of antibiotics. He reports that he feels well and his sputum production and exercise tolerance have returned to his baseline. He received the pneumococcal vaccine 2 years ago at the time of his COPD diagnosis.

A. Knowing that several pathogens can lead to a COPD exacerbation, including pseudomonas, influenza, and *Haemophilus influenzae* type B, what preventive therapy do you recommend at this time?

CASE 27-5. A 38-year-old man with a smoking history presents to your office with a 6-month history of slowly progressive dyspnea on exertion. Physical exam reveals a barrel-chested man with a prolonged expiratory phase and scattered wheezes on chest auscultation. Chest radiograph and PFT are consistent with a diagnosis of COPD.

A. What laboratory test might be helpful in determining an etiology for his symptoms?

CASE 27-6. A 70-year-old man with a history of severe COPD comes to you with complaints of night-time insomnia and anxiety. His current medications include albuterol, ipratropium (Atrovent), prednisone, and theophylline, and they have been stable for several weeks. Physical exam reveals a resting pulse of 90 beats/min and a fine tremor in his outstretched hands. Your differential diagnosis includes hyperthyroidism, hypoglycemia, an acute coronary syndrome, or elevated levels of theophylline.

A. What test do you order next?

LUNG CANCER

▶ ETIOLOGY

Each year, 170,000 new cases of lung cancer are diagnosed in the United States. Although lung cancer is the second most prevalent cancer in both men and women, behind prostate cancer and breast cancer, respectively, it remains the leading cause of death from cancer for both men and women. It is a disease of smokers because roughly 80% of lung cancers are related to smoking. Smoking is also a risk factor for many other conditions, including COPD, coronary artery disease, peripheral vascular disease, and other cancers. Given this, it is no wonder that patients with lung cancer also have other comorbidities and can require surgical management for their lung cancer and for other diseases. The purpose of this section is to outline the diagnosis and staging of lung cancer, review basic treatment strategies, and highlight how the patient with lung cancer requires special attention when presenting with a surgical disease that is not related to the lung cancer.

▶ EVALUATION

How do lung cancer patients present?

The patient with lung cancer presents with two types of complaints: local lung disease and systemic manifestations.

The symptoms of localized lung disease include shortness of breath, cough, hemoptysis, chest pain, and fever. Hemoptysis is a particularly worrisome symptom. Elderly patients with a long smoking history who present with hemoptysis should be assumed to have lung cancer until proven otherwise and should undergo a thorough evaluation to find the source of hemoptysis.

Another typical initial presentation is the patient who presents with fever, productive cough, and a chest radiograph infiltrate that does not improve with antibiotic therapy or improves initially and then worsens again when antibiotic therapy is discontinued. This so-called postobstructive pneumonia occurs when an endobronchial obstruction from tumor allows purulent secretions to pool behind it, making clearance of these secretions impossible and the resulting pneumonia difficult to treat.

What are the systemic manifestations of lung cancer?

Systemic manifestations of lung cancer occur when local invasion or metastatic cancer is present. The symptoms of local invasion include the superior vena cava (SVC) syndrome, Pancoast's syndrome, Horner's syndrome, and clavicular lymphadenopathy.

SVC syndrome occurs when extrinsic compression or invasion of the SVC by tumor or related thrombosis blocks venous return from the head and upper extremities back into the right atrium. This impedance to venous return results in headache and venous congestion with facial edema and plethora. Initially, these symptoms and signs may occur only after the patient has lain flat for several hours such as when sleeping overnight. The facial puffiness may resolve quickly in this early case, often within a couple of hours. As the tumor advances, so does the obstruction, and the symptoms become more severe and constant.

Tumor invasion from an upper lobe into the brachial plexus as it courses from the neck through the shoulder, with or without involvement of the cervical sympathetic chain, causes Pancoast's syndrome. Severe shoulder or arm pain and brachial plexus neuropathies are the main findings of this syndrome. Horner's syndrome may occur as part of Pancoast's syndrome or by itself when apical tumor invasion or malignant lymphadenopathy involves the nerves of the cervical sympathetic chain. Signs of Horner's syndrome in its full form include unilateral facial anhidrosis (i.e., loss of sweating), ptosis, and miosis. The full expression of Horner's syndrome, however, rarely is seen with lung cancer. Horner's syndrome from lung cancer can be accompanied by hoarseness. The presence of hoarseness signals recurrent laryngeal nerve involvement with unilateral vocal cord paralysis. When vocal cord paralysis is present, the tumor is no longer resectable.

Metastatic disease may present with symptoms from malignant invasion of other organs or from symptoms of paraneoplastic syndromes. Metastatic disease to the bone or liver can cause local bony pain or abdominal pain, respectively. Metastases to the brain can cause headache, seizure, or focal neurologic deficits. The paraneoplastic syndromes are found with the neuroendocrine active tumors of small cell carcinoma of the lung. These syndromes include the syndrome of inappropriate antidiuretic hormone release (SIADH), Cushing's syndrome, cerebellar ataxia, dementia syndromes, and sensorimotor neuropathies. Other symptoms common with advanced lung cancer include fatigue, malaise, and cachexia.

How is lung cancer diagnosed and staged?

Once a patient presents with a clinical history suggestive of lung cancer, the goal of further work-up is to diagnose the type of lung cancer and accurately estimate the extent of disease. Once these factors are known, the patient can be appropriately staged and therapeutic decisions made. The work-up begins with a careful history and physical examination of the patient, looking for signs of local or metastatic spread. Evidence of disease spread radically changes both therapeutic options and prognosis.

Chest radiography should be obtained concurrently with the initial history and physical exam. The chest radiograph can give preliminary information on the size and number of pulmonary nodules, it can hint at hilar adenopathy suggestive of local metastasis, and it can reveal the presence of a cancer-related postobstructive pneumonia. If these first steps lead to a likely cancer diagnosis, the next step is to verify the malignant diagnosis and begin the evaluation of its extent.

The precise diagnosis of malignancy can be made only by obtaining and analyzing tissue. With lung cancers, procuring tissue can be done in several ways. The least invasive of these methods is by cytologic confirmation of malignancy from a sputum sample. Other means of obtaining tissue for diagnosis include fine-needle aspiration of a pulmonary nodule under CT guidance, malignant lymph node fine-needle aspiration or biopsy, or bronchoscopic biopsy of a central lesion. As tissue diagnosis is pursued, the patient should also undergo preliminary tests to determine the extent of disease.

Determining which tests are needed to evaluate disease spread depends on the findings up to this point in the work-up. All patients with suspected lung cancer should undergo CT scanning of the thorax and abdomen. Chest CT delineates the local spread of disease by defining which lung lobes are involved; how large the main mass is; whether there are local satellite lesions and where they are located; whether there is suspicious hilar adenopathy; and whether other structures such as the pleura, pericardium, or great vessels are involved. Abdominal CT evaluates the liver and adrenal glands for the presence of metastasis. Patients with musculoskeletal complaints should undergo bone scanning to look for bony metastasis. Any patient with focal neurologic complaints, altered mental status, persistent headache, or seizure should undergo CT of the head to evaluate for brain metastasis. Serum sampling for elevated calcium, aspartate aminotransferase (AST), and alkaline phosphatase levels and for anemia can hint at underlying metastatic disease. In some cases, positron emission tomography can help evaluate the extent of disease. However, its exact role in the diagnosis and staging of lung cancer has yet to be defined.

Once the results of the history, physical exam, laboratory studies, imaging, and tissue diagnostic studies are available, the patient can be staged clinically according to the most recent revision of the International Staging System. This system relies on the TNM nomenclature, where *T* refers to the size of the primary tumor and its location, *N* refers to any possible lymph node involvement, and *M* is used to denote the presence or absence of metastatic disease. From this classification, the stage of disease can be deduced and the 5-year survival with therapy can be inferred.

If the history, physical exam, imaging studies, and chemistries suggest that the patient has a clinically low stage and a potentially resectable lung cancer, the next step is either mediastinoscopy or video-assisted thoracotomy. Rarely, these tests acquire tissue for diagnosis, but the usual goal of these tests is to verify that there is no locally invasive disease that would preclude the patient from a curative surgery. It also allows for further pathologic staging, which can refine therapeutic options and better estimate 5-year patient survival. In a subset of cases, these procedures can be bypassed and the patient can proceed directly to lung resection. For a summary of the International Staging System for lung cancer, refer to Table 27–1.

▶ TREATMENT

The treatment options available to patients with lung cancer depend on the type of cancer present and on the depth of its invasion. Four main types of lung cancer exist. These include squamous cell carcinoma, adenocarcinoma, large cell (anaplastic) carcinoma, and small cell (oat cell) carcinoma. For prognostic and therapeutic reasons, squamous cell carcinoma, adenocarcinoma, and large cell carcinoma are grouped together and referred to as non-small cell lung carcinoma (NSCLC). This categorization is possible because these different histologic types have similar clinical courses and responses to therapy. These cancers make up approximately 80% of all primary lung cancers, whereas small cell carcinoma makes up the remaining 20%.

What are the treatment options?

Treatment options include surgery, radiation therapy, and chemotherapy. Which treatment is offered depends on the type of cancer (small cell vs. NSCLC) and the stage of disease. A detailed review of lung cancer treatment options is beyond the scope of this chapter. Refer to Table 27–2 for estimates of 5-year survival with treatment by stage of disease.

What are the prognoses for lung cancer?

Traditionally, NSCLC has a more indolent course and better response to therapy than small cell carcinoma, and stages I, II, and, rarely, IIIA disease is surgically curable. Patients with more advanced-stage disease have a poor prognosis and small hope of long-term survival. These patients may benefit from palliative chemotherapy and radiation therapy, but this is controversial. However, more than half of patients with NSCLC have extrapulmonary disease at presentation and a concomitant 5-year survival of less than 10%. Only 20% of patients with NSCLC present with surgically curable disease. High TNM staging, poor performance status, weight loss of more than 5% of body weight, and, possibly, male gender each conveys a poorer prognosis for NSCLC.

Small cell carcinoma is an aggressive cancer and is almost always metastatic at the time of diagnosis and not surgically resectable. Risk factors for a worse prognosis with small cell lung cancer include poor performance status, younger age, elevated low-density lipoprotein, and hemoglobin less than 11 g/dL. Small cell lung

TABLE 27–1

AJCC TNM Staging System for Lung Cancer

Primary Tumor (T)

TX   Primary tumor cannot be assessed, or tumor proven by the presence of malignant cells in sputum or bronchial washings but not visualized by imaging or bronchoscopy

T0   No evidence of primary tumor

Tis   Carcinoma *in situ*

T1   Tumor 3 cm or less in greatest dimension, surrounded by lung or visceral pleura, without bronchoscopic evidence of invasion more proximal than the lobar bronchus,[*] (i.e., not in the main bronchus)

T2   Tumor with any of the following features of size or extent:
         More than 3 cm in greatest dimension
         Involves main bronchus, 2 cm or more distal to the carina
         Invades the visceral pleura
         Associated with atelectasis or obstructive pneumonitis that extends to the hilar region but does not involve the entire lung

T3   Tumor of any size that directly invades any of the following: chest wall (including superior sulcus tumors), diaphragm, mediastinal pleura, parietal pericardium; or tumor in the main bronchus less than 2 cm distal to the carina, but without involvement of the carina; or associated atelectasis or obstructive pneumonitis of the entire lung

T4   Tumor of any size that invades any of the following: mediastinum, heart, great vessels, trachea, esophagus, vertebral body, carina; or separate tumor nodules in the same lobe; or tumor with malignant pleural effusion[**]

[*]*Note*: The uncommon superficial tumor of any size with its invasive component limited to the bronchial wall, which may extend proximal to the main bronchus, is also classified T1.

[**]*Note*: Most pleural effusions associated with lung cancer are due to tumor. However, there are a few patients in whom multiple cytopathologic examinations of pleural fluid are negative for tumor. In these cases, fluid is nonbloody and is not an exudate. Such patients may be further evaluated by videothoracoscopy (VATS) and direct pleural biopsies. When these elements and clinical judgment dictate that the effusion is not related to the tumor, the effusion should be excluded as a staging element and the patient should be staged T1, T2, or T3.

Regional Lymph Nodes (N)

NX   Regional lymph nodes cannot be assessed

N0   No regional lymph node metastasis

N1   Metastasis to ipsilateral peribronchial and/or ipsilateral hilar lymph nodes, and intrapulmonary nodes including involvement by direct extension of the primary tumor

N2   Metastasis to ipsilateral mediastinal and/or subcarinal lymph nodes(s)

N3   Metastasis to contralateral mediastinal, contralateral hilar, ipsilateral or contralateral scalene, or supraclavicular lymph nodes(s)

Distant Metastasis (M)

MX   Distant metastasis cannot be assessed

M0   No distant metastasis

M1   Distant metastasis present

Note: M1 includes separate tumor nodule(s) in a different lobe (ipsilateral or contralateral).

continued

Table 27–1. AJCC TNM Staging System for Lung Cancer *continued*

Stage Grouping

Occult Carcinoma	TX	N0	M0
Stage 0	Tis	N0	M0
Stage IA	T1	N0	M0
Stage IB	T2	N0	M0
Stage IIA	T1	N1	M0
Stage IIB	T2	N1	M0
	T3	N0	M0
Stage IIIA	T1	N2	M0
	T2	N2	M0
	T3	N1	M0
	T3	N2	M0
Stage IIIB	Any T	N3	M0
	T4	Any N	M0
Stage IV	Any T	Any N	M1

Used with the permission of the American Joint Committee on Cancer (AJCC), Chicago, Illinois. The original source for this material is the *AJCC Cancer Staging Manual, Sixth Edition* (2002) published by Springer-Verlag New York, www.springer-ny.com.

TABLE 27–2

Lung Cancer: Survival with Treatment by TNM Stage

Stage	TNM Subset	5-Year Survival (%)	
		Clinical TNM	*Pathologic TNM*
1A	T1, N0, M0	61	67
1B	T2, N0, M0	38	57
IIA	T1, N1, M0	34	55
IIB	T2, N1, M0	24	39
	T3, N0, M0	22	38
IIIA	T3, N1, M0	9	25
	T1–3, N2, M0	13	23
IIIB	T4, N0–2, M0	7	—
	Any T, N3, M0	3	—
IV	Any T, any N, M1	1	—

Adapted from Mountain CF: A new international staging system for lung cancer. Chest 89:225–233, 1986.

cancer has a dismal prognosis, and palliative therapy to improve the quality of remaining life is the only reasonable therapeutic option.

How does a diagnosis of lung cancer affect decision making for other surgical diseases?

The surgeon, faced with the patient with known lung cancer who is presenting with an additional surgical disease, has several considerations to ponder when evaluating the risks and benefits of a surgical procedure. The first of these considerations is how urgent and necessary is the procedure, given the patient's health status and lung cancer history. If the lung cancer will severely debilitate the patient or take the life of the patient before the other untreated surgical disease would, then there is little justification for offering the procedure.

Another consideration is what additional risk of procedure is levied on the patient with lung cancer. Patients with lung cancer are frequently long-time smokers. Smokers can have additional medical problems such as COPD, coronary artery disease, and other vascular disease that could potentially increase their risk of postoperative morbidity and mortality. Additionally, the consequences of lung cancer itself can lend to increased risk for postoperative mortality. An example of this is found in the cachectic lung cancer patient who has hypoalbuminemia. Hypoalbuminemia is an independent prognostic indicator and, when present, correlates with an increased mortality.

The ability to weigh all of these considerations adequately and to convey the true risks and benefits of surgery to the patient with lung cancer requires knowledge by the surgeon of the basic staging, prognosis, and treatment of lung cancer. The surgeon also needs to know the risks, benefits, and expected result of any other surgical procedure as well as how to accurately predict the postoperative risk conveyed by any other comorbidities that the lung cancer patient may have. A surgeon with this knowledge base will be able to offer efficacious therapy to lung cancer patients with minimal risk for a bad outcome.

K E Y   P O I N T S

▶ Lung cancer is the second most common cancer in both men and women.

▶ Lung cancer is the first cause of cancer death in men and women.

▶ The two major divisions of lung cancer are non-small cell (adenocarcinoma, squamous cell, and large cell [anaplastic]) and small cell (oat cell) carcinoma.

▶ NSCLCs have a better prognosis.

CASE 27-7.

A 60-year-old male smoker presents with complaints of right shoulder pain, tingling paresthesias of the right upper extremity, and blurred vision. Physical exam reveals asymmetrical pupils with a right-sided ptosis, clavicular adenopathy, and right upper extremity sensory loss.

A. What lung cancer syndrome is this, and what are the characteristics of other atypical presentations of lung cancer?

CASE 27-8.

A 53-year-old woman presented 6 weeks ago with fever, productive cough, and a right lower lobe infiltrate. Antibiotic therapy initially improved her symptoms. She returns now complaining of continued cough, fever, and new abdominal pain. Laboratory tests are remarkable for an elevated AST and a mild anemia. Further work-up reveals a NSCLC.

A. What is her most likely clinical stage at diagnosis?

CASE 27-9.

A 45-year-old male smoker presents for possible resection of a pulmonary nodule. While taking the history, the patient admits to a 15 kg-weight gain in the last 3 months and persistent fatigue. Physical exam reveals a moon-faced, obese male with ecchymoses over his forearms and striae across his abdomen.

A. What is the most likely type of lung cancer that he has?

PNEUMONIA

▶ ETIOLOGY

Pneumonia is a common infectious disease. It is the leading cause of death from an infectious disease and the sixth leading cause of death in the United States. It occurs when pathogens infect the normally sterile distal air spaces of the lungs.

What is the pathophysiology of pneumonia?

The lung maintains the sterility of the alveolar air spaces with a host of defenses. These defenses start with the hairs that line the nasal passages and trap larger airborne particles as they are inhaled. Further on in the nasopharynx, pharynx, and larynx, the mucosa is coated with antimicrobial opsonins such as IgA and fibronectin and ringed with lymphatic tissue rich with infection-fighting leukocytes. Mucus-producing cells and ciliated cells line the pharynx, larynx, trachea, and bronchi. The continually produced mucus traps any deposited particulate matter, and the ciliated cells' beating moves this mucus upward into the pharynx where it is either expectorated or swallowed. Sneezing, coughing, and glottic closure reflexes further protect the airways from the entry of particulate matter.

The distal air spaces contain opsonin-rich fluid and alveolar macrophages, which clear the potentially infectious agents that reach this area. Infection-fighting polymorphonucleocytes and lymphocytes also inhabit the distal air spaces. The alveolar interstitium contains lymphatics that drain the interstitium back to lymph nodes so that any pathogen infecting the distal air spaces can be presented and an inflammatory response initiated. It is the inflammatory response that is responsible for the signs and symptoms of pneumonia.

Pulmonary pathogens infect the alveolar spaces and cause pneumonia through three possible routes. The most common of these is aspiration of pathogens that inhabit the upper airway. Aspiration of upper airway secretions occurs in up to half of normal adults during sleep. Patients with impaired consciousness from medications, alcohol, or illness or with neurologic impairment aspirate more frequently and with higher inocula than normal subjects. Mechanical obstructions with nasogastric tubes, nasal trumpets, and endotracheal tubes also increase the risk for aspiration.

Although the distal air spaces are sterile, the more proximal oral and nasopharyngeal air spaces are not. Bacteria, viruses, and fungi, depending on the season of the year and on the health and location of the affected individual, inhabit these areas. Normal hosts carry the potential pulmonary pathogens *Streptococcus pneumoniae*, *Haemophilus influenzae*, *Staphylococcus aureus*, *Moraxella catarrhalis*, and *Streptococcus pyogenes*. In normal community-dwelling hosts, gram-negative bacterial colonization is rare. However, the prevalence of gram-negative bacterial colonization increases with hospitalization, worsening debility, age, heavy alcohol use, diabetes, and communal living. Anaerobic bacteria also colonize the upper respiratory tract in the gingival crevices and plaque of the teeth. Edentulous patients, for this reason, are less susceptible to anaerobic infections.

The second route of pulmonary infection is through inhalation of aerosolized pathogens. Particles 3 to 5 μm in diameter are small enough to be inhaled directly into the distal air spaces, bypassing the defenses of the upper respiratory tract. These particles carry one or two pathogens and are capable of initiating infection. Organisms that cause infections via this route include *Mycobacterium tuberculosis*, influenza viruses, *Legionella pneumophila*, *Coccidioides immitis*, and *Histoplasma capsulatum*.

The final route of pulmonary infection is hematogenous spread. Patients with infective endocarditis, septic thrombophlebitis, or indwelling lines are at risk for developing pulmonary septic emboli and pneumonia from their concurrent infections.

▶ EVALUATION

What historical points are important in the evaluation of pneumonia?

With pneumonia, identifying the causative pathogen and instituting appropriate therapy quickly are the keys to successful treatment. However, current diagnostic tests cannot identify the pathogen in many cases, nor do they identify the pathogen prior to the initial prescription of antibiotic therapy. Therapeutic decisions must be made empirically based on the likely pathogen. The history and characteristics of the patient are important in identifying the likely pathogen and instituting successful empirical therapy.

Children are susceptible to *S. pneumoniae*, *H. influenzae*, and viruses such as respiratory syncytial virus and influenza A and B. Normal adults living in the community typically contract pneumonia from *S. pneumoniae*, *Mycoplasma pneumoniae*, *L. pneumophila*, and *Chlamydia pneumoniae*. Hospitalized adults or adults in communal living situations are more likely to have gram-negative infections. Immunocompromised patients such as those with human immunodeficiency virus (HIV), chronic steroid use, or immunosuppressive states from organ transplantation or chemotherapy can be infected with rarer pathogens such as *Pneumocystis carinii* (PCP), *Nocardia asteroides*, *Stenotrophomonas maltophilia*, *M. tuberculosis*, cytomegalovirus, or *Aspergillus*. Patients from the Midwest or Southwest United States can contract the fungal infections histoplasmosis and coccidioidomycosis, respectively. Finally, bird fanciers are susceptible to psittacosis infections.

What symptoms are suggestive of pneumonia?

The classic symptoms of pneumonia include fever, cough, and purulent sputum production. More systemic symptoms such as headache, myalgias, malaise, and gastrointestinal upset are common. Severe infections or infections in patients with underlying pulmonary disease cause shortness of breath or even respiratory distress.

Previously, pneumonia was classified into two syndromes: typical and atypical. Typical pneumonia was characterized by acute onset of productive cough, fever, and dyspnea. Atypical pneumonia was more indolent with a dry cough and more systemic symptoms such as headache, myalgias, and nausea. Classification of these syndromes was thought to be useful to separate patients based on the pathogens that caused these different presentations. However, recent studies have failed to show the usefulness of this classification system, and the classification of pneumonia as typical or atypical is falling out of favor.

What physical findings are suggestive of pneumonia?

Vital sign abnormalities found in pneumonia include fever, tachycardia, tachypnea, and, in severe cases, hypotension. Oxygen saturation may be low depending on the severity of disease and on any underlying pulmonary pathology. Hosts able to mount an inflammatory response have more physical exam findings. Immunocompromised patients or elderly patients who are incapable of brisk inflammatory responses may not mount a fever or have signs of pneumonia other than an altered sensorium. Chest exam in hosts who can mount an inflammatory response can show localized decreased breath sounds, dullness to percussion, tactile fremitus, egophony, rales, and rhonchi. Signs of dehydration from fever and poor oral intake such as orthostasis, dry mucous membranes, and poor skin turgor may be present. Patients with lung abscesses may have halitosis as a sign of their underlying anaerobic infection. Certain infectious agents such as measles and varicella viruses show characteristic rashes.

What laboratory studies are helpful in the diagnosis of pneumonia?

Leukocytosis is common but not necessary in patients with pneumonia. Leukopenia, especially in immunocompromised patients, is also seen. Chemistry findings in pneumonia can include hyponatremia from SIADH or hypernatremia from dehydration. Worsening hyperglycemia is often seen in infected diabetic patients.

Sputum Gram stains and cultures can be helpful in identifying the infecting organism, but how helpful they are remains controversial. The controversy surrounds the sensitivity and specificity of the test. A sputum Gram stain and culture requires the patient to cough secretions from the distal air spaces into the oral pharynx and then expectorate the secretions into a specimen cup. The upper airways and oral pharynx are colonized with bacteria, many of which can be pathogenic. These colonizers can interfere with the test either by making the true pathogen difficult to identify or by overgrowing the culture medium and hiding the true pathogen. Delays in the specimen's reaching the lab or mishandling of the specimen can further decrease the utility of the test. Regardless, a good sputum sample that contains more than 25 polymorphonucleocytes per high-power field and fewer than 10 epithelial cells can yield diagnostic information.

ABGs are helpful to identify patients with respiratory failure and in need of hospitalization or intensive care unit (ICU)-level care. Severe pneumonia can cause hypoxia and a respiratory acidosis.

What are the radiographic findings in pneumonia?

Chest radiography in pneumonia can reveal localized opacification that is characteristic of bacterial pneumonia or the diffuse infiltrates that are typical of viral or PCP pneumonia. Infiltrates located in the bases or in the posterior segments of the upper lobes are typical of aspiration pneumonia. Upper lobe opacities are characteristic of reactivation tuberculosis. Lucent areas with air-fluid levels within opacified areas signify lung abscess. Pleural effusions can signal the presence of a parapneumonic process or empyema.

Plain radiography is the test of choice for diagnosis and following the progression of pneumonia, although there are limitations with its use. The severity of disease on radiograph does not predict the severity of disease clinically because patients with impressive infiltrates on radiograph can have minimal symptoms and vice versa. Also, a patient with clinically resolved pneumonia may not clear radiographic infiltrates for up to 6 weeks.

Chest CT is a useful adjunct to plain radiography. It can help separate lung consolidation from pleural effusions and help rule out other disease processes that can mimic or cause pneumonia such as lung cancer, sarcoidosis, and pulmonary edema.

What other tests are helpful for the identification of pathogens?

In the patient with critical illness from pneumonia, persistent symptoms despite antibiotic therapy, or recurrent symptoms after treatment, further diagnostic work-up is indicated. Options for work-up include bronchoscopy, transtracheal aspiration, percutaneous needle aspiration, open lung biopsy, and serologic testing.

Bronchoscopy allows direct visualization of the airways and the recovery of pulmonary material with less nasopharyngeal contamination than sputum Gram staining and culture. Alveolar fluid can be sampled either with the protected brush method or by bronchoalveolar lavage. With the protected brush method, a sheath-covered brush is passed into the lung parenchyma, uncovered, and then passed over the airway mucosa. The brush is then retracted back into its sheath and removed for analysis. Bronchoalveolar lavage entails passing the distal end of the bronchoscope down the divisions of the pulmonary tree until the tip wedges. After wedging of the tip, boluses of saline are flushed into the distal lung and then aspirated back. This sample is then centrifuged for Gram staining and culture. Finally, bronchoscopy can be used to biopsy lung parenchyma for further diagnosis of pneumonia or other pulmonary processes. Bronchoscopy can improve the diagnostic yield, but it cannot reveal the pathogen in every case. Patients on antibiotics are much less likely to have a diagnostic bronchoscopy.

Transtracheal aspiration and percutaneous needle aspiration with their high risk for complications are rarely used. Transtracheal aspiration involves percutaneous sampling of tracheal secretions by perforating the cricothyroid membrane, whereas needle aspiration entails passing a thin needle through the chest wall into a consolidated area using CT guidance. These procedures carry significant risks such as pneumothorax and bleeding.

Open lung biopsy is performed if other tests have been nondiagnostic or if the involved lung segment cannot be sampled with other techniques. It allows direct sampling of air space secretions and tissue with recovery of more tissue than can be sampled with bronchoscopic biopsy. Lung biopsy can be done with a traditional thoracotomy or with the less invasive video-assisted techniques.

Serologic studies can be performed for various pathogens. Testing for *Legionella* species, cytomegalovirus, endemic fungi, and other organisms completes the diagnostic testing and complements sputum studies and bronchoscopy.

▶ TREATMENT

How is pneumonia treated?

Ideally, pathogen-directed antimicrobials should be prescribed. However, initial therapy based on the history of the patient should begin prior to the return of sputum cultures. Several organizations have developed guidelines for treating pneumonia. The most recent published guidelines for community-acquired pneumonia come from the American Thoracic Society (ATS). These guidelines recommend therapy based on the patient's comorbidities (cardiopulmonary disease), severity of pneumonia (requiring outpatient care, hospitalization, ICU monitoring), and risk for drug-resistant or more virulent organisms (*Pseudomonas*, drug-resistant pneumococci). The ATS used combinations of these categories to develop four treatment groups.

The first of these groups includes adults treated as outpatients who have no significant comorbidities. Empirical therapy of this group aims at covering the most common pathogens that infect this group, including *S. pneumoniae*, *M. pneumoniae*, *C. pneumoniae*, and *H. influenzae*. Antibiotics recommended for empirical therapy for this group include the macrolides, azithromycin or clarithromycin, or the less expensive antibiotic doxycycline.

The second category includes patients treated as outpatients but who have significant cardiopulmonary disease or disease-modifying risk factors such as nosocomial infections, older age, alcoholism, exposure to day-care centers, or other immune-suppressive illnesses.

These patients are at risk for the pathogens encountered by the first group but additionally have increased risk for gram-negative infections, drug-resistant pneumococcal infections, and anaerobic infections. An antipneumococcal fluoroquinolone or combination therapy with a β-lactam plus a macrolide or doxycycline is recommended for this disease category. Antipneumococcal fluoroquinolones include ciprofloxacin, ofloxacin, levofloxacin, sparfloxacin, gatifloxacin, and moxifloxacin. The availability of levofloxacin, ciprofloxacin, and gatifloxacin as oral agents makes these the preferred quinolones for outpatient therapy.

Hospitalization for treatment of pneumonia in today's cost-saving climate indicates that the patient has risk factors, clinical indicators, or laboratory findings that suggest a more virulent course and increased risk of mortality from this pneumonia. Alternatively, the patient may be unable to comply with outpatient treatment for a variety of reasons. Inpatients not requiring ICU care should have a step up from the oral outpatient regimens to regimens that contain IV antibiotics. Inpatients without comorbidities or risk factors for gram-negative or drug-resistant pneumococcal infections should receive IV azithromycin. Alternative regimens include monotherapy with an antipneumococcal fluoroquinolone or combination therapy with doxycycline and a β-lactam antibiotic.

Inpatients with comorbidities or risk factors for drug-resistant pneumococcal infections or gram-negative infections should receive an IV β-lactam such as cefotaxime, ceftriaxone, ampicillin/sulbactam, or high-dose ampicillin in addition to a macrolide or doxycycline. An alternative regimen is an IV antipneumococcal fluoroquinolone. Levofloxacin has equivalent bioavailability whether it is given intravenously or orally. This feature allows early transition to oral therapy and can shorten hospital stay in appropriate patients.

The third category of patients requiring ICU admission have fulminant disease and often are infected with virulent pathogens such as *S. pneumoniae* (including drug-resistant pneumococci), *Legionella*, *S. aureus*, *H. influenzae*, enteric gram-negative bacteria, and *Pseudomonas aeruginosa*. Patients with immunosuppression from other diseases such as HIV or from immunosuppressive medications are at additional risk for viral infections, opportunistic infections, and infections with endemic fungi. The guidelines offer therapy recommendations for patients with and without risk factors for *P. aeruginosa* infections. Risk factors for pseudomonal infections include malnutrition, structural lung disease such as bronchiectasis, prolonged corticosteroid therapy, and recent use of broad-spectrum antibiotics.

Patients without risk factors for pseudomonal infections should receive an IV β-lactam in addition to either an IV macrolide or an IV fluoroquinolone. Patients with risk factors for pseudomonal infection should be prescribed two antipseudomonal antibiotics plus an antibiotic with *Mycoplasma* and *Legionella* coverage. Examples of such regimens include an antipseudomonal β-lactam (cefepime, ceftazidime, imipenem, meropenem, piperacillin/tazobactam) and an IV fluoroquinlone. A second alternative is three-drug therapy with an

IV antipseudomonal β-lactam plus an aminoglycoside and either an IV macrolide or antipseudomonal fluoroquinolone.

The fourth group are those patients with nosocomial pneumonia, which is defined as pneumonia contracted by patients living in communal living situations such as hospitalized patients or patients residing in skilled nursing facilities. These patients are at increased risk for aspiration and for gram-negative or drug-resistant bacterial infections. Initial antibiotic therapy should cover these possibilities. Antifungal therapy should be considered in patients with a new pneumonia while undergoing broad-spectrum antibiotic therapy, in immunocompromised patients with persistent fevers despite antibiotic therapy, and in those patients with positive fungal blood cultures.

Once diagnostic tests indicate a likely pathogen, therapy can be directed toward eradicating that pathogen. Diagnostic information also may encourage treatment of a pathogen not suspected on initial clinical evaluation, such as a viral or fungal pneumonia.

The goal of pneumonia therapy is not only eradication of the infecting organism but also symptomatic relief. Various medications can be used to make the patient more comfortable, including antipyretics, antiemetics, and cough suppressants.

What are the surgical considerations in the treatment of pneumonia?

Pneumonia is a known postoperative complication of many surgical procedures, and pneumonia can increase the risk of surgical morbidity and mortality if it is present preoperatively for certain procedures such as thoracotomy. Vigilance for the signs and symptoms of pneumonia and prompt institution of therapy improve the outcome for surgical patients.

Another important consideration is where a surgical patient with pneumonia should be monitored. This is especially important when busy operating and clinic schedules limit the surgeon's time with any given patient. Patients requiring mechanical ventilation, who have septic shock requiring pressor therapy, who have an increase in the size of their pulmonary infiltrates by 50% within 48 hours, or who have acute renal failure in the absence of chronic renal failure should be monitored in the ICU. Other patients with less clear indications such as a respiratory rate greater than 30 breaths/min, a Pao_2/Fio_2* ratio of less than 250, bilateral or multilobar pneumonia, systolic blood pressure less than 90 mm Hg, or a diastolic blood pressure less than 60 mm Hg should be considered for ICU admission. This is especially true for postoperative patients who may still have a nasogastric tube in place, who may be taking sensorium-altering narcotics for pain relief, and who may have difficulty with performing pulmonary toilet.

---

*Fio_2 is fraction of inspired oxygen.

> ### K E Y   P O I N T S
>
> ▶ Pneumonia is an infection of the alveolar air space via aspiration, inhalation, or hematogenous spread of infectious agents.
>
> ▶ The diagnosis of pneumonia should be suspected in patients with fever, elevated white blood cell count, and changed sputum.
>
> ▶ Empirical treatment should be based on the overall medical fitness of the patient and whether the infection is community acquired versus nosocomial.

CASE 27–10. You are called to see a healthy 60-year-old old man admitted today from home in anticipation of his radical prostatectomy for prostate cancer. The patient reports that he has had a 3-day history of productive cough, fever, and malaise. He attributes it to a cold that he caught from his wife. He would like some cough syrup and a sleeping pill. You review his vital sign log and examine him. He has a low-grade temperature but otherwise has normal vital signs. He appears flushed and mildly diaphoretic but otherwise well. He coughs through your attempt to auscultate his chest, but you think you hear rales in his right lower lung field. A chest radiograph confirms your suspicion and reveals an infiltrate in his right base.

A. What is appropriate antibiotic therapy for this patient?

CASE 27–11. You are called to see a 46-year-old woman for oxygen desaturation. She has been hospitalized for 8 days after undergoing an emergent open cholecystectomy for gangrenous cholecystitis. Her postoperative course has been complicated by respiratory failure requiring mechanical ventilation. You evaluate the patient and note that she has a low-grade temperature today and that her oxygen saturations have fallen to 92% from 100% while her ventilator is set to deliver an FiO_2 of 40%. Her chest exam has coarse rhonchi throughout. Her suction canister attached to her endotracheal tube contains purulent secretions. You review

continued

CASE 27–11. *continued*

her lab reports and chest radiograph and note that she has a
persistent leukocytosis and bilateral basilar infiltrates that
have progressed since her morning chest radiograph. You
diagnose a nosocomial pneumonia.

A. What is appropriate antibiotic therapy for this patient?

CASE 27–12. A 62-year-old male smoker presents
to you with a 3-month history of productive cough, malaise,
and weight loss. He has been unable to work for the last week
because of his symptoms. He has received two courses of
antibiotic therapy for a right middle lobe infiltrate. With each
course of antibiotics his symptoms have improved, only to
recur with discontinuation of the antibiotics. His last course
completed a little over 1 week ago. The patient is otherwise
healthy and takes only an aspirin because "another doctor
told me it was good for me." He is frustrated at his illness and
seeks more therapy so he can return to his job at a nursing
home. His physical exam reveals a thin man in no apparent
distress. Vital signs, including his temperature, are normal.
Lung exam is notable for rhonchi over the right anterior
chest. Chest radiograph reveals obliteration of the right heart
border by a right middle lobe infiltrate.

A. What should your next step be?

RESPIRATORY FAILURE

▶ ETIOLOGY

Respiratory failure is the final common pathway of many pulmonary
and some nonpulmonary diseases. It is also a common complication
of surgery. Respiratory failure can be divided into two categories: oxygenation failure and ventilatory failure. Understanding of these pathologic processes requires an understanding of normal lung function.

How do normal lungs function?

The lungs help with many physiologic processes. The lung's alveolar surfaces provide the interface between air and blood, allowing

for oxygenation of the blood to take place. These surfaces also allow the diffusion of carbon dioxide from blood to air space that, when followed by exhalation, allows the body to expel the CO_2 entirely. CO_2 is not only a waste product of the body's metabolism but also a regulator of the body's acid-base status. By expelling CO_2, the lungs contribute to maintaining the body's acid-base homeostasis. This is particularly true in acute conditions because the lungs can quickly regulate serum CO_2 and thus serum pH, whereas the other organs important for acid-base homeostasis, the kidneys, cannot. Finally, the lungs serve as a reservoir of air for the bony bellows of the chest and as such supply the airflow that allows for phonation and speech.

How does failure to oxygenate occur?

Oxygenation failure occurs if a pathologic process disrupts the alveolar interface between air spaces and the blood in the pulmonary capillary bed and prevents oxygenation. There are two major processes that can do this. The first is an increase in dead space within the lung. *Dead space* is defined as areas of lung that are ventilated with air but that do not have perfusion by pulmonary capillaries. Examples of diseases that cause oxygenation failure by increasing dead space include emphysema and pulmonary embolus.

The second process that leads to oxygenation failure is an increase in shunting. *Shunting* is defined as any process that leads to mixing of nonoxygenated blood with oxygenated blood before it enters the systemic circulation. It can occur when there are areas of the lung that continue to be perfused by pulmonary capillaries but receive little or no ventilation. Shunting can be caused by diseases of the air spaces within the lung such as acute respiratory diseases, pulmonary edema, or pneumonia or by diseases that divert blood away before it reaches the lungs. Examples of this include a patent foramen ovale, other intracardiac defects such as ventricular septal defects, or hepatic failure.

Patients who present with acute oxygenation failure complain of dyspnea. In mild cases, this may be only with increasing exertion, but patients with more severe failure may present with dyspnea at rest and tachypnea. In extreme cases, patients present with cyanosis, obtundation, and hemodynamic instability as a result of profound hypoxia. Patients with chronic oxygenation failure from diseases such as emphysema and obesity hypoventilation syndrome may be relatively symptomless despite their hypoxia.

How is oxygenation failure detected?

Detection of oxygenation failure relies on measurements of the Pao_2 and on the percutaneously detected oxygen saturation (Sao_2). The Pao_2 is measured by obtaining an ABG from the radial or femoral artery. Errors in measurement can occur if venous blood is mistakenly sampled or in cases of extreme leukocytosis.

Sao_2 is detected by using a sensor placed on the skin to detect the wavelength of blood in superficial vessels. This wavelength depends on the amount of oxygen bound to the hemoglobin found in red blood cells. This measurement of oxygen saturation, with the help of the oxyhemoglobin dissociation curve, allows for estimates of the Pao_2 continuously without the need for a needle stick. Errors in measuring Sao_2 occur if the sensing device is not calibrated correctly, if the patient has dark skin, or if the probe is unable to detect a pulse because of low perfusion of superficial vessels or because of failure of the probe to stick to the skin. Pulse oximetry is also inaccurate when measuring patients with very low Pao_2.

How is oxygenation failure treated?

Treatment of oxygenation failure aims at increasing the oxygen delivery to the blood. Increasing the delivered Fio_2 is the first step. In spontaneously breathing patients, this can be done with various oxygen delivery devices, including nasal cannula, simple face masks, and Venturi masks. Mechanical ventilation can also be used to improve oxygenation as respiratory failure progresses. Not only can the delivered Fio_2 be 100% on the ventilator but manipulation of airway pressures by the ventilator can also improve oxygenation.

The most important aspects of treating oxygenation failure are diagnosing and treating the underlying cause. This is especially true of oxygenation failure caused by shunting, because shunting responds poorly to the previously mentioned therapies.

How does failure to ventilate occur?

Ventilatory failure occurs when the lungs cannot exhale CO_2 adequately, resulting in increases in serum CO_2 and respiratory acidosis. Diseases that interfere with the bellows function of the chest wall and lungs cause ventilatory failure. Lung pathology that restricts airflow or causes obstruction such as COPD, asthma, and pulmonary fibrosis are examples of this. Ventilatory failure from chest wall dysfunction can be seen in the neuromuscular diseases such as myasthenia gravis, amyotrophic lateral sclerosis, and Guillain-Barré syndrome. It can also be seen in conditions that disfigure the chest wall, such as kyphoscoliosis, severe osteoporosis, and traumatic flail chest. A final mechanism that is commonly seen in surgical patients is respiratory depression secondary to medications. Narcotics and benzodiazepines are common culprits due to their heavy use for perioperative pain control and amnesia.

How is ventilatory failure detected?

The CO_2 retention and respiratory acidosis of ventilatory failure can be insidious and difficult to detect. Patients, especially those with chronic CO_2 retention, can be asymptomatic or have mild symptoms such as headache. Breathlessness is rarely a prominent symptom. However, in advanced ventilatory failure, as in profound oxygenation failure, patients can present with obtundation and hemodynamic instability.

Physical exam findings in ventilatory failure are those specific to the individual diseases that caused the ventilatory failure. They include the wheezing, barrel chest, and prolonged expiration of the obstructive diseases (COPD and asthma). Kyphoscoliosis, osteoporosis, and flail chest show chest wall deformities, and the neuromuscular diseases are remarkable for muscular wasting and weakness.

Confirmation of ventilatory failure relies on ABGs. Acute ventilatory failure shows an elevated $Paco_2$ with a low pH, whereas a chronic compensated state shows the elevated $Paco_2$ but a normal or near-normal pH. In intubated patients, an end-tidal CO_2 can be used to monitor for hypercarbia and ventilatory failure. This sensor on the ventilator tubing measures CO_2 at the end of exhalation. This end-tidal CO_2 under normal physiologic conditions comes directly from the alveolar space and as such is in equilibrium with the alveolar capillary CO_2. Under these conditions end-tidal CO_2 approximates arterial CO_2.

Ventilatory failure eventually leads to hypoxia, but this is a late finding after hypercarbia and respiratory acidosis are advanced. For this reason, pulse oximetry is a poor means of monitoring patients at risk for ventilatory failure.

How is ventilatory failure treated?

Treatment of ventilatory failure improves the bellows function of the chest. Most often this is in the form of positive-pressure ventilation. Devices such as biphasic positive airway pressure (BiPAP) machines and ventilators can overcome the weakness of the neuromuscular diseases, add extra push in those with restrictive disease or deformities, and allow stenting open of the airways in the obstructive diseases. Treatment of respiratory depression caused by medications may require temporary positive-pressure ventilation with a mechanical ventilator as the drug effects are allowed to wear off or are reversed with antidotal agents.

What are the surgical considerations of respiratory failure?

Respiratory failure in postoperative patients is defined as respiratory compromise requiring 48 hours or more of mechanical ventilation postoperatively. Surgical patients can have oxygenation or ventilatory failure related to comorbid diseases or as a result of the surgery itself. Risk factors for the development of postoperative respiratory failure include age, type of surgery, type of anesthetic, underlying malignancy, underlying respiratory disease, need for emergent surgery, poor preoperative functional status, and tobacco use. Patients undergoing abdominal aortic repair, thoracic proce-dures, upper abdominal procedures, and peripheral vascular pro-cedures are at the highest risk.

Prevention of postoperative respiratory failure relies on preoper-ative evaluation and treatment and postoperative pulmonary toilet. In patients who smoke and are undergoing elective procedures, smoking cessation should be encouraged preferably at least 8 weeks in advance of the procedure. Patients with unexplained dyspnea or other respiratory symptoms preoperatively should be evaluated and treated for previously undetected pulmonary pathol-ogy prior to surgery. Patients with known respiratory illnesses should be optimized prior to surgery and not have active acute pulmonary symptoms at the time of the operation unless the surgery is emergent. Postoperatively, prevention of pulmonary complica-tions and respiratory failure relies on pulmonary toilet. In intubated patients this entails suctioning and fastidious attention to infection prevention with hand washing and good patient oral care. Extubated patients require adequate pain control, encouragement to clear secretions, incentive spirometry, and continued treatment of any preexisting pulmonary diseases.

K E Y   P O I N T S

▶ The two categories of respiratory failure are oxygenation failure and ventilation failure.

▶ Oxygenation failure is caused by increased dead space or shunting.

▶ Ventilation failure is caused by chest wall dysfunction, airflow restriction, or respiratory depression.

CASE 27–13. You are called to see a 27-year-old woman who has been admitted to the ICU for monitoring after having postpartum hemorrhage earlier in the day. During her resuscitation the patient received 10 units of packed red blood cells, 4 units of fresh frozen plasma, a six-pack of platelets, and 5 L of crystalloid. With this resuscitation and with emergent embolization of her pelvic vasculature, the patient has had a stable hematocrit and hemodynamic status for the last 6 hours. She now complains of shortness of breath, especially when trying to lie flat to sleep, and her nurse has noted that the patient has an oxygen saturation of 88% on room air. You examine the patient and

continued

CASE 27–13. *continued*

note tachypnea, tachycardia, and rales throughout her posterior chest. You order a chest radiograph and it shows diffuse fluffy infiltrates. You diagnose volume overload with pulmonary edema from the patient's massive resuscitation.

A. What is your first step in treatment?

CASE 27–14. You are called to see the patient in Case 27–13 for obtundation. You find the patient unresponsive. A quick look at her vital signs reveals that she has a respiratory rate of 6 breaths/min and an oxygen saturation of 86% on 4 L of oxygen by nasal cannula. You urgently call for the respiratory therapist and take a moment to speak with the patient's nurse. He reports that the patient had improved with the oxygen therapy to an oxygen saturation of 98% and was able to lie flat. However, the patient complained of residual pelvic pain and had received a dose of 4 mg of IV morphine and 1 mg of IV lorazepam about 30 minutes ago. The nurse has already sent an ABG, and the results of it return as you place a bag mask over the patient's face to assist her respiration. The pH is 7.22, the P_{CO_2} is 58, and the P_{O_2} is 56.

A. What should you do next?

CASE 27–15. You are an anesthesiologist and have just completed a long case in the operating room. The case was that of a 78-year-old man who underwent an emergent repair of a ruptured abdominal aortic aneurysm under general anesthesia. The patient was in the operating room for several hours and required large-volume resuscitation with blood products and crystalloid during the procedure. The general surgery attending physician asks you to extubate the patient prior to his departure from the operating room.

A. What would be your response?

PULMONARY THROMBOEMBOLISM

▶ ETIOLOGY

Venous thromboembolism encompasses a wide clinical spectrum of disease from asymptomatic distal venous thrombosis to life-threatening pulmonary embolism (PE). It hospitalizes 250,000 people each year in the United States. It also develops in patients already hospitalized: patients hospitalized for surgery, congestive heart failure, or malignancy are at increased risk for developing thromboembolism.

What are the risk factors leading to thromboembolism?

More than 100 years ago, Virchow proposed the triad of hypercoagulability, venous stasis, and local trauma as a source of venous thromboembolism. Time has proven him right. Patients with any of a multitude of inherited or acquired hypercoagulable states, those sustaining trauma or undergoing surgery, and those with either forced or elective immobility are at increased risk for thromboembolic disease.

Several inherited hypercoagulable disorders increase the risk for thromboembolic disease. Among these are the predispositions caused by mutations in the genes encoding the proteins of the clotting or fibrinolytic cascade. One of these, factor V Leiden, is estimated to play a role in one fifth of the cases of PE and to be a major factor in cases of recurrent thromboembolic disease. Factor V Leiden is a point mutation in factor V that makes it resistant to deactivation by activated protein C and allows inappropriate propagation of the clotting cascade. Another mutation that affects the function of a clotting factor is the 20210A mutation of prothrombin. Inherited factor deficiencies in the fibrinolytic cascade of protein C, protein S, and antithrombin III also promote venous thromboembolism. Dysfibrinogenemia rounds out the list of inherited risk factors.

The acquired risk factors for venous thromboembolism constitute a large and heterogeneous list. These risk factors directly reflect Virchow's triad. Trauma to blood vessels from traumatic injury or surgery increases risk. Increased risk also comes from stasis, as seen in the higher likelihood of venous thromboembolism in patients with paralysis, polycythemia, congestive heart failure, or forced immobility. Finally, hypercoagulability from hypertension, obesity, pregnancy, smoking, current oral contraceptive use, malignancy, advancing age, and antiphospholipid syndrome increase risk.

Other risk factors for venous thromboembolism result from a mixture of inherited and acquired causes. These include vitamin B_6

deficiency, folate deficiency, hyperhomocystinemia, vitamin B_{12} deficiency, high factor VII levels, and high fibrinogen levels. Non-O blood type and high von Willebrand's factor levels can also increase risk but only in the setting of elevated factor VIII levels.

▶ EVALUATION

What are the signs and symptoms of thromboembolic disease?

Patients with thromboembolic disease can be asymptomatic or can have symptoms from limb- or life-threatening disease. With deep venous thrombosis (DVT), the classic symptoms are calf pain, lower extremity edema, venous distention, and a positive Homans' sign (calf pain with forced dorsiflexion of the foot). However, less than one third of patients with DVT have these symptoms. Other symptoms of DVT can include redness of the leg or, in cases of limb-threatening DVT, tenseness of the leg with cyanosis (phlegmasia cerulea dolens). DVT also occurs in the upper extremities, often at sites of current or previous indwelling central venous catheters, and causes ipsilateral extremity edema.

Like DVT, PE can have a varied clinical presentation. Although DVT is a prerequisite for the development of PE, patients diagnosed with PE rarely have the signs or symptoms of DVT. However, 20% to 30% of patients with known DVT develop symptomatic PE, whereas an additional 30% develop asymptomatic PE. The symptoms of PE include shortness of breath and pleuritic chest pain. The chest pain can also have a dull character. Life-threatening PE can present with cardiovascular collapse and with a patient in pulseless electrical activity. Other than the possible concurrent exam findings of DVT, the exam findings of PE are few and occur in life-threatening cases. Examples include the findings of right ventricular strain and pulmonary hypertension as seen with jugular distention, sternal heave, and a prominent split S_2 on chest auscultation.

What are the laboratory findings in pulmonary thromboembolism?

ABG analysis is a must in patients suspected of PE. In mild cases, a respiratory alkalosis with a mild hypoxia may be present. ABGs may be normal. However, in severe cases profound hypoxia with a low Pao_2 can occur. Other laboratory abnormalities can include a leukocytosis, elevated D-dimers, and elevated fibrinogen levels. Other than D-dimer measurement, these tests are not useful for the diagnosis of thromboembolic disease. D-dimer assays are useful in ruling out the disease because a normal test result has a high negative predictive value.

What are the ECG findings of pulmonary thromboembolism?

The most common ECG abnormality in PE is sinus tachycardia. The classic triad of an S wave in I and a Q wave in III with a T-wave abnormality in III is rarely seen. Other abnormalities can include a right bundle branch block and signs of right ventricular strain.

What are the radiographic findings of pulmonary thromboembolism?

A normal chest radiograph is the most common radiographic finding in patients with PE. However, when pulmonary infarction occurs with PE, pleural-based pyramid-shaped opacities can appear peripherally.

What other studies are used for the diagnosis of thromboembolism?

Studies used for the diagnosis of DVT include ascending venography, impedance plethysmography, Doppler ultrasonography, CT angiography, and magnetic resonance (MR) angiography. Impedance plethysmography and ascending venography are the reference standards for the diagnosis of DVT, but they are rarely used for clinical diagnosis. The most common diagnostic tests today are Doppler ultrasonography and CT angiography. Doppler ultrasonography uses real-time ultrasound with color Doppler of the venous flow to search for DVT. This test is most sensitive for detecting DVT in the compressible veins of the thigh and less sensitive in detecting pelvic or calf DVT. Its benefits are its noninvasiveness and high sensitivity for detecting proximal DVT. The downside of ultrasound is it requirement for trained personnel to carry out and interpret the test.

CT angiography is becoming more common as a diagnostic test for DVT and PE. Most institutions include a scan of the pelvis and upper thighs while performing chest CT angiography looking for PE. The benefits of this scan are its ease of administration and its ability to concurrently look for DVT and PE. Compared to the other diagnostic tests, CT angiography is better at evaluating the vessels of the abdomen and pelvis for thrombosis. Its downsides are the need for nephrotoxic contrast to complete the scan, its cost, and the danger of transport to the scanner for some critically ill patients. MR angiography has many of the features of CT angiography, but its expense and limited availability have limited clinical experience with it.

Tests for the diagnosis of PE include ventilation/perfusion scintigraphy ($\dot{V}/\dot{Q}$ scanning), CT angiography, MR angiography, and pulmonary angiography. All of these tests have been found useful for the diagnosis of PE, and all have noted drawbacks. Which test is best for the diagnosis of PE in any given patient depends on patient and institutional characteristics. MR angiography is a relatively new and expensive modality. Clinical experience with it is limited. Pulmonary angiography is the gold standard test for the diagnosis of PE. It is not a first-line test because of its invasive nature and its risk for major complications such as bleeding, stroke, and renal insufficiency. Most institutions today look to CT angiography or V̇/Q̇ scanning as the initial test for diagnosing PE. Both tests require trained personnel to interpret them, and this can affect the sensitivity and specificity of the test at any given institution.

V̇/Q̇ scanning is most reliable when clinical suspicion is high or low. Compared to CT angiography, V̇/Q̇ scanning takes longer and requires participation by nonintubated patients, but it does not require contrast dye injection. The results of V̇/Q̇ scanning may be difficult to interpret in patients with underlying pulmonary pathology or abnormalities on their chest radiograph. CT angiography offers the benefits of speed, limited need for patient participation, and the ability to diagnose DVT when compared to V̇/Q̇ scanning. It is the better test for those with abnormal chest radiographs or preexisting pulmonary disease.

► **TREATMENT**

What is the preferred treatment for thromboembolic disease?

Anticoagulation is the preferred treatment for thromboembolic disease. Multiple agents are now available for anticoagulation including the heparins, heparinoids, direct thrombin inhibitors, and warfarin (Coumadin). Patients suspected or diagnosed with DVT or PE should be started on an agent for immediate anticoagulation if there are no contraindications to anticoagulation. Warfarin alone is not recommended for initial treatment of thromboembolic disease because this agent takes several days to induce full anticoagulation even if the prothrombin time becomes prolonged in the first few days. This is true because warfarin quickly depletes factor VII with its 6-hour half-life but does not deplete prothrombin for days because of prothrombin's 5-day half-life. It is prothrombin depletion that induces effective anticoagulation in patients on warfarin. For this reason, it is recommended that patients remain anticoagulated with another agent for 5 days as warfarin therapy is begun.

The choices for immediate anticoagulation include unfractionated heparin, low-molecular-weight heparin (LMWH), danaparoid, hirudin, and argatroban. Unfractionated heparin has been the traditional choice for immediate anticoagulation. It is administered by giving an initial bolus (5000 to 10,000 units) followed by an IV drip titrated to keep the activated partial thromboplastin time between 60 to 80 seconds. LMWH has gained popularity now that studies have indicated its safety and efficacy for the treatment of DVT and PE. It is easy to deliver and does not require laboratory monitoring like unfractionated heparin does. It can be given in once- or twice-daily subcutaneous injections. If necessary, factor Xa levels can be followed to gauge its effectiveness.

The currently available heparinoid is danaparoid, and the direct thrombin inhibitors are hirudin and argatroban. More of these agents are in development. The main indication for these three agents is for anticoagulation in patients with thromboembolic disease who have known or presumed thrombocytopenia due to heparin. Warfarin is the only oral agent available for anticoagulation. It inhibits the synthesis of vitamin K–dependent clotting factors II, VII, IX, and X. Though given daily, it may take more than a day to see the anticoagulation changes reflected in the International Normalized Ratio (INR) due to the half-life dependent depletion of affected clotting factors. Usually, a target INR of 2.0 to 3.0 is aimed for inpatients taking warfarin.

The amount and duration of anticoagulation for thromboembolic disease are areas of active research. Some patient subsets such as those with antiphospholipid syndrome, those with malignancy-related thrombosis, or those with recurrent thromboembolic disease require longer or even life-long anticoagulation. Additionally, those with thromboembolism related to antiphospholipid syndrome require higher levels of anticoagulation. Traditionally, longer durations of anticoagulation have shown benefit in reducing morbidity and mortality from thromboembolic disease with little increased risk in major bleeding.

How is pulmonary embolism avoided in a patient with DVT and an absolute contraindication to anticoagulation?

In patients with contraindications to anticoagulation, mechanical barriers placed in the inferior vena cava can reduce the embolic load in patients with known lower extremity DVT or PE. These devices (Greenfield filter, bird cage) do not prevent embolus or propagation of DVT or have any prophylactic effect in patients with upper extremity DVT. Insertion of these devices introduces some risks, such as causing further emboli, inferior vena cava perforation, and intravascular device migration. They can be used alone in patients with absolute contraindications to anticoagulation or with anticoagulants in patients with life-threatening thromboembolic disease and no contraindications to anticoagulation.

Another therapeutic option for thromboembolic disease is thrombolytic therapy. Thrombolytic therapy with streptokinase or tissue plasminogen activator can be given systemically through IV administration or introduced into the thrombosis locally with catheter-based techniques. Current guidelines recommend thrombolytic therapy for cases of PE causing hemodynamic compromise or right ventricular failure. Thrombolytic therapy can be administered for cases of DVT as well.

The final therapeutic option for PE is embolectomy. Embolectomy can be performed via open surgical techniques on the pulmonary arteries or via percutaneous catheter-directed techniques. The high mortality of these procedures truly makes them the therapy of last resort.

How do I administer prophylaxis against thromboembolism?

Most patients who die from PE do so within 30 minutes of the embolism, too little time to institute adequate anticoagulation. Therefore, prophylaxis for thromboembolic disease is crucial for those at risk. Prophylaxis can be accomplished with medications and with mechanical devices. The mechanical devices include compression stockings and sequential compression devices. Most of these devices are fashioned to fit over the calves and thighs, but devices for the feet and upper extremities are available. Pharmacologic prophylaxis can be accomplished with subcutaneous unfractionated heparin or LMWH injections. For patients with known or presumed thrombocytopenia from heparin, danaparoid, hirudin, and argatroban can be given. In special circumstances, such as in cancer patients with indwelling central lines, low-dose warfarin is recommended. Which type of prophylaxis to give depends on the estimated risk for thromboembolic disease in each individual patient. Guidelines for prophylaxis exist for several patient subsets, the most notable of which are those patients undergoing surgery on their hip or lower extremities.

What are the surgical considerations of thromboembolism?

Thromboembolic disease is of special concern to the surgeon. Surgical patients, with the exception of the young patient undergoing a minor procedure, are at increased risk for the development of DVT and PE. Surgery itself increases the risk for thromboembolic disease. The requirements of surgery can increase that risk further. The immobility during the surgery and during the recovery from surgery fosters thrombosis. Indwelling lines placed for the administration of fluids, antibiotics, and pain medications can serve as a nidus for thrombosis. Surgical patients often have preexisting illnesses (malignancy, hypertension, obesity) or habits (smoking) that increase their risk further. Astute surgeons recognize this and place their patients on adequate prophylaxis and keep an eye out for the development of thromboembolic disease.

Treatment of DVT or PE in surgical patients can be especially difficult. Anticoagulating postoperative patients with new anastomoses and surgical incisions can induce major bleeding. Not anticoagulating postoperative patients with new thromboembolism can be life threatening. Determining the risk of bleeding versus worsening thromboembolism requires careful consideration of the risk of both. These considerations should involve the surgical team and, often, an intensivist or pulmonologist.

Surgical patients with a history of thromboembolism within the 3 months prior to surgery or who are undergoing current anticoagulation for thromboembolism should remain anticoagulated with heparin or LMWH up to the time of surgery and should be taken off warfarin. Heparin or LMWH should be discontinued 6 hours preoperatively and should not be restarted until at least 12 hours postoperatively.

Prophylaxis is essential in surgical patients because almost all surgical patients have considerable risk for thromboembolism. Fear of postsurgical bleeding often halts the surgical team from giving pharmacologic prophylaxis after certain procedures (neurosurgery) or when there is an epidural catheter in place. This fear seems unwarranted, and pharmacologic prophylaxis can be given. If an epidural catheter is in place, good communication between surgical and anesthesia team members about the appropriate time to remove the catheter prevents hematoma formation.

K E Y   P O I N T S

▶ Surgical patients are at an increased risk for both DVT and PE.

▶ PE should be suspected in patients who are short of breath with or without chest pain.

▶ Anticoagulation and/or vena caval filters are the mainstay of therapy.

CASE 27–16. An 18-year-old woman presents to the emergency department with a 1-day history of shortness of breath. She notices that she now has difficulty walking from her bedroom to the bathroom without feeling faint and panting for breath. She is an exchange student who recently flew to the United States from England to begin school. She is otherwise healthy, and her only medications are oral contraceptive pills. On physical exam, her heart rate is 110 beats/min, her blood pressure is 95/42 mm Hg, and her respiratory rate is 24 breaths/min. On pulse oximetry her oxygen saturation is 92% on 4 L of oxygen via nasal cannula. Other than her tachypnea and tachycardia, her physical exam is unremarkable. Her chest radiograph shows no apparent

continued

CASE 27–16. *continued*

disease, and her ABG reveals a pH of 7.46, P_{CO_2} of 32, and P_{O_2} of 64 on 4 L via nasal cannula.

    A. What step would you take next?

CASE 27–17. The patient from Case 27–16 is eventually taken to the CT scanner for a CT angiogram of her chest. This test reveals a heavy clot burden in bilateral pulmonary artery distributions but no signs of thrombus in the veins of her legs. An echocardiogram reveals right ventricular dilation with markedly elevated estimated pulmonary artery pressures. Despite these findings, the patient remains comfortable and alert with oxygen therapy, with tachycardia and mild hypotension as the only signs of her massive pulmonary embolus.

    A. What step would you take next?

CASE 27–18. You are called to see a 66-year-old man with recently diagnosed colon cancer. The patient is hospitalized for a lower gastrointestinal bleed thought to be attributable to his colon cancer. The patient is feeling better today after receiving 2 units of packed red blood cells for his gastrointestinal bleed, but he noticed that his right leg is swollen compared to his left. He also notes pain in his calf with ambulation. He would like a pain medication for his calf discomfort. His vital signs are stable and without abnormality, and his oxygen saturation is 99% on room air. You order an ultrasound of his right leg, and the results confirm your suspicion that he has a DVT in that leg.

    A. What do you do next; is systemic anticoagulation warranted?

28

Endocrine Surgery

The field of surgical endocrinology includes the evaluation and treatment of patients either with aberrations of endocrine function or who present with a mass of unknown etiology in an endocrine gland. For clarity, this chapter is organized by specific endocrine gland.

ADRENAL DISORDERS

▶ ETIOLOGY

Which problems of the adrenal gland require surgical consultation?

Patients are referred for surgical consultation for the following reasons:

1. A mass in one or both adrenal glands is seen on computed tomography (CT) or magnetic resonance (MR) imaging.
2. The patient has symptoms of overproduction of an adrenal hormone.

What is meant by the term *adrenal incidentaloma*?

This term refers to masses noted in the adrenal gland found on MR imaging or CT done for another reason. It is estimated that somewhere between 0.4% and 5% of all CT scans done will show such lesions. These lesions may be myelolipomas, adrenocortical adenomas, pheochromocytomas, metastases from nonadrenal neoplasms, or rarely, adrenocortical carcinomas. Evaluation of the mass requires determination of whether it has hormonal function, whether it can represent malignancy of the adrenal gland, or whether it represents metastasis from another site.

What are the indications for operating on an incidentaloma?

Incidentalomas should be removed if they are secreting a hormone excessively or if they are larger than 6 cm in diameter. Nonfunctional lesions between 4 and 6 cm may be either removed or closely observed for changes in size. Most benign cortical adenomas are small (between 1 and 2 cm).

▶ EVALUATION

How is hormonal activity evaluated?

As with all evaluations, a thorough history and physical examination are required. Screening laboratory studies should look for primary aldosteronism, Cushing's syndrome due to cortical adenoma, and pheochromocytoma.

Primary aldosteronism can be screened for by obtaining a serum potassium level and checking blood pressure. Normal potassium level and normal blood pressure essentially rule out this disease. If the patient is hypertensive and hypokalemic while taking diuretics, the diuretics should be stopped and the potassium replaced. If the potassium remains low despite aggressive replacement and cessation of diuretics, further evaluation should be done for primary aldosteronism.

Cushing's syndrome is screened with a low-dose dexamethasone suppression test. A single oral dose of dexamethasone (1 mg) is given at 11:00 PM, and then plasma cortisol is measured at 8:00 AM the next morning. In a normal person, the plasma cortisol level should be lower than 5 µg/dL. Patients with Cushing's syndrome generally have cortisol level higher than 20 µg/dL. If this test suggests Cushing's syndrome, a 24-hour urine is collected for 17-hydroxycorticosteroids and urinary free cortisol, and a plasma adrenocorticotropic hormone (ACTH) level is obtained to confirm the diagnosis.

Pheochromocytoma must be ruled out prior to any consideration of operation for an adrenal mass. All patients being evaluated for operation, regardless of other symptomatology, should have a 24-hour urine study for vanillylmandelic acid, norepinephrine, epinephrine, normetanephrine, and metanephrine to document that the incidentaloma is not a pheochromocytoma.

▶ TREATMENT

What are the surgical options for adrenalectomy?

The adrenal gland can be approached from a posterior, flank, or transabdominal incision. The operation may be done either open or laparoscopically. Either a transperitoneal flank approach or a posterior retroperitoneal approach may be used to perform laparoscopic adrenalectomy. The latter has distinct advantages in patients who have had prior abdominal surgery.

Relative contraindications to laparoscopic adrenalectomy include pheochromocytoma or known malignancy.

CARCINOIDS AND OTHER NEUROENDOCRINE (APUD) TUMORS

▶ **ETIOLOGY**

What is a neuroendocrine tumor?

The neuroendocrine tumors, or APUDomas,* are a group of gastrointestinal tract neoplasms that are capable of taking up and decarboxylating biogenic amines or their precursors. These tumors are thought to originate from embryonic endodermal cells. This is a heterogeneous grouping of tumors that differ in their clinical behavior; may or may not have hormonal function; and may be benign or malignant, familial, or sporadic. Insulinomas are the most common islet cell tumor. Among malignant islet cell tumors, gastrinomas are the most common.

Where are these tumors found?

The cells that make up these tumors are most likely to be found in the foregut and midgut. Therefore, the most likely places to find these tumors are in the islet cells of the pancreas, the proximal duodenum, and the antrum of the stomach.

What are the characteristic features of an insulinoma?

The insulinoma is the most common islet cell tumor. Insulinomas are usually less than 2 cm in diameter, and 80% to 90% are benign. Patients who have them present with significant hypoglycemia that can manifest as seizures, lethargy, sweating, anxiety, or palpitations. Patients with this tumor do not tolerate fasting, and many present with a history of weight gain. To diagnose this disorder it is necessary to demonstrate that the patient has severe hypoglycemia and elevated insulin levels.

What is Zollinger-Ellison syndrome?

Zollinger-Ellison syndrome is a syndrome characterized by excess gastrin secretion that manifests clinically as severe peptic ulcer disease associated with a gastrin-secreting tumor of the pancreas or duodenum.

---

*APUD = *a*mine *p*recursor *u*ptake and *d*ecarboxylation.

What are the characteristic features of a gastrinoma?

Gastrinomas occur in patients of all ages and twice as often in men as in women. Patients present with symptoms attributable to gastrin excess, including heartburn, epigastric pain, diarrhea, and dysphagia, and a majority of them (>90%) have peptic ulcer disease. The ulcers are most commonly found in the proximal duodenum, but some patients have ulcers in multiple sites or in uncommon sites such as the jejunum or the distal duodenum. The diarrhea associated with this disease is secretory, characterized by multiple watery stools occurring independent of meals. A history of nocturnal diarrhea is typical of a secretory diarrhea.

What are some other APUD tumors?

Glucagonomas, vasoactive intestinal polypeptide–secreting tumors (VIPomas), somatostatinomas, and pancreatic polypeptide–secreting tumors (PPomas) are the next most common functioning APUD tumors. It is possible for pancreatic islet cell tumors to produce non-gastrointestinal hormones such as parathormone, ACTH, or serotonin, but these are extremely rare.

What is a carcinoid tumor?

Carcinoids are tumors that derive from chromaffin cells that contain and secrete serotonin (5-hyroxytryptamine [5-HT]). Eighty-five percent of carcinoids are found in the intestine and are classified by location into those deriving from foregut, midgut, or hindgut. Rarely, carcinoids may be found in the bronchus, and patients with multiple endocrine neoplasia type 1 (MEN 1) may have thymic carcinoids. The location determines to some extent what the tumor is likely to secrete and whether it is associated with the typical carcinoid syndrome. Midgut carcinoids are most likely to secrete 5-HT and tachykinins, causing the classic carcinoid syndrome with liver or lung metastasis. Foregut tumors may secrete 5-HT or ACTH but are associated with an atypical carcinoid syndrome when malignant. These tumors are less likely to metastasize to liver and more likely to have bony metastases. Hindgut tumors are sometimes found incidentally at appendectomy. They rarely secrete 5-HT and are almost never associated with carcinoid syndrome.

What is carcinoid syndrome?

Carcinoid syndrome occurs in less than 10% of patients with carcinoid tumors. It occurs when 5-HT is secreted into the systemic venous drainage, escaping hepatic degradation of the hormones. This produces the clinical syndrome of periodic abdominal pain, flushing, wheezing, and diarrhea. Long-term effects include pellagra dermatosis and cardiac valvular fibrosis.

How is the diagnosis of insulinoma made?

Diagnosis is made by measuring glucose, insulin, proinsulin, and C-peptide levels following a 72-hour fast. (Some patients cannot tolerate fasting this long. Generally, glucose and insulin levels are checked every 4 to 6 hours during the fast, and the patients are observed closely in a hospital setting. If the patient becomes symptomatic before 72 hours has elapsed, the postfast blood levels are drawn at that time.)

A postfast serum glucose less than 45 mg/dL with an insulin level higher than 5 μU/mL, an immunoreactive insulin-to-glucose ratio greater than 0.3, and an elevated proinsulin level are diagnostic. C-peptide level should be elevated, and the ratio of proinsulin to insulin should be greater than 0.25. The latter two tests discriminate between insulinoma and excessive insulin due to exogenous insulin overdose. Intraoperative ultrasound is helpful in finding these tumors intraoperatively, and surgical removal is the treatment of choice.

How is the diagnosis of gastrinoma made?

Diagnosis requires the demonstration of an elevated fasting serum gastrin greater than 100 pg/mL and elevated basal acid output greater than 15 mEq/hr (unless the patient has had a prior antrectomy). Because H_2 blockers and proton pump inhibitors raise gastrin levels by reducing acid secretion, it is important that patients stop taking these medications before the diagnostic work-up. Once a patient is found to have elevated gastrin and elevated basal acid output, the diagnosis can be confirmed with a secretin stimulation test. This test is done by giving 2 U/kg of secretin as an intravenous bolus and then measuring serum gastrin levels at 2, 5, 10, and 15 minutes. An increase in serum gastrin to greater than 200 pg/mL confirms the diagnosis.

How are gastrinomas localized?

Localization of these tumors can be challenging. Most gastrinomas (75% to 80%) are found in the so-called gastrinoma triangle (duodenum and pancreas). However, the literature reports gastrinomas being found in other areas quite remote from the triangle, such as in the ovary or in the heart. Unlike insulinomas, which are usually benign, about 60% of gastrinomas are malignant, and localization also involves identifying sites of metastases (which can be functional). As a general rule, pancreatic gastrinomas metastasize more often to liver than do duodenal tumors; duodenal tumors are more likely to have lymph node metastases. In the past, selective venous sampling and angiography were the modalities of choice, but because of cost, invasiveness, and the availability of scintigraphy, they no longer represent the first line of localization. Currently, the primary imaging test for gastrinoma is the somatostatin receptor scan. Radiolabeled somatostatin analog binds with high affinity to the somatostatin-2 receptor, which is present in most gastrinomas. There are about 20% of gastrinomas that lack this receptor, and sometimes very small tumors are not imaged. However, overall, it has high sensitivity and specificity for gastrinomas. CT scanning is helpful to identify lesions that are greater than 1 cm but is less specific than scintigraphy. At operation, intraoperative ultrasound may be helpful in localizing pancreatic lesions, and intraoperative endoscopy is used for duodenal lesions.

▶ TREATMENT

What is the treatment for an isolated functional APUDoma?

The treatment of an isolated functional APUDoma is surgical resection when possible. Surgical cure is rarely possible in the setting of metastatic disease. Symptoms of carcinoid syndrome may be controlled with serotonin inhibitors, interferon, other chemotherapeutic agents, or somatostatin. The long-acting version of somatostatin (octreotide) has particular success in treating symptoms of diarrhea and flushing.

THYROID

▶ ETIOLOGY

What is a goiter?

A goiter is any benign enlargement of the thyroid gland. Goiters may be diffuse, as in Graves' disease; multinodular and not hyperfunctioning; or multinodular and functioning (toxic multinodular goiter [Plummer's disease]). When goiters get large enough to extend into the mediastinum, they are referred to as *substernal goiters*.

What are the risk factors for thyroid cancer?

Ionizing radiation to the neck (particularly if it is given early in life) and a family history of thyroid cancer are the main evidence-based risk factors.

What are the types of thyroid cancer?

About 85% of thyroid cancers are well differentiated. Of these well-differentiated cancers, about 85% to 90% are papillary or a follicular variant of papillary carcinoma, and about 10% to 15% are follicular cancers. The follicular cancers can be further subdivided into microinvasive, macroinvasive, and Hürthle cell cancers. Of the remaining 15% of cancers, about 8% are medullary cancers, 4% are lymphomas, 2% are anaplastic, and 1% are metastases from primary tumors in other locations.

What are the features of the well-differentiated carcinomas?

These tumors are derived from thyroid follicular epithelial cells. Papillary tumors are the most common type; metastasize most frequently to adjacent lymph nodes or to lung; and have an excellent prognosis, independent of whether lymph node metastases are present. Follicular tumors are more likely to have hematogenous metastases, especially to bone and less commonly to liver and brain. Overall, patients with T1 to T3 lesions and lymph nodal involvement have an average 30-year survival of about 95%; in the absence of nodal involvement there is a 99% 30-year survival. When distant metastases are present, there is a 30% to 35% 30-year survival rate. Except for the Hürthle cell variant of follicular carcinoma, most well-differentiated thyroid cancers take up radioactive iodine (RAI). This modality is therefore used both diagnostically (to identify sites of metastasis) and therapeutically (to provide focal radiation to residual thyroid and metastases).

What are some features of medullary thyroid cancer?

Medullary carcinoma of the thyroid (MTC) derives from calcitonin-producing parafollicular cells (C cells), which are of neural crest origin. These tumors can occur sporadically or in association with several familial syndromes (familial MTC, MEN 2a, and MEN 2b). Because of its association with MEN 2, pheochromocytoma should be ruled out in any patient presenting with MTC. The behavior of this tumor is somewhat more aggressive than the well-differentiated thyroid cancers. Reported mortality is about 40% at 10 years. Serum calcitonin is the best marker for this disease and is used to detect recurrent or persistent disease. Carcinoembryonic antigen (CEA) can also be elevated. When CEA is elevated preoperatively, it also can be used as a marker for recurrence. This tumor disseminates both by local extension and hematogenously. When there is suspicion of recurrence, sestamibi (octreotide) scintigraphy may be helpful to localize metastatic disease.

What are the multiple endocrine neoplasia (MEN) syndromes?

MEN syndromes result from the development of tumors in multiple endocrine organs in characteristic combinations. These syndromes are distinct genetic entities. They tend to be familial, following mendelian autosomal dominant genetics, but may be sporadic (especially MEN 2b). The tumors may be benign or malignant and may occur at the same time or sequentially. A listing of the MEN syndromes is shown in Table 28–1. The abnormalities in each gland can range from hyperplasia to adenoma to carcinoma.

▶ EVALUATION

What laboratory tests are necessary?

Surgery for thyroid disease is performed for diagnosis, relief of symptoms of hyperfunction, or alleviation of the mass effect of a growing tumor. Laboratory examination to evaluate function includes a serum thyroid-stimulating hormone and a free thyroxine. Other specific markers such as thyroglobulin, calcitonin, or CEA are often helpful in following patients with a diagnosis of thyroid cancer.

What is done to evaluate a solitary thyroid nodule?

A palpable thyroid nodule is best initially evaluated by fine-needle aspiration (FNA) cytology. This distinguishes between a benign colloid nodule and a cellular aspirate suspicious for thyroid cancer. An FNA that reveals follicular cytology cannot distinguish between a follicular tumor and a papillary tumor with follicular variant.

TABLE 28–1	
Multiple Endocrine Neoplasia (MEN) Syndromes	
Syndrome	**Characteristics**
MEN 1	Parathyroid hyperplasia
	Pancreatic islet cell neoplasm
	Pituitary adenoma (anterior gland, usually prolactinoma)
MEN 2a	Medullary thyroid carcinoma (or C-cell hyperplasia)
	Pheochromocytoma (or adrenal medullary hyperplasia)
	Parathyroid hyperplasia
MEN 2b	Medullary thyroid carcinoma (or C-cell hyperplasia)
	Pheochromocytoma (or adrenal medullary hyperplasia)
	Parathyroid hyperplasia (rarely clinically significant)
	Mucosal neuromas
	Marfanoid facies

▶ TREATMENT

What are the indications for thyroidectomy?

Reasons to remove goiters include symptoms of dysphagia, dyspnea, or orthopnea, hyperfunction uncontrolled with medications, or cosmesis. About 8% of large goiters contain a focus of thyroid cancer. This is roughly the incidence of incidental thyroid cancer in the general population and is not a reason per se to operate on a large goiter.

Thyroidectomy is also done for lumps in the neck suspicious for thyroid cancer and occasionally for Graves' disease.

When is surgery done for hyperthyroidism?

Surgery is an option in cases of Graves' disease and in those patients with toxic multinodular goiters; however, these entities respond well to treatment with RAI, which is currently preferred. Surgery is limited to cases where there is suspicion of malignancy, in pregnant patients, or in those patients who are intolerant to antithyroid medications (which are generally given to render the patient euthyroid prior to RAI treatment).

PARATHYROID

▶ ETIOLOGY

What are some causes of hypercalcemia?

Some of the most common causes of hypercalcemia are listed in Table 28–2. The most common cause of hypercalcemia in the

TABLE 28–2

Causes of Hypercalcemia

Hyperparathyroidism
Thiazide diuretics
Sarcoidosis and other granulomatous diseases
Malignant neoplasms
Hyperthyroidism
Lithium use
Estrogens
Hypervitaminosis A or D
Paget's disease of bone
Immobilization
Familial hypocalciuric hypercalcemia
Renal insufficiency

ambulatory population is primary hyperparathyroidism. Malignant neoplasms can cause hypercalcemia by several mechanisms: (1) by making tumor-associated substances that accelerate or initiate bone resorption, for example, osteocyte activation factor associated with lymphomas; (2) by locally stimulating osteoclasts, thereby causing local bone destruction (breast cancer); and (3) by making parathyroid hormone (PTH)-like substances that mediate bone resorption (solid tumors such as small cell carcinomas of lung, hypernephromas, or some squamous cell tumors).

What are the clinical features of primary hyperparathyroidism?

Primary hyperparathyroidism can present as apparently asymptomatic elevation of calcium in the presence of elevated PTH levels, as bone disease, or as recurrent nephrolithiasis. Symptoms, when present, may be those of hypercalcemia (fatigue, anorexia, nausea, confusion, depression, constipation, polyuria, polydipsia, or cardiac dysrhythmias) or may be related to bone loss (bone pain, weight loss, pathologic fractures) or nephrolithiasis (renal colic).

What is secondary hyperparathyroidism?

Secondary hyperparathyroidism occurs when PTH is produced excessively as a response to a condition that causes partial or complete resistance to the normal metabolic action of PTH. Some of the causes of secondary hyperparathyroidism are summarized in Table 28–3. The most common cause of secondary hyperparathyroidism is chronic renal failure.

▶ EVALUATION

How is primary hyperparathyroidism diagnosed?

The diagnosis is made by documenting elevated serum calcium levels with a concomitant elevation of PTH levels. PTH levels are usually measured with an assay of intact PTH. If there is a need for diagnostic confirmation, a 24-hour urine collection demonstrating increased calcium excretion can be obtained.

Should localization studies be done for primary hyperparathyroidism?

This is a controversial issue. However, many experienced endocrine surgeons would not routinely do localization on patients undergoing a first exploration and who have not had prior operations in the neck. For patients who have had prior neck operations or for patients undergoing minimally invasive parathyroidectomy,

TABLE 28-3

Causes of Secondary Hyperparathyroidism

Cause	Mechanism
Chronic renal failure	Reduced concentrations of $1,25(OH)_2D$
	Phosphate retention due to reduced excretion of PO_4
	Decreased absorption of calcium from the gut
	Decreased skeletal responsiveness to PTH
Osteomalacia	Vitamin D deficiency
Pseudohyperparathyroidism	Nonresponsive PTH receptors

PTH, parathyroid hormone.

noninvasive imaging using ultrasound, CT, sestamibi scan, or MR imaging can be done. Because none is definitive, a positive consistent finding in two studies warrants proceeding to surgery. If all are negative, one can consider digital angiography to more definitively provide localization prior to operation.

▶ TREATMENT

What is the treatment for acute hypercalcemia?

The primary treatment for acute hypercalcemia is saline diuresis. Patients should have a Foley catheter placed and a central venous pressure monitor (if there is any history or risk for congestive heart failure). Normal saline is then administered intravenously until the extracellular fluid volume is restored. Diuretics should *not* be given until the patient is euvolemic because this may actually drive the calcium up if volume has not been adequately restored. Infusion rates of 300 to 500 mL/hr are often needed to rapidly lower the serum calcium level. It is important to monitor magnesium and potassium levels during this treatment because these electrolytes are likely to be lost during this rapid diuresis.

What is the treatment for primary hyperparathyroidism?

The treatment for primary hyperparathyroidism is surgery. The extent of operation is determined by the etiology of the hyperparathyroidism. Most patients have parathyroid adenomas caused by a single abnormal gland (85%), about 10% have parathyroid hyperplasia involving all four parathyroid glands, about 1% to 3% have double adenomas, and 1% to 3% have parathyroid carcinoma. Simple excision of the enlarged parathyroid is usually curative when the disease is caused by a solitary adenoma. When there is hyperplasia involving all four glands, 3 ½ gland resection is the preferred initial management.

Parathyroid carcinoma is a diagnosis often made at the operating table. It is uncommon but should be suspected when there is a palpable parathyroid, an extremely high serum calcium level, a very hard gland, and especially when the enlarged parathyroid is invading surrounding structures. The treatment of choice is en bloc resection.

What are the indications for operation for secondary hyperparathyroidism?

Secondary hyperparathyroidism is usually managed medically. Indications for surgery are failure of medical management, leading to persistent signs and symptoms, including the following:

Calcium/phosphorus product >70
Pathologic fractures
Hypercalcemia in patients who are candidates for renal
    transplants or who have functioning transplants
Symptoms of secondary hyperparathyroidism (bone pain,
    calciphylaxis, severe pruritus)

K E Y   P O I N T S

▶ Endocrine diseases that require surgical evaluation and treatment often occur as a result of hyperfunctioning of a gland or a symptomatic or incidentally discovered mass.

▶ Adrenal masses need to be surgically removed if they are larger than 6 cm or are functional.

▶ APUDomas are a heterogeneous group of neuroendocrine tumors that cause symptoms by secretion of hormones.

▶ The test of choice for localization of gastrinomas is scintigraphy.

▶ The initial evaluation of a solitary thyroid mass is FNA.

▶ Thyroid cancer is common, but the majority of cases are well differentiated and have a good prognosis following treatment.

▶ Hyperparathyroidism may be caused by primary hypersecretion of PTH or by a secondary condition resulting in decreased sensitivity to PTH.

CASE 28–1.
A 65-year-old man was evaluated by CT scan following a minor motor vehicle accident, and a 5-cm mass was noted in his right adrenal gland. Other than hypertension, which is well controlled with beta-blockers, he is healthy.

A. What work-up is appropriate?
B. What are the indications for surgery in this patient?

CASE 28–2.
A 32-year-old man presents to his primary care physician with a recently discovered mass on the right side of his neck.

A. How is this patient initially evaluated?
B. What studies are necessary?
C. If cancer is detected, what is the appropriate treatment?

29

Gastrointestinal Surgery

APPENDICITIS

Appendicitis is a common disorder affecting 7% of the population. Although it generally occurs in younger patients (5 to 30 years old), it can occur at any age. Undiagnosed appendicitis can lead to perforation of the appendix, which may lead to significant morbidity and possibly death. It is therefore imperative that you understand how to evaluate patients for possible appendicitis.

▶ ETIOLOGY

What is the etiology of appendicitis?

The appendix is a tubular structure extending off the proximal cecum. Although the appendix is dispensable, it does play a minor role in the immune system because it contains lymphoid tissue and secretes immunoglobulins. Appendicitis occurs when the appendix becomes obstructed, typically at its base. Obstruction can develop after a viral infection, secondary to lymphoid hyperplasia, or from blockage by a fecalith (stool concretion) or foreign body. Although obstructed, this tubular structure continues to secrete mucus, leading to distention and bacterial overgrowth. Increased intraluminal pressure prevents venous outflow, leading to ischemia of the tissue. Ischemia enables bacterial invasion of the mucosa and the development of septic necrosis. If left untreated, the appendix can perforate, leading to generalized peritonitis and sepsis.

▶ EVALUATION

How does appendicitis present?

Abdominal pain is the most frequent symptom of appendicitis and is often associated with fever, nausea, anorexia, and occasional vomiting. Other symptoms are listed in Table 29–1. Classically, patients have pain that starts in the periumbilical area and later shifts to the right lower quadrant near McBurney's point.

TABLE 29–1

Frequency of Symptoms in Appendicitis

Symptoms and Signs	Frequency (%)
Abdominal pain	>95
Anorexia	>90
Elevated temperature	>80
Nausea	90
Vomiting	75
Pain migration (periumbilical shift to right lower quadrant)	50
Elevated white blood cell count	80
Higher proportion of neutrophils	95

McBurney's point is located at the junction of the middle and outer thirds of the line joining the umbilicus to the anterior superior iliac spine (Fig. 29–1). In the normal setting, the intestine is insensate to touch and inflammation. As the appendix becomes distended, in the case of appendicitis, somatic pain develops and is referred to the midline (i.e., periumbilical area) via T10 to T12 nerves. This causes the initial pain associated with appendicitis, which is crampy and difficult for patients to describe. When the inflammation

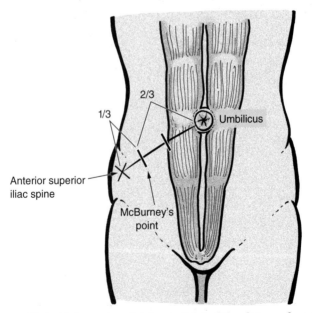

Figure 29–1. McBurney's point is one third of the distance from the right anterior superior iliac spine and the umbilicus.

progresses and extends through the visceral wall, the parietal peritoneal nerves become involved in the local inflammation, which produces right lower quadrant pain and tenderness. This second type of pain is generally constant, sharp, and progressive in intensity.

Following the onset of pain, patients then develop mild nausea, vomiting, or constipation. Various combinations of these gastrointestinal (GI) complaints can occur, and most patients are anorexic. Abdominal pain that starts after a period of copious vomiting is unlikely to be from appendicitis; instead, gastroenteritis or another etiology should be considered. Patients with appendicitis commonly have a low-grade temperature (99.5°F to 101.5°F). Temperatures greater than 102°F are unusual unless the appendix has already perforated. Table 29–1 lists the frequency of signs and symptoms seen with appendicitis. However, fewer than 50% of patients present with a pattern of symptoms classic for appendicitis; in those questionable cases, laboratory and radiologic tests should supplement a thorough history and physical exam.

What are the important features of the physical exam?

Patients with appendicitis usually appear ill. They often lie still on the examining table and are found curled on their side with hips flexed. Patients should identify the location of greatest discomfort, and the examination should start away from this area, in a different abdominal quadrant, and work toward the affected area. The examiner usually elicits marked right lower quadrant tenderness, which may be accompanied by a facial grimace. The presence and location of voluntary or involuntary guarding should be noted. Guarding is due to abdominal wall muscle contracting in response to palpation. Percussion tap tenderness can be a sensitive method for eliciting signs of local peritonitis. A mass may be felt on examination. All women should have a pelvic exam performed to evaluate for pelvic pathology such as pelvic inflammatory disease and ovarian torsion. A rectal exam should also be performed to evaluate for diverticulitis or large pelvic abscess. Several additional signs that are helpful in the diagnosis of appendicitis are listed in Table 29–2.

TABLE 29–2

Additional Signs of Appendicitis

Sign	Description
Rovsing's sign	Pain felt in right lower quadrant resulting from palpation of left lower quadrant
Psoas sign	Increased pain from passive extension of right hip (stretches iliopsoas muscle, which the appendix may overlie)
Obturator sign	Pain produced by passive internal rotation of flexed thigh (pelvic appendix)
Dunphy's sign	Increased pain with coughing

What laboratory tests are important?

Laboratory tests are used as a guide for the diagnosis of appendicitis. All female patients of childbearing age should receive a pregnancy test. White blood cell count can also aid in the diagnosis of appendicitis, because most patients (80%) have a mild leukocytosis with a greater proportion of polymononuclear cells. A normal white blood cell count doesn't rule out appendicitis, whereas a markedly elevated value suggests perforation. Urinary evaluation should always be included to rule out urinary infection or kidney stone. Electrolytes should be obtained for patients who report a significant history of vomiting or diarrhea. When the diagnosis is in question, it is reasonable to include liver function tests (LFTs) and serum amylase and lipase.

What radiographic tests are important?

When the history, physical exam, and laboratory values are suggestive of appendicitis, there is little need for radiologic examinations. However, further testing should be considered when the diagnosis is in question or for women of childbearing age. Gynecologic pathology can present in similar fashion to appendicitis, and the best test for distinguishing between the two is a pelvic ultrasound. For example, an ultrasound can identify a ruptured ovarian cyst or tubo-ovarian abscess, the management of which may not require an operation.

Computed tomographic (CT) scan is a highly accurate test for diagnosing appendicitis (98% sensitivity and 98% specificity), but it is currently overused and often is unnecessary. CT scan is an expensive and time-consuming test that can delay surgical exploration. CT also subjects the patient to radiation. Despite these drawbacks, CT scans can be informative when the diagnosis is unclear or in older patients (age >50 years) who have a higher likelihood of other pathologies such as diverticulitis or cancer. Another test, used less frequently now than in the past, is a barium enema. An appendix that fills completely with barium rules out appendicitis as a diagnosis. If the appendix doesn't fill, appendicitis may or may not be present. For this reason, CT scan with contrast has largely supplanted the use of barium enema in the radiographic diagnosis of suspected appendicitis.

▶ TREATMENT

How is appendicitis treated?

When a physician suspects appendicitis, surgical consultation is obtained. Antibiotics are given once the decision has been made to proceed with surgery. Second-generation cephalosporin, given intravenously, provides adequate gram-negative and anaerobic bacterial coverage. Both laparoscopic and open procedures are excellent options for the treatment or evaluation of appendicitis. The laparoscopic approach may be preferred when the diagnosis is in question. Advantages of laparoscopic appendectomy include shorter convalescence and smaller incisions. Reported complications and outcomes for both approaches are equivalent, as are total costs.

For an open appendectomy, a transverse incision is made through McBurney's point. The external oblique, internal oblique, and transversus abdominis muscle are encountered and split along the direction of their fibers. The posterior fascia and peritoneum are entered. On exploration, the appendix may be acutely inflamed (suppurative), gangrenous, or perforated. Perforated appendicitis can present as an inflammatory phlegmon, a walled-off abscess surrounding the perforation, free pus throughout the peritoneum, or any combination of the three.

Operative management should be individualized. For acute appendicitis, the base of the appendix is generally not involved and an appendectomy is sufficient. If marked infection or necrosis involves the cecum, a more extensive resection may be necessary. This could include a "wedge cecectomy" or rarely an ileocecectomy with a primary anastomosis. Care should be taken to deloculate intestinal interloop abscesses, especially near the ileocecal junction, which can be a source of postoperative intestinal obstruction. This is done by delivering 10 to 20 cm of distal ileum into the wound for inspection, as well as carefully palpating the pelvic cavity and omentum. Free pus in the peritoneum should be irrigated with saline. If there is a considerable amount of pus at exploration, the surgeon will decide whether the skin of the wound should be left open. These wounds have a 20% to 40% chance of becoming infected if closed at the operation. A closed-suction drain is reserved for cases where a well-defined abscess cavity is found.

What if a normal appendix is found during exploration?

If a normal appendix is found during the operation, an appendectomy is still performed. The morbidity is low, and this eliminates the possibility of having the same diagnostic dilemma at a later time if the patient presents again with similar symptoms. It is important to inform the patient that the appendix was removed in this situation. When a normal appendix is found, a thorough exploration must be performed to identify the source of the pain. In women, both ovaries should be visualized. The surgeon should palpate the cecum, ascending colon, and sigmoid colon for a mass or diverticulitis. The small bowel at the ileocecal junction should also be inspected for abnormalities, including masses or evidence of inflammatory bowel disease (IBD). Also, the surgeon should examine the distal small bowel from the ileocecal junction for 2 ft to evaluate for a Meckel's diverticulum. The gallbladder should also be inspected for signs of inflammation. If the appendix is normal in the presence of diffuse purulent peritonitis, identification of the source of infection may mandate a formal midline laparotomy.

K E Y   P O I N T S

▶ Appendicitis is a common cause of abdominal pain.

▶ Pain typically precedes other symptoms.

▶ Consider gynecologic causes of pain in women of childbearing years.

▶ Radiologic tests should supplement a thorough history and physical examination when the diagnosis is in question.

▶ Prompt surgical treatment is curative.

CASE 29–1. A 20-year-old woman presents with a 1½-day history of periumbilical pain that has localized to the right lower quadrant. She denies a history of similar pain and notes some nausea. Her temperature in the clinic is 100.5°F, and she appears uncomfortable. Physical examination is notable for marked right lower quadrant tenderness and some discomfort on the right side during pelvic exam.

    A. What other questions are important to ask about her history?
    B. What else would you ask about her abdominal pain?
    C. Generate a differential diagnosis list.
    D. What laboratory tests would you order?
    E. Would you order a pelvic ultrasound or CT scan?

CASE 29–2. A 9-year-old boy presents with a 2-day history of lower abdominal pain. He has had some diarrhea and vomiting. His mother noted tactile fevers at home. On examination, he looks quite ill and has diffuse abdominal tenderness and guarding, which is greater on the right side.

    A. What details about his pain are important to discern?
    B. What laboratory tests do you need?
    C. What are you concerned about that has already occurred?
    D. Do you need radiologic tests prior to calling the surgical consultant?

ANAL DISEASE

What is the anatomy of the anus?

Anal Canal

The anal canal begins a few centimeters proximal to the dentate line and ends at the anal verge (Fig. 29–2). The anal canal is about 5 cm in length. Histologically, the proximal end of the anal canal is the point at which the columnar epithelium of the rectum becomes transitional epithelium. This epithelium changes to a stratified squamous variety at the dentate line. The dentate line is a clearly observed, undulating line near the midpoint of the anal canal. It is at this location that the anal crypts are found. Anal glands secrete mucus into the anal crypts by way of anal ducts. The distal end of the anal canal is the anal verge, which is the point where the stratified

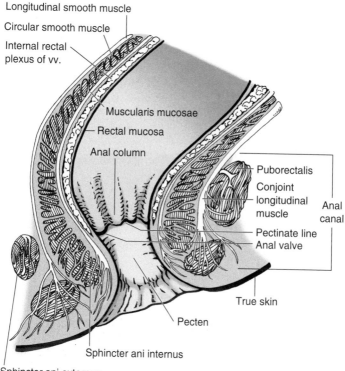

Figure 29–2. The anal canal. (From O'Rahilly R: Basic Human Anatomy: A Regional Study of Human Structure. Philadelphia, WB Saunders, 1983, p 305.)

squamous epithelium becomes true skin. It is marked by the presence of hair follicles and sweat glands. The *anoderm* is a term used to describe the zone between the dentate line and the anal verge.

Nerve Supply

Autonomic nerves supply the rectum and upper anal canal, whereas somatic nerves supply the lower anal canal and perianal skin. For this reason, rectal tumors and polyps can be biopsied without anesthesia. Internal hemorrhoids are also innervated by the autonomic nervous system; therefore, they can be treated without anesthesia using simple fixation techniques.

Blood Supply

Arterial Route. The blood supply of the rectum and anal canal comes from the terminal branches of the inferior mesenteric artery that form the superior hemorrhoidal (rectal) artery. The superior hemorrhoidal artery branches into the right and left branches, and the right branch divides into an anterior and posterior branch. The classic hemorrhoidal plexus are located at the left lateral, right anterolateral, and right posterolateral locations. The middle hemorrhoidal (rectal) arteries are direct branches from the internal iliac arteries. The inferior hemorrhoidal (rectal) arteries are branches of the pudendal arteries, which also arise from the internal iliac arteries.

Venous Route. The venous drainage of the anorectal region consists of the superior hemorrhoidal veins, which drain into the portal venous system, and the middle and inferior hemorrhoidal veins, which drain into the caval system via the internal iliac veins.

Lymphatics

Lymphatic drainage of the rectum travels along the internal iliac vessels as well as the aorta. Lymphatic drainage of the anal canal follows the internal iliac vessels but also may travel through channels located in the inguinal region.

Muscles

Internal Sphincter Muscle. The internal anal sphincter is smooth involuntary muscle and is simply the terminal thickening of the inner visceral smooth muscle layer of the rectal wall. The internal sphincter plays an important role in fecal continence.

External Sphincter Muscle. The external anal sphincter is skeletal muscle and thus under voluntary control. There is a distinct anatomic plane between the internal and external sphincters, and it is occupied by the longitudinal connective tissue fibers that are continuous with the outer longitudinal muscle of the rectum. The external anal sphincter is arbitrarily separated into the subcutaneous, superficial, and deep components.

Puborectalis Muscle. The puborectalis muscle is the deep component of the external anal sphincter. It is a significant muscle in terms of maintaining fecal continence. The puborectalis muscle originates and inserts on the pubis after encircling the rectum at the anorectal junction. When contracted, the puborectalis muscle creates a 90-degree angle between the anal canal and rectum. Puborectalis relaxation allows the anorectal angle to approach 180 degrees, which in combination with relaxation of the other components of the external anal sphincter allows defecation.

▶ **ETIOLOGY**

What are some common anal complaints?

Anal Pain

Pain in the anal area is a common symptom of anal disease. It is critical to determine the nature of the pain. Is the pain sharp? Does it come on with bowel action? How long does it last after a bowel action? Is it associated with a lump? Did the pain start suddenly (common with a thrombosed hemorrhoid)? Sharp pain with, and lasting after, a bowel movement is usually associated with an anal fissure. It is also critical to note whether the pain is aggravated by coughing or sneezing. Often patients who have an abscess around the rectum, especially if it is an intrasphincteric abscess, have horrible pain on coughing and sneezing.

There are several benign levator ani muscle spasm syndromes that can cause rectal pain as well. The most common is called *proctalgia fugax*. Patients often describe a cramping or gnawing pain 1 or 2 inches up inside the rectum, which occasionally awakens them at night. It is not associated with any anal pathology.

There are referred pains to the anorectum as well, and one must question the patient carefully regarding pain that radiates out into the buttocks or down the leg. Often this may indicate a referred pain to the anal area coming from an entrapment syndrome in the lower back.

Anal Lump

When inquiring about a lump, it is important to know whether it has come on suddenly, if it is tender, whether it is associated with any redness or a fever, and whether there is a protrusion from the anal canal. When the patient admits to a protrusion, ask whether it spontaneously returns to the anal canal or if the patient has to manually replace it.

Anal Itching

Anal itching is common and is usually seen with poor anal hygiene or with condylomata acuminata. It is often seen following the use of broad-spectrum antibiotics. It may be associated with a discharge.

Anal Discharge

There are several types of anal discharge. Generally, a purulent discharge is associated with an abscess, a bloody discharge is associated with the rupture of a thrombosed hemorrhoid, and a whitish or mucus discharge is associated with a rectal villous tumor. Other conditions, such as proctitis, can present with blood and mucus mixed together.

Anal Bleeding

Anal bleeding is probably the most common symptom in patients with anal disease. A great deal of information can be obtained from a thorough questioning of the nature of the bleeding. It often indicates what examination the patient needs at that particular moment. Is the blood seen only on the toilet tissue; streaked on the stool; mixed with the stool; associated with clots, pain, or mucus? Does it drip in the toilet water, expel with "spurting," and so forth?

▶ EVALUATION

How do I prepare the patient?

Preparation for examining a patient with an anorectal problem depends on whether the patient has an acute, painful condition. If so, no preparation is required. In a patient with a chronic condition, it is customary to prepare the patient with 1 or 2 Fleet Phospho-Soda enemas taken approximately 1 to 2 hours before the exam is scheduled. Antibiotic preparation is not indicated, except for patients who may have an artificial heart valve in place.

How do I proceed with the examination?

Although examination is everyday practice to the doctor, to the patient it is an unusual event. An unhurried demeanor, taking time to listen to the patient's story, and explaining in advance the sequence of the examination and what the patient may feel at each stage helps allay anxiety. The room should be well heated, and the patient should be comfortable on the examining table.

Three positions are in general use for examining the anorectum: left lateral, knee-chest (prone jackknife), and lithotomy. The choice is largely determined by the habit and training of the clinician.

Inspection

Inspection is critical since a great deal of information can be obtained by simply viewing the perianal area. One can diagnose perianal pruritus, and 90% of anal fissures can be diagnosed by gently moving the anal tissues. Hidradenitis (an infection in the apocrine sweat glands), anal tumors, pilonidal disease, and condylomata acuminata are also readily apparent on simple inspection of the perianal area. Laxity of the anal orifice can also be ascertained by just a simple inspection. The patient is then asked to strain to demonstrate any prolapsing hemorrhoidal tissue or rectal mucosal prolapse.

Digital Exam

Digital examination starts on the outside of the anal canal. The clinician looks for induration in the perianal tissues, such as would be found with a fistula in ano, as well as tenderness and swelling. The digital examination of the anal canal should be carried out carefully and slowly, with a well-lubricated finger.

Anoscopic Exam

Direct visual examination of the anal canal is usually carried out with a small anoscope. If the patient has a painful condition, the clinician should insert the anoscope away from the pain in the anal area. If the patient has an acute abscess, the patient should be examined under anesthesia. The obturator in the slotted anoscope can be removed in each quadrant, thereby allowing you to view each quadrant easily. One should never turn the anoscope without the obturator in place.

Proctoscopic Exam

Proctoscopic examinations can be carried out with either a rigid or flexible sigmoidoscope. One must keep in mind that there is a 90-degree angle between the anal canal and the rectum when one is introducing the scope. The clinician should use a minimal amount of air in insufflating the rectum. Flexible sigmoidoscopy, using a 60-cm-long flexible endoscope, also allows for the detection of lesions in the sigmoid colon. It can be performed easily in an outpatient setting with one or two cleansing phospho-soda enemas. The clinician is able to biopsy through the scope with ease. Insufflated air should be removed from the colon just before withdrawal of the scope.

Colonoscopy

Colonoscopy is the most accurate method of investigating the large bowel mucosa and has the advantage over barium enema that tissue can be obtained for histologic examination. However, it is more time-consuming, and in 15% to 20% of patients complete examination of the colon may not be possible. Colonoscopy is indicated where the results of a barium enema examination are equivocal or where symptoms remain unexplained after a normal radiograph of the colon. Accuracy of colonoscopy and barium enema in the right side of the colon are similar for cancer, but the colonoscope is superior in identifying smaller lesions. Colonoscopy may be useful to monitor disease and to detect the onset of recurrent cancers in patients at risk. It permits biopsy of lesions through the whole colon, as well as removal of polyps. Colonoscopic snare polypectomy is the treatment of choice for the majority of colonic polyps. Approximately 95% are amenable to this method of treatment. Contraindications for polypectomy include a polyp with a base wider than 2.5 cm or a polyp in which malignant change is strongly suspected. Full bowel preparation is essential for colonoscopy. The examination is usually done as an outpatient procedure. Sedation is usually required.

What other studies may be performed?

Anorectal ultrasound is commonly used to stage rectal cancers and evaluate the perirectal area for involved lymph nodes. It is also helpful in evaluating complicated anorectal fistulas.

Occasionally, magnetic resonance (MR) imaging may be indicated if a fistula is complex or recurrent. In recent years, the anorectal physiology lab has been most helpful in studying problems such as constipation related to the pelvic floor. One of the common causes of constipation is outlet obstruction caused by inappropriate puborectalis muscle function. This can be diagnosed with cine-defecography and electromyography in a pelvic floor laboratory. Many women with rectoceles, if properly studied, may benefit from biofeedback therapy and thereby forego an unnecessary surgical procedure.

A pelvic floor laboratory is also helpful in diagnosing Hirschsprung's disease and evaluating patients with incontinence.

ANAL PRURITUS

▶ ETIOLOGY

What is the cause of anal pruritus?

Pruritus ani is a symptom, not a disease, and occurs in many conditions. Irritation or soreness should be distinguished from pain. When the condition becomes chronic, the skin becomes thick and lichenified. The most common cause of anal pruritus is poor anal hygiene. Other causes of pruritus ani include infections, dermatologic conditions, anorectal conditions, diarrheal states, and neoplasia.

▶ EVALUATION

How should the patient be evaluated?

Evaluation of a patient with pruritus ani starts with an accurate history. In addition to questions about anal hygiene, the patient should be asked about recent antibiotic use.

▶ TREATMENT

How is the patient with anal pruritus treated?

It is important to review proper perianal hygiene with the patient. Patients must be instructed to cleanse the anal canal carefully and to remove any bits of stool that are in the creases of the anal canal. The perianal area can then be treated with a barrier cream, such as Calmoseptine, often preceded by a short course of hydrocortisone cream. Frequently these patients are also treated with an antifungal agent, such as clotrimazole (Lotrimin) 1% cream. If the pruritus ani persists, skin punch biopsies should be taken under local anesthesia to rule out rare causes, such as Bowen's disease, Paget's disease, or psoriasis.

HEMORRHOIDAL DISEASE

▶ CLASSIFICATION

How are hemorrhoids classified?

Hemorrhoids are a common problem and are usually manifest by symptoms of pain, itching, or irritation in the anal area. Hemorrhoids traditionally have been classified using the following scheme:

First degree: no detectable prolapse
Second degree: spontaneous reducing of prolapse
Third degree: detectable prolapse requiring manual reduction
Fourth degree: permanent prolapse

▶ ETIOLOGY

What is the difference between an internal and an external hemorroid?

Internal hemorrhoids occur proximal to the dentate line. External hemorrhoids occur distal to the dentate line and are covered by squamous epithelium. A thrombosed external hemorrhoid is actually an intravascular thrombosis rather than a perianal hematoma. An external skin tag results from the spontaneous resolution of a thrombosed hemorrhoid. Mixed hemorrhoids are the combination of both internal and external hemorrhoids and are due to looseness of the rectal mucosa, which allows them to prolapse out of the anal aperture. Strangulated hemorrhoids are prolapsed hemorrhoids in which the blood supply is compromised due to sphincter spasm. Progression of this condition results in gangrenous hemorrhoids.

▶ TREATMENT

The treatment of hemorrhoids is directed solely toward those that are symptomatic. Asymptomatic hemorrhoids require no therapy.

How are internal hemorrhoids treated?

Treatment varies depending on the degree. First- and second-degree hemorrhoids (the most common symptom of which is bleeding) can usually be managed with dietary regulation, such as adding bulk to the diet. If bleeding is a problem, banding or infrared coagulation can be used to treat the hemorrhoid. Patients with third-degree hemorrhoids usually are considered for operative resection. If symptoms cannot be relieved by applying a ligature to the internal hemorrhoidal complex as an outpatient procedure, surgical excision may be indicated. Fourth-degree hemorrhoids, those with permanent prolapse, must be treated with surgical excision.

How are external hemorrhoids treated?

External hemorrhoids usually are symptomatic when they cause pain or become thrombosed. Radical elliptical excision under local anesthesia is the treatment of choice. If the patient presents with a subacute or resolving thrombosed hemorrhoid, usually only reassurance and education regarding the hemorrhoid condition are indicated. The patient should return for a full examination later when he or she has less pain.

How are mixed hemorrhoids treated?

The treatment of mixed hemorrhoids is directed toward the most symptomatic component. If patients have to manually replace their hemorrhoids, surgical excision is usually indicated.

How are strangulated hemorrhoids treated?

Hemorrhoidectomy on an urgent basis is usually mandatory. Usually, patients are admitted to the hospital for approximately

24 hours to make certain that their pain control is adequate. The operation may be done under general anesthesia, regional anesthesia, or local anesthesia with sedation.

Approximately 2% of patients undergoing hemorrhoidectomy have a complication requiring a subsequent return to the operating room, namely an unhealed wound, bleeding, or anal stenosis.

ANORECTAL SUPPURATIVE DISEASES

Abscess

Anorectal infections often have two phases: an "acute" abscess phase and a "chronic" fistula in ano. In 30% to 60% of cases, anorectal abscesses do not lead to fistulas.

When diagnosing acute abscess, one must always keep in mind the diagnoses of hidradenitis suppurativa, pilonidal abscess, and anorectal Crohn's disease. The majority of acute abscesses originate in the anal glands, of which there are 4 to 10. The anal glands are located around the circumference of the anal canal at the level of the dentate line. Most of the glands are located in the posterior midline. The patient with an abscess presents with acute pain and swelling in the anal region. Malaise and pyrexia are common.

Do not rely on antibiotics to cure the abscess. They are useful as an adjunct to surgery only in select patients, namely, patients with a prosthetic heart valve or those who are immunosuppressed or diabetic. Delay of surgical drainage allows extension of the abscess to form a more complex type of fistula or risks systemic sepsis, distant abscesses, septic shock, and even death.

Most acute abscesses can be drained under local anesthesia as an outpatient procedure. The incision should be made as close to the anal verge as possible in case a fistula develops. Certain abscesses that do not have an external component have to be examined and drained in the operating room.

Once drainage has been established, one then must consider the possibility of a fistula's developing. Usually the patient is requested to come back to the clinic for examination in 7 to 10 days. One can do a bidigital examination and feel the induration of the fistula's tract. The recent introduction of anal ultrasound with hydrogen peroxide injection of the fistula's tract is especially helpful in outlining the anatomy of the fistula's tract. Complex fistulas or previously operated fistulas may even require MR imaging examination to delineate the relationship of the tracts to the anal sphincter. In the patient who has had an abscess drained without obvious signs of fistula development, microscopic fistula may still be present, leading to a recurrence.

Fistula in Ano

This condition usually presents as a noticeable discharge from the external opening of the anal canal. Differential diagnosis of fistula in ano includes hidradenitis, pilonidal disease, simple perianal suppurative disease, and infected sebaceous cysts.

There are four main classes of fistula in ano:

Intersphincteric: most common
Transsphincteric: second most common
Supersphincteric: rare
Extrasphincteric: trauma or systemic disease

The usual relationship of the cutaneous openings relative to the anal orifice is described by Goodsall's rule (Fig. 29–3).

Successful treatment involves an operative procedure that accurately defines the course of the fistula and then deals with the tract and the internal and external openings. Spontaneous healing of a fistula in ano is rare.

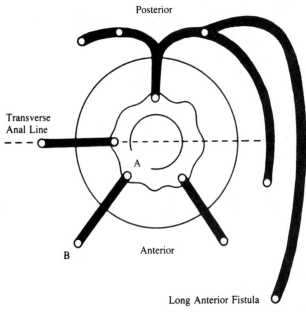

Figure 29–3. The internal orifice is labeled A. The rule predicts that if a line is drawn transversely across the anus, an external opening (B) anterior to this line will lead to a straight radial tract, whereas an external opening that lies posterior to this line will lead to a curved tract and an internal opening in the posterior commissure. The long anterior fistula is an exception to the rule. (From Sabiston D [ed]: Textbook of Surgery: The Biological Basis of Modern Surgical Practice, 15th ed. Philadelphia, WB Saunders, 1997, p 1041.)

The classic operation for fistula in ano is the lay-open technique. This involves transection of a portion of the sphincteric mechanism. For high transsphincteric fistulas and suprasphincteric fistulas, staged operations with a seton and a combination of endoanal flaps are often used.

Patients who are being considered for corrective surgery for fistula in ano must be informed that there may be some alteration in their control of gas and liquid stool following surgery.

Fistulas in Inflammatory Bowel Disease

Fistula in ano is seen in patients with Crohn's disease and can be difficult to manage. Frequently, if fistulas involve a significant amount of the sphincter mechanism, a seton is placed and may be left in permanently. Often the fistula can be so extensive that the patient is essentially incontinent, and a proctectomy is necessary.

Pilonidal Disease

Pilonidal disease is an infection of the skin and subcutaneous tissue located over the sacrococcygeal region in the gluteal cleft. Hair shafts can grow into the subcutaneous tissue. Midline intergluteal skin holes communicate with the subcutaneous cavities. Infection of these cavities and the surrounding skin causes pilonidal disease. The disease is generally one of four varieties: (1) an acute abscess, (2) recurrent abscesses, (3) chronic abscess and draining sinus, or (4) unhealed surgical wound. The appropriate treatment for any abscess is incision and drainage under local anesthesia. The patient needs to be followed in case a persistent pilonidal sinus develops. If the patient has evidence of chronic disease with nodularity and several sinus tracts, excision of the involved tissue is indicated.

Anal Fissure

An anal fissure is a common clinical entity. It is a break or a "tear" in the stratified squamous epithelium of the distal anal canal. The majority of anal fissures are located in the posterior midline. If it is located laterally, one must think of Crohn's disease, human immunodeficiency virus (HIV), or a malignancy of the anal canal. If Crohn's disease is suspected, a complete evaluation of the GI tract is indicated. Other rare causes of anal fissure include syphilis, tuberculosis, and leukemia.

The classic symptoms of an anal fissure are extreme pain, usually brought on during defecation, associated with red blood that may streak the stool or be present on the toilet tissue. Patients frequently avoid defecation because of the pain. The pain has been described as a feeling of passing glass during defecation. Examination reveals a classic posterior ulcer in the anoderm. A chronic anal fissure usually has associated scar tissue and hypertrophied anal papillae at the dentate line. There may be an external skin tag that is frequently called a *sentinel pile*.

Initial management is usually warm tub baths, a high-fiber diet with psyllium fiber, and an anesthetic cream containing hydrocortisone. Medical therapy is directed at softening the stool and releasing the pressure of the internal sphincter. Topical nitrates have been used with variable success. The proposed mechanism of action for nitroglycerin paste has been to reduce the anal sphincter pressure as well as increase the anal blood flow.

Surgical treatment for anal fissure has always been aimed at reducing the resting pressures of the anal canal. Anal dilation has been used for many years and is a simple procedure. The disadvantage is that it may lead to irreversible fecal incontinence in more than 10% of the patients. Lateral internal sphincterotomy is perhaps the most common surgical procedure for the treatment of anal fissure. It is usually done under local anesthesia with sedation. The healing rate is better than 90%. Temporary incontinence has been documented but usually resolves in several months. Permanent incontinence occurs in approximately 5% to 6% of patients.

Hidradenitis Suppurativa

Hidradenitis suppurativa is an infection of the apocrine sweat glands. The infection can be localized or spread in an intradermal fashion. The dermal sinus tracts can be quite extensive. Hidradenitis suppurativa may be mistaken for an anal fistula. Treatment for an acute abscess is the same as any other abscess, with incision and drainage after local anesthesia. Definitive treatment involves excision and may occasionally require plastic surgical techniques for wound management. Antibiotics do not prevent recurrence.

PROLAPSE OF THE RECTUM

▶ ETIOLOGY

What is rectal prolapse?

Rectal procidentia, or complete rectal prolapse, means that the full thickness of the rectal wall circumferentially protrudes through the anal canal. On rare occasions, the prolapse can become incarcerated with vascular compromise, which is a surgical emergency. Most patients with rectal prolapse have a defect in the pelvic floor muscles with a diastasis of the levator ani muscles and a weakening of the endopelvic fascia. On radiograph they show a loss of the normal horizontal position of the rectum. At the time of surgery, an abnormally deep cul-de-sac of Douglas is noted. Often, these patients have a markedly redundant colon, particularly the sigmoid colon. A significant number of these patients are incontinent and have a patulous, weak anal sphincter.

▶ EVALUATION

How is rectal prolapse diagnosed?

This condition is diagnosed by asking patients to strain, which reveals complete prolapse through the anal aperture. If patients have signs of incontinence, their anorectal function should be studied carefully, since this may alter surgical therapy. If they also are troubled with constipation, which is frequent, it is important to evaluate their colonic motility with a transit time study because this information may also impact the decision regarding surgical therapy.

▶ TREATMENT

How is rectal prolapse treated?

Abdominal Operations. Many abdominal operations have been advocated for rectal prolapse. Most of them involve some form of fixation of the rectum to the periosteum of the sacrum. This may or may not be combined with a bowel resection, depending on the redundancy of the colon. The initial step in the genesis of a prolapse is the intussusception of the sigmoid colon into the upper rectum. Any operation that prevents this intussusception prevents a recurrence. The most common operation done in the United States involves an abdominal proctopexy with or without a sigmoid resection. Occasionally, with the patient with an atonic colon, a subtotal colectomy and an abdominal proctopexy may be required.

Perineal Operations. Perineal operations have been advocated for rectal prolapse for many years. The most common one is a rectosigmoidectomy with a coloanal anastomosis.

ANAL CANCER

▶ ETIOLOGY

What is anal cancer?

Carcinoma of the anal canal differs from rectal carcinoma histologically and in its treatment. Anal canal epidermoid carcinoma involves either the transitional epithelium of the proximal anal canal or the stratified squamous epithelium of the distal anal canal. Based on histology, it may be termed a *cloacogenic, basaloid carcinoma,* or *squamous carcinoma*. Patients may present with pain, a mass, and bleeding.

▶ EVALUATION

How is anal cancer detected?

On examination, the mass may be visible on inspection at the anal opening or detected only by digital and anoscopic exam. Biopsy confirms the diagnosis.

▶ TREATMENT

How is anal cancer treated?

In contrast to rectal carcinoma, treatment most often does not require radical resection. Anal canal carcinoma most often is managed with combination chemotherapy and radiation therapy. An abdominoperineal excision is usually required if the patient fails therapy with chemotherapy and radiation therapy.

Carcinomas involving the perianal skin beyond the anal verge are typical skin cancers: squamous cell carcinoma, melanoma, and basal cell carcinoma. Treatment for these skin cancers is excisional. Perianal Paget's disease is in situ anal adenocarcinoma. Bowen's disease is an in situ squamous carcinoma. These patients present with a longstanding anal pruritus. Biopsy yields a diagnosis, and effective treatment involves excision of all involved skin.

SEXUALLY TRANSMITTED DISEASE

Sexually transmitted diseases (STDs), involving more than 50 organisms, continue to increase worldwide. The accurate diagnosis and treatment of STDs of the anorectum can be difficult because patients often harbor more than one organism. Distinguishing between what is acting as a pathogen and what has merely colonized the anorectum is not always easy.

Condylomata Acuminata

Anal condylomata acuminata, or anal warts, are caused by the human papillomavirus. They are most often acquired by sexual contact. Presenting symptoms include pain, bleeding, itching, and a discharge or the mere presence of topical nodules. Examination reveals anal warts that vary in size and extent. Some patients develop a dysplastic lesion as well as an invasive squamous cell carcinoma.

Treatment involves biopsy of representative lesions and destruction of the remaining lesions. Recurrence is high, and counseling the patients and their sexual partners is advised.

Gonorrhea

Gonorrhea is likely the most common STD affecting the anorectum. It is caused by the gram-negative intracellular diplococcus *Neisseria gonorrhoeae*. Anorectal gonorrhea almost uniformly results in a thick yellow mucopurulent discharge from the anus. Sigmoidoscopy often reveals a proctitis extending to no more than about 10 cm from the anal verge. Diagnosis is made by culturing the organism. First-line treatment is now a single intramuscular injection of 250 mg of ceftriaxone, followed by doxycycline 100 mg orally twice a day for 7 days.

Chlamydia trachomatis Infection

Chlamydia trachomatis is the most common sexually transmitted bacterial infection worldwide. Symptoms of anorectal infection include pain, tenesmus, and fever. Sigmoidoscopy reveals a severe granular proctitis with mucosal friability and frank ulceration. Diagnosis is made with a biopsy of the inflamed mucosa. Treatment is with oral tetracycline or erythromycin 500 mg four times a day.

Syphilis

Primary anal syphilis caused by the spirochete *Treponema pallidum* is largely a disease of homosexual men. Diagnosis is by demonstration of the corkscrew-shaped yellow-green spirochetes on dark-field examination. Treatment is with a single dose of 2.4 million units of long-acting benzathine penicillin.

Herpes Simplex

Anogenital herpes simplex virus (HSV) infection is caused in most cases by HSV-2, with only about 10% being caused by HSV-1. The symptoms include minor local irritation, burning, and paresthesias in the anorectal area. A painful proctitis has also been noted. On examination, tiny red vesicles are typically seen and may be clustered or scattered in the perianal skin. Diagnosis is made with a Papanicolaou smear or a positive Tzanck preparation. Treatment of an acute infection is with acyclovir.

HIV

Surgery for anorectal disorders remains among the most common procedures performed in HIV-positive individuals. The anorectal conditions that affect HIV-positive patients generally fall into one of two broad categories: either a routine condition that occurs in the general population or a disorder that is unique to the HIV-positive individual. Treatment plans must take into consideration the effect of repetitive anoreceptive intercourse on sphincter function, the presence of diarrhea, and prior sphincter-cutting surgery. Anal condyloma is the most common anorectal condition seen in HIV patients.

There is a high incidence of anal intraepithelial neoplasia (AIN) in HIV patients. Although there is controversy surrounding the management of AIN in the HIV patient, the tendency is to observe these patients carefully at 3-month intervals rather than excising excessive anal tissue. Cytomegalovirus (CMV), acid-fast bacilli, and HSV may cause ulcers in the immunosuppressed patient. Despite a thorough search for a causative factor, a specific etiology cannot be identified in up to 50% of the HIV-positive patients with anorectal ulcers.

K E Y   P O I N T S

▶ The anal canal, beginning at the dentate line and ending at the anal verge, is about 5 cm in length.

▶ Bleeding is the most common symptom in patients with anal disease.

▶ The treatment of symptomatic hemorrhoids depends on the type and severity of the disease.

▶ Anorectal abscesses require surgical drainage.

▶ Many types of STDs can affect the anal canal.

CASE 29–3. A 25-year-old woman presents with a painful perianal mass. On examination, the area is erythematous, exquisitely tender, and fluctuant. The mass is subsequently drained in the operating room and diagnosed as a perirectal abscess. Six weeks later, the patient returns with foul-smelling discharge from a sinus tract to the left of the anus.

   A. What exam is necessary for evaluation of this problem?
   B. What is the most probable diagnosis, based on this patient's symptoms?
   C. What are the treatment options?

BILIARY TRACT

The majority of the symptoms that warrant surgical consultation result from obstruction and/or inflammation at some point in the biliary tract.

▶ ANATOMY AND PHYSIOLOGY

What is bile?

Bile is synthesized in the liver. It consists of an emulsion of bile salts, cholesterol, lecithin, and bile pigment (bilirubin). Bile functions to aid in digestion and absorption of fats in the intestine and to transport and excrete products of metabolism (bilirubin, cholesterol, phospholipids). Bile secretion, particularly in response to a fatty meal, is increased by secretin, cholecystokinin (CCK), vasoactive intestinal peptide (VIP), and gastrin.

What are the structure and function of the biliary tract?

The biliary tract is responsible for storage, transport, and secretion of bile into the intestine. The biliary tract consists of the tiny biliary canaliculi, intrahepatic bile ducts, extrahepatic bile ducts, the gallbladder, and the ampulla of Vater (Fig. 29–4). The extrahepatic bile ducts exit the underside of the liver as right and left hepatic ducts and merge to become the common hepatic duct. The gallbladder sits under the liver in the gallbladder fossa and is drained by a small cystic duct inferomedially, which then enters the common hepatic duct. The cystic duct enters at a variable point along the common hepatic duct, which then becomes the common bile duct. The common bile duct continues into the head of the pancreas, where it usually joins with the pancreatic duct and empties into the second portion of the duodenum, medially. The terminus of the bile duct is called the *ampulla of Vater,* and efflux of bile is controlled at this site by the sphincter of Oddi.

What is the gallbladder?

The gallbladder is a hollow organ that acts as a reservoir for the storage and concentration of bile. It receives bile via the cystic duct. Increased pressure in the bile duct relative to the gallbladder ensures filling. Gallbladder contraction is stimulated by meals via the release of CCK, motilin, secretin, gastrin, and cerulein, particularly in response to a fatty meal. Although the gallbladder is rich in vagal innervation, sectioning of the vagus nerve does not alter hormonal-stimulated contraction. The gallbladder is not an essential organ. One percent to 1.5% of patients have digestive symptoms after cholecystectomy. These symptoms are usually mild.

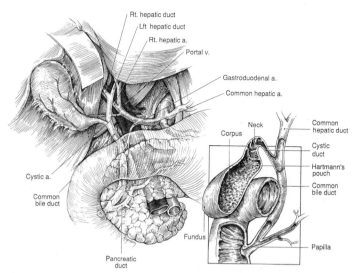

Figure 29–4. Anatomy of the biliary system and its relation to surrounding structures. (From Sabiston D [ed]: Textbook of Surgery: The Biological Basis of Modern Surgical Practice, 15th ed. Philadelphia, WB Saunders, 1997, p 1118.)

What is the enterohepatic circulation?

The enterohepatic circulation is the normal active re-uptake of bile salts in the terminal ileum for recycling in the liver. Resorption of bile salts is a passive function elsewhere in the intestine. Normal enterohepatic circulation allows for recycling of about 2 g of bile salts six times daily, with about 0.5 g being lost in the intestine. The loss is matched by hepatic synthesis. Patients with disruption of the enterohepatic circulation (i.e., ileal resection or bile duct obstruction) may experience diarrhea or malabsorption. Over time, though, increased hepatic synthesis and increased jejunal and colonic absorption of bile salts may ameliorate these symptoms.

What is the triangle of Calot?

The triangle of Calot is an important surgical landmark consisting of the cystic duct inferolaterally, the common hepatic duct inferomedially, and the inferior border of the liver superiorly. Variability in the anatomy of the hepatobiliary blood supply and the ductal structures is common, and this area deserves great respect from surgeons (see Fig. 29–4).

▶ ETIOLOGY

What are some of the terms used to describe biliary pathology?

Cholelithiasis—stones in the gallbladder
Choledocholithiasis—stones in the bile ducts
Cholecystitis—acute or chronic inflammation of the gallbladder
Gallbladder hydrops—chronic obstruction of the gallbladder resulting in dilation of the gland
Biliary colic—recurrent pain in the right upper quadrant associated with cholelithiasis
Ascending cholangitis—severe infection resulting from obstruction of the bile ducts
Jaundice—a build-up of bilirubin in the blood stream resulting in yellow skin and sclerae

What causes gallstones?

Gallstones are common. Precise reasons for gallstone formation remain elusive but appear to be due to an imbalance in the bile constituents and solubility, leading to precipitation of bile as sludge or stones. Most stones form in the gallbladder. By the age of 75 years, about 35% of women and 20% of men will have developed gallstones. Not all are symptomatic. Factors predisposing to gallstone formation include genetics (familial, certain geographic regions, and ethnic groups), pregnancy, rapid and significant weight loss (including after surgery for obesity), diabetes, obesity, gender (female tendency), biliary stasis, or inflammation. Pigmented stones (bilirubin) are common in patients with hemolytic conditions such as thalassemia, sickle cell states, and hemolytic anemias. Most gallstones are mixed or cholesterol stones; 20% to 30% are primarily pigmented stones. Roughly 15% contain enough calcium to be visible on a plain radiograph or CT scan.

The components of bile (bile salts, cholesterol, lecithin, and bilirubin) make up an emulsion. Both bile pigment and cholesterol are poorly soluble in aqueous solution, and the bile salts and the lecithin form micelles to keep them in solution. This arrangement is tenuous at best, and various factors may cause the cholesterol or bile pigment to precipitate out of solution. Figure 29–5 demonstrates the narrow balance between the components to achieve solubility. An excess of one or the other insoluble ingredients can cause precipitation leading to stone formation. Thus, there are two common components of gallstones: cholesterol and bilirubin. The components are usually mixed but may be relatively pure in settings of greatly increased cholesterol or bilirubin secretion. Bilirubin can precipitate with calcium, creating the insoluble salt calcium bilirubinate.

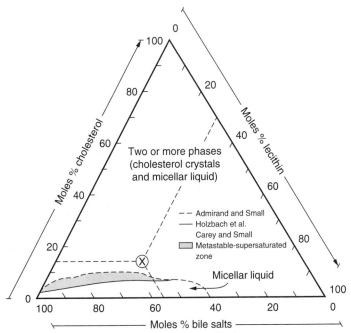

Figure 29–5. Determination of cholesterol saturation index (CSI). Tricoordinate-phase diagram for representing by a single intersecting point (x) relative concentrations of cholesterol, lecithin, and bile salt in bile. In this scheme, relative concentration of each lipid is expressed as a percentage of the sum of the molar concentrations of all three. This manipulation permits representation of the relations between three constituents in two dimensions, the water content being invariant at, say 90% (10% wt/vol solids). In this figure, for example, at point x, the relative concentration of bile salt from its coordinate is 55% (indicating 55% of the sum of all three lipids), whereas that for lecithin is 30% and that for cholesterol is 15%. The range of concentrations found consistent with a clear, aqueous micellar solution is limited to a small region at the lower left. A solution having the composition represented by the point x, on the other hand, would initially be visually turbid and contain precipitated forms of cholesterol crystals in addition to bile salt-mixed micelles. Last, a solution represented by a point falling in the shaded area below the dashed line would be unstable (i.e., meta-stable, supersaturated), meaning that by prediction it would be initially clear (micellar). Within a short time, however, various precipitated forms of cholesterol crystals would form, and such a solution would then be visually turbid, similar to all solutions above the dashed line. (From Sleisenger MH, Fordtran JS [eds]: Gastrointestinal Disease: Pathophysiology, Diagnosis, Management, 3rd ed. Philadelphia, WB Saunders, 1983, p 435.)

How do gallstones cause symptoms?

Gallstones cause symptoms when they obstruct some portion of the biliary tree. The spectrum of disease includes biliary colic, chronic cholecystitis, acute cholecystitis, and choledocholithiasis with or without associated cholangitis. Intermittent cystic duct blockage causes biliary colic. Blockage of the gallbladder combined with inflammation results in acute or chronic cholecystitis. Blockage of the bile ducts may cause pain and jaundice and lead to mild, moderate, or severe and life-threatening ascending cholangitis. Blockage of the pancreatic duct, or passage of a gallstone through the ampulla of Vater, may lead to mild, moderate, or severe and life-threatening pancreatitis.

What is biliary colic?

Biliary colic is a symptom complex occurring when the gallbladder or bile duct contracts against a stone or other obstruction. Right upper quadrant or epigastric pain is episodic, rapid in onset, and spiking in nature and resolves with the relaxation of the contraction. Classic symptoms of biliary colic are caused by gallbladder stones. The pain often follows meals, especially those rich in fatty content. The pain begins within 2 hours of the meal and may last for several hours.

What is chronic cholecystitis?

Chronic cholecystitis results from recurrent bouts of biliary colic almost invariably due to gallstones. Chronic or intermittent obstruction of the gallbladder causes changes in the gallbladder wall that can be seen pathologically as scarring, loss of mucosa, and the occasional extension of bile glands beyond the muscularis (Rokitansky-Aschoff sinuses). Chronic cholecystitis may also result in functional changes to the gallbladder with inability to adequately concentrate bile and poor filling and contraction on functional studies. Symptoms may include biliary colic; abdominal, chests or back pain; or simply a vague pain in the right upper quadrant after eating.

What is acute cholecystitis?

Acute cholecystitis results from infection or inflammation of the gallbladder; 90% to 95% of the cases result from obstruction of the cystic duct. Signs and symptoms include pain, fever, and occasionally mild jaundice, secondary to hepatic inflammation, dysfunction, and stasis. The clinical presentation of acute cholecystitis may range from a mild illness, with low-grade fever and leukocytosis, to a severe septic illness with gangrene of the gallbladder, bacteremia, and sometimes even perforation of the gallbladder. The right upper quadrant is markedly tender to palpation. Laboratory abnormalities may include mild elevations in serum bilirubin and alkaline phosphatase and variable elevation of the white blood cell count. Occasionally, serum amylase, alanine aminotransferase, and aspartate aminotransferase are elevated. The pain associated with acute cholecystitis may be epigastric or right sided. It may also radiate to the back, between the scapulae.

What is Murphy's sign?

Murphy's sign is a clinical finding. The patient inhales while the examiner palpates the right upper quadrant. A positive Murphy's sign results from patients' halting their inspiration during the exam. Often tenderness is encountered, but it is not necessary for a positive test. A positive Murphy's sign is an indication of inflammation somewhere in the right upper quadrant. Although classically described with acute cholecystitis, it may also be present in cases of acute hepatitis, colitis, right-sided pyelonephritis, and pancreatitis. A more sensitive approach is to perform the exam under ultrasound guidance, termed *ultrasonic Murphy's sign*. The ultrasound probe is placed directly over the gallbladder during the test. A positive ultrasonic Murphy's sign is highly specific for acute cholecystitis.

Can acute cholecystitis occur in the absence of stones?

Yes. Acalculous cholecystitis constitutes about 5% of cases of acute cholecystitis. This disease is commonly seen in patients who are seriously ill from some other source, such as burns or trauma or following other operations. Other predisposing factors include sepsis, prolonged parenteral nutrition, starvation, and multiple blood transfusions. The incidence is increased in patients with collagen vascular disease such as sarcoidosis, polyarteritis nodosum, and lupus erythematosus.

What is hydrops of the gallbladder?

Hydrops results from complete obstruction of the cystic duct and dilation of the gallbladder. The gallbladder fills with mucus, and the term *white bile* is used to describe it. Hydrops is frequently painful, and the gallbladder is often palpable.

What is a porcelain gallbladder?

A porcelain gallbladder has calcium in the gallbladder wall and is a risk factor for gallbladder cancer. Often, the gallbladder is visible on plain films or CT. Porcelain gallbladder is one of the indications for cholecystectomy in the absence of stones or biliary symptoms.

What is emphysematous cholecystitis?

This is a radiographic finding of gas in the wall of the gallbladder. It is associated with severe acute cholecystitis.

What is a Courvoisier's gallbladder?

Courvoisier's gallbladder is the finding of a massive, palpable, non-tender gallbladder. Courvoisier's gallbladder results from chronic obstruction of the common bile duct. This is usually seen in patients with carcinoma and progressive narrowing of the bile duct. Nontender distention is rarely seen due to gallstone disease, which is associated with acute obstruction of the duct.

What is choledocholithiasis?

About 10% to 15% of patients with gallbladder stones may develop choledocholithiasis (common duct stones). Stones in the gallbladder may migrate down the cystic duct into the bile duct and lodge there or pass through the ampulla into the duodenum. Persistent common bile duct stones may continue to grow until they cause symptoms by obstructing the bile duct. Infrequently, stones may form primarily in the bile duct.

Stones in the bile duct may be asymptomatic or may cause biliary colic, partial or complete biliary obstruction with associated jaundice, cholangitis, or pancreatitis. The severity of the symptoms is directly related to the degree of obstruction, pressure in the biliary tree, presence or absence of infection, and degree of pancreatic irritation or disruption. Complete biliary ductal obstruction is associated with severe pain and hyperbilirubinemia (≤ 15 mg/dL).

What is ascending cholangitis?

Ascending cholangitis is a clinical syndrome whose hallmarks are biliary obstruction, increased pressure in the biliary tree, and infected bile. The obstruction may be due to intraluminal stones, prior surgical injury, trauma, or stricture of benign or malignant origin. The presentation of ascending cholangitis may range from mild fever, jaundice, and right upper quadrant pain to a fulminant, life-threatening condition associated with septic shock and death. In its severe form, cholangitis remains one of the true surgical emergencies, requiring immediate decompression of the bile ducts to alleviate bacteremia and shock.

What is Charcot's triad?

Charcot's triad is a clinical syndrome consisting of jaundice, right upper quadrant pain, and fever associated with acute ascending cholangitis. It is present in two thirds of the cases.

What is Reynold's pentad?

Reynold's pentad is a clinical syndrome that adds hypotension and mental status changes to the Charcot's triad. It is seen in cases of severe ascending cholangitis.

What causes bile duct strictures?

Strictures of the bile duct may be benign or malignant. Benign strictures are most commonly associated with gallstones and associated inflammation or injury to the bile ducts during biliary surgery (laparoscopic cholecystectomy). Other benign causes include trauma, pancreatitis, cholangitis, inflammatory diseases, or congenital abnormalities.

Malignant bile duct strictures may originate in the biliary tract or in any of the adjacent structures (i.e., lymphoma, pancreas, stomach or duodenum, liver substance). All strictures of the biliary tract should be considered malignant until proven otherwise.

What is gallstone ileus?

Gallstone "ileus" results when a large gallstone erodes though the wall of the gallbladder and into the small intestine. The ileus results from the stone's becoming lodged somewhere in the intestine (usually the ileocecal valve) and causing intestinal obstruction. Findings on plain films may include evidence of bowel obstruction, a stone in the right lower quadrant, or air in the biliary tree.

What forms of cancer can form in the biliary tract?

Malignant neoplasms occur in all parts of the biliary tract. Gallbladder cancer makes up 4% of all cancers of the alimentary tract, 75% of the cases presenting after the 6th decade of life. Although the etiology is unknown, risk factors include female gender, a history of cholelithiasis (present in 70% to 90% of cases), and porcelain gallbladder. Most of the tumors are adenocarcinoma and are found incidentally at the time of cholecystectomy.

Cancer of the bile ducts (cholangiocarcinoma) is uncommon, accounting for less than 0.5% of alimentary cancers, and is usually adenocarcinoma. Etiologic relationships are not clear, but bile duct stones are common, and in Asian patients, a history of infestation with *Ascaris* or *Clonorchis* is often present. There is also an increased incidence of cholangiocarcinoma in patients with long-standing ulcerative colitis. Tumors found in the most distal duct are called *ampullary carcinomas*. Those occurring at the bifurcation of the right and left hepatic ducts are termed *Klatskin's tumors*, and those originating in the liver are called *intrahepatic cholangiocarcinoma*.

What is sclerosing cholangitis?

Sclerosing cholangitis is an inflammatory disease affecting the bile ducts. It presents as fibrosis and narrowing and may affect both intrahepatic and extrahepatic ducts. The disease may be idiopathic, but as many as 70% of cases are associated with ulcerative colitis. Other associated diseases include Peyronie's disease, retroperitoneal or pancreatic fibrosis, or pancreatitis. The disease may present with vague right upper quadrant pain, weight loss, jaundice, or cholangitis. Progression may lead to cirrhosis, portal hypertension, and hepatic failure. Definitive treatment is liver transplantation. Disease limited to extrahepatic ducts may be treated with excision of the ducts and hepaticojejunostomy.

▶ EVALUATION

What historical points and examination findings are important?

The history and physical exam are the starting points of any evaluation for abdominal pain. Specific attention to the biliary tree includes questions regarding prior biliary disease or surgery, jaundice, dark urine or light stool, alcohol consumption, prior hepatitis or exposure to it, drug use, weight loss, pregnancy, and family history of gallstones. Physical exam should detect icterus or jaundice, stigmata of alcohol abuse, as well as the presence of abdominal tenderness, mass, or fluid (ascites).

What laboratory tests are used in the evaluation of biliary disease?

The most helpful laboratory tests are the complete blood cell count (CBC), liver panel, amylase, lipase, and coagulation profile. The CBC helps differentiate acute from chronic cholecystitis and determine the severity of infection or inflammation of the biliary system. The liver panel provides information regarding ductal obstruction (hyperbilirubinemia, alkaline phosphatase) and hepatocellular inflammation (transaminase elevation is much higher in cases of hepatitis than biliary disease). Pancreatic enzyme measurement aids in the diagnosis of pancreatitis. Many patients with acute or chronic biliary disease have coagulopathy secondary to liver dysfunction, infection, and malnutrition. A viral panel for hepatitis A, B, and C may also be helpful.

How is biliary colic evaluated?

Biliary colic is a symptom suggestive of and associated with gallstones. Ultrasound, CBC, and LFTs are obtained. The ultrasound report must be checked for the presence or absence of gallstones, ductal dilation, gallbladder wall thickening, and pericholecystic fluid. When stones are documented by ultrasound and there is no ductal dilation or jaundice, patients with recurrent biliary colic who are fit for surgery should be referred for cholecystectomy (most often laparoscopic). Occasionally, stones are not seen on ultrasound in patients with classic signs and symptoms. Oral chole-cystogram or HIDA scanning with a fatty meal may provide solid evidence of biliary disease. Elevation of the alkaline phosphatase level or the LFTs also suggest gallbladder disease in patients with biliary colic and cholecystectomy should be considered.

What imaging modalities are used to evaluate biliary disease?

Ultrasound of the right upper quadrant is the most helpful, most cost-effective, and least invasive imaging study for evaluation of bil-iary disease. Gallbladder stones, when present, are identified 90% to 95% of the time as echogenic foci. A contracted (chronically ill) gallbladder may be seen. Gallbladder wall thickening and peri-cholecystic fluid (signs of acute inflammation) can also be detected, though with less accuracy. Ultrasound is effective at identifying bil-iary ductal dilation, either intrahepatic or extrahepatic (common duct). Occasionally a stone is seen in the common duct, or a mass may be detected in the gallbladder or the ampullary region. Ultrasonography is less helpful in very obese patients or in patients with lots of bowel gas.

Plain abdominal radiographs are rarely indicated or helpful in the evaluation of biliary disease. Only 15% of gallstones are radiopaque.

Abdominal CT scanning is less accurate than ultrasound for detection of gallbladder stones but is highly effective at demon-strating extrahepatic or intrahepatic ductal dilation, masses any-where in the biliary tree or pancreatic region, presence of significant pancreatitis, and inflammation or fluid in or around the gallbladder.

An oral cholecystogram may confirm the presence of gallstones occasionally not seen by ultrasound. This study also may provide evidence of gallbladder dysfunction after a fatty meal or CCK stim-ulation. An oral dose of an iodinated compound is administered in the evening. The following morning a plain radiograph is taken. The gallbladder, if normal, should be opacified as the compound is secreted into the bile and taken up by the gallbladder. Failure to visualize the gallbladder indicates cystic duct obstruction. Contrast in the gallbladder may outline and demonstrate gallstones. Incomplete emptying after a fatty meal is evidence of dysfunction and chronic cholecystitis, especially if associated with pain. This study has been largely supplanted by ultrasonography but remains extremely accurate.

What is a HIDA scan?

A hepatobiliary iminodiacetic acid (HIDA) scan is a nuclear medicine study often used to evaluate the biliary tract. A radiolabeled sub-stance along with an iminodiacetic (IDA) compound (technetium-99 in conjunction with 2,6-dimethyl acetanilid) is injected intravenously. The radioisotope is excreted into the bile by the liver and taken up by the gallbladder. The liver is visible in 5 to 10 minutes, and the bile ducts and gallbladder are visible soon thereafter. Nonvisualization of the gallbladder is nearly always due to cystic duct obstruction. Nonvisualization of the gallbladder is diagnostic in a patient with right upper quadrant pain and a clinical picture of acute cholecystitis. Absence of radioactive tracer in the duodenum suggests biliary ductal obstruction. Dynamic study of the gallbladder may be performed during and after a fatty meal or CCK stimulus allowing calculation of a gallbladder ejection fraction. Patients must fast prior to examination, and false-positive studies (e.g., nonvisualized gallbladder) are possible in critically ill patients whose livers are dysfunctional or whose gallbladders may be chronically distended and dysfunctional from starvation and multisystem disease.

What is endoscopic retrograde cholangiopancreatography (ERCP)?

Endoscopic retrograde cholangiopancreatography (ERCP) is an invasive study that allows imaging and manipulation of the biliary tree (and pancreatic ducts) using upper GI endoscopy. Prone positioning and conscious sedation are required. The endoscope is passed into the duodenum where the ampulla is identified and cannulated. Video-imaging and fluoroscopy are used. The biliary tree may be imaged and biliary anatomy and pathology defined. Stones in the duct may be retrieved with balloons and baskets, thereby relieving obstruction. Strictures may be dilated or stented. Neoplasms may be biopsied or brushed for diagnosis. A sphincterotomy at the ampulla may be performed to allow a wider opening for ductal drainage. ERCP may be combined with endoscopic ultrasonography. ERCP has revolutionized the management of biliary disease by allowing less invasive treatment options than traditional surgical approaches. In skilled hands complications are uncommon (3% to 10%), but if they occur they may be significant (pancreatitis, cholangitis, bleeding, perforation, complications of conscious sedation).

What is a cholangiogram?

A cholangiogram is performed by access to the bile ducts (by ERCP, by intraoperative cannulation of the cystic duct or common bile duct, or by transhepatic approach) and instillation of radiopaque contrast material. It is the ideal way to evaluate the intraluminal anatomy of the bile ducts and to identify regions and sources of obstruction.

What is transhepatic cholangiography (THC)?

Transhepatic cholangiography (THC) is performed by passage of a thin needle through the abdominal wall into the liver and then into the intrahepatic bile ducts under CT or ultrasonic guidance. A catheter is passed into the duct and contrast material is instilled to define ductal anatomy by fluoroscopy or plain radiography. Biliary drainage may be accomplished by leaving catheters in place. Complications of THC are more common than with ERCP; therefore, this procedure is reserved for patients who are not candidates for ERCP or in whom ERCP was not successful (i.e., inability to cannulate the ampulla). Complications may include pain, bleeding, bile leak, sepsis, hemobilia, and catheter dislodgment.

How is a patient with suspected gallbladder cancer evaluated?

Carcinoma of the gallbladder should be included in the differential diagnosis of patients presenting with right upper quadrant pain, weight loss, and jaundice. Nausea, vomiting, and a palpable gallbladder may be present.

After a thorough history and physical examination, evaluation should at the least include a CBC, liver panel and coagulation profile, chest radiograph, and CT scan of the abdomen and pelvis. Most gallbladder cancers are discovered incidentally at the time of cholecystectomy or in the postoperative pathology specimen. If carcinoma is realized during a laparoscopic operation, the procedure should be converted to an open laparotomy. If carcinoma is discovered in the pathology specimen, a full laboratory panel in addition to staging CT scan is indicated. If gallbladder carcinoma is suggested on routine ultrasound, this should be followed by CT scanning with operative strategy based on staging.

How is a patient with suspected bile duct cancer evaluated?

Cancer of the bile ducts most commonly presents with ductal obstruction and jaundice. Symptoms of nausea, vomiting, malaise, fatigue, anorexia, and weight loss are common. Jaundice is often "painless" or may be associated with a dull or severe aching in the epigastrium or back. Hyperbilirubinemia may be profound (≤ 20 mg/dL), and patients report dark urine and clay-colored stool. After a thorough history and physical examination, lab survey should include a CBC, LFT panel, coagulation profile, chest radiograph, and CT scan of the abdomen and pelvis.

▶ TREATMENT

How is chronic cholecystitis treated?

Chronic cholecystitis is really a pathologic diagnosis. Patients usually have a history of chronic, intermittent biliary colic or repeated episodes of mild, acute cholecystitis and biliary colic. Symptoms may be severe or minimal.

Patients should undergo the same work-up outlined for biliary colic, and those fit for surgery should be referred for cholecystectomy after the diagnosis is made and appropriate work-up is completed.

Are there reasons to remove the gallbladder in cases of asymptomatic cholelithiasis?

The mere presence of gallstones is not an indication for cholecystectomy. Diabetic patients, those with sickle cell disease, and patients with gallstones larger than 2 cm have an increased risk of developing symptomatic and complicated cholecystitis. Findings of a porcelain gallbladder or large or definite polypoid growth in the gallbladder should lead to cholecystectomy because both are associated with findings of gallbladder carcinoma. Asymptomatic patients with gallstones who are contemplating surgery for morbid obesity should undergo cholecystectomy at some point. In the absence of specific risk factors, the risk of "prophylactic" cholecystectomy probably exceeds that of nonoperative management.

What are the advantages and disadvantages to a laparoscopic versus open approach to cholecystectomy?

Both laparoscopic and open cholecystectomy provide definitive treatment and cure for most patients with symptoms thought due to gallstones. There are significant differences between the two procedures, however. Open cholecystectomy (even through a small incision) is more painful. Hospitalization usually lasts 2 to 4 days. Narcotic requirements are higher, and return to full physical activity is quite a bit longer. On the other hand, complication of injury to the bile ducts is lower in open procedures. This is particularly true for complicated cholecystectomies (e.g., acute cholecystitis, gangrene of gallbladder). The "reported" incidence of common duct injury is 1/150 to 200 laparoscopic cholecystectomies and 1/500 to 800 open operations. After laparoscopic cholecystectomy, patients are discharged later in the day, or more commonly, the following day. Return to work and full physical activity is sooner. Although operating room costs are higher with laparoscopy, hospital costs overall are lower due to shorter stays. The vast majority of cholecystectomies are now performed laparoscopically and are converted to open operations for intraoperative problems or for unclear anatomy.

How is acute cholecystitis treated?

Acute cholecystitis is both a clinical and pathologic diagnosis. Hospitalization is usually indicated for intravenous (IV) hydration, pain control, antibiotic therapy, laboratory survey, and confirmatory ultrasound. The ultrasound report should be checked for documentation of stones, determination of ductal dilation, wall thickening, and fluid around the gallbladder. Early cholecystectomy should be recommended to those fit for surgery. Patients should be informed that there is a higher chance of a laparoscopic procedure's being converted to an open procedure for their safety. Patients who are critically ill and not fit to tolerate cholecystectomy may be treated by percutaneous cholecystostomy. Common bile duct stones may be removed at the time of cholecystectomy or with preoperative or postoperative ERCP.

What is a common bile duct exploration (CBDE)?

There are a number of ways to evaluate and treat disorders of the bile ducts (i.e., stones, infection, benign or malignant neoplasms, or strictures). Prior to ERCP, the standard treatment modality for common duct pathology was common duct exploration. This technique remains an excellent diagnostic and therapeutic tool.

Prior to or during cholecystectomy, bile duct stones may be suspected or demonstrated. They may be obstructing the bile ducts or causing cholangitis. During cholecystectomy, the bile ducts may be imaged using intraoperative ultrasound or intraoperative cholangiography.

Common duct exploration may be performed during open or laparoscopic surgery. When done with laparoscopic techniques, the cystic duct is usually used for access. This makes it difficult to work on the bile ducts proximal to this entry point. Open CBDE commences with a longitudinal incision on the common duct. Stay sutures are placed. The duct may be flushed with irrigation, explored with gentle forceps or balloon catheters, or inspected with a flexible endoscope (choledochoscope). After stones are removed, the duct is usually closed over a T-tube and a drain is left. T-tube cholangiography is performed 2 to 6 weeks later to verify clearance of stones and ductal patency, emptying, and integrity. If clear, the T-tube is removed in the office. If obstruction of the bile duct cannot be relieved during the operation, a biliary bypass may be fashioned to provide biliary decompression (choledochoduodenostomy, choledochojejunostomy). Owing to excellent ERCP techniques, CBDE is uncommon and tends to be reserved for patients who have failed or are not candidates for ERCP.

What is a cholecystostomy tube?

Occasionally, patients with acute cholecystitis are critically ill and too sick to tolerate either an anesthetic or an operative procedure. The gallbladder may be decompressed by placement of a tube directly into it through the abdominal wall using ultrasound or CT guidance and local anesthesia. In concert with antibiotics and critical care management, the elimination of infected bile under pressure leads to resolution of symptoms. The tube may remain indefinitely in those patients for whom subsequent elective cholecystectomy is too risky.

How is choledocholithiasis treated?

Stones in the common bile duct may cause symptoms from obstruction, inflammation, or infection. These may present as pain, jaundice, cholangitis, or gallstone pancreatitis. Ductal stricture may occur. When common duct stones are discovered before or during cholecystectomy, the duct may be evaluated and cleared by pre-operative or postoperative ERCP or intraoperative common duct exploration. If a stone is impacted at the ampulla and ERCP is not successful, surgical treatment is indicated. Options include duodenotomy and sphincteroplasty with stone removal or biliary bypass using a choledochoduodenostomy or choledochojejunostomy.

How is gallstone pancreatitis treated?

Gallstone pancreatitis is thought to occur as a result of a gallstone passing through the ampulla of Vater and causing obstruction, irritation, or inflammation of the pancreatic duct. This may result in pancreatitis ranging in severity from a very mild and brief inflammatory illness to a severe and fulminant necrotizing, septic, and fatal illness.

Mild pancreatitis is treated with bowel rest, IV fluid, and observation. If the etiology is thought to be gallstone pancreatitis, cholecystectomy is indicated when the pancreas "cools off" (i.e., amylase and lipase approach normal levels). Moderately severe pancreatitis is treated also with bowel rest. The pancreas may stay inflamed for weeks, and parenteral nutrition may be indicated. CT scanning of the abdomen is an excellent imaging technique to define the degree of pancreatic inflammation or disruption as well as the possibility of pancreatic necrosis or secondary infection. Cholecystectomy is indicated when the pancreas inflammation has resolved. Severe gallstone pancreatitis requires intensive care management, supportive nutrition, bowel rest, and occasionally prophylactic antibiotics. Most cases are treated nonoperatively. If pancreatic sepsis is demonstrated or highly suspected, débridement and abdominal decompression may be indicated. The role of early ERCP for severe pancreatitis is controversial.

How is ascending cholangitis treated?

Ascending cholangitis occurs in the setting of bile duct obstruction, secondary infection of bile, and increased pressure in the biliary tree from ongoing secretion of bile into an obstructed system. Patients may present with Charcot's triad or Reynold's pentad.

Ultrasound demonstrates dilated ducts and gallbladder stones in most cases. In its severe form this represents one of the true surgical emergencies. After rapid resuscitation and stabilization with fluids and antibiotics, immediate bile duct decompression is mandated. This is accomplished most often by ERCP. If emergent ERCP is not available or is unsuccessful, a second option is transhepatic cholangiography and decompression (THC). If this is not available or is unsuccessful, open common duct exploration should be immediately performed. When the duct is opened, pus issues forth. After removal of the common bile duct stones, T-tube drainage is indicated. Patients often stabilize immediately and dramatically after biliary decompression. Delayed or immediate cholecystectomy may be performed depending on the clinical status of the patient. Antibiotic therapy should be broad and aimed at the most common pathogens (*Escherichia coli*, *Klebsiella*, *Proteus*, *Bacteroides* species). Milder cholangitis may respond well to antibiotics and IV fluids, allowing less emergent duct clearance and cholecystectomy.

Are there nonsurgical treatments for gallstones?

Yes, but they are neither as effective nor as safe as elective cholecystectomy. Symptomatic patients with gallstones who are truly not surgical candidates may take oral medications to dissolve their stones (chenodeoxycholate and ursodeoxycholate). These agents tend to work well only for small cholesterol stones; take 6 to 12 months to effectively dissolve the stones; work 50% of the time; and require large daily doses, making compliance poor. Liver toxicity may occur. Stones recur after cessation of therapy. In Europe, lithotripsy is used occasionally for gallstones. Interventional techniques (radiologic) may be used with minimal anesthesia to access the gallbladder and remove or dissolve stones. Common duct stones are usually managed by ERCP with sphincterotomy. In high-risk patients with cholelithiasis, it is hoped that their gallstones will pass into the duodenum if they exit the gallbladder. In this group, the risk of complicated cholecystitis or common duct problems may be lower than the risk of general anesthesia and cholecystectomy.

How are benign biliary strictures treated?

Most benign strictures are secondary to injury from laparoscopic cholecystectomy. Other causes of benign strictures include persistent common duct stones, pancreatitis, sclerosing cholangitis, pyogenic cholangitis, and retroperitoneal fibrosis. If injury is recognized at the time of cholecystectomy, the duct should be repaired or treated by hepaticojejunostomy. If strictures are found late, they should first be defined anatomically by cholangiography (ERCP or THC). CT scan may be indicated. Unless obviously benign and iatrogenic, strictures should be presumed malignant. Benign strictures may be amenable to balloon angioplasty and/or stenting via ERCP. If these are unsuccessful, the best option is probably with biliary bypass (such as choledochoduodenostomy, choledochojejunostomy, or hepaticojejunostomy).

How is gallbladder cancer treated?

The treatment of gallbladder carcinoma depends on the stage of the tumor. Most of these neoplasms are discovered incidentally at the time of laparoscopic cholecystectomy. If carcinoma of the gallbladder is discovered during laparoscopy, the operation should be converted to a laparotomy and operation tailored to the findings. Potential contaminated (seeded) port sites should be excised. If the tumor is found in the pathology specimen, CT scanning should be done for staging. Many patients present with unresectable disease and metastasis. The treatment of gallbladder cancer has evolved along with the increasing safety of hepatic resection. Stage I disease (limited to the gallbladder wall) is treated by cholecystectomy alone. Survival for in situ disease is nearly 100%. Stages II and III cancers require aggressive segmental liver resection or wedge resection. Stage IV disease in the absence of distant metastasis may also be treated with aggressive resection, with some patients surviving 5 years. Unresected gallbladder carcinoma is uniformly fatal. Aggressive surgical treatment of stages II, III, and sometimes IV disease has led to 5-year survival rates of 10% to 50%. There is no established role for either chemotherapy or radiation therapy.

How is cancer of the bile duct treated?

Cancers of the bile duct are usually adenocarcinomas. They may occur at the head of the pancreas and duodenum (ampullary carcinoma), at the biliary confluence under the liver (Klatskin's tumors, extrahepatic cholangiocarcinoma), or in the liver (intrahepatic cholangiocarcinoma). These are not responsive to either chemotherapy or radiation therapy. CT scanning is the imaging modality of choice. ERCP may be helpful in delineating ductal anatomy and patency or obstruction. Some centers advocate the use of MR imaging (MR cholangiopancreatography) to evaluate the ductal anatomy. Endoscopic ultrasound may be helpful for staging and tissue diagnosis. Many patients present with unresectable disease, and palliation is indicated. Patients with possibly resectable tumors should undergo exploratory laparoscopy or laparotomy and, if found resectable, are treated with aggressive surgery. The goal is to achieve complete resection with negative microscopic margins (R0 resection). Tumor site dictates the type of operation. Ampullary lesions are resected by pancreaticoduodenectomy. Klatskin's tumors require bile duct resection and hepaticojejunostomy. Intrahepatic tumors require partial hepatectomy. Surgical mortality continues to decline with better technique and postoperative care, and survivors are more common.

K E Y   P O I N T S

► Most symptoms associated with biliary tract pathology are related to obstruction and/or inflammation.

► Bile is used to digest fat and to aid in the transport of lipid-soluble toxins and nutrients.

► Gallstones are common but not always symptomatic.

► The most appropriate initial study to assess the anatomy of the biliary tract is right upper quadrant ultrasound.

► Ascending cholangitis is a life-threatening infection and requires rapid relief of the biliary obstruction and application of antibiotics.

CASE 29–4.
A 24-year-old woman presents with a history of several episodes of right upper quadrant pain. These episodes usually follow eating cheese or fried foods. The pain lasts about 2 to 4 hours and usually goes away by itself. However, she has been seen in the emergency department twice and has been treated with narcotics both times.

   A. What evaluation is necessary?
   B. Her symptoms are caused by gallstones. What treatment options are available?

CASE 29–5.
A 59-year-old man who has known cholelithiasis presents to the emergency department with a 12-hour history of severe abdominal pain.

   A. What is the differential diagnosis?
   B. What evaluation is warranted?
   C. The patient is determined to have gallstone pancreatitis. What is the initial treatment?
   D. When should an operation be performed?

CASE 29–6. A 42-year-old woman, who underwent laparoscopic cholecystectomy 6 months earlier, presents to the emergency department with jaundice, abdominal pain, and fever.

A. What is the likely cause?

B. How should she be evaluated?

C. What are the treatment options for retained (secondary) common bile duct stones?

CASE 29–7. The patient in Case 29–6 is hospitalized, awaiting ERCP. She suddenly develops severe shaking chills and exhibits mental status changes. Her temperature spikes to 39.8°F, and she becomes hypotensive.

A. What is the likely cause?

B. What are the treatment options?

CASE 29–8. A 67-year-old man presents with a 6-month history of weight loss, progressive jaundice, and vague nausea. He denies significant pain but states that his appetite is gone.

A. How should he be evaluated?

B. The patient is diagnosed with a mass in his right upper quadrant. What additional work-up is necessary?

C. What are the treatment options?

INTESTINAL OBSTRUCTION: PREOPERATIVE AND POSTOPERATIVE MANAGEMENT

Management of intestinal obstruction is an important, commonly encountered entity in general surgery. Understanding the causes, consequences, and management of this problem is fundamental to the care of surgical patients.

▶ ETIOLOGY

What are the types and causes of intestinal obstruction?

Intestinal obstruction can be classified by location, as in small bowel versus large bowel obstruction, and may be further subdivided by mechanistic descriptors, such as *extrinsic*, *intramural*, and *intraluminal processes*.

In the small bowel, *extrinsic* processes include adhesions, incarcerated hernias, metastatic tumor encasement, and incorporation of bowel into abscess cavities. *Intramural* causes, such as Crohn's disease, lymphoma, primary carcinoma, and stenosis due to radiation enteritis, can also obstruct the small intestine. Finally, diseases such as gallstone ileus, foreign body ingestion, and intussusception are examples of *intraluminal* causes of small bowel obstruction.

Large bowel obstruction can occur as a result of *extrinsic* encasement (e.g., "frozen abdomen/pelvis"); *intraluminal* blockage from fecal impaction; and a number of *intramural* mechanisms, including colon cancer, colonic volvulus, complicated diverticulitis and Crohn's disease, and strictures resulting from ischemic colitis and radiation enteritis.

A "closed-loop" obstruction is one in which both inflow and outflow of the compromised bowel are blocked. Incarcerated hernia, a loop of bowel torsed around an adhesive band, cecal or colonic volvulus, and obstructing colon cancer in the presence of a competent ileocecal valve all are examples of closed-loop obstructions.

▶ EVALUATION

What are the presenting signs and symptoms?

The chief complaint of any type of intestinal obstruction is diffuse, poorly localized, crampy abdominal pain. This pain originates from the stretch receptors in the visceral peritoneum innervated by the autonomic nervous system. Whereas pain due to small bowel obstruction tends to be intermittent or colicky and may be relieved by vomiting, large bowel obstruction usually causes constant pain.

Depending on the location and type of obstruction, nausea and vomiting can occur early, late, or not at all. Proximal small bowel obstruction results in frequent, large-volume, bilious vomiting, whereas distal small bowel obstruction results in low-volume, low-frequency, progressively feculent vomiting. Emesis infrequently results from obstruction of the colon or rectum and is feculent when present. Obstipation, or the inability to have flatus, is usually present in obstructions of the midgut and hindgut but may not be present in foregut obstruction.

On physical exam, abdominal tenderness and distention are the most prominent features. Proximal obstructions may result in mild epigastric or periumbilical tenderness, whereas more distal obstruction causes diffuse and progressive tenderness to palpation. Distention is usually absent in proximal small bowel obstruction and more marked in distal small bowel and large intestinal obstruction.

Bowel sounds can be hypoactive, hyperactive, or absent depending on the level and longevity of the obstruction and the presence or absence of bowel ischemia.

In the special case of a closed-loop obstruction, pain is progressive and rapidly worsening, vomiting may be prominent, tenderness is diffuse, and distention and obstipation may not be present.

What pathophysiologic changes accompany bowel obstruction?

Intestinal gas (mostly swallowed air) and fluid accumulate in the obstructed bowel. The disruption of the environment of the normal intestinal flora may result in worsening peristalsis, and bacterial endotoxins may stimulate mucosal secretions, increasing the luminal fluid content. When luminal pressure exceeds 20 cm H_2O, absorption is inhibited and secretion of salt and water increases. Whereas closed-loop obstructions may result in intraluminal pressures higher than 50 cm H_2O, most open-loop obstructions generate pressures of 8 to 12 cm H_2O, suggesting that hypersecretion may not significantly impact fluid accumulation in open-loop obstructions.

When luminal pressure rises, intestinal blood flow initially increases. In addition, enzymatic breakdown of the bowel contents increases the intraluminal osmolarity. These simultaneous changes favor the flow of extracellular fluid into the bowel lumen. Later, as luminal pressure continues to rise and the bowel wall becomes edematous, intestinal blood flow becomes compromised. As gas and fluid accumulate, the migrating myoelectrical complex of the intestinal musculature is disrupted, leading to a pattern of disorganized contractions.

The physiologic consequences of a closed-loop obstruction evolve rapidly. As high intraluminal pressure develops, the mucosa becomes disrupted and the bowel wall becomes more edematous.

As the mural venous and then arterial pressures are exceeded by the intraluminal pressure, intense inflammation, gangrene, and perforation can develop. Unless this perforation is contained by the omentum or other surrounding structures, frank peritonitis can occur.

In an open-loop obstruction, the patient's ability to vomit allows for some intestinal decompression. As the patient loses gastric, bilious, and pancreatic secretions through emesis, however, a different pathophysiology takes place. This is classically described as a *hypochloremic, hypokalemic metabolic alkalosis*. The alkalosis results from both the loss of gastric acid and, perhaps more significantly, the exchange of hydrogen for sodium in the renal tubules, in the kidney's effort to correct the patient's dehydration. This process results in what is termed a *paradoxical aciduria*.

What other diagnoses should be considered?

Abdominal pain, distention, and vomiting can accompany many intra-abdominal conditions, such as appendicitis, cholecystitis, biliary colic, perforated peptic ulcer, and diverticulitis. In addition, these inflammatory processes can result in an ileus that may mimic the signs and symptoms of bowel obstruction. However, a clear history and physical exam as well as initial laboratory findings usually suffice to distinguish these entities from intestinal obstruction.

What are the typical radiologic findings associated with intestinal obstruction?

In patients with suspected intestinal obstruction, initial radiographs should include plain films with the patient in flat, upright, and lateral decubitus positions. Typical findings include multiple dilated (>3 cm) loops of small bowel on the flat film and multiple air-fluid levels on the upright and/or decubitus films. Usually, no air is seen in the colon unless the obstruction is incomplete or complete but early. The absence of these findings should be considered with caution, since a closed-loop obstruction of the small bowel may contain fluid and very little gas and may not be apparent on plain films. In acute colonic obstruction, significant dilation of the proximal colon occurs at 8 to 10 cm, whereas the sigmoid is considered dilated at 4 to 5 cm in diameter.

Contrast studies, including small bowel follow-through and contrast enema, have specific indications and contraindications. In the case of incomplete small bowel obstruction that fails to resolve after several days of conservative therapy with fluid hydration and nasogastric suction, a small bowel follow-through may confirm the diagnosis and localize the site of blockage. In addition, water-soluble contrast agents, which are hyperosmotic, may pull fluid from the edematous bowel wall into the intestinal lumen and help resolve the obstruction. In cases where the clinical findings and plain films are typical of complete bowel obstruction, or when strangulation or perforation is suspected, contrast studies are contraindicated. Barium suspensions, although providing the best visualization of the bowel lumen, can cause intense peritonitis if the bowel wall has been disrupted, so barium should not be used if perforation or gangrene is suspected.

▶ TREATMENT

How is intestinal obstruction treated?

The basic initial treatment of bowel obstruction involves bowel rest and fluid resuscitation. Restriction of oral intake and placement of a nasogastric tube for decompression help alleviate symptoms caused by swallowed air and refluxing fluid proximal to the site of obstruction. Fluid resuscitation is guided by the patient's clinical appearance, level of electrolyte or acid-base imbalance, and urine output. Occasionally, invasive monitoring devices such as a pulmonary artery catheter may be indicated to properly resuscitate patients with underlying cardiac, pulmonary, or renal diseases. Although the usefulness of antibiotics in patients who are treated conservatively has yet to be clearly demonstrated, broad-spectrum antibiotics should be given when the decision to operate has been made.

When should patients have surgery?

In general, patients who have rapidly evolving symptoms (within minutes to hours, suggesting a closed-loop obstruction) and those with symptoms of strangulation or perforation should be brought to the operating room immediately. Other indications for surgery include the development of peritoneal findings, persistent fever, elevated white blood cell count, decreased urine output, metabolic acidosis, and failure to resolve symptoms with conservative management for 24 to 48 hours.

Another consideration is the past surgical history of the patient. Whereas some obstructions due to adhesions from previous surgeries may resolve with bowel rest alone, in patients with de novo obstruction (i.e., without a history of prior laparotomy), surgery is usually necessary to resolve the obstruction and diagnose the cause.

How should patient care continue in the postoperative period?

Postoperatively, attention should be paid to clinical confirmation that the obstruction has been relieved. Nasogastric tube output should decrease, bowel sounds should return, and the patient should begin to have flatus and bowel movements as peristalsis returns. Once bowel function is evident, the patient may undergo a trial of clamping of the nasogastric tube for 4 to 6 hours. If the patient tolerates this trial without becoming nauseated or experiencing vomiting, the nasogastric tube can be removed and a diet of clear liquids initiated. As the diet is gradually advanced to full liquids, soft solids, and finally to a regular diet, IV fluids are tapered.

In the absence of signs of bowel function, a recurrent obstruction owing to unlysed adhesions, an internal hernia, or some other undiagnosed cause must be considered and should be managed in a fashion similar to the initial presentation. If the patient is unable to tolerate oral or enteral nutrition over a 7- to 10-day period, peripheral or central parenteral nutrition should be instituted.

K E Y   P O I N T S

▶ When evaluating a patient with bowel obstruction, first distinguish between a complete obstruction, which would require urgent operative intervention, and a partial obstruction, which usually can be managed conservatively.

▶ Conservative management of bowel obstruction consists of nasogastric drainage, restriction of oral intake, IV fluid resuscitation, and serial abdominal examinations.

▶ Prolonged restriction of oral intake should prompt implementation of parenteral nutrition.

CASE 29–9. A 53-year-old woman who underwent a right hemicolectomy 2 months earlier presents to the emergency department with a 6-hour history of vague abdominal pain and a 3-hour history of intermittent vomiting of food, then bilious fluid.

    A. What is your differential diagnosis?
    B. What tests should you order?

CASE 29–10. A 67-year-old man with a history of exploratory laparotomy with splenectomy and ventral hernia repair has been admitted with a diagnosis of small bowel

continued

CASE 29–10. *continued*

---

obstruction. After 2 days of fluid resuscitation and nasogastric decompression, he continues to have abdominal pain and has not had flatus or a bowel movement.

   A. Under what circumstances should this patient be taken to the operating room?

   B. The patient undergoes an exploratory laparotomy and lysis of adhesions. On postoperative day 5 the patient's nasogastric tube output is decreasing but he has scant bowel sounds and has yet to have flatus or a bowel movement. What do you do?

DIVERTICULAR DISEASE OF THE COLON

▶ **ETIOLOGY**

What is diverticular disease?

A diverticulum is an abnormal saccular protrusion of the bowel wall. Most left-sided colonic diverticula are called "false" or "pseudo" because they do not contain all three layers of the bowel wall. In these diverticula herniation of the mucosa occurs through the muscular layer at points of penetration of the vasa recta. Diverticula can also form in the cecum and ascending colon. These congenital right-sided diverticula are often "true" diverticula and contain all three layers of the bowel wall similar to a Meckel's diverticulum. On rare occasions, diverticula can be found occupying the entire colon. An aggregation of diverticula is called *diverticulosis*, which is an *asymptomatic* state discovered incidentally during endoscopy or contrast enema. Diverticular disease is a *symptomatic* state that occurs when the diverticula become inflamed, bleed, rupture, obstruct, or fistulize. Diverticular disease can be either simple or complicated.

How do patients with diverticular disease present?

In simple diverticulitis the inflammation is mild and the perforation is walled off by pericolonic fat, preventing extension to the peritoneal cavity. These patients present with left lower quadrant pain and low-grade fever. In complicated diverticulitis the inflammation is severe, and perforation leads to an abscess or diffuse peritoneal contamination. These patients may present in extremis with high fever, tachycardia, hypotension, and shock. If the inflammatory process is chronic, it may result in a narrowing of the colonic lumen. These patients present with obstructive symptoms like nausea, vomiting, and constipation.

What is a colovesical fistula?

A chronic inflammatory state in the colon can lead to fistula formation. Because the sigmoid colon is near the bladder and other pelvic organs, a tract can form from the colon to these organs. A fistulous connection between the colon and the bladder (colovesical fistula) is the most common fistula seen, but colovaginal, colocutaneous, and coloenteric fistulas also occur. A colovesical fistula should be suspected in patients with chronic urinary tract infections that fail to respond to appropriate antimicrobial therapy. Other common complaints include lower abdominal pain, dysuria, urinary frequency, hematuria, pneumaturia, and rarely fecaluria.

Can patients have significant bleeding from diverticulitis?

Significant lower GI hemorrhage can result from an inflamed diverticulum that has eroded and ruptured the vasa recta. Classically, the presentation is that of an otherwise healthy patient who feels the urge to have a bowel movement and passes a large amount of bright red blood or maroon-colored stool. Bleeding stops spontaneously in approximately 70% of cases; 30% continue to bleed and require emergency operative management.

▶ EVALUATION

History and physical examination are crucial aspects in the evaluation of the patient with diverticular disease. When the history and physical exam are clearly consistent with diverticular disease, additional tests may not be necessary.

What laboratory tests are helpful?

When indicated, certain laboratory tests may help confirm or rule out diverticular disease but should not be viewed as diagnostic. A CBC with differential may show a leukocytosis with a left shift in the patient with abscess or phlegmon. In the bleeding patient, a decreased hematocrit is seen. Urinalysis may be helpful in the patient suspected of having a colovesical fistula.

What radiographic studies are helpful?

Abdominal and upright chest radiographs can demonstrate free air and other causes of abdominal pain. Contrast enema, ultrasound, and CT scanning all have a role in the diagnosis of diverticular disease. Contrast enema and ultrasound have their limitations, so CT is the preferred method. Features of diverticulitis on CT include free intraperitoneal air, colonic diverticula, bowel wall thickening, soft-tissue density in the pericolonic fat or mesentery representing phlegmon, and intraperitoneal fluid collections suggesting abscess. A CT scan may also show an air-fluid level in the bladder supporting the diagnosis of a colovesical fistula.

Is there a role for endoscopic evaluation?

Colonic endoscopy is generally contraindicated in the setting of acute diverticulitis. Air insufflation may convert a sealed perforation to a free leak. Occasionally, limited sigmoidoscopy is necessary to rule out IBD. In cases of hemorrhage flexible sigmoidoscopy may be useful to localize the bleeding site.

▶ TREATMENT

Once the diagnosis of simple (versus complicated) diverticular disease is established, treatment algorithms can be initiated. In general, patients with simple diverticular disease can be treated medically, whereas patients with complicated disease usually require a surgical approach. Simple diverticulitis, which is present in 75% of cases, is not associated with complications, and most patients respond to medical therapy. In the absence of systemic symptoms and signs, patients with mild abdominal tenderness may be treated on an outpatient basis. Medical therapy includes oral antibiotics that cover anaerobic and gram-negative organisms (e.g., metronidazole and/or ciprofloxacin). Treatment for 10 to 14 days, with follow-up after completion of antibiotic therapy, is a standard approach. Patients who manifest fever, leukocytosis, inability to eat, and significant abdominal tenderness should be hospitalized for IV fluid hydration and antibiotics. Immunocompromised patients and diabetics can mask symptoms and should be admitted to the hospital and followed closely.

What is the role for percutaneous drainage in a patient with an abscess?

Patients who present with perforation and a contained abscess should be considered for CT-guided percutaneous drainage. After IV fluids and antibiotics are started and the patient is hemodynamically stable, the patient's films should be reviewed by an interventional radiologist. If the localized sepsis can be adequately drained and controlled by placement of a percutaneous catheter, the patient may be able to avoid emergent surgery that carries an inherently high morbidity and mortality. This approach may also obviate the need for temporary stoma placement and therefore a second operation.

What are the indications for surgery in a patient with diverticulitis?

Emergent/Urgent. Patients with evidence of diffuse peritonitis or with ongoing hemorrhage with hemodynamic instability should be explored immediately. Patients who fail to improve after conservative treatment, manifested by increasing pain, spreading peritonitis, or worsening leukocytosis, may need urgent exploration.

Elective. An elective operation should be offered to patients who have had one episode of complicated diverticular disease, such as abscess, obstruction, hemorrhage, or fistula. Patients who have had two confirmed episodes of acute diverticulitis severe enough to require hospitalization should be considered for elective resection. A subset of patients should be considered for surgical therapy following just one attack: young patients (age <45 years), immunocompromised patients, and patients with connective tissue disorders.

What operation should be done in an emergency setting?

The basic principles in approaching these patients include control of sepsis, resection of diseased tissue, and restoration of intestinal continuity with or without a protective stoma. The following are three basic options:

1. A two-stage operation, where resection and colostomy are performed at the initial operation (Hartmann procedure), followed by a second operation at a later date that restores intestinal continuity
2. A two-stage operation that involves resection, anastomosis, and proximal diversion performed at the initial operation, followed by a second operation at a later date that restores intestinal continuity
3. A single-stage operation that involves resection and primary anastomosis

The decision as to which approach to take is made at the time of surgical exploration and depends on many factors. Stoma sites should be marked preoperatively when possible.

What are the contraindications to primary anastomosis?

A primary anastomosis should not be performed if there is uncertain viability of the bowel, generalized feculent peritonitis, diffuse purulent peritonitis, an immunocompromised state, malnutrition, or severe anemia. A Hartmann procedure should be performed in these circumstances. A subset of patients fall into the category of mild systemic illness, chronic abscess cavity, and minimal fecal load and can be considered for resection, primary anastomosis, and protective temporary loop ileostomy.

What is an on-table lavage?

An *on-table lavage* refers to an intraoperative method of removing the colonic fecal load in a patient who has not had a preoperative bowel preparation. A Foley catheter is placed into the cecum through the appendiceal stump. Instillation of warm saline through the catheter flushes out stool to an open distal segment of colon that has been connected to a piece of large-bore corrugated plastic tubing. This technique is applied when the only contraindication to primary anastomosis is a proximal fecal load. In properly selected patients this technique may avoid the need for a stoma.

What is the surgical approach toward elective resection of sigmoid diverticulosis?

Ideally one should wait 6 to 8 weeks after the last attack of diverticulitis to perform an elective operation. The evening before surgery the colon should be prepared with ingestion of either 2 to 4 L of polyethylene glycol solution or 90 mL of sodium phosphate. In addition, 2 g of metronidazole and neomycin should be given orally. Preoperative ureteral stent placement should be considered in patients who have had a significant inflammatory response to their diverticulitis. The patient is placed on the operating table in the synchronous position to allow access to the perineum. After mobilization of the upper rectum, sigmoid, and left colon, the left ureter should be identified. The diseased colon is identified, and the appropriate mesentery is taken. The distal resection margin should always be the proximal rectum, which is recognized by the convergence of the tenia. The proximal resection margin should include the thickened disease bowel. It is not necessary to remove all the diverticula. Recurrent diverticulitis rarely occurs in the proximal colonic segment, but there is increased likelihood for recurrence if the distal margin includes retained sigmoid colon. A primary anastomosis can almost always be performed in the elective setting.

What operation do I offer a patient with a colovesical fistula?

Patients with colovesical fistulas can usually be managed with a one-stage operation. At operation the fistula tract is identified and taken down. The involved colon is resected and a primary anastomosis is performed. If the fistulous opening to the bladder is identified, it is closed primarily. If the opening to the bladder cannot be identified, which is often the case, a Foley catheter should be left in place for 7 to 10 days after surgery.

How do I treat a patient with symptomatic right-sided diverticular disease?

Right-sided diverticular disease may be isolated or seen with universal diverticular disease. Diverticular disease of the cecum and ascending colon presents at a younger age and is more common in Asians. Right-sided diverticulitis mimics acute appendicitis with symptoms of right lower quadrant pain, nausea, and vomiting. Features that may distinguish it from acute appendicitis include a prolonged and less acute presentation. Moreover, fever, anorexia, and vomiting occur less often. A right lower quadrant mass may be encountered on physical exam in cecal diverticulitis. When this inflammatory mass is discovered at laparotomy, it may be difficult to distinguish it from a carcinoma, so a formal right hemicolectomy should be performed in this circumstance. Diverticulectomy alone can be performed if the diagnosis is clear. Nonoperative management follows the same principles of left-sided disease.

K E Y   P O I N T S

▶ History, physical exam, and selective use of laboratory and radiographic tests are essential for accurate diagnosis.

▶ Complications of diverticular disease include obstruction, hemorrhage, fistula formation, abscess, and purulent or fecal peritonitis and often require surgical therapy.

▶ Simple diverticular disease is often treated medically.

▶ Percutaneous drainage of an infected fluid collection may convert a two-stage operation into a single stage.

▶ Surgical approach depends on multiple factors.

CASE 29–11. A 56-year-old diabetic man comes to the emergency department complaining of abdominal distention, fever, and worsening left lower quadrant pain for 2 weeks. His examination is remarkable for a temperature of 102°F, heart rate of 115 beats/min, and localized peritoneal irritation in the left lower quadrant.

A. What further history should you elicit?
B. What tests should be ordered?
C. How should this patient be managed?
D. What if he fails conservative treatment?

ESOPHAGEAL MOTILITY

What is "normal" swallowing?

Swallowing is a complex process to transport food or liquid boluses from the mouth to the stomach. It requires proper coordination of the oropharynx, the upper esophageal sphincter (UES), the esophageal body, and the lower esophageal sphincter (LES). It involves both voluntary and involuntary muscle contractions. A swallow is instigated by the voluntary movement of a bolus of food to the back of the throat. The larynx is elevated and the epiglottis closes to protect the trachea from aspiration of food or liquid, and the soft palate is also elevated to prevent food from entering the nasal passages. This phase of swallowing, in spite of its complexity, takes only 1 to 1.5 seconds. Once the bolus reaches the posterior pharynx, the UES responds by relaxing to allow passage of the bolus into the body of the esophagus, followed by contraction to prevent regurgitation. A peristaltic wave then propagates down the esophageal body at approximately 3 to 4 cm/sec, allowing the bolus of food to complete the esophageal phase of swallowing in around 9 seconds. Once the peristaltic wave reaches the LES, the LES responds with relaxation followed by contraction, allowing passage of the bolus into the stomach and preventing subsequent reflux of gastric contents into the esophagus.

When the process is working correctly, it requires minimal conscious thought in spite of being extremely complex and rapid. When it is disrupted at any level, it creates a distressful clinical situation that affects patients profoundly. There is a complex interaction of adrenergic and cholinergic nerves that play a part in swallowing. Stress, which often accompanies swallowing disorders for obvious reasons, can exacerbate symptoms considerably. Disruption at any point of the process can lead to dysphagia (difficulty swallowing) or odynophagia (painful swallowing).

▶ ETIOLOGY

What are the common causes of dysphagia?

With the complexity of the process of swallowing it is not surprising that the list of etiologic factors that can cause dysphagia is long (Table 29–3). The process of swallowing involves neural input to regulate both voluntary and involuntary muscles that must then make coordinated and well-timed movements. The esophagus is anatomically near a number of organs within a relatively small and constrained space. Each step of swallowing is so dependent on the perfect coordination of the steps before and after that the slightest dysfunction at any level leads to complete disruption of the process. Both in the neck and in the mediastinum, the esophagus

TABLE 29–3

Causes of Dysphagia

Mechanical
Endoluminal
   Esophageal carcinoma
   Esophageal webs
   Foreign body
   Benign tumors
Extraluminal
   Thyromegaly
   Lymphadenopathy
   Cervical spine osteophytes or severe cervical lordosis
   Congenital vascular anomalies
   Dilated or tortuous aorta
   Pericarditis or mediastinitis

Neurogenic: Central Nervous System Disease
Amyotrophic lateral sclerosis
Multiple sclerosis
Parkinson's disease
Huntington's chorea
Sydenham's chorea
Dysautonomia
Tabes dorsalis
Cerebrovascular accident
Basilar artery thrombosis
Aneurysm with brain stem compression
Tumors of the brain stem or base of the skull
Closed head trauma

Muscular
Primary esophageal motility disease
   Achalasia
   Hypertensive upper esophageal sphincter ± Zenker's diverticulum
   Diffuse or segmental esophageal spasm
   Nutcracker esophagus
   Hypertensive lower esophageal sphincter
Secondary esophageal motility disease
   Scleroderma
   Systemic lupus erythematosus
   Polymyositis dermatomyositis
Motor end plate disease
   Myasthenia gravis
   Tetanus
Metabolic myopathy
   Thyrotoxicosis
   Hypothyroidism

Iatrogenic
Laryngectomy
Thyroidectomy
Parathyroid exploration
Tracheostomy
Thoracic surgery
Irradiation

Gastroesophageal Reflux Disease

is vulnerable to compression by surrounding organs. Benign and malignant esophageal neoplasms can cause intrinsic obstruction. Inflammation in the esophagus can lead to stricture formation or may cause motility problems when present chronically. The symptoms and health problems associated with severe dysphagia are considerable, but only some of the etiologies are treatable surgically.

What are the causes of a painful swallowing?

Although dysphagia from any etiology can be perceived as painful swallowing, most commonly odynophagia is associated with severe esophagitis of viral, fungal, or erosive origin. Patients at risk for infectious esophagitis include those who are chronically debilitated, immunosuppressed, or on systemic steroids or prolonged antibiotic treatment. Sudden onset of odynophagia in a patient with any of these risk factors should prompt a work-up that includes upper endoscopy. *Candida* esophagitis is the most common cause of sudden odynophagia; however, in acquired immunodeficiency syndrome (AIDS), viral etiologies (CMV, Epstein-Barr virus, HIV, HSV) as well as unusual bacterial infections must be considered. Those at risk for erosive esophagitis include patients with longstanding untreated gastroesophageal reflux disease (GERD). Chronic esophagitis can lead to measurable abnormalities in esophageal motility, which can reverse once the inflammation is treated. It can also lead to anatomic stricture formation or, in the case of GERD, intestinal metaplasia (Barrett's esophagus) or eventually malignant transformation of the gastroesophageal junction.

▶ EVALUATION

The key to the proper surgical management of patients with motility disorders is a thorough work-up. A comprehensive GI motility lab that includes facilities for upper endoscopy, esophageal manometry, 24-hour pH monitoring, static barium swallow, and video-cine-esophagram aids in the definition or the pattern of dysmotility. This allows us to predict which patients are likely to benefit from surgery and what type of surgery should be performed.

What radiologic studies help in the evaluation of dysphagia?

Typically dysphagia is categorized by the anatomic site (i.e., cervical vs. thoracic dysphagia) or the underlying type of dysfunction (i.e., obstructive vs. primary muscular dysfunction). A careful history of the patient's symptoms may help define the problem. A barium swallow can be used to rule out mechanical intraluminal or extraluminal obstruction of the esophagus. Patients with radiographs that suggest esophageal neoplasm should be worked up immediately with upper endoscopy and biopsy. Specific anatomic abnormalities may suggest (or are sometimes diagnostic for) underlying primary motility disorders. For example, the presence of a bird-beak deformity suggests achalasia, and Zenker's diverticulum suggests UES spasm (Figs. 29–6 and 29–7). Hiatal or paraesophageal hernias (Fig. 29–8) are characterized by their radiographic appearance.

The information that can be obtained from static films is enhanced greatly by obtaining a video-cine-esophagram. This study adds the ability to evaluate direct physiologic information regarding what is a dynamic process (swallowing). The leakage of contrast into the trachea indicates an impaired ability to protect the airway. The coordination of the process can be evaluated grossly, and abnormalities associated with failure in coordination of swallowing such as Zenker's diverticulum (associated with nonrelaxation of the UES) can be identified. The atonic nature of classic achalasia can be distinguished from vigorous achalasia, and the classic bird-beak deformity can be seen.

Although a wealth of information is found in plain radiographic images of the esophagus, it does not replace physiologic quantita-

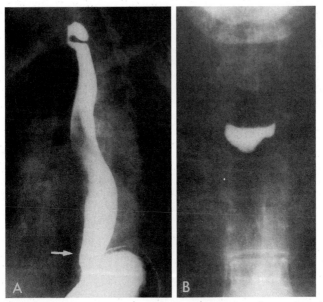

Figure 29–6. *A*, Zenker's diverticulum in a patient with an associated "patulous cardia" *(arrow)* and asymptomatic gastroesophageal reflux without esophagitis. *B*, Residual barium in the 2.5-cm pouch (anteroposterior view). (From Orringer MB: Extended cervical esophagomyotomy for cricopharyngeal dysfunction. J Thorac Cardiovasc Surg 1980;80:669.)

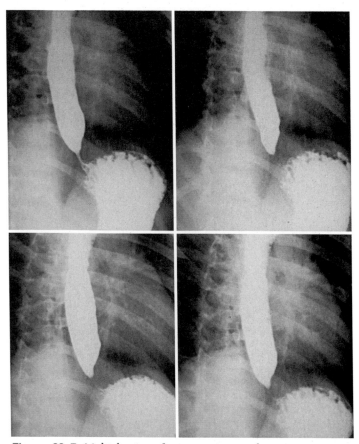

Figure 29–7. Multiple views from one cine-esophagram in a patient with early achalasia showing a persistent bird-beak taper at the esophagogastric junction and impaired esophageal emptying. (From Sabiston D [ed]: Textbook of Surgery: The Biological Basis of Modern Surgical Practice, 15th ed. Philadelphia, WB Saunders, 1997, p 718.)

tive testing in all cases. In cases where esophageal neoplasms are identified as the cause of the dysphagia, barium swallow and a CT scan of the chest and abdomen are an essential part of the preoperative work-up. The barium swallow is often the first test done and defines the level of the neoplasm, which can be important in planning surgery. The CT scan is important to staging and helps identify those patients who may benefit from neoadjuvant chemotherapy/radiation therapy. It gives information about lymph node involvement or potential invasion of adjacent structures. Additional information can be obtained by endoscopy, which can demonstrate the exact depth of penetration or involvement of

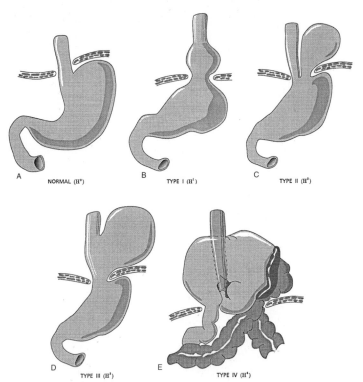

A   NORMAL (H⁰)   B   TYPE I (H¹)   C   TYPE II (H²)

D   TYPE III (H³)   E   TYPE IV (H⁴)

Figure 29–8. *A,* Normal position of the gastroesophageal junction. A defective sphincter is present when pathologic reflux occurs. *B,* Small sliding hiatal hernia (type I). *C,* Type II hernias show an esophagogastric junction in a normal position with a hernia alongside the esophagus in the mediastinum. *D,* Type III hernias are paraesophageal with the esophagogastric junction in the chest. *E,* Type IV hernias are the massive herniation of stomach and of other abdominal organs into the mediastinum. (From Sabiston D [ed]: Textbook of Surgery: The Biological Basis of Modern Surgical Practice, 15th ed. Philadelphia, WB Saunders, 1997, p 775.)

adjacent organs. An abdominal CT scan is included to assess the spread to the liver or perigastric and perihepatic nodes.

What are esophageal manometry and pH monitoring?

Manometry involves the placement of a catheter with multiple channels in the esophagus to simultaneously measure the intraluminal pressures at the physiologic sphincter of the UES, within the body of the esophagus, and at the LES with each swallow. This allows the quantitative physiologic characterization of the motility patterns that accompany wet swallows as well as the correlation of symptoms with the activity in the esophagus. The position and length of the sphincters as well as their function can be measured. Information about the coordination of swallowing and the propagation of a peristaltic wave can help define specific motility disorders and tailor surgical interventions to fit a particular patient's anatomic and physiologic disease. The manometric features of specific motility disorders are listed in Table 29–4.

Another type of catheter that measures intraluminal pH at various levels of the esophagus can be placed. Patients may keep the catheter in place for up to 24 hours, noting on a symptom diary any times when they experience chest pain or heartburn. The number of episodes and the amount of time spent at a pH less than 4 are scored and correlated to the patient's symptom diary, then compared to norms in the population to give a score called the *De Meester score*. Higher scores denote a greater degree of reflux and a greater chance that fundoplication (the surgical treatment for reflux) will give relief of symptoms. There is some degree of reflux that can be documented in normal subjects.

The addition of these objective quantitative measures of esophageal function has allowed us to compare patients with defined motility disorders and has also allowed surgeons to closely monitor the physiologic effects of surgical interventions so that we can refine surgical techniques and improve surgical outcomes.

What does the pH monitoring add to the manometry?

Patients with severe reflux and esophagitis may exhibit manometric findings (particularly in the distal esophagus) that suggest a motility problem. Most mild abnormalities reverse spontaneously with treatment of the reflux. Therefore, particularly in patients that are hard to classify or those with only mild esophageal dysfunction, the pH monitoring studies may help predict those patients who will be helped by antireflux surgery. There should be some hesitation to proceed with antireflux surgery in patients with severe dysmotility of the esophageal body in conjunction with reflux. Some of these patients are in the midst of an evolving motility disorder and will have progressive dysphagia after a fundoplication.

Which patients should undergo endoscopy?

Any patient with an intrinsic obstructing mass should undergo endoscopy and biopsy promptly. This is also true for patients with stricture at the LES and the radiographic appearance characteristic of achalasia, since occasionally a longstanding stricture can undergo malignant transformation. Usually malignant lesions have

TABLE 29-4

Manometric Features of Normal and Abnormal Esophageal Motility

Normal
LES: pressure 15–25 mm Hg
LES: normal relaxation with swallowing

Normal Esophageal Body Peristalsis
Mean amplitude of peristaltic wave 30–100 mm Hg
Simultaneous contractions after 10% of wet swallows
Monophasic waveforms
Duration 2–6 seconds
Good progression of wave with no repetitive contractions

Achalasia
LES normal or increased (> 45 mm Hg)
Absent LES relaxation with swallowing
Aperistalsis of the esophageal body
Intraesophageal basal pressure greater than intragastric pressure

DES
Simultaneous (nonperistaltic) contractions
   Repetitive ≥ 3 peaks
   Increased duration > 6 seconds
Spontaneous contractions: not initiated in oropharynx
Intermittent normal contraction
Contractions may be high amplitude

Vigorous Achalasia
Esophageal motility as in DES
Absent or reduced LES relaxation

Nutcracker Esophagus
Mean amplitude >180 mm Hg
Increased duration > 6 sec
Normal peristaltic sequences

Hypertensive LES
Normal esophageal peristalsis
LES > 45 mm Hg with normal relaxation

Hypertensive UES
Normal esophageal peristalsis
UES > 45 mm Hg ± normal relaxation with swallowing

Nonspecific Esophageal Motility Disorders
Absence of peristalsis with normal LES pressure and relaxation
   or
Abnormal peristalsis
   Abnormal waveforms
   Isolated simultaneous or spontaneous contractions
Normal LES

DES, diffuse esophageal spasm; LES, lower esophageal sphincter; UES, upper esophageal sphincter.

a more irregular shape, but it is best to be sure before surgical intervention for achalasia. Intraoperative endoscopy to monitor the adequacy of myotomy is extremely helpful. Patients with odynophagia should undergo endoscopy with biopsy to allow proper treatment of infectious esophagitis. In addition, any patient who has had long-standing GERD with little or no relief from medical therapy should have endoscopy to rule out premalignant changes in the distal esophagus (Barrett's esophagus). These patients need monitoring following antireflux surgery to ensure that the distal esophagus returns to normal once the reflux is eliminated.

▶ TREATMENT

What are the treatment options for the primary esophageal motility disorders?

The treatment options for esophageal motility disorders need to be tailored to the specific pattern of dysmotility.

GERD

Patients with GERD usually respond to medical treatment with a combination of acid-blocking and promotility agents. The proton pump inhibitors are the most effective medical treatment; however, there are some patients who do not tolerate the side effects. These are relatively new medications, and little is known about the safety of long-term or lifetime use. The valve function of the LES and gastroesophageal junction can be improved with a hiatal repair and fundoplication. These surgical manipulations return the distal esophagus to the abdominal cavity, restore the angle of His, and increase the effective pressure of the LES. A 360-degree wrap (Nissen) is done in patients who have completely normal motility of the esophagus, whereas a 270-degree (Toupet) wrap is more appropriate for patients who have problems with peristalsis in the esophageal body to prevent postoperative dysphagia.

Achalasia

Patients with achalasia respond transiently to bougie dilation or botulinum toxin injection to the LES. Surgical results have been excellent with this disorder. A thoracoscopic or laparoscopic approach is used to divide the muscular layers of the LES along its entire length. The adequacy of the myotomy is monitored with an endoscope and carried onto the stomach for a short distance. An antireflux procedure is then performed to reconstruct the angle of His. Most patients have some degree of reflux postoperatively if they undergo pH monitoring, but the procedure gives excellent relief from dysphagia (>95%) and related symptoms. Most patients are asymptomatic in terms of the reflux.

Diffuse Esophageal Spasm/Nutcracker Esophagus

Medical therapy consists of dietary modifications, including five or six soft meals daily and treatment with hydralazine or anticholinergic medications. Patients in whom medical therapy fails benefit from an extensive esophageal body myotomy done through a thoracoscopic or thoracic approach. The myotomy extends from just below the aortic arch along the body of the esophagus. For those patients with an abnormal LES in addition to spasm, the myotomy is carried further onto the body of the stomach to ensure that they are able to swallow postoperatively. An antireflux procedure is combined with the myotomy to restore the angle of His. Relief of symptoms is achieved in 90% of patients postoperatively.

Hypertensive LES

Hypertensive LES is treated similar to achalasia by myotomy of the LES. Surgical results are similar when the dysfunction is confined to the LES. However, in about half of cases, there is associated dysfunctional motility of the esophageal body. Careful review of the manometry can select those patients who will do well with a localized myotomy of the LES (Heller myotomy) versus those who will require a more extensive myotomy.

Nonspecific Esophageal Motility Disorders

This group of patients may represent motility disorders that have not fully evolved, because many will exhibit specific patterns (most commonly diffuse esophageal spasm) later. However, many never progress to a specific motility disorder. If the patients have documented reflux and esophagitis in addition to a minimal motility disruption, it is worth doing an antireflux procedure to see if the pattern of dysmotility improves once the distal esophagus is no longer exposed to acid. However, complete wraps or tight hiatal repairs should be avoided, because some of these patients have progressive dysmotility and symptoms can become worse after a 360-degree wrap.

Secondary Esophageal Motility Disorders

Patients with dysmotility secondary to reversible conditions, such as hyperthyroidism or hypothyroidism, should undergo treatment of the underlying condition to improve swallowing. Patients with stroke or other progressive neurologic disorders rarely have significant improvement after the acute recovery, and treatment should include support of nutritional needs by alterations in diet. In cases where the patient shows no improvement and continues to lose weight, feeding gastrostomy or jejunostomy may be needed. Elderly patients or those who have nonspecific esophageal motility after a prolonged illness occasionally have improvement of symptoms after their nutritional status is restored and can have the feeding tube removed after demonstrating an ability to support their nutritional needs through oral intake.

Iatrogenic Dysphagia

The underlying cause of the dysphagia should be identified. For example, patients who have had surgical procedures to the oropharynx or cervical esophagus may have a stricture that is amenable to bougie dilation. Occasionally a rotation flap is needed to open a surgical stricture. In all cases where the surgical procedure was for malignancy, recurrent tumor should be ruled out. Patients who have undergone procedures in the neck can have recurrent laryngeal nerve injuries. They may interpret the discomfort of coughing, and being unable to protect the airway fully, as difficulty in swallowing. A full evaluation with cineesophagram, direct laryngoscopy, and a swallowing evaluation may help sort this out so that appropriate therapy can be instituted. If airway protection is an issue, medialization of the affected vocal cord may allow more normal swallowing. Many patients benefit from speech pathology and diet modifications to improve swallowing.

SUMMARY

Our understanding of esophageal motility disorders has greatly improved due to advances in diagnostic tools. The advent of minimally invasive techniques has made procedures more appealing, thus increasing the number of referrals for surgery to help with the management of this difficult problem. Success of surgical therapy for motility disorder depends not only on the surgeon's skill but also on accurate diagnosis, so that patients who will benefit from surgery can be identified and the appropriate procedure selected. The presence of a dedicated multidisciplinary GI motility laboratory aids both with the diagnosis and precise definition of specific disorders and with the monitoring of the success of therapy.

K E Y   P O I N T S

▶ Normal esophageal motility is a complex process, and understanding of normal physiology helps in the evaluation of disordered swallowing.

▶ The evaluation of dysphagia requires careful analysis of information obtained from the history and physical examination and anatomic information from radiographs and physiologic data.

▶ Careful tailoring of surgical intervention to the specific abnormality improves patient outcome.

▶ Participation of surgeons who treat esophageal disorders in multidisciplinary teams that include gastroenterologists and a GI motility lab helps improve outcomes of surgical treatment.

CASE 29–12. A 20-year-old second-year medical student presents with 3-month progressive dysphagia beginning with solids and becoming progressively worse. He has had a 15-lb weight loss and had woken up at night with undigested food on the pillow. He has a barium esophagram that shows a mega-esophagus with air-fluid levels and a typical bird-beak deformity. He has finals in 1 week and does not wish to undergo surgical repair because it has the potential to make him miss his exams.

     A. What is the most likely diagnosis?
     B. What nonsurgical treatment options are available to him? How do they affect the eventual surgical procedure?

GI CANCER

▶ **ETIOLOGY**

What is the etiology of GI cancer?

Most cancers of the GI tract arise from the mucosal lining of the various organs and therefore by definition are carcinomas. These neoplasms result from alterations in somatic DNA, creating cells that no longer observe the normal rules of growth. They proliferate without control, have no limit on life span, invade their neighbor's territory, and spread to other organs, ultimately causing the death of the host-patient. Multiple gene mutations must occur in the progression from normal mucosa to an invasive, metastatic carcinoma. These mutations include activation of growth genes such as *KRAS* and/or loss of tumor suppressor genes such as *TP53*. An individual born with these gene mutations has an enhanced susceptibility to cancer, because fewer somatic mutations must occur to complete neoplastic progression. The cause of these gene mutations is unknown. GI carcinomas usually invade the wall of the viscus where they arise, penetrate lymphatics, and spread to regional lymph nodes, and then travel to other organs. Cancers of the GI tract most commonly metastasize to the liver, presumably because of portal venous drainage. GI carcinomas can also spread to other tissues by direct extension. Surgical resection is preferred therapy, but all too often, regional or distant spread of the cancer precludes effective removal of the disease.

Cancers can also arise from the mesenchymal structures of the GI tract, including fibrous supporting tissue, blood vessels, fat, and muscle tissue. These tumors are sarcomas and exhibit the same malignant behavior as carcinomas but have a different biology. Irrespective of tissue of origin, these cancers are grouped as GI stromal tumors (GISTs). They spread to contiguous organs and the liver and lung but rarely to lymph nodes. The natural history of the disease is more indolent than that of carcinoma, and some GISTs are susceptible to gene-based therapy. Standard treatment is complete surgical removal.

There is a large amount of lymphoid tissue in the GI tract, and it also can undergo malignant degeneration. GI lymphomas most commonly arise in the stomach or small intestine, and like other non-Hodgkin's lymphomas they are considered systemic diseases. Surgical resection of the primary tumor followed by systemic chemotherapy is generally the treatment of choice.

Neuroendocrine tumors (NETs) appear throughout the gut, the most common being carcinoid tumors which are APUD (*a*mine *p*recursor *u*ptake and *d*ecarboxylation) tumors. Carcinoids appear most often in the appendix, rectum, and small intestine but are seen in the stomach as well. They can be either benign or malignant. Malignant carcinoids metastasize to the liver and produce bioactive amines, including serotonin. Carcinoid syndrome (flushing and diarrhea) is caused by the secretion of serotonin into the systemic circulation from deposits of metastatic carcinoid tumor in the liver. Their biology and treatment are complex. Pancreatic endocrine tumors are also NET and APUD tumors. They are uncommon but produce florid syndromes related to the particular bioactive amine they secrete, including insulin (profound hypoglycemia), gastrin (severe gastric and duodenal ulceration), and vasoactive intestinal polypeptide (profuse diarrhea). Surgical resection is the preferred treatment.

What are the common GI cancers?

GI cancers are a major health problem and a common cause of cancer death. Carcinoma of the colon and rectum is overwhelmingly the most common GI cancer in the United States, with 200,000 cases occurring annually, predominantly in patients older than 50 years of age. Untreated, colorectal carcinoma obstructs the large intestine, bleeds, spreads to liver and contiguous organs, and causes painful death. The disease is amenable to early diagnosis using screening colonoscopy in populations at risk. If colorectal carcinoma is found early, the cure rate is high. A distant second in incidence in the United States is pancreatic carcinoma, at 35,000 cases annually. It is, nevertheless, a miserable disease that is rarely diagnosed early and therefore infrequently cured. Pancreatic carcinoma arising in the head of the pancreas obstructs the common bile duct (producing jaundice) and/or the duodenum (causing gastric outlet obstruction). Regional spread to visceral nerves causes considerable pain. Liver failure from metastatic disease is a frequent cause of death. Gastric cancer is next in frequency (21,000 cases per year) and behaves in a fashion similar to pancreatic cancer, except that gastric ulceration and bleeding provide an opportunity for earlier diagnosis. Carcinomas arising at the gastroesophageal junction have shown a rapid rise in incidence over the last several years. Constriction of the distal esophagus produces difficulty swallowing, which leads to the diagnosis.

Carcinomas also occur throughout the remainder of the GI tract including the proximal esophagus, duodenum, small intestine, gallbladder, bile duct, ampulla of Vater, liver, and anus. Bleeding, pain, or obstructive symptoms in any of these areas may indicate the presence of a carcinoma.

Lymphomas produce similar symptoms and must be considered in the differential diagnosis of abdominal masses and GI bleeding. GISTs are uncommon and present as an abdominal mass confirmed to be tumor on an abdominal imaging study.

Cancers from other sites frequently metastasize to the GI tract, in particular the liver. Most patients dying from metastatic cancer have liver metastases. Less common, but florid in their manifestations, are metastases to the small intestine from lung cancer, malignant melanoma, and ovarian carcinoma. The latter produces bulky tumors on the surface of the intestine that, in late stages, cause obstruction. In contrast, metastatic cancer to the bowel from GI carcinomas creates a significant ileus and poor bowel function even when tumor burden is low. Lung carcinoma and malignant melanoma produce tumors in the bowel wall that bleed and act as a lead point for intussusception and obstruction (an otherwise uncommon cause of bowel obstruction in adults).

Why is there a high death rate associated with GI cancers?

The high mortality in patients with GI cancer is due to the fact that these tumors become well established and may significantly invade lymphatics before causing symptoms. Pain in the GI tract is mediated by neural stretch receptors and slow transmission pain fibers. Surgically, GI viscera can be incised with a blade or the electrocautery without causing pain as long as the bowel or other organ is not distended or distorted. In contrast to the parietal peritoneum, the wall of GI viscera has an absence of fine touch discrimination and well-localizing pain receptors. Therefore, invasion of the wall of a viscus by a malignant neoplasm is painless until the tumor invades visceral nerves, and localizing sensations are poor unless the tumor irritates the parietal peritoneum. Abdominal viscera are rich in lymphatic channels that provide a ready route of spread for GI carcinomas. These cancers tend to be indolent in their growth rate but relentless in progression and spread of the disease. In this regard, they are biologically aggressive.

Classic symptoms of GI cancers such as bleeding or obstruction or weight loss are generally manifestations of advanced disease. Early diagnosis of GI cancers is not common in the absence of routine screening. Except for regular colonoscopy to identify colorectal carcinoma in high-risk populations, screening for GI cancers in the United States has not been of high yield. Because gastric carcinoma is common in Japan, use of upper GI endoscopy as a screening test in that country appears to have had a favorable impact on survival from that disease.

What conditions are associated with GI cancers?

There is a marked worldwide variation in the incidence of various GI cancers. Gastric carcinoma is common in Japan and much less frequent in the United States. Hepatitis B is endemic in Taiwan and China and is associated with a high risk of hepatocellular carcinoma. Esophageal carcinoma is relatively frequent in Iran. Western Europeans and Americans have a relatively high incidence of colon carcinoma. First-generation immigrants to the United States usually maintain the risk associated with their country of origin.

A past history of any cancer, particularly breast carcinoma, is a risk factor for GI cancer. Approximately 3% of patients with any cancer develop a second primary cancer. Smoking is associated with increased incidence of all cancers, including those of the GI tract; in particular, esophageal and gastric cancers are more common in smokers and in alcoholics. Achlorhydria is associated with an increased risk of gastric carcinoma.

Alcoholism and chronic hepatitis B and C leading to cirrhosis of the liver have a role in development of hepatocellular cancer. Chronic ulcerative colitis is associated with an increased risk of colon carcinoma; patients who have had extensive active ulcerative colitis for longer than 10 years have a 20% risk of developing colon carcinoma. Adenomatous polyps of the colon are common by age 70 and are associated with development of colon carcinoma unless removed. HIV infection is a risk factor for development of anal carcinoma.

A family history of more than one first-degree relative with colorectal carcinoma, particularly if the onset was before the age of 50, is a risk factor for development of the disease. There are several inherited predispositions to the development of GI cancer. These syndromes constitute about 5% of the spectrum of GI cancers but are important to recognize because of autosomal dominant inheritance, the high risk of early onset of the disease, and the need to consider prevention strategies (Table 29–5).

▶ EVALUATION

What are common symptoms and physical findings in patients with GI cancers?

As indicated earlier, GI cancers are usually asymptomatic when small. Unless the cancer bleeds or obstructs the bile duct, esophagus, or the intestine, it is usually relatively large when discovered. Vague persistent symptoms of early satiety, change in bowel habits, loss of appetite, or poorly localized, ill-defined abdominal pain in a reliable patient may signal the presence of a GI cancer. Pain from the liver or pancreas is steady; pain from the bowel is crampy and intermittent. Classic pain patterns include gnawing pain in the epigastrium radiating straight through to the back from invasion of celiac nerves by pancreatic cancer, burning epigastric pain, and early satiety from gastric cancer, radiation of pain to the right shoulder from gallbladder or liver cancer irritating the diaphragm, crampy lower abdominal pain from colon carcinoma, and painful

TABLE 29–5

Inherited Predisposition to Gastrointestinal Cancer

Syndrome	Gene	Manifestation
Familial adenomatous polyposis (FAP)	*APC* gene	Multiple colonic polyps, colon carcinoma in 3rd decade of life
Hereditary nonpolyposis colon carcinoma (HNPCC)	*MLH1* gene and others	High incidence of early-onset colon carcinoma
Peutz-Jeghers	*STK11* gene	Pigmented mucosal lesions, diffuse intestinal polyps, and gastrointestinal cancers
Multiple endocrine neoplasia, type 1	*MEN1* gene	Pancreatic islet cell tumors
Familial gastric cancer	*CDH1* gene	Gastric carcinoma

urge to defecate with an incomplete sense of emptying the rectum (tenesmus) caused by rectal carcinoma.

Patients presenting with advanced GI cancers have considerable weight loss; are cachectic, anorexic, fatigued; and may have considerable pain. Associated symptoms may include vomiting, jaundice, and/or blood in the stools. Patients with such florid symptoms usually have a palpable abdominal mass or rectal tumor and possibly a suspicious lymph node in the left supraclavicular fossa (Virchow's node) from cancer having traversed the thoracic duct. The liver may be palpably enlarged from metastatic tumor; the abdomen may be distended from ileus or ascites.

Cancer must be high on the list in the differential diagnosis of colon obstruction. Older patients presenting with acute peritonitis may have perforated a gastric or colon cancer. Gastric outlet obstruction from cancer causes vomiting of undigested food. Small bowel obstruction as a presentation of a previously undiagnosed cancer is less common but can occur from intussusception of a small bowel tumor, kinking of the bowel from a cancerous adhesion, or direct compression from an external tumor. Partial obstruction of the bowel may produce diarrhea from bacterial overgrowth. Patients with obstructive jaundice and a palpable gallbladder (Courvoisier's gallbladder) have pancreatic or periampullary cancer until proven otherwise. GI lymphomas may cause systemic symptoms of fever, chills, night sweats, and weight loss similar to lymphomas in other locations. Anal cancers present as a bleeding, painful, visible mass, or ulceration. GIST lesions may cause few symptoms and simply present as a large palpable abdominal tumor. Many are found incidentally on abdominal imaging for some other purpose.

What questions should I ask a patient?

Patients presenting with abdominal pain, blood in the stools, abdominal mass, or weight loss of more than 10 lb (or any of the other symptoms listed earlier) should be asked how long the symptoms have been present and whether the symptoms have become progressively worse. The location of pain and where it radiates can help direct the work-up (lower abdomen for colon; periumbilical area for small bowel; epigastrium for stomach, pancreas, liver and gallbladder; mid-back for pancreas; right shoulder for gallbladder and liver). Associated symptoms such as a persistent change in bowel habits (colon cancer), change in character of stools (decrease in caliber of stool from rectal cancer or change in color from obstruction of bile duct or bleeding), or markedly diminished appetite are informative. It is useful to know the nature of the patient's past GI complaints and whether any of the associated conditions listed earlier are present. A significant family history for GI cancer may heighten suspicion that cancer is the cause of the patient's complaint. Questioning the patient regarding food intake may reveal that a swallowed bolus "hangs up" or causes pain in the substernal area or epigastrium (esophageal cancer) or that undigested food is regurgitated (gastric outlet obstruction from gastric, duodenal, or pancreatic cancer). Pruritus or dark urine may call attention to jaundice. Knowing that the patient has changed his or her activities of daily living due to the symptoms adds significance to the complaint. Has the patient had relatively recent diagnostic studies such as endoscopy, contrast imaging of the bowel, or CT or MR scans?

When should a patient undergo further investigation?

Persistence of any of the symptoms discussed earlier or physical findings should be investigated.

Anemia, particularly the iron deficiency type, should direct attention to the GI tract. Occult or overt GI bleeding requires that cancer be excluded as a cause. Similar attention should be given to changes in liver enzymes or increased bilirubin. Physician instinct or patient concern that symptoms are caused by cancer, particularly in patients older than 50 years of age or those with significant family histories, should be given attention.

What diagnostic procedures are useful?

A careful history and thorough physical examination directed to the issues described earlier, plus routine blood and serum studies (CBC, chemistry panel to include liver enzymes, and test for occult blood in the stool) should produce a working hypothesis and list of differential diagnoses that guide the rest of the diagnostic work-up. Initial blood tests should also include serum tumor markers, such as carcinoembryonic antigen (CEA), CA 19-9, and α-fetoprotein (AFP), which roughly correlate with extent and type of tumor (CEA for colorectal carcinoma and liver metastases, AFP for hepatocellular carcinoma, CA 19-9 for pancreatic and biliary carcinoma).

Direct visualization of the gut by endoscopy is a productive next step in diagnosis. If esophageal, gastric, or duodenal carcinoma is suspected, upper GI endoscopy and biopsy are indicated. Similarly, full colonoscopy and biopsy should be performed for suspected colon or rectal carcinoma. Cancers of the biliary tree may be identified by ERCP. This procedure also provides opportunity to palliate obstructive jaundice by placement of a stent. Air contrast barium studies may substitute as a first diagnostic procedure but do not provide a tissue diagnosis, and the residual barium may complicate other imaging studies. If these tests are nondiagnostic and the patient has significant anemia and occult blood in the stool, small bowel tumors should be sought by a barium upper GI study and small bowel follow-through using an enteroclysis technique (drug-induced laxity in the bowel that enhances visualization of tumor).

Next in diagnostic sequence is contrast CT or MR imaging of the abdomen and pelvis, which provide excellent anatomic detail and can demonstrate tumors greater than 1 cm in the liver or pancreas, enlarged lymph nodes, some small bowel tumors, and peritoneal implants greater than 1 cm. Ultrasound imaging identifies tumors in the liver, pancreas, and peritoneum, but CT and MR imaging give much better anatomic detail. Endoscopic ultrasound (ultrasound probe attached to an endoscope) is effective for determining the depth of penetration of accessible tumors (i.e., rectum, esophagus, stomach, duodenum, and bile duct) and is therefore a useful staging technique.

The size and extent of GI cancers, as well as the presence or absence of metastatic disease, can be defined with these studies. Tumors not accessible by endoscopy can be sampled by CT or ultrasound image–guided percutaneous needle biopsies. Although associated with a risk of hemorrhage, core biopsies that obtain approximately 50 mg of tissue are preferred to fine-needle aspiration biopsies that obtain individual cells. Neither technique is useful for diagnosing lymphoma.

How are GI cancers staged?

Defining the stage of a patient's cancer guides treatment and estimates prognosis and is therefore important in decision making. Stage determined by diagnostic studies is termed *clinical stage.* Staging based on information obtained at surgery and the final pathology report is the pathologic stage of the cancer. The preferred system for cancer staging is the TNM classification, where T is tumor (size and depth of penetration), N is regional lymph node status, and M is presence or absence of metastases to distant lymph nodes or other organs. The following is a generalization for GI cancers:

Stage I: cancer is confined to the visceral wall and <2 cm in size (T1, N0, M0)

Stage II: cancer has spread through the visceral wall and is >2 cm in size (T2, N0, M0)

Stage III: cancer has spread to regional lymph nodes (any T, N1, M0)

Stage IV: cancer has spread to distant lymph nodes or other organs (any T, any N, M1)

As a rule, stages I and II cancers have a reasonable chance for cure, stage III cancers have a high risk for recurrence, and stage IV cancers are usually incurable.

▶ TREATMENT

The starting point for treatment of GI cancers is confirmation of the diagnosis and the clinical stage of the patient's disease. A comprehensive treatment plan should be formulated. Because cancer treatment is multidisciplinary, review of the diagnostic material and treatment plan at a tumor board or in consultation with medical and radiation oncologists is useful and in the best interest of the patient. To whatever extent possible, relieve symptoms such as pain, nausea, or diarrhea. Correct severe anemia and consider the patient's nutritional status. Address the patient's fears and concerns. Be direct, honest, and empathetic in answering patient questions. Be aware and sensitive to what the patient wants to know and what the patient interprets from your communication. Be mindful of cultural differences. Sensitive communication with the cancer patient is one of the finest tests of physician behavior.

What are the important surgical aspects of the treatment of GI cancer?

A complete surgical resection of the patient's tumor is usually the only chance for cure of virtually all GI cancers (anal carcinoma is an exception). The very biology of the disease, including lymphatic and distant spread of tumor cells, dictates that "complete surgical removal" is a relative term. Complete eradication of cancer cells from the patient's body is probably dependent on host response factors and the adaptation mechanisms of the cancer cells themselves. Nevertheless, a thorough surgical resection of all visible and palpable tumor, with the margins of the resection free of cancer cells on histologic examination, is curative for a substantial percentage of stages I and II GI cancers, and even for stage III disease when regional lymph nodes can be effectively removed. Direct extension of a carcinoma to an adjacent organ does not preclude cure, if the cancer can be completely resected.

The operative approach should be carefully planned using all available imaging studies and a thorough knowledge of the anatomy involved. The surgeon usually strives for a 5-cm margin of uninvolved bowel or stomach both proximal and distal to gastric or intestinal cancers and sufficient resection of bowel mesentery to remove the mesenteric lymph nodes at risk. Lesser margins (but histologically tumor free) must be accepted for cancers of the liver and pancreas. Hepatocellular cancer most commonly occurs in patients with cirrhosis who tolerate surgery and liver resection poorly. Surgical opportunity is limited in these cases.

Partial resection (so-called debulking) of GI cancers is an exercise in wishful thinking and generally not helpful (see subsequent discussion of indications for palliative surgery). Therefore, the treatment team must carefully determine preoperatively that the patient's situation offers a reasonable opportunity for curative resection. Exquisite judgment must be exercised to determining whether the potential benefit (cure or extended palliation) from resection of a cancer warrants the risk and morbidity of the procedure (i.e., esophagectomy or pancreaticoduodenectomy in an elderly, debilitated patient).

Preoperative control of medical problems and good preparation for surgery, including mechanical cleansing of the colon, are essential. Careful execution of the surgical procedure by an experienced team improves overall survival rates from cancer. This is accomplished by a reduction in complications and overall better selection of patients. Patients who survive surgical complications may yet have prolonged debility that may delay the start of other therapies.

Indications for palliative surgery for GI cancers include relief of obstruction of the common bile duct, gastric outlet, or small or large bowel and control of bleeding. However, consideration of the mortality and morbidity risk and the debilitating aspects of a surgical procedure is important when assessing a patient for palliative surgery. For example, an operation to relieve small bowel obstruction in a patient with diffuse bulky peritoneal cancer implants and extensive previous abdominal surgery all too often adds enterocutaneous fistulas to the patient's situation, without relieving the obstruction.

For certain tumors, including colon and rectal carcinoma, carcinoid tumors, and NETs of the pancreas, resection of liver metastases provides extended survival and a low, but consistent, cure rate (30% at 5 years for colorectal metastases). The metastatic disease must be confined to the liver, the primary tumor must be controlled, the liver tumors must be resectable by standard techniques, and the patient must be able to undergo the operation safely.

What are the important aspects of radiation treatment of GI cancer?

Radiation therapy in sufficient doses is highly effective for destroying even bulky cancer, but its use in the abdomen is hampered by dose tolerance of the bowel and the liver. The small intestine becomes dysfunctional and scarred at doses higher than 50 Gy, and radiation hepatitis and progressive fibrosis of the liver begins at 30 Gy. For virtually all GI cancers, doses higher than this (~60 Gy) are required for eradication of cancer cells. Thus, radiation therapy in doses sufficient to kill GI cancer cells is poorly tolerated. As a corollary, radiation therapy cannot be given in sufficient doses to eliminate unresectable GI cancer or residual tumor from an ill-conceived debulking procedure. In specific situations radiation therapy is valuable as an adjunct treatment for control of undetected microscopic deposits of tumor extending beyond the limits of the surgical resection and for relief of pain.

The anatomy of the deep pelvis complicates the resection of rectal carcinomas. There is considerable manipulation of the tumor in dissection, and the bony pelvis limits the lateral extent of resection. Using techniques to limit radiation dose to the small bowel, radiation therapy given either before or after resection of rectal carcinomas improves local control of the cancer. 5-Fluorouracil, a chemotherapeutic drug, appears to sensitize carcinoma cells to radiation and is usually given in conjunction with radiation therapy. Data suggest that preoperative radiation therapy (50 Gy) in combination with chemotherapy improves local control and survival for esophageal carcinoma. Postoperative radiation and chemotherapy reduce pain and extend survival for unresectable pancreatic carcinoma. Even with the dose limitations required, radiation therapy for bulky liver metastases provides palliative pain relief. The same is true for recurrent or unresectable cancer in the pelvis.

What are the important chemotherapeutic aspects of the treatment of GI cancer?

5-Fluorouracil in combination with leucovorin given for several months after resection of stages II and III colon and rectal carcinomas improves survival, as established by several clinical trials. Unfortunately, there is no other proven effective adjuvant therapy for GI cancers. Approximately 70% of anal carcinomas can be cured without surgery by combined treatment with chemotherapy and radiation therapy. Chemotherapy may be given following resection of GI lymphomas or as alternative therapy for unresectable disease. Reasonable palliation may be obtained from chemotherapy for recurrent or unresectable gastric, pancreatic, colon, and rectal carcinoma. For GIST, the molecular therapy Gleevec (imatinib mesylate) is effective in shrinking bulky tumors that carry the *c-kit* gene mutation.

K E Y   P O I N T S

▶ GI cancer is a disease of somatic DNA-creating cells that proliferate without control, have no limit on life span, invade their neighbor's territory, and cause death of the host-patient.

▶ Symptoms of weight loss, anemia, anorexia, early satiety, abdominal pain, cramping, bloating, or palpable abdominal or pelvic mass suggest the presence of a GI cancer.

▶ After history and physical examination, upper or lower GI endoscopy, abdominal imaging by CT scan, and biopsy are the most effective methods of diagnosis.

▶ Preferred treatment of GI cancers is complete surgical resection of the tumor and regional lymph nodes.

CASE 29–13. A 72-year-old man reports mild, crampy, abdominal pain referred to the lower abdomen that is worse after meals. He notes some decrease in the caliber of his stools and a 10-lb weight loss over the last 4 months. Hematocrit is 29; stool is positive for occult blood.

    A. What diseases would you consider?
    B. What studies would you order?
    C. If the diagnosis is cancer, how would you treat him?

CASE 29–14. A 59-year-old woman complains of fatigue, epigastric pain radiating through to her back, 12-lb weight loss, and the recent onset of jaundice and pruritus. Abdominal exam shows a palpable, mildly tender gallbladder.

    A. What diagnosis is most likely?
    B. What diagnostic studies would you order?
    C. How would you treat a cancer causing these symptoms?

INFLAMMATORY BOWEL DISEASE

▶ **ETIOLOGY**

What is inflammatory bowel disease?

The term *inflammatory bowel disease* (IBD) has come to denote two clinically distinct diseases: mucosal ulcerative colitis (MUC) and Crohn's disease. Many theories on the causation of IBD have been considered, including infections, allergic, environmental, psychological, genetic, and autoimmune derivations. However, no one cause has held up under the scrutiny of multiple scientific studies, so that a combination of factors seems more likely than a single cause.

CROHN'S DISEASE

What are the demographics of Crohn's disease?

The incidence of Crohn's disease is highest in United States, Europe, Israel, and Australia. The incidence of Crohn's disease ranges from 1 to 7 per 100,000 population per year. It is less prevalent in blacks and

Asians. There is a family history in 7% to 14% of cases. There is a relatively high incidence among Ashkenazi Jews. There is no predilection for gender. There is a bimodal age distribution, with incidence peaking in both the 2nd and 4th decades.

▶ EVALUATION

What are the patterns of Crohn's disease?

Crohn's disease is a chronic inflammatory condition that can affect any part of the GI tract from the mouth to the anus. The typical clinical patterns can be classified into three groups: ileocolic, small bowel, and colonic disease. Approximately 40% of patients have involvement of the distal ileum and proximal colon (ileocolic disease), about 25% to 30% involve the small intestine alone, and about 25% involve the colon alone. Approximately 5% of patients with Crohn's disease present with clinical findings that do not correlate with the three typical patterns. In this atypical group, the disease can primarily affect the stomach, duodenum, or perineum or can present with extraintestinal manifestations that precede bowel symptoms by months or years.

What are the pathologic findings in Crohn's disease?

Crohn's disease affects the intestinal wall transmurally. The earliest macroscopic pathologic manifestations are small aphthous ulcers. These are shallow, 1- to 3-mm-wide ulcers with white bases. With progression of disease, these ulcers become deeper and confluent and fissures tend to develop. These linear ulcers and transverse fissures around areas of intact mucosa give the luminal surface a "cobblestone" appearance. Noncaseating granulomata occur in the bowel wall and are one of the key features differentiating Crohn's disease from MUC. Because Crohn's disease extends transmurally, penetrating ulcers and fissures may lead to a wide variety of septic complications such as abscess and fistula formation to adjacent organs.

How can Crohn's disease be recognized in the operating room?

In its classic form, Crohn's disease of the small bowel is easily recognizable. The involved segment, which is usually just proximal to the ileocecal valve, is indurated and thick walled. Extensive fat wrapping may be observed, a phenomenon in which mesenteric fat extends circumferentially around the diseased bowel. Skip lesions affecting small bowel occur in 20% of cases. In small bowel disease there is severe serositis or a "corkscrew" appearance of the serosal vessels and thickening of the mesenteric margin. The proximal bowel above the strictured segment commonly is dilated owing to chronic obstruction. The mesentery of involved small bowel is quite thickened and often contains large lymph nodes, most commonly located in the distribution of ileocolic and superior mesenteric vessels.

In Crohn's colitis, patchy or uniform ulceration and thickening of the bowel wall may be seen with varying degrees of fat wrapping or skip lesions. However, this is not always the case, and the full extent of disease may be best judged by colonoscopy.

How do patients with Crohn's disease present?

The onset of Crohn's disease is usually slow, nonspecific, and insidious, which contributes to a delay in diagnosis. The typical presenting symptoms include abdominal pain, diarrhea, and weight loss. However, because patients with Crohn's disease may develop inflammation anywhere along the GI tract, the clinical features on presentation are diverse and depend directly on the location of inflammation (Table 29–6).

Abdominal pain, which is the most common symptom, is usually crampy and intermittent. Continuous or episodic diarrhea following meals is typical. Stools are usually liquid or semisolid. Chronic obstruction and inflammation in the diseased segment lead to malabsorption, especially in severe small bowel disease (jejunoileitis). Diminished food intake, which may alleviate abdominal discomfort and diarrhea, contributes to malnutrition, vitamin deficiencies, and weight loss. Children with extensive Crohn's disease often have growth retardation. Low-grade fever may be present in all patterns of Crohn's disease. Adolescents may present with fever of unknown origin, diarrhea, and abdominal pain with or without GI contrast abnormalities or growth retardation. High fever is often associated with intra-abdominal abscesses or peritonitis. Perianal pain and drainage are due to fissures or complex fistulas and abscesses in the perianal area. Anorectal pathology is more frequently observed in patients with Crohn's colitis (50% to 75%) but is also seen in 10% to 25% of patients with ileocolic and small bowel disease. The anemia seen in Crohn's disease is most often an iron deficiency or megaloblastic anemia due to vitamin B_{12} and folic acid deficiency. Anemia can be more profound in Crohn's colitis associated with hematochezia.

TABLE 29–6

Typical Patterns of Presentation of Crohn's Disease

Site of Disease	Frequency (%)	Signs and Symptoms
Ileocolic	40	Abdominal pain, diarrhea, fever, enteric fistulas and abdominal mass, weight loss
Small bowel (jejunoileitis)	25–30	Abdominal pain, diarrhea, fever, enteric fistulas and abdominal mass, weight loss, steatorrhea, growth retardation, malabsorption
Colonic	25	Hematochezia, mucus, diarrhea, weight loss, fever

What are the complications of Crohn's disease?

Crohn's disease may also present in the form of intestinal complications or symptoms directly related to these complications (Table 29–7).

What is toxic megacolon?

With acute, severe attacks of colitis, dilation of the colon may occur. Usually the patient has a history of colitis of several months or years of duration. Occasionally toxic colitis or megacolon is the initial manifestation of the disease. Patients are systemically ill with tachycardia, fever, leukocytosis, hypoalbuminemia, and signs of localized or generalized peritonitis. Dilation of the colon, especially the transverse colon or splenic flexure, completes the picture.

What are the extraintestinal manifestations of IBD?

Both Crohn's disease and MUC are associated with a spectrum of extraintestinal manifestations (Table 29–8) that can involve nearly every system in the body. As many as 30% to 40% of patients with IBD have at least one extraintestinal manifestation. Most of these conditions respond to the therapy for the intestinal disease, with the exception of hepatobiliary disease and ankylosing spondylitis. These manifestations may be the primary reason that the patients seek medical care, and timely diagnosis of the underlying bowel condition may depend on their recognition.

TABLE 29–7

Intestinal Complications of Crohn's Disease

Small bowel obstruction
Internal fistula
    Enteroenteric: ileocolic or ileoileal being the most common type
    Enterovesical: ileovesical being the most common type
    Enterovaginal
Abscess
    Intra-abdominal
    Pelvic
    Intramesenteric
    Retroperitoneal
    Psoas
Large bowel obstruction due to strictures or cancer
Toxic megacolon
Hemorrhage: uncommon
Free perforation: uncommon
Obstructive uropathy due to phlegmon and abscess
Anorectal complications
    Stricture
    Complex fistulas and abscesses
    Rectovaginal fistula

TABLE 29–8

Extraintestinal Manifestations of Inflammatory Bowel Disease

Skin
  Aphthous stomatitis
  Erythema nodosum
  Pyoderma gangrenosum
Liver
  Primary sclerosing cholangitis
  Adenocarcinoma of the bile ducts
  Pericholangitis
Joints
  Arthralgia
  Arthritis
  Ankylosing spondylitis
Eyes
  Uveitis
  Iritis
  Episcleritis
Renal
  Nephrolithiasis

How do I diagnose and work up patients with Crohn's disease?

Any patient with chronic recurrent abdominal pain, diarrhea, and weight loss should be evaluated for Crohn's disease. Physical findings of perineal (fissure, ulcer, large elephant ear skin tags, anorectal stricture, complex anorectal fistulas, abscesses), abdominal (tenderness, fistula, mass), or extraintestinal involvement may be helpful.

Laboratory studies are usually nonspecific. Anemia, hypoalbuminemia, steatorrhea, elevated sedimentation rate, and white blood cell count are common.

Barium studies (small bowel series, enteroclysis, barium enema) can be helpful in the diagnosis of Crohn's disease. Ulcers, fissures, and cobblestone appearance are early findings. Fistulas, abscesses, skip lesions, and strictures of the small bowel come later. Distention of the bowel proximal to narrowed areas and separation of the bowel loops owing to thickened bowel wall and mesentery may also be seen. Later in the course, Kantor's "string sign" may occur due to narrowing of the intestinal lumen, most commonly seen in terminal ileum.

CT scan and ultrasound have diagnostic and therapeutic value, especially in cases with acute presentation with complications of the disease. CT- or ultrasound-guided drainage of abscess prior to definitive surgical resection is valuable in lessening activity of disease.

Upper GI endoscopy may reveal esophageal, gastric, and duodenal involvement. Colonoscopy reveals diseased areas (aphthous ulcers, internal fistulization, strictures, skip lesions, and cobblestoning) in the colon and the terminal ileum. Biopsy of these areas may show features of Crohn's disease, especially granuloma formation. Noncaseating granuloma, which is considered by most clinicians as the pathognomonic finding of Crohn's disease, can be found on biopsy in 10% to 20% of cases.

What is the differential diagnosis of Crohn's disease?

Irritable bowel syndrome, appendicitis, acute ileitis, lymphoma, intestinal tuberculosis, MUC, carcinoma of the small bowel, ischemia, infectious colitis, and metastatic lesions are some of the principal differential diagnoses to consider when evaluating a patient with suspected Crohn's disease. Acute ileitis, usually associated with *Yersinia enterocolitica* infection, may evolve into Crohn's disease in 15% of cases and presents a diagnostic challenge for appendicitis. For this reason incidental appendectomy is recommended to prevent the future misdiagnosis of appendicitis in these patients unless obvious Crohn's disease is present. This scenario has been rare, in our experience.

▶ TREATMENT

What is the treatment for Crohn's disease?

Despite the introduction of new drugs and surgical alternatives, there is still no cure for Crohn's disease. The aims of treatment are to maintain nutritional support, provide symptomatic relief, and reduce and prevent further bowel inflammation.

The initial therapy for uncomplicated Crohn's disease is nonoperative and includes nutritional and pharmacologic therapy. Many patients with Crohn's disease are malnourished and have weight loss. A low-residue, high-protein diet (elemental diet) may improve the nutritional status of such patients. If the patient is not able to tolerate food, total parenteral nutrition is occasionally valuable. Elemental diets are also used as an adjunct in the management of growth failure in prepubertal children and short bowel syndrome. There is no clear evidence supporting the role of preoperative total parenteral nutrition.

The mainstays of medical therapy for Crohn's disease are 5-aminosalicylic acid (5-ASA) products (sulfasalazine, mesalamine, olsalazine), steroids to induce remission, antibiotics, and immunosuppressive agents. Mesalamine is used for small bowel and colonic disease. Sulfasalazine and olsalazine are reserved for colonic disease due to their site of action after degradation. 5-ASA products and steroids are the most commonly used products for reducing symptoms and obtaining remission in active disease. Steroids are not used to maintain remission. Immunosupressives, such as azathioprine and 6-mercaptopurine, are valuable in the management of Crohn's disease. They have a steroid-sparing effect and also help close intestinal and perineal fistulas. However, the response is delayed, commonly requiring 3 to 6 months of treatment before a benefit occurs. Cyclosporine is another immunosuppressive that has been used in Crohn's disease; however, controversy exists due to serious potential side effects and limited effectiveness. Ciprofloxacin and metronidazole are also effective in the management of perineal infections due to fistulas and abscesses and may be useful for patients with active Crohn's colitis.

Recently a new immunosuppressive (infliximab, an antitumor necrosis factor α derivative) has been successfully used in the management of Crohn's disease that is refractory to conventional treatment. The initial concern of increased risk of lymphoma noted in clinical trials has not been apparent with its commercial use. The role of this medication in maintaining long-term remission needs to be proven. Currently mesalamine and azathioprine are the two agents that have demonstrated effectiveness in maintaining patients in remission.

About 75% to 90% of patients with Crohn's disease ultimately require one or more operations in their lifetime. The most common indications for surgery are intestinal obstruction, septic complications (abscesses, internal and external fistulas, toxic megacolon, and free perforation), and the failure of medical treatment. Intestinal obstruction may present acutely and can be partial, high grade, or complete. Fistulas are the most common septic complications, followed by abscesses and phlegmon. About 10% to 25% of patients with Crohn's disease need surgery because of a poor response to medical therapy. Surgery is indicated to avoid long-term steroid administration and its potential side effects.

Because Crohn's disease is chronic and recurrent, surgeons must keep in mind the long-term outlook for the patient. Surgery is effective for relieving complications but does little to alter the progress of disease. Small intestine is a precious resource, and conservation is therefore imperative, since massive and repeated resections can lead to short bowel syndrome. The key principle in patients with Crohn's disease is to limit the surgery to correction of the current complication. Crohn's disease without intestinal obstruction or perforation is not an indication for surgery.

Several types of operation are used in the surgery of Crohn's disease. These vary depending on the disease location (Table 29–9). For small bowel disease, conservative resection of the diseased segment with primary anastomosis is the preferred surgical procedure. Remove diseased segments with margins of 2 to 5 cm. There is no added value to use frozen sections to assess the status of margins. Wide margins of resection confer no advantage to the patient and are unnecessary. If an inflammatory mass and phlegmon adheres to vital structures, such as iliac vessels, or if removal would necessitate massive amount of small bowel resection, it may be necessary to bypass the involved segment with ileotransverse bypass or to create a diverting stoma (ileostomy or jejunostomy) rather than resect the involved segment. Bypass procedures, with

TABLE 29-9

Types of Operations for Crohn's Disease

Surgical Procedure	Location of Disease
Intestinal resection with or without anastomosis	
Ileocolic resection	Ileocolic
Small bowel resection	Small bowel
Total proctocolectomy with end ileostomy	Colon, perineum
Total abdominal colectomy with ileorectal anastomosis	Colon
Segmental colectomy	Colon
Bypass procedure	
Ileotransverse	Ileum and colon
Gastroduodenostomy or gastrojejunostomy	Duodenum
Ileostomy	Perineal with septic complications
Strictureplasty	Duodenum, ileum and colon, and small bowel

the exception of the treatment of duodenal Crohn's disease, are not used definitively because the diseased segment may develop future complications, including malignancy. Ileostomy alone is used infrequently, except to divert the fecal stream in severe perineal Crohn's disease. A temporary ileostomy is used when bowel resection is required in the presence of factors adverse to anastomotic healing. For patients with multiple strictures of the small bowel or for patients with short bowel syndrome, intestinal conservation may be achieved by surgically widening the stricture, a procedure called *strictureplasty*. This avoids multiple or extensive resections.

What is the prognosis of Crohn's disease?

Crohn's disease is incurable, and treatment strategies are developed around this fact. The risk of reoperation is greatest in the first 5 postoperative years. About 40% to 70% of patients require at least one additional procedure by 15 years. Most frequently recurrence involves the segment of bowel proximal to the site of anastomosis. Adverse factors affecting the rate of recurrence are tobacco use and presence of a bowel anastomosis. To a slight extent, prophylactic 5-ASA may delay recurrence.

Is there any increased risk of cancer in patients with Crohn's disease?

Patients with Crohn's disease carry an approximately 50% increased risk of developing intestinal malignancies. The most common intestinal malignancies are colorectal and small bowel cancer (usually ileal). For small bowel cancer, efforts have been made to identify preventable risk factors, including surgically excluded bowel loops (bypassed segments), chronically obstructed unresected disease, and chronic fistulous disease. The risk of colorectal cancer in Crohn's colitis is approximately three times that of the normal population. However, this risk is markedly lower than that in patients with MUC.

MUCOSAL ULCERATIVE COLITIS (MUC)

What are the demographics of MUC?

The incidence of MUC is highest in United States, Europe, Israel, and Australia. MUC, like Crohn's disease, occurs more frequently in Jews and less frequently in blacks and Asians. The incidence rate for MUC ranges from 5 to 10 per 100,000 population per year. There is a slight female predominance in contrast to Crohn's disease. However, like the Crohn's disease, it has a bimodal age distribution, with a peak occurring in both the 2nd and 6th decades.

▶ EVALUATION

What is the pathology of MUC?

MUC is an inflammatory disease of the colon of unknown etiology and characteristically is a mucosal disease. Unlike Crohn's disease, the mucosa is usually inflamed continuously without any skip lesions. The disease is variable in the extent and severity of involvement of the colon. In its most limited extent it may affect only the distal rectum. In its most extensive form the entire colon is involved (pancolitis). Total colonic involvement is accompanied by extension of mucosal inflammation with secondary changes into the distal terminal ileum in 10% to 20% of patients (so-called backwash ileitis). The spectrum of severity ranges from inflammation so mild that it is undetectable except by biopsy to severe ulceration leading to perforation or hemorrhage. The process of ulceration and granulation followed by re-epithelialization may lead to polypoid lesions that are not neoplastic and referred to as *pseudopolyps* or *inflammatory polyps*. Distal colon ulcerative colitis may involve only the rectum (proctitis) or may involve both the sigmoid colon and the rectum (proctosigmoiditis). The prognosis for those with distal colon MUC appears to be good for the majority of patients. Approximately 30% of MUC patients have disease limited to the rectum. In 40%, the disease extends above the rectum, and the remaining 30% develop pancolitis at their first attack.

What is the pattern of presentation in patients with MUC?

MUC often evolves into one of two patterns: (1) acute, early onset with severe symptoms, or (2) an indolent, chronic, and recurrent pattern with chronic illness, malnutrition, and steroid dependency. When operation is necessary, it is usually because of the severity of one of these two patterns.

What are the most common presenting signs and symptoms in patients with MUC?

The cardinal symptom of MUC involving any portion of the colon is rectal bleeding (hematochezia). This is present in 80% to 90% of patients at the onset of their disease. Diarrhea is present at onset in more than 80% of patients. Diarrhea may vary from less formed stools to the passage of small amounts of mucopus and blood as frequently as every few minutes. Rectal bleeding and diarrhea can be accompanied by tenesmus, rectal urgency, and anal incontinence, depending on the severity of the disease. Patients may also present with cramping abdominal pain and variable degrees of fever, vomiting, weight loss, and dehydration.

During an acute attack of ulcerative colitis, dehydration, hypotension, abdominal tenderness, and distention are predominant symptoms. In rare cases extraintestinal manifestations, such as pyoderma, arthropathy, or thromboembolic events may be the initial presenting symptoms. Fistulas, anal abscesses, and skin tags are uncommon in MUC patients, and the presence of these findings should raise the suspicion of Crohn's disease. However, anal canal fissures can be seen in up to 15% of patients with MUC secondary to frequency, urgency, and straining.

What are the complications of MUC?

Extraintestinal manifestations, cancer, dysplasia, fulminant colitis, toxic megacolon, perforation, and hemorrhage are the major complications related to MUC. In general, extraintestinal features parallel the activity of colitis and usually can be treated adequately by medical therapy. With the exception of hepatic complications and ankylosing spondylitis, they usually respond to proctocolectomy.

Acute, severe attacks of MUC—so-called fulminant or toxic colitis—may occur as the first manifestation of the disease (15%) or during the course of longstanding illness. This presentation is characterized by frequent, bloody bowel movements, high fever, and abdominal pain. Patients are profoundly ill with tachycardia, fever, leukocytosis, and hypoalbuminemia of varying severity. Signs of localized or generalized peritonitis may be present. Toxic megacolon is a further complication of toxic colitis, in which a plain radiograph film of abdomen shows a colon diameter of 5 cm or more. The mortality of patients with toxic megacolon may be as high as 20% to 30%. Toxic megacolon may also be associated with Crohn's colitis and infectious colitis such as amebiasis and *Clostridium difficile* colitis.

Bowel perforation may occur with or without colonic dilation. If a free perforation occurs, it has a high mortality rate. Abdominal colectomy and ileostomy is the procedure of choice.

Hemorrhage requiring emergency transfusion is an uncommon complication of ulcerative colitis and usually occurs with fulminant disease.

How do I diagnose and work up patients with MUC?

Any patient who presents with rectal bleeding with mucus, diarrhea, and abdominal pain should be evaluated for MUC. Physical examination findings can be normal. Blood can be found on digital rectal exam. Abdominal tenderness, distention, and hypoactive bowel sounds are features of toxic colitis. Signs and symptoms of extraintestinal manifestation can also be helpful.

Abnormalities of laboratory tests in MUC parallel the extent and the severity of the bowel disease. Anemia, leukocytosis, hypoalbuminemia, elevated sedimentation rate, and electrolyte imbalance usually accompany severe colitis. Hypokalemia and metabolic acidosis can be particularly severe as the result of diarrheal loss of potassium and bicarbonate. Stool cultures should be taken.

An abdominal radiograph series is part of the evaluation of patients with moderate and severe colitis to detect colonic dilation or perforation. This is especially important for patients who are taking steroids whose abdominal exam may not reflect the severity of intra-abdominal pathology.

Barium enema is contraindicated in patients with acute fulminant colitis, because perforation and barium peritonitis may occur. With longstanding MUC, there is a loss of haustral markings. The colon narrows and shortens and assumes the appearance of a rigid, contracted tube, the so-called lead pipe appearance. Pseudopolyps and strictures can also be seen in longstanding disease. Presence of colonic stricture with MUC should arouse suspicion of cancer, and the patient should be referred for surgical consultation.

Endoscopy is the most accurate method for both diagnosis and determination of the extent of the disease. Sigmoidoscopy is essential because disease involves the rectum in more than 90% of cases. Colonoscopy should be done in all other patients to determine the extent of the disease or if sigmoidoscopy is not diagnostic. In longstanding disease, surveillance colonoscopy with biopsies is valuable to diagnose cancer or dysplasia. Colonoscopy should not be done in patients with toxic megacolon or fulminant colitis.

Early in the course of MUC the mucosa manifests edema and friability, with bleeding on minor trauma. With progression or increasing severity a granular, spontaneously hemorrhagic mucosa appears, with overlying mucopurulent exudate. The lumen is narrowed and straightened, and the normally thin mucosal folds are lost. In the most severe presentation, the mucosa is diffusely inflamed, hemorrhagic, and ulcerated. Biopsy is helpful to confirm the diagnosis. Pseudopolyps can also be seen.

What is the differential diagnosis of MUC?

Differential diagnoses of MUC include diverticulitis, ischemic colitis, lymphoma, collagenous colitis, and infectious causes. Diverticulitis and ischemic colitis have a segmental pattern of involvement quite unlike the usual distribution of MUC. Collagenous colitis presents with watery diarrhea in middle-aged women, with normal endoscopic but pathognomonic biopsy findings of thickened collagen deposits under the mucosa.

Infectious causes also should be excluded prior to steroid therapy. These include amebiasis, CMV, *E. coli*, *Shigella*, *C. difficile*, *Campylobacter jejuni,* and AIDS-related GI infections. The most important differential of diagnosis of MUC is Crohn's disease. Certain clinical, radiologic, pathologic, and endoscopic features help differentiate the two. Nevertheless, 10% to 15% of cases cannot be differentiated and are called *indeterminate colitis*. Comparisons of various features of Crohn's disease and MUC are summarized in Table 29–10.

▶ TREATMENT

What is the medical treatment for MUC?

Most patients with MUC can be managed medically. However, pharmacologic therapy for MUC is not curative. The mainstays of

---

TABLE 29–10

Comparison of Features of Crohn's Disease and Mucosal Ulcerative Colitis (MUC)

	Crohn's Disease	MUC
Clinical Pattern	Can affect any part of the digestive tract. Perineal disease and external fistulas are common.	Proctitis and/or colitis only. Perineal disease and fistulas are internal and very rare.
Pathologic/ Endoscopic/ Radiologic Features	Segmental, skip lesions, strictures, ileal and small bowel involvement, and rectal sparing are common. Cobblestone appearance Transmural disease, fibrosis, and granulomas are common. Crypt abscesses are rare.	Continuous, strictures are uncommon and usually associated with malignancy. Rectal sparing and small bowel involvement are rare. Pseudopolyps are common. Mucosal disease: disease may involve all the layers of bowel wall only in severe disease. Crypt abscesses are common.

medical therapy for MUC are similar to Crohn's disease and include 5-ASA products (sulfasalazine, mesalamine, olsalazine), steroids, antibiotics, and immunosuppressives. Medical treatment of patients with MUC can be subdivided into early (or acute) treatment and a later (or maintenance) therapy. As in Crohn's disease, the treatment of MUC starts with general and supportive therapy. Reduced activity, bed rest, and a lactate-free diet are advisable.

Sulfasalazine has been used in the treatment of MUC for almost 60 years and is of particular value for mild to moderate disease. The usual dose is 4 g daily, with a maintenance dose of 2 g daily. In the last decade, there have been attempts to separate sulfasalazine into its components and use the therapeutically active 5-ASA portion and eliminate the sulfapyridine portion to minimize the side effects related to it. This has been accomplished with the introduction of mesalamine or olsalazine type of products, which are currently being used in the management of active disease to achieve remission and as maintenance therapy. A topical form of these 5-ASA products is used as a suppository or enema to achieve remission in cases of more distal disease. Steroids are used to treat acute and severe cases of MUC. Steroids are effective in achieving rapid, short-term remission. The usual concept has been to use the drug for a relatively short course of therapy, often prednisone, in doses of 40 to 60 mg per day, then tapering the doses gradually over a period of 1 to 3 months. In severe disease, steroids may be administered intravenously, often in conjunction with IV feeding.

Topical steroid enema or suppository also can be helpful in the management of active proctitis or proctosigmoiditis. Immunosuppressives, such as azathioprine and mercaptopurine, have been used in the management of active disease. They have steroid-sparing effect. Unfortunately, their slow action, often requiring 3 to 6 months, is a significant disadvantage. Cyclosporine is another immunosuppressive that is effective for patients who do not respond to steroids. Unlike the other immunosuppressives, it has a rapid onset of action.

Controlled trials have shown that chronic administration of 5-ASA products orally or topically reduces relapse rates. Topical steroids may also be helpful as maintenance therapy in patients with proctitis or proctosigmoiditis. This is also true for immunosuppressives such as cyclosporine, azathioprine, and mercaptopurine. Systemic steroids have no place in maintaining long-term remission in the management of MUC.

What is the surgical treatment of MUC?

Unlike Crohn's disease, MUC can be completely cured with surgical therapy. Emergency operation is indicated for acute problems that are refractory to medical therapy. Urgent operation is indicated in the following circumstances:

Free perforation or signs of general peritonitis
Severe, localized peritonitis indicating imminent perforation
Septic shock
Massive hemorrhage
Increasing colonic dilation
Clear deterioration of patient's condition over 24 hours after initial
    resuscitation

Abdominal colectomy with ileostomy is the procedure of choice in
these conditions. Emergency colectomy has an overall mortality
rate of 5%. Most of these deaths are related to perforation, which
has a 40% mortality rate.

The most common indication for elective operation in patients
with MUC is failure of medical therapy. Total proctocolectomy with
ileal pouch anal anastomosis is the elective operation of choice
in most patients. In this procedure the entire colon and rectum
are removed and the ileum is made into a reservoir and anastomosed to the anal canal. The other elective procedures include total
proctocolectomy and creation of a Brooke (end) or continent (Kock
pouch) ileostomy, subtotal colectomy with ileostomy, or ileorectal
anastomosis. These procedures are done in circumstances when
restorative proctocolectomy with ileal pouch anal anastomosis is
not feasible. Total proctocolectomy and Brooke (end) or continent
(Kock pouch) ileostomy is done in patients with poor anal sphincter
pressures or cancer of the lower third of rectum, or if the patient is
elderly. Subtotal colectomy with ileostomy is done in cases of diagnostic dilemma of Crohn's disease versus MUC, patients on large
doses of steroids, or patients with toxic colitis. In these situations
the rectum is preserved to minimize the operative risk associated
with pelvic dissection and a pouch procedure. Subtotal colectomy
with ileorectal anastomosis is rarely performed today.

For many years the only surgical therapy of significant value was
total proctocolectomy with permanent ileostomy. With the development of pelvic pouch procedures, however, the willingness of patients
to accept colectomy has greatly increased. Pelvic pouch procedures
have indeed become a significant therapeutic advance in the management of patients with MUC. Most patients believe that ileoanal
anastomosis gives a better quality of life than does an ileostomy.

Is there an increased cancer risk in patients with MUC?

Patients with MUC have a 20% to 30% risk of developing colorectal
cancer within 20 years of diagnosis. The cancer risk relates to both
the extent of colonic involvement and the duration of disease. Risk
of colorectal cancer is also another major indication for surgery in
patients with MUC. Prophylactic colectomy without proof of dysplasia (precancerous lesions) or cancer is controversial. However,
yearly colonoscopy with random biopsies of the whole colon is

strongly recommended after 10 years of disease. Detection of dysplasia is an indication for total proctocolectomy regardless of the disease activity.

What is the prognosis of MUC?

Unlike Crohn's disease, MUC can be completely cured with total proctocolectomy. About 10% to 25% of patients require colectomy after a severe presentation. The remainder usually respond to medical therapy at the time of the initial presentation. The long-term prognosis of MUC is good, and the mortality rate is low.

K E Y   P O I N T S

▶ The term *IBD* encompasses two clinically distinct entities: Crohn's disease and MUC.

▶ Because Crohn's disease can involve any part of the GI tract, presenting symptoms can be quite variable.

▶ Any patient with chronic recurrent abdominal pain, diarrhea, and weight loss should be evaluated for IBD, especially Crohn's disease.

▶ Patients with MUC usually present with rectal bleeding and diarrhea.

▶ Unlike Crohn's disease, MUC can be cured by surgery.

▶ Both Crohn's disease and MUC may be associated with debilitating extraintestinal manifestations.

CASE 29–15.   A 21-year-old woman college student presents with a history of intermittent, crampy lower abdominal pain for the last 6 months. She also complains of episodes of loose bowel movements, usually after meals. She states that if she eats less, her symptoms are considerably improved. She has noted a 15-lb weight loss during this period. She has no history of foreign travel. None of her family or acquaintances have similar symptoms.

  A. What are the possible diagnoses?
  B. What are the steps of evaluation?

CASE 29–16. A 35-year-old man with a history of MUC since the age of 16 was doing well on medical management of the disease. Three months ago, he began to notice decreased caliber of his stools. This persisted for several weeks until the last 2 weeks, during which time he noted only loose stools. He has also noted a 20-lb weight loss over the last 6 months and states that he "has no appetite."

    A. What is the likely diagnosis?
    B. What are the steps of evaluation?

SURGICAL LIVER DISEASE

▶ **ETIOLOGY**

What is the risk of surgery on a patient with liver disease?

Patients with liver disease who undergo surgery are at increased risk of perioperative morbidity and mortality. The Child's-Pugh classification (Table 29–11) is used to assess the severity of liver impairment. For patients undergoing major surgery, those in Child's class A have a less than 1% risk of death; those in Child class B have a 10% risk of death; and, those in Child's class C have a 50% risk of death. Thus, a careful risk-benefit analysis is required when considering major surgery for patients with significant liver disease (Child's classes B and C).

TABLE 29–11

Child's-Pugh Classification

Parameter	Points		
	1	**2**	**3**
Albumin (g/dL)	>3.5	2.8–3.5	<3.5
Bilirubin (mg/dL)	<2	2–3	>3
PT (sec above normal)	<4	4–6	>6
Ascites	None	Mild	Moderate
Encephalopathy	None	Some	Severe

Class A = 5–6 points; Class B = 7–9 points; Class C = 10–15 points.

What is cirrhosis?

Cirrhosis, a leading cause of death and disability worldwide, is an irreversible fibrotic change to liver parenchyma that occurs after protracted liver injury from hepatitis B, hepatitis C, and heavy alcohol use. Less common causes of cirrhosis include primary biliary cirrhosis, hemachromatosis, autoimmune disease, α_1-antitrypsin deficiency, and drugs.

A major complication of cirrhosis is portal hypertension (high pressure in the portal venous system). Portal hypertension results in the development of esophageal varices, portal hypertensive gastropathy, and rectal varices. All of these manifestations of portal hypertension may result in life-threatening GI bleeding. About a third of patients with cirrhosis bleed from their varices within 2 years of discovery of the varices. More than two thirds of patients who have bled from varices will rebleed within 2 years. Mortality of acute variceal bleeding is between 20% and 50%.

▶ TREATMENT

What is the management of portal hypertension and variceal bleeding?

The primary treatment for acute variceal bleeding is endoscopic sclerotherapy and IV infusion of octreotide. If bleeding continues, a Sengstaken-Blakemore tube can be placed in the esophagus to tamponade bleeding varices. However, balloon tamponade is only a temporary measure and has the potential of severe complications of esophageal and gastric necrosis and perforation. After nonoperative control of acute variceal bleeding, noncardioselective betablockade with propranolol or nadolol can be used to reduce the risk of rebleeding (~30% chance of rebleed in 2 years), but long-term survival is variable.

If acute variceal bleeding is refractory to medical management, the patient should be considered for a portal-systemic shunt. The goal of shunt placement is to reduce the pressure in the portal system. A transjugular intrahepatic portal-systemic shunt (TIPS) can be placed by an interventional radiologist and is less invasive than a surgical shunt. Hepatic encephalopathy is a potential complication of TIPS, but this complication is usually medically treatable.

What are the indications for emergent surgical shunt placement?

The indications for emergent surgical shunt placement are failure of medical management including endoscopic sclerotherapy, pharmacotherapy, and TIPS. Elective shunt placement can be considered in a patient with adequate hepatic reserve who has failed multiple TIPS.

What is the difference between "selective," "nonselective," and "partial" shunts?

Surgical shunts can be classified into nonselective, selective, and partial types. Nonselective shunts decompress the whole portal venous system and are more easy to place but do not maintain hepatic perfusion. Selective and partial shunts are designed to maintain hepatic perfusion.

What are the indications for a nonselective shunt?

Indications for total, nonselective portal systemic shunts include acute Budd-Chiari syndrome (hepatic vein thrombosis or obstruction), uncontrollable variceal bleeding refractory to medical treatment modalities, and patients with colonic or stomal varices. In the end-to-side portacaval shunt (Fig. 29–9), the portal vein is divided and the proximal end anastomosed to the inferior vena cava. This shunt decompresses the portal system but does not decompress hepatic sinusoids, and thus ascites is not cured. In side-to-side total portal systemic shunts, an anastomosis is created between the portal vein (or one of its major tributaries) and the inferior vena cava (or one of its major tributaries). To be a total shunt, the connection has to be greater than 1 cm in diameter. Physiologically, TIPS is a side-to-side shunt. These shunts decompress the portal system as well as the hepatic sinusoidal venous beds, and thus there is alleviation of ascites. This type of shunt is the procedure of choice because it avoids the liver hilum and thus simplifies subsequent liver transplantation, if indicated. Because nonselective shunts do not preserve hepatic perfusion, hepatic encephalopathy can develop postoperatively.

When is it appropriate to use a selective or partial shunt?

Selective variceal decompression with a distal splenorenal shunt (DSRS) provides selective decompression of gastroesophageal varices. The DSRS is formed by anastomosing the distal end of the splenic vein to the left renal vein. The DSRS is effective in controlling variceal bleeding in patients with nonalcoholic cirrhosis. However, it worsens ascites and thus is contraindicated in patients with uncontrollable ascites.

Like selective shunts, partial shunts are designed to maintain hepatic perfusion. A partial shunt (e.g., Sarfeh shunt) is a small-diameter (<1 cm) interposition portacaval shunt using a polytetrafluoroethylene graft, with ligation of the coronary vein and collateral vessels. These shunts have rebleeding and survival rates comparable to nonselective shunts. They also have a lower rate of encephalopathy compared with nonselective shunts.

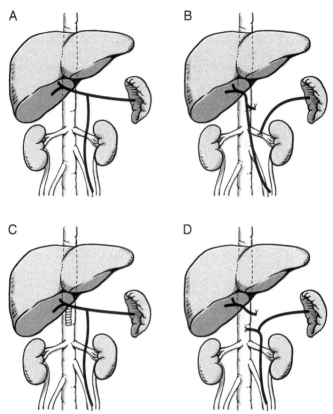

Figure 29–9. Surgical vascular shunts used in portal hypertension. *A,* Normal portal venous anatomy. *B,* Selective distal splenorenal shunt. *C,* Small bore side-to-side portacaval shunt (Sarfeh shunt). *D,* Nonselective end-to-side portacaval shunt.

LIVER TUMORS

▶ ETIOLOGY

What is the most common liver tumor?

The most common form of primary liver cancer is hepatocellular carcinoma (HCC). HCC, sometimes referred to as *hepatoma*, is one of the most common malignancies in the world, with a concentration in sub-Saharan Africa and Southeast Asia. The tumor is less common in America, Europe, and North Africa. The incidence of HCC is strongly linked to the prevalence of hepatitis B virus (HBV) infection, and there is strong epidemiologic and molecular biology evidence to support the causal relationship between HBV infection and the development of HCC. Diseases that are associated with chronic liver injury such as hemochromatosis, α_1-antitrypsin deficiency, and primary biliary cirrhosis are also associated with an increased risk of developing HCC. In the United States, HCC is rarely seen in patients younger than 60 years of age, whereas in the rest of the world it is frequently seen in individuals younger than 40 years of age.

What type of benign liver tumors are there?

The most common types of benign liver tumors are hemangiomas, focal nodular hyperplasia, and adenomas. Cavernous hemangiomas are the most common and occur most frequently in women in their 4th decade of life. If large enough, hemangiomas may create an arteriovenous shunt that eventually leads to high-output congestive heart failure as well as a consumptive coagulopathy. Hemangiomas usually present as an asymptomatic abdominal mass but may also cause abdominal pain if the tumor encroaches on adjacent organs. Hemangiomas may be evaluated with abdominal ultrasound, abdominal CT scan with IV contrast, MR imaging, isotope-tagged blood cell scans, or hepatic angiography. Percutaneous biopsy of hemangiomas is not safe because of the risk of major hemorrhage.

Indications for surgical resection of hemangiomas are local symptoms or systemic effects such as heart failure. Whereas small hemangiomas may be treated with local nonanatomic wedge resection, large hemangiomas require hepatic resection along anatomic planes.

Focal nodular hyperplasia may represent a response to injury rather than a true neoplasm. It is usually asymptomatic and discovered incidentally. A few patients present with a mass, abdominal discomfort, and, rarely, bleeding. It occurs in both men and women, usually in their 2nd to 5th decade of life. These tumors are found near the free edge of the liver and appear nodular and scarred. A wedge biopsy should be performed on these lesions to rule out malignancy. Whereas small lesions may be excised with a wedge resection, large ones should be left alone.

Hepatic adenomas are more common in women who take oral contraceptives (progesterones and estrogens). Oral contraceptive use also increases the risk for necrosis or rupture of the adenoma. About half of patients present with an asymptomatic abdominal mass found on physical exam or imaging study, and the other half present with abdominal pain. In cases of tumor rupture, patients may present in shock. Ultrasound, CT scan, and hepatic angiography are obtained to evaluate hepatic adenomas. Treatment of small and asymptomatic hepatic adenomas is controversial. Some advocate the cessation of oral contraceptives and watchful waiting. Others recommend surgical excision if the adenoma is persistent or if the woman desires to get pregnant. Large (>5 cm) and symptomatic tumors should be removed via a segmentectomy or lobectomy. Recurrence after resection is rare. The risk for transformation into HCC is also rare.

▶ EVALUATION

How do I evaluate a patient with suspected HCC?

The most common symptom of HCC is weight loss. Other symptoms and signs such as jaundice, weakness, dull and constant right upper quadrant or epigastric pain, hepatomegaly, palpable mass, or bloody ascites may also be present. Laboratory findings in patients with HCC may include an elevated serum alkaline phosphatase, an elevated bilirubin, positive hepatitis B or C virus serologic tests, or an elevated AFP level. Ultrasound is an inexpensive and accurate method of detecting HCC. A CT scan allows the exact determination of the location and dimensions of the tumor. Because most HCC tumors are supplied by the hepatic artery, hepatic artery angiography can accurately delineate the vascular anatomy of these tumors that may be useful information for the surgeon in selected cases. Metastatic work-up should be performed in all patients with potentially resectable disease or who are transplantation candidates and should include a CT scan of the chest, abdomen, and pelvis and nuclear medicine bone scan.

Can other tumors metastasize to the liver?

Metastatic neoplasms of the liver are much more common than primary liver cancer. Metastases confined to the liver are primarily seen in colorectal cancer. Most patients are asymptomatic but may present with weight loss, anorexia, fatigue, abdominal pain or mass, jaundice, and fever. Patients with carcinoid tumor metastatic to the liver have the carcinoid syndrome (intermittent flushing and diarrhea). Diagnosis of metastatic disease of the liver is with laboratory tests (LFTs, CEA, gamma-glutamyltransferase) and imaging with abdominal CT scan.

▶ TREATMENT

What is the treatment of HCC?

Untreated HCC portends a dismal prognosis. Median survival of untreated HCC is about 1.6 months. However, with surgical and nonsurgical treatment, survival at 5 years can be increased to 50%. Improvements in therapies have allowed long-term survival for those with minute HCC (<3 cm in diameter). Though surgical resection is the treatment modality that offers the greatest survival rate, other modalities are available for those with advanced disease, poor liver reserve, or poor operative risk. These include transcatheter arterial embolization, cryoablation, radiofrequency ablation, and percutaneous ethanol injection.

HCC is amenable to resection if the remaining hepatic mass has adequate functional reserve, if the resection is technically feasible, and if there is no evidence of extrahepatic spread. Indications for orthotopic liver transplantation in the HCC patient vary from center to center but generally include unresectable tumors (due to inadequate functional reserve or technical feasibility of resection) less than 5 cm, minimal intrahepatic tumor dissemination, and absence of extrahepatic spread.

Partial hepatic resection for HCC can be classified as anatomic or nonanatomic. The boundaries of anatomic resections are determined by the segmental blood supply of the liver. Nonanatomic resections disregard the segmental anatomy of the liver and are mostly reserved for small, peripheral lesions.

Adequate hepatic reserve is essential for patients undergoing partial hepatic resection for HCC. The Child's-Pugh classification provides a quick method of estimating the preoperative hepatic reserve and risk of perioperative morbidity of these patients.

What are indications for surgical resection of colorectal cancer metastases?

Indications for surgical resection of colorectal cancer metastases to the liver are fewer than four tumors, no extrahepatic disease, and ability to obtain a 1-cm margin. Anatomic resection more commonly provides adequate margins, but nonanatomic wedge resections are possible with small peripheral metastases.

More than three quarters of patients have extrahepatic recurrence after resection of colorectal cancer liver metastases. Patients who underwent resection of liver metastases with adequate margins have only a small chance of recurrence in the liver. Patients with unresectable liver metastases may undergo palliative hepatic artery chemotherapy infusion, cryoablation, chemoembolization, or radiotherapy.

LIVER INFECTIONS

What causes a hepatic abscess?

Hepatic abscesses may be bacterial, parasitic (usually amebic), or fungal. With the advent of antibiotic therapy, bacterial or pyogenic abscesses have become rare. Currently, bacterial or pyogenic abscesses usually result from a direct extension of a bacterial infection from adjacent organs, such as the gallbladder, or hematogenous spread via the portal vein from appendicitis, or diverticulitis, or via the hepatic artery from distant sources such as a pneumonia or bacterial endocarditis. Organisms in pyogenic hepatic abscesses are usually of enteric origin (e.g., *E. coli*, *Klebsiella pneumoniae*, *Bacteroides,* and enterococci). The mortality of hepatic abscesses is 15%. Mortality is higher in patients with coexistent malignancy or advanced infection.

Patients with bacterial abscesses have high fever, malaise, rigors, jaundice, epigastric or right upper quadrant pain, and referred pain to the right shoulder. Marked leukocytosis, anemia, and elevated alkaline phosphatase are usually present. Abdominal ultrasound and abdominal CT scan are used to evaluate hepatic abscesses. Bacterial abscesses are multiple in about half of cases. Treatment of bacterial abscesses includes IV antibiotics to cover enteric gram-negative and anaerobic organisms as well as percutaneous or surgical drainage.

How do amebic liver abscesses differ?

Patients with amebic abscesses (caused by *Entamoeba histolytica*) have a presentation similar to those with bacterial abscesses, except that the onset is more gradual. Amebic abscesses are usually solitary. Diagnosis of amebic abscesses is by serologic tests and imaging. Treatment of amebic abscesses is with metronidazole. Complications of bacterial and amebic abscesses include intrahepatic spread of the infection, systemic sepsis, and abscess rupture. Failure of initial treatment may indicate bacterial superinfection of amebic abscesses.

What is an echinococcal disease of the liver?

Echinococcus granulosus and *Echinococcus multilocularis* are tapeworms that can cause hydatid disease of the liver, which is rare in North America. The dog is the definitive host and humans are intermediate hosts. Patients acquire *Echinococcus* eggs by ingesting contaminated food. The egg is digested in the duodenum and yields an embryo that travels to the liver via the portal venous system. Hydatid cysts grow slowly and cause symptoms when they become large or cause biliary obstruction or portal hypertension. Cysts may spontaneously rupture, causing abdominal pain and anaphylaxis. Diagnosis is by serologic testing and imaging with abdominal ultrasound and CT scan. Treatment is with preoperative albendazole followed by operative cyst drainage. Operative cyst drainage is performed with care to prevent dissemination of the organism that leads to peritoneal seeding and anaphylaxis.

K E Y   P O I N T S

▶ The Child's-Pugh classification is a measure of hepatic reserve. It may be used to evaluate preoperative patients with a history of liver disease or patients scheduled for liver resection.

▶ Patients with advanced liver disease (Child's classes B and C) are at increased risk for liver-related perioperative complications.

continued

▶ The primary treatment for bleeding esophageal varices caused by portal hypertension is medical: endoscopic sclerotherapy, octreotide infusion, and balloon tamponade (if necessary).

▶ If available, TIPS placement should be considered in patients with intractable variceal bleeding.

▶ HCC is a common solid malignancy worldwide, especially in areas where HBV is endemic.

▶ Metastatic disease of the liver is more common than primary liver cancer.

▶ Bacterial hepatic abscesses are usually caused by enteric organisms.

CASE 29–17. A 50-year-old Asian man with a history of hepatitis B complains of malaise, weight loss, and abdominal pain. His physical exam is unremarkable; it is pertinently negative for stigmata of chronic liver disease. Laboratory tests are significant for mildly elevated liver transaminase levels, a markedly elevated AFP, and a normal CEA.

    A. What is the differential diagnosis of this patient's complaints?
    B. What imaging tests would aid in the diagnosis?
    C. What are the treatment options?

CASE 29–18. A 30-year-old woman taking oral contraceptives complains of right upper quadrant pain. She is otherwise in good health and has no history of liver disease or viral hepatitis and no recent travel history. She denies weight loss, malaise, or anorexia. Her physical exam is positive for right upper quadrant tenderness and no mass. She has normal LFTs and mild leukocytosis. Right upper quadrant ultrasound reveals findings consistent with acute cholecystitis. There is also a 2-cm lesion seen in the free edge of the right lobe of the liver.

    A. What is the differential diagnosis of this liver lesion?
    B. What should be the management of this lesion?

CASE 29–19. A 14-year-old boy presents with a 1-week history of right lower quadrant pain, high fevers, sweats, and malaise. He has marked leukocytosis, elevated LFTs, and a CT scan that shows perforated appendicitis and multiple small lesions in the liver.

    A. What most likely represents the liver lesions?
    B. What is the management of these lesions?

PANCREATIC DISORDERS

PANCREATIC INFLAMMATORY DISORDERS

▶ ETIOLOGY

What is pancreatitis?

Pancreatitis is an inflammatory process of the exocrine pancreas. The inflammation can be triggered by different noxious stimuli and can express itself in a variety of clinical forms, beginning with acute versus chronic. The more common acute form has been described as a "burn" of the retroperitoneum. A combination of phenomena generates cellular damage and triggers an inflammatory process that affects the gland and peripancreatic tissues. These phenomena include activation of digestive enzymes within the pancreatic acinar cells (usually focal, less commonly diffuse) and/or the leakage of pancreatic juice into the peripancreatic area through a ductal disruption (usually from a side branch). In the acute form the gland returns to its normal state, but in the chronic form permanent fibrotic changes are seen.

What triggers inflammation of the pancreas?

Many risk factors have been associated, indirectly or directly, with pancreatic inflammation. Table 29–12 lists those implicated in the development of pancreatitis. In a few cases, a risk factor cannot be identified (i.e., idiopathic pancreatitis). With new imaging modalities many cases of idiopathic pancreatitis have been ultimately shown to be caused by intraductal pancreatic neoplasms.

    The most common etiology is cholelithiasis, followed by alcohol abuse. The passage of stones through the ampulla of Vater has been clearly identified with the development of acute pancreatitis. Small stones and gravel or sludge are most commonly implicated.

TABLE 29–12

Risk Factors for Pancreatitis
Gallstones
Alcohol abuse
Hyperlipidemia
Pancreas divisum
Papillary stenosis
Neoplasms
Drugs
Hypercalcemia
Operative intervention
Burns
Cardiopulmonary bypass
Scorpion venom
Viral infections
Endoscopic retrograde pancreatography

Alcoholic pancreatitis is usually seen after many years of heavy drinking, although it can present after isolated episodes of heavy alcohol abuse. The mechanism of damage associated with alcohol abuse is not clearly identified, but recently it has been discovered that these patients may have a genetic disposition to pancreatitis if they drink alcohol and smoke tobacco.

What is the difference between acute and chronic pancreatitis?

Acute and chronic pancreatitis are two different disease processes involving the same basic mechanism of inflammation of the acinar cells. A useful analogy to understand the difference between these two processes is that of forest fires. Crown fires are those that spread rapidly, burning the top of trees and shrubs. They can be dramatic and extensive but are short lived and leave behind a forest that can recover. Ground fires, on the other hand, appear following long periods of drought and burn the dried organic deposits below the surface with little, if any, flame. They can burn for long periods, killing the root structure of the forest and permanently scarring the land. Acute pancreatitis is like a crown fire, dramatic and devastating at times; it is usually short lived, allowing in most instances a full recovery with no permanent damage of the pancreatic structure. Chronic pancreatitis is a more insidious and long-lived process that destroys the glandular structure of the pancreas, permanently scarring the gland and, at times, the surrounding tissue.

Acute pancreatitis is characterized by the systemic inflammatory response that is triggered with the process, taking a severe and devastating form in 10% to 15% of cases. Chronic pancreatitis is characterized by scarring of the pancreas after symptomatic relapsing pancreatitis or subclinical smoldering pancreatitis.

How does acute pancreatitis present?

Typically patients give a history of sudden onset of moderate to severe abdominal pain followed by nausea and vomiting, frequently associated with a recent meal. Severe, continuous burning or stabbing pain in the epigastrium, radiating through to the back, is characteristic. Patients present with varying degrees of systemic compromise mainly related to fluid third spacing into the retroperitoneum.

They can exhibit tachycardia, hypotension, oliguria, or acute hypoxemia. Abdominal exam is characterized by epigastric or diffuse bilateral upper quadrant tenderness, distention, and decreased or absent bowel sounds. Tenderness can be mild to severe, on occasions presenting as an acute abdomen. Rarely, dramatic signs such as periumbilical or flank ecchymosis (Cullen's or Grey Turner's signs) are present. Associated signs of biliary tract disease, such as jaundice or cholangitis, can also be present.

How will chronic pancreatitis present?

The chronic form of the disease is characterized by progressive, slow destruction and fibrosis of the pancreas due to persistent or repeated insults. It usually presents as recurrent attacks of acute pancreatitis of varying severity, mixed with asymptomatic periods. Weight loss and malnutrition may occur. Asymptomatic periods are initially common and can be of months or years but will progressively shorten. Eventually, continuous pain and exocrine insufficiency ensue. After 5 or 6 years of disease, insulin deficiency may be present. At times the initial presentation is in the late stage of the disease with exocrine insufficiency and malabsorption, without abdominal pain, and with or without diabetes. Chronic pancreatitis can also initially present with local complications, such as pseudocyst or biliary and/or duodenal obstruction simulating a pancreatic head neoplasm. In most patients chronic pancreatitis is related to alcohol addiction, so addictive personalities will be encountered that need to be addressed.

▶ EVALUATION

How is acute pancreatitis diagnosed?

No diagnostic test has sufficient sensitivity or specificity in the diagnosis of pancreatitis. A combination of the clinical picture, identification of risk factors, laboratory data, and imaging studies gives the necessary clues to identify this disease.

The most frequent laboratory abnormality is an elevated serum amylase or lipase level. Their absolute value in plasma has no correlation with the severity of the attack. Serum elevations of lipase persist longer than amylase. Associated laboratory abnormalities may include leukocytosis, elevated LFTs (with an obstructive pattern), and evidence of hemoconcentration. Electrolyte abnormalities may include metabolic acidosis and hypocalcemia.

Plain radiographs can show indirect signs of retroperitoneal inflammation, such as elevated diaphragms and poor inspiration, or localized ileus due to peripancreatic irritation of the gut (a sentinel loop or a colon cut-off sign). Underlying chronic pancreatitis may be associated with calcifications in the area of the pancreas.

Abdominal ultrasound can identify gallstone disease and may show inflammation of the pancreas. CT scan can give a clear picture of the pancreatic inflammation, although this is rarely necessary to establish the diagnosis. CT is important to grade the severity of pancreatitis.

In certain instances, the diagnosis is established at the time of abdominal exploration. Swelling and inflammation within the lesser sac are evident, together with intraperitoneal foci of fat saponification characteristic of enzymatic activation and fat digestion.

What is the clinical course of acute pancreatitis?

In most instances acute pancreatitis resolves within 24 to 72 hours after onset. In 10% to 20% of cases it does not improve, and this predicts a severe course. Full-blown systemic inflammatory response syndrome (SIRS) with subsequent development of multisystem organ failure (MSOF) occurs. Characteristically, respiratory failure ensues first, together with hemodynamic compromise. Sequential organ system failures can follow. Another form of severe disease appears in some patients who present with minimal systemic compromise but persistent abdominal pain and failure to thrive that can persist for days or weeks. The severest form of this disease is associated with the development of necrosis of the gland and/or peripancreatic tissue.

The clinical course of severe pancreatitis has an early phase that is dominated by the manifestations of SIRS. Early morbidity and mortality are related to this process. The late phase of the disease is characterized by septic complications that ensue in the debilitated individual. Local complications associated with retroperitoneal inflammation or necrosis characterize this phase. Infection of the necrotic tissue is associated with increased mortality. This phase may persist for several weeks.

Disruption of the pancreatic ductal system with ongoing leak of activated pancreatic enzymes is implicated as a central event in the evolution of severe pancreatitis. When sought, disruption can be demonstrated in two thirds of patients with severe pancreatitis.

Can the severity of pancreatitis be predicted?

Acute pancreatitis is a complex and multifactorial process that is difficult to predict. However, several scoring systems have been developed to estimate the clinical course on diagnosis. These scoring systems have a clear value in the comparison of management strategies. They can also raise suspicion regarding the need for more intensive monitoring and care. The most common scoring system is Ranson's criteria (Table 29–13). Image scoring systems, such as the CT severity index (Table 29–14), can give good initial indication of severity of disease and predict morbidity, need for surgery, the presence of a ductal leak, and mortality. Any value greater than 6 is associated with a long hospital stay, higher mortality, and the presence of a pancreatic ductal disruption.

What complications can ensue from acute pancreatitis?

Complications can be classified into early and late. In the early phase, consequences of SIRS and MSOF prevail. In the later phase of the disease both systemic and local complications can be found. Bacterial or fungal superinfection of necrotic tissue has the strongest association with mortality.

Pancreatic ductal disruption, probably occurring early, is responsible for most fluid collections. After a few weeks these become walled off and form pseudocysts or decompress into other organs, such as the colon or bile duct, forming an internal pancreatic fistula. If symptomatic fluid collections are percutaneously drained and not allowed to mature into a pseudocyst, a persistent ductal disruption can lead to an external pancreatic fistula.

TABLE 29–13
Ranson's Prognostic Signs

At Diagnosis
Age > 55 years
WBC > 16,000/mm^3
Blood glucose > 200 mg/dL
LDH > 350 IU/dL
AST > 250 IU/dL

During the Initial 48 Hours
Hematocrit fall > 10%
Blood urea nitrogen increase > 8 mg/dL
Serum Ca^{2+} < 8 mg/dL
Pao_2 < 60 mm Hg
Base deficit > 4 mEq/L
Fluid sequestration > 6000 mL

AST, aspartate aminotransferase; LDH, lactate dehydrogenase; WBC, white blood cell.

TABLE 29-14

Computed Tomography Severity Index

	Points
Image	
Normal pancreas	0
Gland enlargement	1
Peripancreatic inflammation	2
Single fluid collection	3
Multiple fluid collections	4
Presence of Necrosis	
<30%	2
30–50%	4
>50%	6
Total	*10*

When extensive pancreatic necrosis is present, exocrine insufficiency with malabsorption can ensue. The same can happen with insulin production, causing diabetes mellitus. Extrapancreatic local complications can include erosions into surrounding hollow viscous organs such as transverse colon, duodenum, small bowel, or bile duct. These erosions can affect neighboring arteries and result in a pseudoaneurysm. Thrombosis or occlusion (by extrinsic compression) of the splenic, superior mesenteric, or portal veins can occur in response to the inflammation. Biliary or duodenal obstruction due to edema and inflammation or scarring can also occur.

How is chronic pancreatitis diagnosed?

A history of recurrent abdominal pain is characteristic in a patient with exocrine and endocrine pancreatic insufficiency. The patient may not have steatorrhea, yet stool fat studies are abnormal and there is an inability to gain weight. Physical exam may include some abdominal tenderness but is usually unrevealing. Signs of malnutrition may be present. An abdominal mass is uncommon unless a pseudocyst is present. Few or no laboratory abnormalities can be present. During acute attacks amylase and lipase may be only minimally elevated.

Imaging studies can demonstrate typical morphologic changes to the gland. Scattered parenchymal calcifications and pancreatic ductal dilation are characteristic features. Although not the most frequent finding, the appearance of pancreatic ductal "chain of lakes" is classically described. These changes can be evident on plain films, CT scan, or retrograde pancreatography. If all of these studies are normal, the patient does not have chronic pancreatitis and the ever-present abdominal pain is from some other etiology, such as chronic peptic ulcer disease or IBD. On occasion, the etiology is factitious.

▶ TREATMENT

What is the management of acute pancreatitis?

The initial management of acute pancreatitis involves two main strategies: (1) decrease pancreatic exocrine stimulation through bowel rest, and (2) provide necessary supportive care, mainly through aggressive fluid resuscitation. These measures suffice for most attacks of acute pancreatitis. Definitive treatment of associated risk factors, such as gallstones, should be performed during the same hospitalization to prevent recurrent attacks.

With severe disease, intensive monitoring is warranted. Pancreatic necrosis and fluid collections should be sought. It is at this stage that information derived from an abdominal CT scan is important. An aggressive but minimally invasive approach should guide the initial management of severe pancreatitis. All necessary supportive care should be undertaken. Symptomatic drainable fluid collections need to be addressed, usually through a percutaneous approach. This provides significant symptomatic relief and addresses ongoing ductal leaks. Broad-spectrum antibiotic treatment has been found to decrease septic complications in the later phase of the disease. An operative approach toward retroperitoneal necrosis may be necessary in the absence of significant response to less invasive measures. Surgical débridement is indicated when infected necrosis is demonstrated. Necrosectomy is rarely necessary in the initial phase of the disease but can prove life-saving later in the course.

Which are the management strategies for chronic pancreatitis?

The most common problem is abdominal pain, which can be difficult to control, and a team approach is required. Medical management of the exocrine and endocrine insufficiency is combined with modifications of risk factor behaviors, particularly limiting alcohol use. The patient with gallstones should undergo cholecystectomy. Direct interventions are dictated by pancreatic ductal anatomy and aimed at relieving abdominal pain. Main pancreatic duct strictures or stones are mandatory before using endoscopic approaches, such as stenting. When endoscopic approaches fail, surgical treatment may be required to deal with obstructed or distorted ducts through resection or a drainage procedure.

K E Y   P O I N T S

▶ Acute pancreatitis is an inflammatory process involving
  first the pancreas and then the peripancreatic tissue in
  the lesser sac or retroperitoneum. The inflammation
  triggers a systemic inflammatory response.

▶ The most frequent cases of acute pancreatitis are alcohol
  abuse and choledocholithiasis.

▶ When severe, acute pancreatitis has an early phase
  dominated by SIRS and a late phase when septic and
  local complications predominate.

▶ Treatment of acute pancreatitis is directed to the
  supportive management of SIRS and an early approach
  to pancreatic ductal disruptions that perpetuate that
  inflammation.

▶ Chronic pancreatitis is a relentlessly progressive and
  destructive inflammatory process that primarily affects
  the acinar cells and then the ductal system.

▶ Symptoms of chronic pancreatitis include frequent,
  recurrent, severe abdominal pain, malnutrition, glucose
  intolerance, and steatorrhea.

▶ Mixed with the progressive destruction of the gland,
  smoldering inflammation occurs.

▶ Treatment of chronic pancreatitis is designed to identify
  the process, determine the ductal anatomy, and then
  design therapy. A multidisciplinary approach is required.

CASE 29–20. A 55-year-old man who is a chronic
alcoholic complains of steady abdominal pain. He gives a
history of multiple prior bouts of acute pancreatitis in the
past. He states that he stopped drinking alcohol 1 year
earlier, but this did not affect the pain. He also has lost 25 lb
over the last year.

  A. What history is important to obtain?
  B. What is the differential diagnosis?
  C. What steps are involved in the evaluation of this patient?

PANCREATIC DUCTAL DISRUPTIONS

▶ ETIOLOGY

What is pancreatic ductal disruption?

This entity can be a consequence of pancreatitis, trauma, or intervention. At times it can present with no recognizable history of pancreatic disease.

▶ EVALUATION

How do pancreatic disuptions present?

Disruptions can take different clinical forms, but all represent the same basic disease process. Disruption of the ductal system with leak of pancreatic juice can produce internal or external pancreatic fistulas. Internal pancreatic fistulas are most commonly contained within the retroperitoneum and walled off, forming pancreatic pseudocysts. At times a free leak into the peritoneal cavity can manifest as pancreatic ascites. Posterior disruptions can track through the diaphragmatic hiatus into the mediastinum or rupture into the pleural space, presenting as pancreatic pleural effusion. Sometimes erosion into the GI tract forms a pancreaticoenteric fistula. After percutaneous interventions, ductal leaks can form external pancreatic fistulas.

▶ TREATMENT

How are pancreatic ductal disruptions managed?

The successful management of this entity begins with a decision regarding the need for intervention. An incidental finding of a pseudocyst may not warrant intervention in the absence of symptoms. When an asymptomatic pseudocyst is the initial presentation, in the absence of a clear history of pancreatitis or trauma, it is most important to rule out a cystic neoplasm of the pancreas.

The basic principles of fistula management should guide the therapy: to decrease fistula output the physician must eliminate downstream obstruction, ensure adequate drainage of the area, control infection, and provide adequate nutrition.

When pancreatic ductal disruptions are symptomatic, their management should be guided by the ductal anatomy. ERCP is the single most important study to determine the ductal anatomy and then the most appropriate treatment.

A normal main pancreatic duct without demonstrable leak or distal obstruction indicates a high chance of spontaneous resolution or response to minimal intervention such as percutaneous drainage. A demonstrable side leak and/or distal ductal stricture likely responds to a combination of percutaneous drainage and decompressing the pancreatic duct with transampullary stenting. When complete disruption or obstruction of the duct is found, a "disconnected-duct syndrome" is present, and surgical intervention, when possible, is the best treatment strategy. Usually the latter is best achieved through resection of the involved segment of duct or anastomosis to the bowel to provide adequate drainage of the disconnected segment.

CONGENITAL ANOMALIES

What are some clinically important congenital anomalies of the pancreas?

Pancreas Divisum

Pancreas divisum, the most common anomaly, is found in about 5% of normal people. The incidence is higher in patients with idiopathic pancreatitis. It may be a cause of pancreatitis. The divisum portion is derived from the lack of complete fusion of the ducts that drain the ventral and dorsal pancreatic buds. The bulk of pancreatic secretions from the tail, body, and part of the head reaches the duodenum only through the duct of Santorini draining through the minor papilla.

Annular Pancreas

This anomaly is a consequence of abnormal rotation of the ventral pancreatic bud, leaving pancreatic tissue encircling the duodenum. Symptoms are those of duodenal obstruction in infancy or, rarely, in adulthood.

Ectopic Pancreas

These clusters of exocrine tissue can be found in the stomach or duodenum as a submucosal mass, in a Meckel's diverticulum, or in other areas of the GI tract. They are usually incidental findings.

PANCREATIC TUMORS

Neoplastic degeneration of the pancreas occurs most frequently at the level of the ductular epithelium. Next in frequency are neoplasms that originate in the islet cells as endocrine tumors, followed by the heterogeneous group of cystic tumors. Lymphoma can present as an isolated mass in or around the pancreas.

▶ ETIOLOGY

What is ductal adenocarcinoma of the pancreas?

A common malignancy, it represents the eighth most common cancer and the fifth leading cause of cancer death in the United States. Until recently, only 5% of patients diagnosed with this tumor survived 5 years.

No conclusive causative agent has been found. Cigarette smoking has been found to be a significant risk factor. Weaker associations have been identified with the consumption of coffee and alcohol and exposure to organic solvents and petroleum products. Several hereditary disorders predispose to this tumor.

Genetic anomalies associated with these tumors include activation of *KRAS* oncogene, activation of *CERBB2* protooncogene, and/or deletion of *TP53* tumor suppressor gene. The latter is particularly associated with invasive cancer.

No adequate screening tools have been developed.

What are the types of cystic neoplasms of the pancreas?

Three main types of cystic neoplasms are recognized as primary tumors in the pancreas.

Serous Cystadenomas

These are benign tumors with anecdotal reports of malignant degeneration. Frequently large at presentation, they are most commonly found in the area of the head and have a characteristic "honeycomb" appearance with cysts of less than 2 cm. This, together with the less frequent "starburst" appearance with a centrally located calcified scar, is pathognomonic of these tumors. They generally have an indolent course. Resection is indicated when they are symptomatic or rapidly enlarging. Asymptomatic lesions can be closely followed. Biopsy samples only a small portion of the tumor and is risky. If the patient is in good health and there is diagnostic doubt, the lesion is best removed.

Mucinous Cystic Neoplasms

More common in the body and tail of the gland, they also tend to be large at presentation. The appearance differs from serous tumors in that the cysts tend to be larger than 2 cm. They can present as a single macro cyst. The presence of papillary fronds, septa, or eccentric solid components of the wall is pathognomonic. These tumors have a significant malignant potential (~50%). Resection should be the treatment, together with detailed histopathologic analysis, to differentiate the more common and benign mucinous cystadenoma from the aggressive cystadenocarcinoma.

Intraductal Papillary Mucinous Tumor of the Pancreas (IPMT)

IPMTs are mucin-producing tumors that are derived from, and therefore connected to, the pancreatic ductal system. The latter is confirmed during ERCP or intraoperative pancreatography. They are increasingly diagnosed and represent a field defect of neoplastic degeneration of the ductal system. IPMTs are usually symptomatic and frequently present as idiopathic pancreatitis of the elderly with a dilated side branch or main pancreatic duct. They have a malignant potential, with 30% to 40% of cases having an invasive component at the time of diagnosis. IPMTs require resection for adequate treatment.

What are pancreatic endocrine tumors?

These uncommon tumors arise from the islet cells of the pancreas. Most frequently they are nonfunctional, but some can produce gut hormones that can cause specific symptoms (Table 29–15). The diagnosis is usually established through the identification of the clinical syndrome or the presence of a pancreatic mass. In general these tumors have a more indolent course than adenocarcinomas, and long-term survival can be seen even with hepatic metastasis.

What are the characteristics of adenocarcinoma of the pancreas?

About 70% of these tumors arise in the head, neck, and uncinate process, 20% in the body, and 10% in the tail of the gland. Staging is based on the American Joint Committee on Cancer (Table 29–16). The tumor frequently involves neighboring structures by direct extension. In general fewer than 20% of patients have disease confined just to the pancreas, 40% have locally advanced disease, and 40% have distant metastasis.

▶ EVALUATION

How is adenocarcinoma of the pancreas diagnosed?

The most frequent presenting signs and symptoms are weight loss, pain, anorexia, and jaundice. A search for pancreatic malignancy should be sought in the following scenario: nonobese patient, older than 40 years of age, with the recent onset of diabetes mellitus, painless jaundice, or a palpable gallbladder (Courvoisier's sign).

TABLE 29-15

Characteristics of Pancreatic Endocrine Tumors

Tumor: Hormone	Clinical Syndrome	Percentage Malignant
Gastrinoma: gastrin	Peptic ulcers, diarrhea	60–90
Insulinoma: insulin	Hypoglycemia	10–15
VIPoma: vasoactive intestinal peptide	Watery diarrhea, hypokalemia	60–80
Glucagonoma: glucagon	Hyperglycemia, dermatitis	60–70
"PPoma": pancreatic polypeptide	None	>60
Somatostatinoma: somatostatin	Hyperglycemia, steatorrhea, gallstones	90
Nonfunctioning	None	>60

Adapted from Feig BW, Berger DH, Fuhrman GM (eds): The MD Anderson Surgical Oncology Handbook, 2nd ed. Philadelphia, Lippincott Williams & Wilkins, 1999.

Thin-sectioned dual-helical CT scanning with IV contrast timed to the arterial and venous phases provides the most complete information for diagnosis and preoperative staging. Almost all pancreatic cancers are hypodense and can be missed if relying on a CT scan's portal venous phase only. Additional tools that aid in the diagnosis are ERCP and endoscopic ultrasound. Laparoscopy with intraoperative ultrasound can aid in the diagnosis and determination of resectability.

A preoperative tissue confirmation of malignant disease is not necessary to proceed to resection if the following criteria are met: a dilated bile and pancreatic duct, a well-defined hypodense mass in the pancreas, and no CT evidence of stage IVa or IVb disease. Seeking a preoperative tissue diagnosis places the patient at risk for complications of biopsy, offers little help in the management, and potentially delays treatment for resectable disease. However, a tissue diagnosis is mandatory when resection is not an initial viable option and before primary chemotherapy is begun.

▶ TREATMENT

How is adenocarcinoma of the pancreas treated?

Curative resection gives the best chance for long-term survival. Surgical treatment is dictated by the location of the tumor. For lesions in the head of the gland (most common), a pancreaticoduodenectomy (Whipple procedure) is required. Distal pancreatectomy, including splenectomy, is required for lesions in the body or tail of the pancreas. The latter operation is less effective, since tumors in the body or tail tend to be more advanced by the time

TABLE 29-16

AJCC TNM Staging System for Pancreatic Cancer

Primary Tumor (T)

TX	Primary tumor cannot be assessed
T0	No evidence of primary tumor
Tis	Carcinoma *in situ**
T1	Tumor limited to the pancrease, 2 cm or less in greatest dimension
T2	Tumor limited to the pancreas, more than 2 cm in greatest dimension
T3	Tumor extends beyond the pancreas but without involvement of the celiac axis or the superior mesenteric artery
T4	Tumor involves the celiac axis or the superior mesenteric artery (unresectable primary tumor)

Regional Lymph Nodes (N)

NX	Regional lymph nodes cannot be assessed
N0	No regional lymph node metastasis
N1	Regional lymph node metastasis

Distant Metastasis (M)

MX	Distant metastasis cannot be assessed
M0	No distant metastasis
M1	Distant metastasis

*This also includes the "PanInIII" classification

Stage Grouping

Stage	T	N	M
Stage 0	Tis	N0	M0
Stage IA	T1	N0	M0
Stage IB	T2	N0	M0
Stage IIA	T3	N0	M0
Stage IIB	T1	N1	M0
	T2	N1	M0
	T3	N1	M0
Stage III	T4	Any N	M0
Stage IV	Any T	Any N	M1

Used with the permission of the American Joint Committee on Cancer (AJCC), Chicago, Illinois. The original source for this material is the *AJCC Cancer Staging Manual, Sixth Edition* (2002) published by Springer-Verlag New York, www.springer-ny.com.

they are diagnosed. Extended resections including surrounding anatomic structures are still controversial and have not clearly demonstrated a benefit.

The Whipple procedure removes the head of the pancreas together with the duodenal loop and distal common bile duct. The standard resection includes the gastric antrum. A pylorus-preserving variant differs in that the resection is at the level of the first portion of the duodenum, leaving the pylorus and duodenal bulb behind. Reconstruction is performed sequentially through a pancreatic, biliary, and gastric (or duodenal) anastomosis usually to the jejunum. Mortality from pancreatic resections has been reduced to almost zero. Mortality rates, morbidity, and length of stay are steadily improving, as increasing volumes of these procedures are done at each hospital. The most common complication following pancreatic resection is pancreatic anastomotic leak with pancreatic fistula. Other complications are those common to all major surgical procedures.

Exciting adjuvant protocols are being developed for use in the postoperative period and also as primary nonsurgical treatment of advanced disease. Adjuvant treatment includes radiation therapy and radiosensitizing chemotherapy agents (most frequently 5-fluorouracil). Primary treatment for nonresectable disease is currently based on gemcitabine combination drug protocols.

The 5-year survival rate for patients resected with curative intention is now higher than 25% with the newer adjuvant protocols.

How is unresectable or recurrent adenocarcinoma of the pancreas treated?

Common complications of the advanced form of the disease are biliary and/or gastric outlet obstruction and disabling pancreatic pain. Palliation most commonly begins with an endoscopically placed biliary stent to relieve jaundice and allow liver function to return to normal. If endotherapy is not possible, a percutaneous transhepatic biliary tube is placed through the tumor obstruction into the duodenum. Because of new technology, a patient rarely requires operation for just biliary obstruction. Surgical bypass for biliary and/or duodenal obstruction is usually done when the patient is explored with the intent to resect and the disease is found to be unresectable. In patients with unrelenting pain that is no longer controlled by oral narcotics, a celiac alcohol block under fluoroscopic control is highly effective. The unrelenting pain is due to tumor invasion of the celiac axis.

K E Y   P O I N T S

▶ Advanced adenocarcinoma of the pancreas has an extremely poor prognosis. Keys to survival include early diagnosis and aggressive management.

▶ About 70% of adenocarcinomas of the pancreas occur in the head, neck, and uncinate process.

▶ Tumors of the pancreas can mimic other clinical entities such as pancreatitis or pseudocysts. A high index of suspicion and an aggressive diagnostic approach are the keys to any chance of successful prolongation of life with treatment.

▶ Surgical excision is the only route to potential long-term survival.

PEPTIC ULCER DISEASE

For 100 years physicians have been treating peptic ulcer disease without a clear understanding of its etiology. Despite advances in the understanding of gastric physiology, it remains unclear why the upper GI tract in general and the stomach and duodenum in particular are not digested in the presence of pepsin and hydrochloric acid. During the past 30 years major advances in clinical pharmacology, endoscopy, nuclear medicine, and GI research have altered the patterns of diagnosis and treatment of peptic ulcer disease. Unfortunately, healed ulcers recur at a high rate, and newer anti-inflammatory drugs add to the total pool of peptic ulcer disease complications.

▶ ETIOLOGY

What factors influence the development of peptic ulcer disease?

It has often been said that peptic ulcer disease is an entity of the 20th century. By the early 1950s, approximately 5% of all men may have been affected by gastric or duodenal ulceration. Thereafter, there was a dramatic decrease in the incidence of ulcer disease to a low point at approximately the time the histamine H_2 receptor antagonist was discovered. The cause of this decrease is unknown, but it may have been associated with alterations in lifestyle, more accurate diagnostic tests, or perhaps the more frequent use of over-the-counter antacid preparations. Although the etiology of peptic ulcer disease is still unclear, there are at least five major factors that influence its development: (1) acid secretion, (2) pepsin, (3) nonsteroidal anti-inflammatory drugs (NSAIDs), (4) massive acid hypersecretion in Zollinger-Ellison syndrome, and (5) *Helicobacter pylori*.

Experiential and clinical studies of gastric acid secretion have played a major role in evaluating the etiology of peptic ulcer disease. Patients with either duodenal or prepyloric ulcerations are considered gastric acid hypersecreters, whereas patients with pure gastric ulcers have either decreased or normal gastric acid. Although acid is always present in gastric ulceration, the etiology of this disease may rely more on a breakdown of defense mechanisms, the quality of gastric mucus, or perhaps a genetic predisposition for this disease.

What is stress gastritis?

This entity, also known as *hemorrhagic gastritis*, was the scourge of intensive care units in years past but is now rarely seen. The response of the gastric mucosa to unusual stress, such as sepsis, trauma, burns, or prolonged intensive care unit stay, is to initiate a hemorrhagic and ulcerative reaction, usually involving the entire stomach. This results in slow but ongoing hemorrhage and often the demise of the patient. Early results with ongoing gastric lavage and angiographic infusion of vasopressin were occasionally successful, but most patients underwent near-total or total gastrectomy. Unfortunately the combination of emergency surgery and the comorbidity of the primary illness resulted in a high mortality. In the 1960s and early 1970s, empirical observations demonstrated that hourly antacids via the nasogastric tube resulted in complete gastric acid neutralization and caused a dramatic decrease in the incidence of hemorrhagic gastritis. Experimental studies demonstrated that neutralization of acid essentially eliminated back-diffusion of hydrogen ions, which was the culprit in stress gastritis. At the present time the use of H_2 receptor (H_2R) antagonists and proton pump inhibitor (PPI) acid suppression has eliminated hemorrhagic gastritis in intensive care patients. Severely ill or traumatized patients should have their gastric pH monitored and maintained above 6.

How frequently is *H. pylori* associated with peptic ulcer disease?

A recent and exciting discovery is the association between the bacterium *H. pylori* and chronic gastritis, duodenal ulcer, and, perhaps, gastric ulcer. Recent studies have documented the presence of *H. pylori* in up to 90% of patients with duodenal ulcer disease and in approximately 50% of patients with gastric ulcer. Whether this agent is the specific cause of ulceration or simply an associated factor is unknown, but this discovery has certainly altered the treatment of all peptic ulcer disease.

What is Zollinger-Ellison syndrome?

Zollinger-Ellison syndrome is a disease associated with massive gastric hypersecretion, numerous duodenal and jejunal ulcerations, diarrhea, and non-beta islet cell pancreatic tumors. These neoplasms secrete the hormone gastrin, which targets the parietal cell mass of the proximal stomach, producing massive amounts of hydrochloric acid. Before the development of H_2R antagonists and PPIs, the mortality rate from exsanguinating hemorrhage was quite high. The incidence of this syndrome is now low, estimated at 0.1% to 0.2% of all patients with duodenal ulcer disease. The diagnosis is confirmed with an elevated serum gastrin, elevated basal cell secretion, and, if necessary, a positive secretin-infusion test.

▶ EVALUATION

How do patients with peptic ulcer disease present?

The defining symptom of patients with ulcer disease is pain. Duodenal ulcer patients have a gnawing pain that is often relieved by solid food or liquids. Patients with either severe gastritis or gastric ulcer have increased pain on eating with no relief from the further ingestion of food.

How are peptic ulcers diagnosed?

Upper GI endoscopy has played a major role in both the diagnosis and treatment of peptic ulcer disease and its complications. The endoscopist accurately diagnoses whether the ulcerations are duodenal, prepyloric, or gastric. Duodenal or prepyloric ulceration is treated medically, and further endoscopy may not be needed if the symptoms disappear. Gastric ulcers must be biopsied to rule out malignancy, and these patients require surveillance endoscopy to evaluate healing. Although symptoms of gastric ulcer may abate with treatment, a nonhealing ulcer may harbor a small malignancy or may continue to ulcerate, leading to complications. Patients with nonhealing duodenal or gastric ulcers are candidates for surgery.

Blood tests or biopsy tissue may be used to assay for the presence of *H. pylori* or for antibodies against the organism.

▶ TREATMENT

What are the options for medical treatment of peptic ulcer disease?

In patients with duodenal ulcers, excellent acid suppression and relatively high initial cure rates can be achieved by either H_2R antagonists or PPIs. Most of the H_2R drugs must be administered at least twice daily. Many patients can achieve an ulcer cure using PPIs on a once-a-day basis. Patients who have persistent symptoms should be treated either twice a day with PPIs or with a combination of PPI in the morning and an H_2R in the evening. The overnight secretion of acid (on an empty stomach) must be suppressed to achieve adequate palliation or "cure." Overall cure rates as high as 80% to 90% can be achieved after 8 weeks of medical therapy. After cessation of PPI treatment, however, recurrence rates as high as 50% have been documented at 3 to 6 months and 75% at 1 year. Some patients have a recurrence while asymptomatic. Recommendations for maintenance therapy and surveillance for ulcer recurrence remain unclear at this time. Some physicians maintain patients on continual H_2R acid suppression day and night, whereas some use night-time suppression only. Although *H. pylori* remains sensitive to a range of antibiotics, a "standard" treatment program is lacking. Most gastroenterologists use a combination of bismuth tablets for approximately 2 weeks in conjunction with tetracycline or amoxicillin 500 mg four times daily and metronidazole 250 mg four times a day. Recommendations vary as to the frequency of serologic testing or gastric aspiration, and a standard maintenance program has yet to be proposed.

The treatment of gastric ulceration and chronic gastritis remains controversial. Although acid secretion is either normal or reduced in gastric ulcer patients, H_2R and PPI medications are commonly used. Cytoprotective agents have been used in an attempt to increase the early response rate of gastric ulceration. Sucralfate has no effect on either gastric acid or pepsin secretion but does bind to the base of the ulcers, providing a coating against acid injury. In addition, it may stimulate local prostaglandin and mucus production, aiding the healing process. Most physicians recommend daily PPIs in patients on long-term NSAID therapy. Misoprostol is the only commercially available prostaglandin that can adequately protect the gastric mucosa from NSAID-induced injuries. Unfortunately, this medication must be taken four times daily.

What are the options for surgical treatment of peptic ulcer disease?

Although surgery for intractable ulcers has decreased, operations for the complications of bleeding, perforation, and obstruction have remained rather steady and even increased in the case of hemorrhage. This may be due in part to the use of anti-inflammatory drugs in general and NSAIDs in particular.

The modern era of surgery for duodenal and/or prepyloric ulceration began when Dr. Lester Dragstedt performed bilateral truncal vagotomy to abolish basal acid secretion and reduce maximal acid output by approximately 60% on a 24-hour basis. Prior to this physiologic approach, most patients underwent some form of gastric resection, often including resection of the pylorus and a portion of the duodenum.

How does the surgeon choose which operation to perform?

Table 29–17 lists the accepted operations for peptic ulcer disease, their recurrence rates, and the incidence of postgastrectomy syndromes or adverse effects following either vagotomy or gastric resection. In choosing an operative approach, the surgeon must balance the cure rate with the potential for early and late complica-

TABLE 29–17

Operations for Peptic Ulcer Disease

Operation	Recurrence (%)	Postgastrectomy Syndromes (%)
Vagotomy, pyloroplasty	5–8	15–20
Vagotomy, antrectomy	1–3	15–20
Proximal gastric vagotomy	10–15	0–5
Subtotal gastrectomy	2–4	15–20

tions. These decisions must take into consideration the patient's age and overall medical condition and whether the operation is an elective, urgent, or emergency procedure. Elective operations can be performed with mortality rates of 1% to 2%. On the other hand, emergency procedures, especially for hemorrhage, carry a mortality of 10% to 20%, usually as a result of operating on a patient who is often both hypovolemic and hypotensive.

Why is truncal vagotomy often performed with a pyloroplasty?

Because bilateral truncal vagotomy delays gastric emptying, especially of solid food, a gastric-emptying procedure (pyloroplasty) is performed concomitantly. Truncal vagotomy and pyloroplasty can be done with extremely low mortality and morbidity and results in a peptic ulcer cure rate of 92% to 95%. The overall incidence of unfavorable postsurgical side effects, or postgastrectomy syndromes, is approximately 15% to 20%. Table 29–18 lists both the classic and more modern postgastrectomy syndromes. The two most common syndromes are postvagotomy gastroparesis and alkaline reflux or bile gastritis caused by retrograde bile flow through the pyloroplasty. The rare syndromes of dumping and postvagotomy diarrhea are self-limiting in most cases and severe in only 1% to 2% of patients. Truncal vagotomy and pyloroplasty has become a standard ulcer operation not only for elective surgery but also in emergency situations when a definitive procedure is indicated.

What is the advantage to performing an antrectomy in addition to truncal vagotomy?

Antrectomy in combination with vagotomy results in the highest cure rate of all surgical procedures for peptic ulcer disease with an acceptable incidence of postgastrectomy syndromes. The antrectomy is usually performed as a hemigastrectomy with gastric recon-

---

TABLE 29–18

Postgastrectomy Syndromes

Alkaline reflux gastritis
Postvagotomy gastroparesis
Dumping
Diarrhea
Afferent limb syndrome
Efferent limb syndrome
Alkaline esophagitis
Gastric remnant carcinoma
Roux-Y gastroparesis syndrome

struction to either the duodenum (Billroth I) or the small intestine (Billroth II). Either procedure is acceptable, and each has a similar incidence of postgastrectomy disorders. In the Billroth II operation, the addition of an enteroenterostomy between the efferent and afferent limbs diverts most of the bile away from the stomach. This is our preferred method of gastric resection, essentially eliminating early bilious vomiting and late alkaline gastritis.

What is a "proximal gastric vagotomy"?

This procedure, also known as "highly selective vagotomy," maintains vagal innervation to the antrum and pylorus. Both the right and left vagus nerves are isolated, and the small vagal branches to the body of the stomach are transected. Vagal innervation of the antrum and pylorus is maintained. Although the recurrence rate has been reported as high as 15% to 20%, preservation of the antral pump and the integrity of the pylorus eliminates most of the postgastrectomy syndromes. Proximal gastric vagotomy remains the procedure of choice for the few cases of elective surgery for duodenal or pyloric ulceration.

How are gastric ulcerations treated differently?

As a general rule, operations for pure gastric ulceration have no physiologic basis because most patients have either normal or decreased acid secretion. Although gastric ulcers can be located anywhere in the stomach, the more common location is on the lesser curve, at the border of the antrum and gastric body. All patients with gastric ulcers undergo at least several endoscopic procedures with biopsies to rule out malignancy and subsequent surveillance to evaluate healing. The main indications for surgery for benign ulcers are nonhealing ulcers, bleeding, and perforation. Gastric resection is the operation of choice. It is doubtful that vagotomy adds anything to the primary gastric resection, so most surgeons do not perform truncal vagotomy for gastric ulcers. We prefer the Billroth II gastroenterostomy with a distal enteroenterostomy. When resection includes both the ulcer and the entire antrum, cure rates higher than 90% should be expected.

How is Zollinger-Ellison syndrome treated?

Prior to the development of H_2R antagonists and PPIs, the only treatment for Zollinger-Ellison syndrome was removal of the target organ of serum gastrin, namely the stomach. Total gastrectomy caused immediate cessation of the diarrhea and eliminated all acid secretion and the lethal complication of hemorrhage from recurrent duodenal ulcers. With the development of drugs that suppressed the massive hypersecretion of gastric acid there was a rapid shift away from surgery for this syndrome. Unfortunately, clinicians were still faced with the fact that islet cell tumors of the pancreas have an overall 10-year mortality of 50%, with most patients dying of metastatic disease. During the last 2 decades advances in high-resolution CTs, angiographic procedures, portal venous sampling techniques for serum gastrin, and radionuclide octreotide scanning have led to increased localization of even tiny gastrinomas and an aggressive surgical approach to resection. Currently, radionuclide octreotide scanning is the most sensitive means of localizing gastrinomas. Approximately 90% of these tumors reside in what is known as the *gastrinoma triangle* encompassing the head of the pancreas, proximal duodenum, celiac axis, biliary tree, and a portion of the left lobe of the liver. The present indications for surgery in Zollinger-Ellison syndrome are either lesions demonstrated on CT exam or radionuclide "hot spots" consistent with gastrinoma, even in the presence of a negative CT. An aggressive surgical approach includes removal of any tumors in the pancreas and duodenum, removal of localized lymph nodes when palpable, and even wedge resections of the liver for either palpable or "hot" lesions demonstrated by octreotide scan. Many patients have undergone second and third operations for recurrent gastrinoma. It appears that the overall survival is increasing, but more time is needed to evaluate the efficacy of this approach.

What are some complications of peptic ulcer disease?

Hemorrhage

Upper GI hemorrhage has been and remains the most life-threatening complication of acute or chronic gastric or duodenal ulceration. This is one of the few complications that requires a multidisciplinary approach involving the physician, endoscopist, invasive radiologist, and surgeon.

Patients presenting with a recent history of acute hemorrhage usually undergo urgent or emergent endoscopy. The gastroenterologist determines the source and location of the bleeding. During the first endoscopic procedure the physician may elect to use epinephrine injection, heater probe, or laser to control the hemorrhage from the ulcer. The incidence of rehemorrhage from a gastric ulcer is far greater than from duodenal or prepyloric ulcers. With rebleeding, the physician must evaluate the overall condition of the patient and decide if further nonoperative therapy is indicated. In high-risk patients, angiographic clotting of the appropriate blood vessels results in the immediate cessation of hemorrhage. The success rate is equal to the ability to catheterize the vessel. The radiologist places coils distally and proximally into the gastroduodenal artery with Gelfoam between the coils in patients with bleeding duodenal or prepyloric ulcers. Bleeding gastric ulcers on the lesser curve of the stomach are treated by clotting of the left gastric artery. In low-risk patients, surgery is indicated for bleeding that persists beyond transfusion of 4 units of packed red blood cells within 24 hours.

Bleeding duodenal or prepyloric ulcers are controlled by performing a generous pyloroplasty, oversewing the ulcers, and if possible, ligating the proximal gastroduodenal artery. Most surgeons also perform a bilateral truncal vagotomy. In view of the high rehemorrhage rate, bleeding gastric ulcers are usually treated by hemigastrectomy or more extensive resection if the ulcer is high on the lesser curve of the stomach.

Perforation

Patients presenting with this acute complication of peptic ulcer disease, even high-risk patients, almost always require surgical intervention. Failure to operate often results in peritonitis, sepsis, and death. Patients presenting to the emergency department with acute abdominal pain should be studied with appropriate radiographs, including an upright chest and flat and upright views of the abdomen. In most cases free air is easily demonstrated. If the diagnosis is not obvious, further evaluation should include an abdominal CT scan with IV and oral contrast agent. In the case of acute perforation, free air is easily recognized, and extravasation of the oral contrast agent may be seen.

Patients undergoing surgery for perforation who have no history of acid suppression or ulcers are usually treated by an omental patch incorporated into the closure of the duodenum. Postoperatively they undergo maximum medical therapy and treatment for *H. pylori*, when appropriate. A definitive procedure, including pyloroplasty through the perforation and truncal vagotomy, is performed if the patient has an ulcer history. Either procedure has a relatively low morbidity and mortality when patients undergo surgery within 8 hours of the acute perforation. In cases of severe peritonitis due to a delay in the diagnosis of a perforated duodenal ulcer, a simple omental patch is almost always successful, regardless of the history. Gastric perforation is almost always treated by gastric resection, in view of the high early recurrence and reperforation rates.

Obstruction

Peptic ulcer disease is often an illness of exacerbations, remissions, and a relatively high recurrence rate when the patient is off acid suppression. Years of ulcer formation in one or several locations can result in a slow but progressive narrowing of the gastric outlet. Most patients can tolerate a remarkable degree of duodenal stenosis, subtly altering their diet to accommodate this deformity. Approximately 20% of ulcer patients present with gastric outlet obstruction. In many patients balloon dilation has been fairly successful in maintaining a relatively normal gastric outlet, thus avoiding surgical intervention. In most patients who undergo surgery, the length of the obstruction is fairly short, and the surgeon performs a pyloroplasty through the obstructed area, followed by a truncal vagotomy. There appears to be an increased incidence of postoperative gastroparesis in these patients, and thus a temporary gastrostomy tube should be placed to avoid prolonged nasogastric intubation. In the presence of a long obstructing segment or inflammatory mass surrounding the duodenum, the preferred surgical treatment is gastric resection (antrectomy) and truncal vagotomy. Gastroenterostomy to bypass an obstructed duodenum is performed in unusual circumstances, where resection might be dangerous.

What are the surgical options to treat recurrent ulcers?

The mainstay of surgery for recurrent ulceration is completion truncal vagotomy with antrectomy or further gastric resection depending on the specific operation performed previously. Many of these patients are found to have had an inadequate vagotomy at prior operation. Table 29–19 lists the primary operations and remedial surgery performed for recurrent ulceration. Zollinger-Ellison syndrome should be ruled out as the cause of recurrence of ulceration prior to surgical consideration. A small percentage of patients undergo extensive subtotal or near-total gastric resection. In these cases, gastric reconstruction is performed by using a 50-cm Roux-Y gastroenterostomy to ensure that no bile refluxes to the small gastric pouch and esophagus. This type of gastroenterostomy is performed when the gastric remnant is less than 25%.

What are the postgastrectomy syndromes?

The term *postgastrectomy syndrome* (see Table 29–18) has been used to characterize the adverse side effects following vagotomy and gastric drainage or gastric resection. In some of the earliest descriptions from the 1890s, surgeons described postoperative bile and food vomiting and what they called "dumping stomach," characterized by rapid transit of a meal. Even in those days, it became obvious that most of these symptoms improved over time.

Currently, the most common syndromes are *postoperative bile vomiting, alkaline reflux gastritis,* and *postvagotomy gastroparesis.* Following either pyloroplasty or gastric resection, bile can easily

TABLE 29-19	
Surgery for Recurrent Ulceration	
Prior Surgery	**Remedial Operation**
Vagotomy, pyloroplasty	Revagotomy, antrectomy
Vagotomy, antrectomy	Revagotomy, subtotal gastrectomy
Proximal gastric vagotomy	Vagotomy, hemigastrectomy
Subtotal gastrectomy	Vagotomy, near-total gastrectomy

reflux back into the stomach. In the presence of gastroparesis, early postoperative bilious vomiting is most troubling to the patient. Chronically, alkaline gastritis results in dramatic inflammation of the stomach, a reddened mucosa, and significant burning abdominal pain. In patients undergoing gastric resection, this syndrome can be prevented by performing a Billroth II reconstruction with distal enteroenterostomy between the afferent and efferent limbs.

Chronic Gastroparesis

The chronic syndrome of gastroparesis results in significant delayed gastric emptying and can be documented by radionuclide gastric emptying studies. Recurrent bezoar formation and retained food are common, and these patients undergo dramatic alterations in their diet. Prokinetic agents, such as erythromycin, have been shown to significantly speed gastric emptying in patients with gastroparesis. Following years of chronic abdominal pain, bezoar formation, and gastric dilation, patients may require further gastric resection to allow an otherwise atonic stomach to empty.

Dumping Syndrome

The dumping syndrome can be provoked or demonstrated in up to 20% of patients undergoing either pyloroplasty or gastric resection. Severe dumping, however, occurs in only 1% of patients following these procedures. The etiology is rapid transit of carbohydrates and sugars into the small intestine, provoking a neurohumoral response resulting in severe tachycardia, sweating, dizziness, abdominal pain, and the urge to recline within 15 to 30 minutes following the ingestion of a meal. Either "tincture of time" and/or dietary manipulation results in improvement in this syndrome in most cases. Less than 1% are considered to have the severe form of this syndrome and require further therapy. The somatostatin analog octreotide essentially eliminates the dumping syndrome but must be taken parenterally before each meal. The recent introduction of long-acting octreotide certainly benefits the small number of patients who require therapy. We have published the results of a small group of patients whose severe dumping syndrome necessitated surgical revision. Conversion of their prior operation to a Roux-Y gastroenterostomy significantly delays gastric emptying by bypassing the duodenal pacemaker. Only a small number of patients, however, require surgical revision for this syndrome.

Postgastrectomy Diarrhea

Postgastrectomy diarrhea is a unique syndrome occurring in less than 1% of patients, resulting in rapid small intestinal transit and numerous (10 to 15) liquid stools a day, irrespective of diet.

Radionuclide and barium studies demonstrate severe rapid transit from the stomach to the right colon. If the syndrome does not abate over time, various surgical procedures are used to slow rapid transit. We have recently demonstrated the efficacy of one or two stapled anastomoses in slowing transit through the small intestine, due to the inhibitory effect of the anastomoses on intestinal electrical activity.

Efferent Limb Syndrome

The efferent limb syndrome is a mechanical disorder caused by scarring of the efferent portion of the gastroenterostomy, leading to symptoms of gastric outlet obstruction and bilious vomiting. Patients with this disorder almost always require surgical intervention.

Afferent Limb Syndrome

The afferent limb syndrome is a unique disorder caused by scarring of the afferent portion of the gastroenterostomy, leading to a massively dilated afferent limb, intermittent bilious vomiting, and the possibility of emergent presentation. Radionuclide biliary scanning usually demonstrates a massively dilated afferent limb. Over time this limb can decompress, with bile pouring into the stomach. CT exam similarly demonstrates dilation of the proximal small intestine and occasionally dilation of the pancreatic and biliary system. Enteroenterostomy between the afferent and efferent limbs decompresses the afferent limb and treats this syndrome. An alternative treatment is resection of the efferent and afferent limbs and creation of a Roux-Y gastroenterostomy.

Gastric Remnant Carcinoma

Gastric remnant carcinoma is a unique and often debated entity. There seems to be an increased incidence of carcinoma in the gastric remnant approximately 20 to 25 years following a previous ulcer operation. Most patients have had a Billroth II resection. A smaller percentage have undergone either gastroduodenostomy or vagotomy with a concomitant drainage procedure. Most clinicians attribute this condition to persistent alkaline reflux gastritis with bile salts bathing the gastric remnant. In patients with chronic alkaline reflux gastritis who undergo either endoscopic surveillance or endoscopy due to symptoms, biopsy of the gastric mucosa has demonstrated dysplastic changes perhaps due to continual irritation by bile salts. Although it is rare, we consider high-grade dysplasia of the stomach to be a potentially premalignant lesion. Such endoscopic findings should be confirmed by further biopsies over a period of months. The finding of gross carcinoma in the gastric remnant necessitates a total gastrectomy.

K E Y	**P O I N T S**

▶ Duodenal and prepyloric ulceration is associated with hypersecretion of gastric acid.

▶ *H. pylori* is found in about 90% of patients with duodenal ulcer disease and in roughly 50% of patients with gastric ulcers.

▶ The defining symptom in patients with ulcer disease is pain.

▶ The initial treatment of uncomplicated ulcer disease is medical therapy.

▶ Patients with nonhealing ulcers or with complications of ulcer disease (bleeding, obstruction, or perforation) are candidates for surgical intervention.

CASE 29–21. A 75-year-old man complains of a steady epigastric pain for the last several months. He states that the pain increases when he eats and thus he has reduced his food intake. He has lost 15 lb in the last 3 months.

    A. What questions would you ask this patient?
    B. How would you evaluate him?
    C. Assuming that the patient is ultimately found to have a gastric ulcer, how would you follow him?

30

Hematology

When is a low hemoglobin level dangerous?

Anemia reduces the arterial oxygen content in direct proportion to the loss of red blood cell mass. As this decrease occurs, oxygen delivery to tissues can be maintained only by increasing cardiac output or oxygen extraction. The ability to maintain organ function with severe anemia varies among individuals; in general, however, there begins to be a measurable *mortality* when the hemoglobin falls below 5 g/dL (hematocrit <15%). Although a hemoglobin of 5 to 10 g/dL may not be immediately life threatening, it can be physiologically significant, and one should be concerned about marginal oxygen delivery to vital organs such as the heart, brain, and kidneys.

How do I tell when anemia is physiologically significant?

Anemia in concert with signs or symptoms of organ dysfunction should be considered significant. Some of these clinical factors can be described as "transfusion triggers." Concomitant hypovolemia should be addressed with the administration of crystalloid solutions. General symptoms of physiologically significant anemia include weakness, easy fatigability, dyspnea, and malaise. Mental status changes can sometimes be due to inadequate oxygen delivery to the central nervous system (CNS), particularly in patients with cerebrovascular disease. Similarly, cardiac symptoms and signs include angina, tachycardia, and electrocardiographic changes in patients with subclinical coronary artery disease. Depressed cardiac function from marginal myocardial oxygen delivery may manifest itself as refractory metabolic acidosis, oliguria, or azotemia.

So, when should I give my patient red blood cells?

Almost all patients with a hemoglobin level of less than 6 g/dL (hematocrit <18%) should be transfused. Possible exceptions to this rule might be young adults without comorbid medical conditions or without symptoms or signs of inadequate oxygen delivery, as described earlier.

Those patients who have a hemoglobin level of 6 to 10 g/dL should be selectively transfused with red blood cells. Indications for transfusion include symptoms and signs mentioned previously; extremes of age (>65 years old, neonates); and coincident cardiopulmonary, vascular, or renal disease.

Most patients with a hemoglobin greater than 10 g/dL do not need a transfusion of red blood cells. Exceptions to this rule might include critically ill patients at high risk for multiple organ failure, patients with persistent signs or symptoms of impaired oxygen delivery, and neonates with severe cardiopulmonary disease.

Do critically ill patients require a higher hematocrit?

It seems conceptually attractive that critically ill patients, who have a higher metabolic demand, might benefit from a higher hematocrit. Studies to date, however, do not demonstrate a benefit across all critically ill patients. In fact, some studies show a higher incidence of complications in patients with a more "liberal" transfusion trigger. This may be due to biologically active substances in stored red blood cells (cytokines and proinflammatory lipids) that could exacerbate critical illness. One exception is elderly patients with acute myocardial infarction, who appear to benefit from transfusion to a hemoglobin greater than 11 g/dL.

Are indications for transfusion different in rapid, acute blood loss?

Yes. Acute blood loss does not result in a change in hematocrit until extravascular fluid or exogenously administered fluid produces hemodilution, so hematocrit alone cannot serve as a transfusion guide. Furthermore, assessment of signs and symptoms of anemia is clouded by the manifestations of hypovolemia. In rapid, acute blood loss, initial support should be 2 L of crystalloid solution; if the patient has persistent hemodynamic abnormalities, red blood cells should then be transfused. It is vital to remember that in patients with acute and ongoing blood loss, the hematocrit cannot be used as the sole indicator for transfusion; indeed, the delay inherent in documenting anemia might be life threatening.

How many red blood cells should I give?

Treatment should be tailored to the physiologic response of the patient. In general, however, 2 units of packed red blood cells are given to an adult with an indication for transfusion. Two units is approximately 500 mL (or about 10% of circulating blood volume), which should be adequate to raise the hemoglobin by 2 g/dL.

How much blood do I give to a child?

The usual dose of red blood cells in children is 20 mL/kg body weight. This corresponds roughly to 25% of the blood volume and should be enough to raise the hemoglobin by 3 or 4 g/dL.

Are there alternative oxygen carriers for patients who refuse transfusion for religious reasons?

Possibly. A number of products are being developed. Although none of these are currently approved for general use by the U.S. Food and Drug Administration, some have been given on a compassionate-use basis outside of clinical trials. Three formulations of polymerized hemoglobin solutions (PolyHeme, Hemolink, and Hemopure) are in the advanced stages of clinical testing. Two of these are derived from human blood, so they may still be shunned by certain groups. Another class of oxygen carriers is the synthetic perfluorocarbons, one of which (Oxygent) is in advanced clinical trials.

When is a low platelet count dangerous?

Platelet counts below 20,000/µL are sometimes associated with spontaneous bleeding and generally should be treated. An exception to this rule is those patients with consumptive coagulopathies, in which transfusion of platelets may not increase the platelet count and may actually exacerbate illness. Patients undergoing invasive procedures should generally have their platelet counts maintained above 50,000/mm^3. Patients with platelet counts less than 100,000/mm^3 have prolonged bleeding times and should be selectively transfused, that is, with clinical evidence of ongoing bleeding or a falling hematocrit. In clinical situations in which any bleeding might be catastrophic (e.g., injury or operation on the CNS), it is preferable to keep the platelet count greater than 100,000/mm^3.

Are there times when a platelet count might be normal, but platelet function is inadequate?

Yes. The most common examples are drug-induced platelet dysfunction. In a patient treated with aspirin or other therapeutic antiplatelet agents and who has evidence of bleeding despite an adequate platelet count, platelet transfusion might be indicated. Other causes of platelet dysfunction include uremia, chronic alcoholism, and certain inherited disorders.

How many platelets should I give? What is a six-pack?

There are two basic types of platelet preparations: random donor platelets and apheresis units. A single "unit" of random donor platelets contains 5.5×10^{10} platelets and is only enough to raise the platelet count by approximately 5000 to 10,000/mm^3 of blood. Thus, the usual dose of random donor platelets is six "units" or a "six-pack" derived from as many as six different donors. Today, the preferred platelet preparation is an apheresis unit (or "PLA") that is derived from a single donor, contains approximately 3.0×10^{11} platelets, and is enough to raise the platelet count by approximately 30,000 to 60,000/mm^3.

Who needs transfusion with fresh frozen plasma (FFP)?

Fresh frozen plasma (FFP) is used to replace clotting factors. Therapy is guided by measurement of the International Normalized Ratio (INR) and partial thromboplastin time (PTT). In general, an INR less than 1.5 is adequate to support hemostasis but should be treated if there is evidence of ongoing bleeding or in instances when any bleeding might be catastrophic. In general, patients in the perioperative period or injured patients with an INR greater than 1.5 should receive FFP. The most common cause of an elevated PTT is the administration of heparin or contamination of the blood specimen with heparin. If a surgical patient does have a PTT greater than 1.5 times control, FFP should be administered.

Are the indications for FFP different in rapid, acute blood loss?

Yes. In general, patients requiring 5 or more units of red blood cells due to acute blood loss have lost so much plasma that they can no longer support adequate hemostasis. Although there is a small amount of residual plasma in packed red blood cells, it is not enough to maintain coagulation. Empirical administration of FFP in cases of major blood loss is thus reasonable. Waiting for laboratory values can result in unacceptable delay. Most blood banks have a "massive transfusion protocol" that incorporates this concept. For every 5 units of red blood cells transfused, 2 units of FFP are reasonable.

What is cryoprecipitate and who needs it?

Cryoprecipitate is a fraction of plasma that precipitates out from FFP when it is at 1°C to 6°C. It is rich in fibrinogen, factor VIII, and von Willebrand's factor (vWF). Thus, patients with low fibrinogen (<100 mg/dL), factor VIII deficiency, or deficits in vWF may benefit from transfusion of cryoprecipitate. The cryoprecipitate derived from 1 unit of FFP is only 10 to 15 mL in volume and is not adequate for replacement of these factors. Generally, 8 to 10 units are transfused.

Specific concentrated factors are also available to treat specific deficiencies, such as hemophilia.

K E Y   P O I N T S

▶ Transfusion triggers for red blood cells are based primarily on clinical factors, not lab tests.

▶ There is general agreement that red blood cells should be administered for a hemoglobin less than 6 g/dL.

▶ The indications for transfusion are different in acute blood loss versus gradual anemia.

▶ Most critically ill patients do not appear to benefit from a hemoglobin greater than 10 g/dL.

CASE 30–1. A 28-year-old helmeted motorcycle rider is brought into the emergency department after being struck at an intersection by a car traveling 40 mph. The patient's vital signs on arrival include a heart rate of 125 beats/min, blood pressure of 85/50 mm Hg, and respiratory rate of 27 breaths/min. He is awake and responsive. He complains that he cannot move his left extremities and has no sensation below his umbilicus. He has an obvious open tibial-fibular fracture on the right, with palpable distal pulses in the right foot.

    A. Why is the patient hypotensive?
    B. How would you treat him initially?
    C. What laboratory studies would you order?

CASE 30-2. The patient from Case 30–1 has been treated initially with 2 L of normal saline and his vital signs favorably respond. His pulse rate drops to 110 beats/min and his blood pressure rises to 108/70 mm Hg. However, while radiographic studies are being obtained, his blood pressure drops to 88/50 mm Hg. The pelvic radiograph shows a fracture of the pubic rami with a wide separation of the pubic symphysis. A lateral thoracic spine film demonstrates a fracture dislocation at T5-T6. His initial hematocrit is 30%.

    A. Why has this patient experienced a recurrence of his hypotension?
    B. How are you going to treat him?

| DISSEMINATED INTRAVASCULAR COAGULATION |

▶ **ETIOLOGY**

What is disseminated intravascular coagulation (DIC)?

Disseminated intravascular coagulation (DIC) has never had a widely accepted definition, which has led to a poor understanding of this process. As the name suggests, DIC results from activation of the clotting cascade within the vascular space throughout the body, regardless of the patient's clinical manifestations.

A general appreciation of the clotting system is necessary to understand DIC. The most important thing to recognize about the coagulation system is that it is not truly a cascade—it is rather a balance. That is to say, there are a number of forces that cause acceleration of the clotting system to enhance clot formation, but there are also a number of factors built into the system to down-regulate or decelerate this same clotting process. These factors help prevent patients from having pathologic thrombosis (deep venous thrombosis [DVT], pulmonary edema [PE], and DIC). Factors that represent the up-regulatory side of the equation include the numbered coagulation factors, thrombin, fibrinogen, calcium, and platelets. Factors that participate in the down-regulation of clotting include antithrombin, proteins C and S, and thrombomodulin. In addition to the up-regulatory and down-regulatory sides of the coagulation system, there is also a system whereby clot, once it is formed, can be cleared: the fibrinolytic system.

How is DIC initiated?

Given that DIC is a disruption in the normal balance of the coagulation system, DIC can start in a number of different ways. The common underlying theme is a hypercoagulable state, following which the patient is subjected to the intravascular release of a clotting stimulus.

The first defined case of DIC was caused by an amniotic fluid embolism. Women at the time of delivery have a somewhat up-regulated coagulation system (hypercoagulable) that helps prevent excessive postpartum bleeding. If a stimulant to clotting were introduced into the vascular space, a rapid, excessive acceleration in the clotting cascade can occur unchecked. Amniotic fluid contains fetal tissue factor, an extremely potent stimulus to the procoagulant forces. When the fluid breaks the placental barrier and enters the maternal circulation, an explosive up-regulation of the coagulation cascade and rapid, unchecked fibrin formation within the mother's blood stream result. As this is occurring, the mother's body is unable to increase the activity of the down-regulatory mechanisms, and so the ability to keep up with this explosive fibrin formation and deposition is rapidly overwhelmed. As clot is deposited in the microcirculation, areas of ischemia result, and the microvascular endothelium begins releasing tissue plasminogen activator, which causes systemic activation of the fibrinolytic system (plasminogen). Once the fibrinolytic system has been activated, clot begins to break down throughout the body. This process not only includes the pathologic microvascular thrombosis but also may include clot that occurred during the child's delivery at the site of placental separation. In fact, any clot is then subject to lysis, and so bleeding may be seen from the nose, at intravenous (IV) sites, or any place recent tissue trauma has occurred.

While this process is ongoing, the fetal tissue factor is continuing to stimulate maternal clot formation, which, in turn, leads to thrombin deposition and thus activation of the fibrinolytic system with clot breakdown and subsequent bleeding. The clinical manifestation of this process then is bleeding, but it must be remembered that this bleeding is the result of excessive clotting, rather than simply an absence of adequate clotting factors (Fig. 30–1).

When and where are the conditions right for DIC?

The first condition that must occur for DIC to result is a hypercoagulable state. There are a number of clinical scenarios where a hypercoagulable state is seen. A patient with hypovolemic shock, for example, has increased catecholamine release that causes perturbation of the platelets. Platelets, in turn, cause enhanced response of the clotting factors. Thus, patients in shock (of any type) are set up for DIC in that they have a hypercoagulable state.

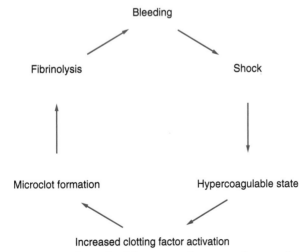

Figure 30–1. The cycle of disseminated intravascular coagulation.

A number of other clinical conditions can produce a hypercoagulable state, such as deficiency of antithrombin or protein C, polytrauma, neoplasm, or the peripartum state.

Once the stage is set with a hypercoagulable state, the introduction of a clotting stimulus into the vascular space results in an uncontrolled procoagulant response. Examples of an intravascular clotting stimulus include amniotic fluid embolism, transfusion of ABO mismatched blood, crush injury of an extremity with tissue factor release, surgical trauma in an area of high tissue factor expression (e.g., brain), or release of gram-negative or gram-positive toxins into the blood stream.

Are there different degrees of DIC?

The most severe and extreme form of DIC was described earlier, with hypercoagulability followed by fibrinolysis, followed by depletion of factors and systemic bleeding.

In its mildest form, DIC may occur with no pathologic bleeding whatsoever. In fact, a small amount of excessive thrombin and fibrin formation may occur but be adequately controlled with the down-regulatory system of proteins C and S and antithrombin. A clinical example is a patient with gram-negative sepsis. If the patient is adequately resuscitated and the infection is controlled appropriately, there may be only mild laboratory evidence of DIC, such as an acceleration in the formation of thrombin, demonstrated by increased thrombin antithrombin (TAT) complexes and D-dimers. This patient's platelet count may be normal, or even increased, and no bleeding would be manifest.

An intermediate form of DIC presents with more significant clotting that is uncontrolled by the down-regulatory mechanisms. Here, microvascular thrombosis does occur, and there is some activation of the fibrinolytic system, but neither proceeds to a level adequate to either compensate for the microvascular thrombosis or result in systemic bleeding. This situation can occur in a patient with gram-negative septic shock when the patient is adequately treated but under-resuscitated. In this case, because the fibrinolytic system has not been active enough to break down the areas of microvascular thrombosis, the microthrombi may plug the capillary beds and lead to ischemia of the end organs. These patients may manifest symptoms of end-organ dysfunction, such as acute renal failure or adult respiratory distress syndrome.

The most severe form of DIC is illustrated in the case of a patient with septic shock (a hypercoagulable state) due to an infected dead extremity (a clotting stimulus). The dead tissue releases bacterial toxins as well as tissue factor into the circulation. The intravascular release of clotting stimulants in the presence of the hypercoagulable state produces severe DIC. The end result is overwhelming activation of the clotting system, with subsequent depletion of the procoagulant factors and full activation of the fibrinolytic system. This patient would have a platelet count that was very low (likely <40,000/mm^3) with a prolonged INR, as well as extremely high TAT and D-dimer levels. Because of the massive systemic activation of the fibrinolytic system, this patient will be bleeding from previously hemostatic sites, and the likelihood of survival in this case is extremely small.

▶ EVALUATION

What are the most important things to do when evaluating a patient for DIC?

The first step when a patient is suspected of having severe DIC is to rule out other causes of bleeding. In the surgical patient, one that is unpleasant to think about but is not infrequently present is the presence of an unligated blood vessel at the operative site. In the patient who is less than 24 hours postoperative, this must be considered the cause of the bleeding until it is excluded.

Once an unligated vessel has been ruled out, other causes can be evaluated. At this time it is reasonable to obtain laboratory studies including a complete blood count, INR, D-dimer, and fibrinogen levels. It is also important to normalize a cold patient's temperature. A cold patient may have bleeding that is independent of a defect in the coagulation system. Because the coagulation process is a series of chemical reactions, cooling of the patient results in slowing of these reactions and thus a decrease in the effectiveness of clotting. If the patient is bleeding and is cold, the way to confirm that indeed the patient's temperature is the cause is to look at the laboratory results. If hypothermia is the sole explanation, then the INR and activated PTT (aPTT) should be normal. When a laboratory receives a blood specimen from a patient, the specimen is warmed to 37°C and then run on a coagulation analyzer. Thus, the lab corrects for the patient's hypothermia. If the INR and the aPTT are prolonged, further investigation should occur.

Attention should be turned to the D-dimer and fibrinogen levels. If the D-dimer levels are low, then the likelihood of DIC is small. This patient may be bleeding secondary to decreased concentrations of specific clotting factors, such as in someone taking warfarin (Coumadin). If, however, the D-dimer levels are very high and the fibrinogen levels are low with prolonged coagulation parameters (aPTT, INR), then it is likely that the patient has severe DIC.

▶ TREATMENT

What can be done for a patient with DIC?

The best hope for patients who are manifesting pathologic bleeding is that the bleeding is not due to severe DIC. To this end, it is important to rule out causes other than DIC (for which treatments may exist) and treat them appropriately. The patient who is hypothermic should be warmed to 37°C, and the patient with a potential missed injury or unligated blood vessel should have this possibility explored to its exclusion. If the patient truly has DIC, the treatment is primarily supportive, with attempts made to reduce the stimulus of both the hypercoagulable state and the clotting initiator.

One of the most common causes of a hypercoagulable state is hypovolemia. Patients with suspected DIC should be aggressively resuscitated to correct the deficiency in the circulating blood volume. As long as hypovolemia persists, the patient's hypercoagulable state will persist as well. Once the patient's hypovolemia has been corrected, attention would be turned to both warming the patient (if he or she is cold) as well as removing the clotting stimulus. The latter may be as simple as stopping the transfusion of a unit of blood that is ABO incompatible or may come through the amputation of a dead or infected extremity. There are a number of different processes that can result in presentation of a clotting stimulus to the vascular space, but all generally are the result of the presence of infected, devitalized, or frankly necrotic tissue.

Thus, the treatment of the DIC is supportive rather than truly therapeutic. That is, today, we remove the factors that stimulate the propagation of DIC rather than provide a specific therapy for the syndrome. Over the past several decades, a number of agents have been advocated for treating DIC. To date, none have been successful in breaking the vicious cycle of DIC. Those that have been tried and failed include heparin, aminocaproic acid (Amicar), antithrombin, and hemofiltration.

K E Y   P O I N T S

▶ DIC results from an imbalance of clotting factor regulation.

▶ Initiation of DIC requires an existing hypercoagulable state and the presence of an intravascular clotting stimulus.

▶ In the first 24 hours following trauma or surgery, active hemorrhage due to a missed injury or inadequate hemostasis must be ruled out first before consideration of other causes of uncontrolled bleeding.

▶ Hypothermia is a cause of uncontrolled bleeding that must be ruled out or treated before consideration of DIC.

▶ DIC is associated with abnormal coagulation indices (elevated INR and decreased fibrinogen).

▶ There is no specific therapy for DIC other than supportive care and the elimination of the hypercoagulable state and/or the clotting stimulus.

CASE 30–3. A 23-year-old man was involved in an auto accident in which he sustained a ruptured spleen and bilateral femoral fractures. He comes to the intensive care unit (ICU) after undergoing splenectomy and rodding of both femurs. He is noted to have an initial hematocrit of 32%, but this drops to 21% over the next hour with associated hypotension. His temperature is 36.1°C, the INR is 1.1, and the aPTT is 27 seconds.

- A. What is the differential diagnosis?
- B. What factors help suggest the correct diagnosis?
- C. What is the appropriate treatment for this patient?

CASE 30–4. A 46-year-old man was admitted to the hospital with a foul-smelling gangrenous right leg. He has had diabetes and peripheral vascular disease for many years. Initially, the patient refused operative intervention for his leg. He subsequently became septic, with hypotension, a temperature to 40°C, and a white blood cell count of 30,000/mm^3. Antibiotic therapy was initiated. On starting the antibiotics, the patient was noted to have bleeding from his IV sites and his nose. In addition, he began to pass melanotic stools. His hematocrit dropped from 41% to 24%, while his INR increased to 3.0. Fibrinogen levels dropped to 50 mg/dL.

- A. What is the most likely explanation for his bleeding?
- B. What is the most appropriate next step in the management of this patient?

INDICATIONS FOR SPLENECTOMY

What is the most common indication for splenectomy?

Blunt abdominal trauma represents the leading indication for splenectomy in the United States. The spleen is the intra-abdominal organ most commonly injured by blunt abdominal trauma. Penetrating trauma and iatrogenic intraoperative injury can also cause splenic injury and can require emergency splenectomy. The spleen rarely ruptures spontaneously, but when it does, an underlying infection or malignancy can usually be identified.

How is splenic injury diagnosed?

One should always suspect a splenic injury in any trauma patient who presents with abdominal pain or distention, left upper quadrant tenderness, palpable left upper quadrant mass (Ballance's sign), hypotension, tachycardia, acute blood loss, anemia, left lower rib fractures, or referred left shoulder pain (Kehr's sign). Any degree of disruption of the splenic capsule, parenchyma, or blood supply is considered a splenic rupture. Ruptures are routinely graded according to the size of a hematoma and/or the depth of a laceration by computed tomographic (CT) scan. Although some surgeons have used the degree of splenic injury in decision algorithms to initiate conservative (nonoperative) treatment plans, such grading systems have not correlated well with successful nonoperative management. Nevertheless, the uniformity created by grading systems allows authors to standardize descriptions so that publications can be meaningfully interpreted.

Should splenic injury be treated operatively or nonoperatively?

Treatment of splenic injuries depends on several factors: etiology and extent of injury, abdominal examination, hemodynamic stability, concomitant intra-abdominal injuries, and transfusion requirements. Approximately 80% of adult patients and 40% of pediatric patients with splenic trauma undergo an exploratory laparotomy for splenectomy or splenic repair. The other 20% of adults and 60% of children can be managed successfully with nonoperative management. Nonoperative management requires less than a grade IV splenic injury as diagnosed by abdominal CT scan, careful observation (usually with ICU admission), frequent abdominal examinations in a neurologically intact patient, and serial hematocrit determinations. Any patient who develops peritonitis, becomes hemodynamically unstable, or requires more than 2 units of blood transfusion must be explored expediently. With respect to patients who undergo laparotomy, roughly 40% require splenectomy and 60% can be managed with splenic preservation. Techniques of splenic preservation include application of topical hemostatic agents, argon beam coagulation, wrapping the spleen in absorbable mesh, partial splenectomy, and débridement of devitalized tissue with hemostasis and tissue reapproximation or suturing (splenorrhaphy).

What is the most common indication for elective splenectomy?

Idiopathic thrombocytopenic purpura (ITP), an acquired syndrome caused by the destruction of platelets exposed to IgG antiplatelet factors, is the most common indication for elective splenectomy.

The spleen not only produces these offending autoantibodies but also serves as the site of platelet sequestration and destruction. Laboratory findings in ITP include a moderate to severe thrombocytopenia with a platelet count always less than 100,000/mm^3, prolonged bleeding time but normal prothrombin and aPTT, and normal or increased numbers of megakaryocytes in a bone marrow aspirate. Platelets may be absent from a peripheral blood smear. Iron deficiency anemia suggests chronic bleeding.

ITP remains a diagnosis of exclusion, occurring in patients without systemic illnesses or medications capable of causing thrombocytopenia. An increased incidence has been noted in patients with human immunodeficiency virus infection, acquired immunodeficiency syndrome, and systemic lupus erythematosus. Clinically, patients present with bleeding gums, epistaxis, ecchymoses, purpura, and/or gastrointestinal or genitourinary bleeding.

Initial therapy for symptomatic ITP consists of steroids gradually tapered over 6 to 8 weeks (usually starting with prednisone 60 mg daily), IV gamma globulin, and occasionally plasmapheresis. This regimen increases the platelet count in 75% of individuals, thereby averting the risk of major hemorrhage, but only 15% to 20% will be cured. Splenectomy should be performed in the following situations:

Thrombocytopenia that does not respond to aggressive medical therapy
Thrombocytopenia that recurs with steroid taper or discontinuation
Side effects from the medical treatment that prove unacceptable
Occurrence of intracranial hemorrhage

Splenectomy produces a sustained remission in 80% of patients. Surgeons must thoroughly search the abdomen for accessory spleens, which most frequently reside near the splenic hilum and pancreatic tail and occur in up to 20% of individuals. If ITP recurs after splenectomy, an unresected accessory spleen should be considered the culprit until proven otherwise. Residual splenic tissue can be located using a technetium-99 sulfur colloid liver-spleen scan.

What is the preferred method of splenic resection?

Laparoscopic splenectomy (LS), as opposed to open splenectomy (OS), has rapidly become the preferred method of splenic resection, especially for ITP spleens, which are normal in size. Figure 30–2 illustrates patient positioning, trocar site placement, and instruments used in an LS. A recent study reviewing 47 splenectomies for ITP (29 LS, 18 OS) showed that the LS group had less intraoperative blood loss, no transfusions, faster recovery of bowel function, earlier oral intake, shorter hospital stay (3 vs. 7 days), and lower total costs compared to the OS group. As a general rule, laparoscopy results in less postoperative pain, decreased narcotic use, earlier return to normal activities, and improved cosmesis over any equivalent open procedure.

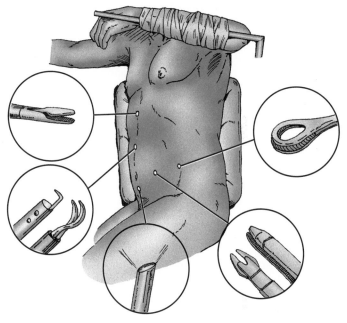

Figure 30–2. Laparoscopic splenectomy: Patient positioning, trocar site placement, and instrumentation. (Adapted from Hiatt JR, Phillips EH, Morgenstern L [eds]: Surgical Diseases of the Spleen. New York, Springer, 1997.)

What is the difference between primary and secondary hypersplenism?

Hypersplenism refers to the presence of cytopenias characterized by sequestration and destruction of cells within the spleen, a normally compensating bone marrow, and correction or amelioration of the condition after splenectomy. Primary hypersplenism, a diagnosis of exclusion, can be reached only when no other cause for the cytopenia can be identified. In contrast, secondary hypersplenism occurs in the presence of a disorder known to cause hypersplenism (e.g., leukemia, autoimmune hemolytic anemia).

How does splenomegaly differ from hypersplenism?

Splenomegaly, diffuse enlargement of the spleen, differs from hypersplenism in that splenomegaly describes a large splenic *size,* whereas hypersplenism describes overactive splenic *function*. For example, 60% of patients with cirrhosis develop congestive splenomegaly, but only 15% develop hypersplenism.

What are hematologic disorders?

Hematologic disorders comprise all benign and malignant diseases with their cell of origin derived from the pluripotent hematopoietic stem cells in bone marrow. These disorders are further categorized based on the affected cell line and include hemolytic disorders (hereditary spherocytosis [HS], thalassemia, sickle cell disease), myeloproliferative disorders (polycythemia vera, chronic myelogenous leukemia [CML], myelofibrosis), and lymphoproliferative disorders (lymphoma, leukemia).

Do hematologic disorders require splenectomy?

The primary hematologic disorders that can require splenectomy include ITP (as discussed earlier), Hodgkin's disease (HD) for staging, HS, and CML.

HD once required splenectomy for accurate staging, but now HD rarely needs more than a peripheral lymph node biopsy, laboratory testing, and radiographic studies for staging.

HS, the most common congenital hemolytic anemia, results from a deficiency in the protein spectrin, which then produces a rigid, nondeformable red blood cell membrane. Splenic destruction of these red blood cells causes anemia, splenomegaly, and jaundice. Chronic hemolysis results in an 85% incidence of pigmented gallstones. Splenectomy cures HS in 100% of patients; cholecystectomy should be performed at the same time if cholelithiasis is detected.

CML has three phases: the chronic phase, the accelerated phase, and the terminal blast crisis. Splenomegaly, the most common physical finding in CML, predicts a poor response to transfusions in patients in the accelerated or blast phases because of splenic sequestration. Splenectomy offers palliation in these patients by decreasing the need for transfusions and relieving pain from symptomatic splenomegaly.

Bleeding esophageal varices caused by splenic vein thrombosis (usually secondary to pancreatitis) are best treated by splenectomy.

Other hematologic disorders that occasionally require splenectomy are listed in Table 30–1.

Which splenic neoplasms require splenectomy?

Benign primary splenic neoplasms, although quite rare, include vascular lesions (angiomas), hamartomas, pseudotumors, and cysts. These lesions require partial or total splenectomy only to prevent spontaneous rupture, alleviate symptoms, or exclude a primary malignancy.

Vascular lesions, with hemangiomas and then lymphangiomas being the most common, can be solitary or multiple, produce hypersplenism, and occasionally rupture. Hamartomas represent developmental anomalies with normal cellular elements creating a focal

TABLE 30-1

Indications for Splenectomy

Always Indicated
Hereditary spherocytosis
Primary malignant splenic tumors

Frequently Indicated
Immune thrombocytopenic purpura
Splenic abscess
Splenic vein thrombosis causing bleeding esophageal varices
Symptomatic primary hypersplenism

Occasionally Indicated
Spontaneous rupture
Trauma
Hematologic disorders including the following:
   Chronic lymphocytic leukemia
   Elliptocytosis with hemolysis
   Hemoglobin H disease
   Idiopathic autoimmune hemolytic disease
   Myelofibrosis
   Nonspherocytic congenital hemolytic anemias (e.g., pyruvate kinase deficiency)
   Thrombotic thrombocytopenic purpura

Rarely Indicated
Congestive splenomegaly due to portal hypertension
Splenic artery aneurysm
Splenic sarcoidosis
Hematologic disorders including the following:
   Severe anemia and thrombocytopenia associated with chemotherapy
   Felty's syndrome (rheumatoid arthritis, splenomegaly, and neutropenia)
   Gaucher's disease (disordered lipid metabolism and splenomegaly)
   Hairy cell leukemia
   Macroglobulinemia
   Non-Hodgkin's lymphoma
   Porphyria erythropoietica
   Primary splenic lymphoma
   Sickle cell anemia
   Systemic mast cell disease
   Thalassemia major

Never Indicated
Asymptomatic primary hypersplenism
Splenic abscess with widespread sepsis
Hematologic disorders including the following:
   Acute leukemia
   Agranulocytosis
   Hereditary hemolytic anemia of moderate degree

disorganized tumor-like pattern. Pseudotumors, which are reactive inflammatory lesions, present a diagnostic dilemma in that they cannot be distinguished from malignant neoplasms unless resected. Parasitic echinococcal (hydatid) cysts require splenectomy. Nonparasitic cysts probably result from developmental anomalies; partial splenectomy is indicated for symptomatic cysts larger than 4 cm.

Malignant primary splenic lesions should always undergo splenectomy. Malignant neoplasms include all of the lymphoproliferative and myeloproliferative hematologic disorders discussed earlier, as well as vascular tumors (hemangiosarcoma, lymphangiosarcoma), sarcomas (e.g., fibrosarcoma, leiomyosarcoma), and malignant fibrous histiocytomas. Metastases (such as breast, lung, melanoma) need not be resected when asymptomatic.

What causes a splenic abscess?

The following clinical conditions can lead to formation of a splenic abscess: hematogenous spread from a remote site of sepsis; direct extension from an infected adjacent organ; splenic trauma resulting in infarction and a secondarily infected hematoma; and direct seeding from IV drug abuse. Splenectomy is essential for cure but is not indicated in the presence of widespread sepsis, where the spleen becomes involved as a terminal manifestation of uncontrollable infection.

K E Y   P O I N T S

▶ **The most common indication for splenectomy is blunt abdominal trauma.**

▶ **The most common indication for elective splenectomy is ITP.**

▶ **Laparoscopic splenectomy has become the gold standard for elective splenic resection.**

▶ **With the exception of HS, hematologic disorders require splenectomy only when medical management fails or splenomegaly causes symptoms.**

CASE 30–5. A 26-year-old man arrives in the emergency department after a high-speed motor vehicle collision. His vital signs are stable. You elicit some mild left upper quadrant tenderness on exam. An abdominal ultrasound detects free fluid in the pelvis, so you get a CT scan that shows a grade II splenic laceration. No other injuries are diagnosed. His hematocrit is 40%.

    A. List five clinical signs that suggest splenic injury in the trauma patient.
    B. Justify your decision to manage this patient nonoperatively.

continued

CASE 30–5. *continued*

C. Name three changes in this patient's clinical course that would make you take him to the operating room immediately.

CASE 30–6. A 42-year-old woman comes into your office complaining of easy bruisability. She has no medical illnesses and takes no medications.

A. Name five clinical signs suggestive of thrombocytopenia.
B. You suspect this patient has ITP. What tests do you order, and what do you expect the results to show if your hypothesis proves correct?
C. You confirm a diagnosis of ITP. How do you plan to treat this patient?

31

Infectious Diseases

NECROTIZING FASCIITIS

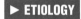 ETIOLOGY

What is necrotizing fasciitis?

Necrotizing fasciitis is a rapidly progressive (in hours) soft tissue infection of the fascia usually due to multiple pathogens. It is characterized by infectious thrombosis of the vessels passing between the skin and deep tissue, eventually producing skin necrosis. Given the rapidity with which it can progress, a high index of suspicion and recognition of such an infection are key to management.

The infection begins with a swollen area that may or may not have erythema. The most common clinical sign is severe pain. These infections are marked by the absence of clear borders or palpable limits. The infection spreads along the fascial planes, causing thrombosis of the penetrating vessels as it spreads. The skin thus becomes devascularized, and over 1 to 3 days the skin may become dusky. Bullae containing yellowish to black fluid may develop and rupture. The bullae and skin necrosis are surrounded by edema and inflammation. The fascial necrosis is usually wider and more extensive than the affected skin indicates. The patient may be febrile and can rapidly become toxic. Anatomically, the infection is marked by a layer of necrotic tissue that is not walled off by an inflammatory process. There is rapid necrosis of the subcutaneous tissue, which leads to deep infection.

What is Fournier's gangrene?

Fournier's gangrene is necrotizing fasciitis of the male perineum. The first sign of infection is often a black eschar on the scrotum.

How is fasciitis differentiated from other skin infections?

Exact categorization of some soft tissue infections may be difficult. Classification must be based on the anatomic structure involved, the clinical picture, and the infecting organism. It is essential not to underestimate the severity of the disease and confuse it with cellulitis, phlebitis, or abscess. Additionally, if necrotizing fasciitis is confused with clostridial myositis or vascular gangrene, overtreatment could lead to the unnecessary loss of limbs. See Table 31–1 for the differential diagnosis of necrotizing soft tissue infections.

Cellulitis is an acute spreading infection of the skin that can involve subcutaneous tissues. It is characterized by erythema, warmth, and tenderness of the affected area. Erysipelas is a cellulitis generally caused by group A streptococci. These superficial spreading, erythematous, and warm lesions are distinguished by their induration and elevated margins. Staphylococcal cellulitis also presents with erythematous, hot, and swollen lesions. However, these lesions can be differentiated from erysipelas by their nonelevated, poorly demarcated margins. Other causes of cellulitis include *Haemophilus influenzae* (characteristic blue-red-purple-red color) and *Vibrio vulnificus* (patients with liver disease and immunocompromised hosts).

Chronic, progressive, superficial gangrene (Meleney's ulcer) usually follows an infection at an abdominal operative wound site. It begins as a local, tender area of swelling and erythema that subsequently ulcerates. The ulcer gradually enlarges, surrounded by a margin or gangrenous skin with an outer edematous area. If not treated, the process will slowly and progressively form an enormous ulcer. Differentiation from necrotizing fasciitis can easily be made by the rate of progression. Necrotizing fasciitis advances rapidly. Meleney's ulcer advances very slowly.

Clostridial cellulitis is a necrotizing clostridial infection of the subcutaneous tissue. The deep fascia, however, is not involved, and myositis is not present. Gas formation is common and can be extensive. As its name indicates, this infection is caused by the clostridial species, usually introduced into the tissue through an inadequately débrided traumatic wound. The incubation period is several days, longer than the 1 to 2 days for clostridial myonecrosis. Although the onset is gradual, the disease may subsequently progress rapidly. Local pain and systemic toxicity are not prominent features of clostridial cellulitis. The skin may show discoloration and edema as well as prominent crepitus.

Much less common, but more serious, than clostridial cellulitis is clostridial myonecrosis. Clostridial myonecrosis (gas gangrene) is a life-threatening, rapidly progressive infection of skeletal muscle by

TABLE 31–1

Differential Diagnosis of Necrotizing Soft Tissue Infections

Cellulitis
Clostridial cellulitis
Chronic, progressive superficial gangrene (Meleney's ulcer)
Clostridial myonecrosis

clostridial bacteria. It occurs after a contaminated muscle injury and occasionally after surgery. The usual incubation period is 2 to 3 days, although it may be as short as 6 hours. The onset is very acute, and pain is the earliest and most important symptom. The pain rapidly increases in intensity and the patient soon becomes toxic appearing, with tachycardia and pale, sweaty skin. Low-grade fever is frequently present. Profound toxemia can occur early and progress to delirium and hemolytic jaundice. Local findings include tense edema and tenderness. The skin lesions found with clostridial cellulitis are not usually present. If the wound is opened, the muscle may be herniated through the opening. The wound has a characteristic foul odor, and a serosanguineous dirty-appearing discharge may escape from the wound. Gas bubbles may be evident. Crepitus may be present but is not as prominent as in clostridial cellulitis.

The infection usually involves a mixed microbial flora, including streptococci, staphylococci, gram-negative bacteria, and anaerobes, especially peptococci, peptostreptococci, and *Bacteroides* species. Clostridia may be present, making the disease resemble clostridial cellulitis (Table 31–2).

The term *necrotizing fasciitis* encompasses two bacteriologic entities. In type I, at least one anaerobic species is isolated in combination with one or more facultative aerobic species such as streptococci (nongroup A) and members of Enterobacteriaceae. In type II, group A streptococci are isolated either alone or in combination with other species, especially *Staphylococcus aureus*. Necrotizing fasciitis can be found in about half the cases of streptococcal toxic shock syndrome.

▶ **EVALUATION**

What are the physical findings?

An area of previous trauma or underlying skin lesion is often discernible. The affected area should be inspected for erythema,

TABLE 31–2

Common Organisms in Necrotizing Fasciitis
Group A streptococci
Other streptococci
Bacteroides
Enterococcus spp
Staphylococcus spp
Peptococcus/Peptostreptococcus
Clostridium spp
Escherichia coli
Proteus mirabilis
Klebsiella spp
Pseudomonas spp

edema, discoloration, ecchymoses, bullae, and dermal gangrene. The borders should not be clearly demarcated. The lesion should be inspected and palpated to determine if it is raised or flat, the latter being consistent with necrotizing fasciitis. Additionally, the presence or absence of crepitus should be determined. Assess for regional lymphadenopathy.

Assess the patient for systemic signs and symptoms of toxicity, including tachycardia, fever, hypotension, pale skin, and diaphoresis.

What are the keys to the diagnosis?

The key to diagnosis of necrotizing fasciitis is having a high index of suspicion. Given the rapidity with which this infection progresses, early diagnosis and initiation of treatment are imperative. The initial diagnosis of necrotizing soft tissue infections should all be treated as a single entity, infectious gangrene, until surgical treatment can be undertaken and further differentiation can be made.

A frozen-section tissue biopsy can help establish an accurate diagnosis earlier. Fine-needle aspiration of suggestive lesions has also been shown to be useful in diagnosis. Computed tomography (CT) or magnetic resonance imaging (MRI) can be useful in determination of the extent of the necrotizing process. However, an acutely ill patient should be treated with immediate surgical débridement and not have treatment delayed by CT or MRI scan.

▶ TREATMENT

What are the goals of surgical débridement?

Treatment includes emergency surgical exploration to define the nature of the process by direct examination of the fascial planes and muscle at the site of infection and to carry out appropriate débridement. At surgery, the finding of edematous, dull gray, and necrotic fascia and subcutaneous tissue confirms the diagnosis. Thrombi in penetrating vessels are visible. Débridement must be thorough with the removal of all avascular skin and tissue. Débridement should extend until only bleeding tissue remains. Where necrotic fascia undermines viable skin, longitudinal skin incisions aid the débridement of fascia without sacrificing excessive amounts of skin. Fournier's gangrene requires extensive scrotal and perineal débridement, but the testicles can usually be preserved. For all types of necrotizing fasciitis, daily return trips to the operating room for careful inspection and further débridement may be necessary for at least 3 to 5 days.

Which antibiotic therapy should be used?

Gram-stained smears and bacteriologic cultures are helpful for diagnosis and species-guided antibiotic therapy. Antibiotics should initially be chosen that cover both aerobic and anaerobic bacteria with adjustments made once the results of Gram stain and culture are available. See Table 31–3 for suggested antibiotic therapy.

When is hyperbaric oxygen therapy indicated?

Hyperbaric oxygen therapy has been advocated for clostridial myonecrosis and suggested as possible treatment for other necrotizing infections. However, no trials exist that prove the effectiveness of hyperbaric oxygen.

TABLE 31–3

Recommended Antibiotics for Polymicrobial Infections

Combination Therapy
Aerobic coverage—combine with a drug having anaerobic activity
   Cephalosporins: cefotaxime, ceftriaxone
   Monobactams: aztreonam
   Quinolones: ciprofloxacin, levofloxacin
   Aminoglycosides: amikacin, gentamicin, tobramycin
Anaerobic coverage—combine with a drug having aerobic activity
   Extended-spectrum penicillins: carbenicillin, mezlocillin, ticarcillin
   Others: clindamycin, metronidazole

Single-Drug Therapy
Aerobic *and* anaerobic coverage
   Beta-lactamase inhibitors: ampicillin/sulbactam, piperacillin/tazobactam,
     ticarcillin/clavulanate
   Cephalosporins: cefotetan, cefoxitin, ceftizoxime
   Carbapenems: imipenem/cilastatin

K E Y   P O I N T S

▶ A high index of suspicion is fundamental to timely diagnosis and treatment.

▶ Extensive testing and imaging are not required or recommended.

▶ Early surgical treatment allows for prompt determination of the extent of the disease process and adequate tissue débridement.

▶ Initiate the immediate administration of antibiotics once the diagnosis is suspected.

CASE 31–1. A 43-year-old man presents to your clinic with a nickel-sized purple lesion on his scrotum that he states he just noticed the previous day. He also complains of pain in the area. He denies any trauma or known infection in the area.

    A. What is your chief clinical concern?
    B. How would you proceed with the work-up?

CASE 31–2. You are the surgical intern on call when you are called to see a patient who underwent abdominal surgery earlier that day who now has increasingly severe abdominal pain around the incision and low-grade temperature to 38.3°C.

    A. What is your differential diagnosis and your chief concern?
    B. What action should you take?

CASE 31–3. A 74-year-old woman with a history of type II diabetes presents to the emergency department with a painful, swollen, erythematous thigh lesion with a central blackened area. You have been called as the surgical consult to see the patient.

    A. What is your chief concern?
    B. What therapy do you initiate immediately?

SEPSIS

▶ ETIOLOGY

What is sepsis?

In 1991, the American College of Chest Physicians and the Society of Critical Care Medicine jointly sponsored a consensus conference that attempted to describe and define the four syndromes of inflammatory response: the systemic inflammatory response syndrome (SIRS), sepsis, severe sepsis, and septic shock (Table 31–4).

SIRS is a widespread inflammation that occurs in patients who have both infectious and noninfectious causes. The findings associated with SIRS include a temperature greater than 38°C or less than 36°C, tachycardia, tachypnea or hypocapnia, and leukocytosis or leukopenia. Sepsis is defined as the subcategory of patients with SIRS who have a documented infection. Severe sepsis indicates that the patient suffers from hypoperfusion with organ dysfunction, and septic shock implies a state of hypoperfusion and persistent hypotension (see Table 31–4).

Although these definitions proposed by the consensus conference have helped to standardize the meaning of these terms, critics have pointed out that these definitions do not separate the syndromes into sufficiently distinct pathophysiologic entities. Furthermore, they define not diseases but rather manifestations of inflammation. Additionally, if more disease-specific, distinct pathophysiologic classifications were used, more successful treatments could be evaluated.

What is the scope of the problem?

Sepsis is the most common cause of death in medical and surgical intensive care units in U.S. hospitals. Sepsis occurs in more than 500,000 patients per year, and only 55% to 65% of septic patients survive. The risk of death increases 15% to 20% with each additional organ system that fails. On average, two organ systems fail during a sepsis episode.

What causes sepsis?

Traditionally, sepsis has been attributed to gram-negative organisms, and much of the research on sepsis has centered on the role of lipid A and endotoxin. However, in the last 10 years, the number

TABLE 31–4	
Key Definitions	
SIRS	Systemic inflammatory response syndrome; widespread inflammation from both infectious and noninfectious causes
Sepsis	Systemic inflammatory response with documented infection
Severe sepsis	Sepsis with hypoperfusion and organ dysfunction
Septic shock	Hypoperfusion and persistent hypotension

of cases of sepsis caused by gram-positive organisms and fungi has increased while the incidence of gram-negative sepsis has remained constant. Approximately 75% to 85% of cases of sepsis can be attributed to gram-negative or gram-positive bacteria. However, in up to 30% of cases, the causative organism cannot be identified. Risk factors for gram-negative bacteremia include diabetes mellitus, lymphoproliferative disorders, liver cirrhosis, burns, and invasive procedures. Risk factors for gram-positive organisms include indwelling vascular catheters, indwelling mechanical devices, burns, and intravenous drug use.

What is the pathophysiology of sepsis?

Sepsis results from an imbalance in the natural host immune system. The normal acute inflammatory response consists of both proinflammatory and anti-inflammatory mediators that work in balance in response to injury or infection. In patients with sepsis, this natural balance is lost, and there is an exaggerated proinflammatory response.

A trigger, such as endotoxin from gram-negative bacteria or cell wall components from gram-positive bacteria, initiates a cascade of proinflammatory mediators called *cytokines*. These cytokines include tumor necrosis factor (TNF), interleukins (ILs), granulocyte-macrophage colony-stimulating factor (Table 31–5), and the interferons.

TABLE 31–5	
Cytokines and Their Actions	
TNF	Activates T cells
	Activates neutrophils and macrophages
	Induces IL expression
IL-1	Induces hepatic acute-phase response
	Induces IL expression
	Inhibits lipoprotein lipase
	Induces shock
IL-2	Promotes lymphocyte proliferation
IL-6	Stimulates production and release of neutrophils
	Induces fever
	Induces hepatic acute-phase response
IL-8	Induces hepatic acute-phase response
	Stimulates release of prostanoids
TNF-α	Induces nitric oxide synthase
	Is a potent vasodilator
GM-CSF	Primes macrophages to produce proinflammatory mediators

TNF, tumor necrosis factor; IL, interleukin; GM-CSF, granulocyte-macrophage colony-stimulating factor.

TNF and IL-1 promote endothelial cell–leukocyte adhesion, the release of protease and arachidonic acid metabolites, and activation of the clotting cascade. Integrins on leukocyte cell membranes are up-regulated, leading to increased adherence of leukocytes and platelets to endothelial cells. This adhesion causes decreased local microvascular perfusion, leading to hypoxia. Tissue hypoxia triggers the release of more cytokines, leading to a cascade effect in the proinflammatory cycle. Additionally, high concentrations of growth factors, cytokines, and oxygen radicals are released locally, leading to fluid losses from the intravascular space to the tissues. As the fluid losses increase, hypovolemia ensues, and the ensuing release of catecholamines and nitric oxide worsens the situation. As increased nitric oxide is produced, the vasodilation increases, leading to reduced peripheral vascular resistance in the setting of intravascular depletion.

Nitric oxide plays a major role in the vasodilation seen in septic shock. Nitric oxide synthase is also implicated in the myocardial depression typical of sepsis. Nitric oxide is also responsible for the decreased vasopressor responsiveness observed in patients with severe sepsis and septic shock. Additionally it has immunomodulating effects and direct cytotoxic potential and may even function as a free radical scavenger. Nitric oxide regulates vasomotor tone in patients with severe sepsis and septic shock. Recognition of the role of nitric oxide in cardiovascular function in septic patients has fostered attempts to modify the concentration of nitric oxide by inhibiting the enzymatic formation of nitric oxide or binding the nitric oxide to hemoglobin and other scavengers. However, none of the strategies to modify the nitric oxide concentration has improved the survival of patients with severe sepsis and septic shock.

Metabolites of arachidonic acid are also important mediators in the inflammatory cascade, leading to fever, tachypnea, and tachycardia. Prostaglandins have local effects, with thromboxane acting as a potent vasoconstrictor and stimulating platelet aggregation. Endogenous opioids act as neuroendocrine mediators, causing respiratory depression, hypotension, and bradycardia. Their exact role in the pathophysiology, however, remains under investigation.

▶ EVALUATION

Tachypnea and hypoxemia are nearly universal in sepsis. Any unexplained respiratory, hepatic, renal, or gastric failure should lead to a suspicion of sepsis. Laboratory data are of limited value in the diagnosis of sepsis. Leukocytosis can be seen, although this can give way to leukopenia. An acidosis usually exists. Blood cultures, taken at two separate times, provide the best evidence for sepsis while identifying the organism. However, positive blood cultures are present in only one third of patients.

What metabolic changes occur during sepsis?

During sepsis, the resting energy expenditure rises 50% to 80% and urinary nitrogen excretion reaches 20 to 30 g/day. Protein synthesis falls and muscle protein catabolism increases, with a subsequent fall in the respiratory quotient, indicating an intense free fatty acid (FFA) oxidation. Plasma glucose, amino acid, and FFA levels increase.

The septic response includes a hyperdynamic cardiac state, reduced peripheral vascular resistance, narrowed arteriovenous oxygen difference, and a lactic acidosis.

How does sepsis result in organ dysfunction?

Recognition and treatment of organ dysfunction are essential in the management of sepsis because it is the total burden of organ failure that leads to morbidity and mortality. Pulmonary dysfunction is often first to occur in sepsis and tends to persist throughout the course of the illness. In sepsis, patients are frequently tachypneic and hypoxic. The demand on the lungs is increased due to lactic acidosis and increased energy expenditure. These factors require an increase in minute ventilation in the context of increased airway resistance and decreased respiratory compliance. Almost 85% of patients with sepsis require ventilatory support, and 50% meet the definition for acute respiratory distress syndrome.

Initially, sepsis is characterized by a physiologic stress response with an increase in cardiac output and decrease in peripheral vascular resistance. As sepsis progresses into shock, cardiac output nearly doubles and peripheral vascular resistance continues to decrease. Myocardial depressant factors reduce contractility, and cardiac output is not able to meet the demands of the extremely low peripheral resistance, leading to worsened hypotension. As the stress on the heart increases, left ventricular failure can result, leading to a low cardiac output state of septic shock. α-Adrenergic drugs can be used to increase systemic vascular resistance as well as increase myocardial contractility and heart rate. Cardiac dysfunction is also associated with down-regulation of the density and function of β-receptors. Many patients with sepsis have left and right ventricular dysfunction, with depressed ejection fraction and ventricular dilation.

Oliguria may occur with sepsis due to hypotension but usually can be corrected with volume repletion. Renal failure requiring dialysis is relatively uncommon provided adequate volume resuscitation occurs. True liver failure is also uncommon, although transient abnormalities in aminotransferases and bilirubin levels are common.

▶ **TREATMENT**

How is sepsis treated?

The basic principles in the treatment of sepsis include prompt treatment of shock, débridement or drainage of infected tissue, and early antibiotic therapy. The mortality rate is 10% to 15% higher for those patients who do not receive prompt, appropriate antibiotic therapy. If the pathogen is unknown, broad antibiotic coverage should be started. Coverage with multiple antibiotics increases the likelihood of empirically covering all possible pathogens. Treatment with a penicillinase-resistant penicillin along with gentamicin or tobramycin is adequate broad coverage. Alternatively, an antipseudomonal cephalosporin or penicillin can be combined with an aminoglycoside. A fluoroquinolone can be substituted if aminoglycoside toxicity is a concern.

Supportive measures include fluid resuscitation and ventilatory and nutritional support. Vasopressor therapy may be necessary but should not replace the use of adequate fluid resuscitation for sufficient preload. Evaluation of tissue perfusion is also a key component to the treatment of a septic patient. Oxygen delivery and consumption must be assessed. Even without evidence of hypotension or lactic acidosis, tissue oxygenation can be inadequate. Adequate oxygen delivery to the cells requires a hemoglobin of at least 9 g/dL. However, attempting to provide supraphysiologic levels of oxygen delivery has not been shown to improve survival in septic patients. Prevention of nosocomial infections, stress ulcers, skin breakdown, and deep venous thrombosis is also critical to the patient's outcome.

Glucocorticoids are potent anti-inflammatory agents and block the pro-inflammatory effects of IL-1 and TNF, as well as inhibiting their release from activated monocytes. Given these properties, glucocorticoids have been tried as a treatment for sepsis. However, several large trials in the 1980s failed to show any benefit to patients with sepsis who received glucocorticoids. In the 1990s, though, the prolonged use of low-dose hydrocortisone or methylprednisolone has been shown in some small studies to reduce the production of cytokines and improve hemodynamics and pulmonary function in patients with septic shock. These findings, however, have not yet been confirmed by a large multicenter trial.

Activated protein C is an endogenous protein that has anti-inflammatory, antithrombotic, and profibrinolytic properties. Normally, activated protein C is converted from the inactive state by thrombin coupled to thrombomodulin. In sepsis, thrombomodulin is down-regulated by inflammatory cytokines, leading to reduced levels of protein C in patients with sepsis. In a recent study, recombinant human activated protein C given to patients with sepsis and organ failure significantly reduced mortality in patients with severe sepsis. However, its use may also be associated with an increased risk of bleeding.

Antithrombin III has also been tested in trials as a treatment of sepsis. Supraphysiologic doses of antithrombin III have been shown in animal studies to have anti-inflammatory as well as anticoagulant activity. However, a randomized trial of intravenous antithrombin III in patients with clinical evidence of sepsis showed no effect on mortality and an increased risk of bleeding.

Other strategies have attempted to interrupt various steps of the inflammatory cascade. Polymyxin B has been tried to inactivate endotoxin without significant reduction in mortality. Efforts to scavenge oxygen radicals have not been shown to be useful clinically. TNF antagonists have also not proved successful. Individual anticytokine therapies have also not been shown in clinical trials to improve mortality, though they have led to physiologic improvement and even survival improvement in some subgroups of patients. Thus, continued investigation of these individual agents, as well as combination therapies, is warranted. Inhibition of nitric oxide synthase has also been investigated as a treatment for sepsis, given the key role that nitric oxide plays in the vasodilation seen in sepsis. By inhibiting nitric oxide synthase, some of the hemodynamic instability should be attenuated. However, the beneficial effects of blocking nitric oxide must be balanced against the negative effects of decreased organ perfusion and cardiac index.

Continuous plasma filtration with the use of sorbents has been proposed as a means of removing multiple inflammatory mediators. Animal studies have shown improved outcomes in septic shock, but clinical studies are still in progress. Continuous arteriovenous and venovenous hemofiltration has been shown to reduce plasma levels of TNF-α, complement, IL-1, IL-6, and IL-8. Further clinical investigation is still needed to assess their role in the treatment of sepsis.

K E Y   P O I N T S

▶ SIRS is widespread inflammation that can occur in patients with infectious or noninfectious disorders.

▶ Sepsis is the subcategory of SIRS patients who have a documented infection.

▶ The risk of death increases 15% to 20% with each additional organ system that fails.

▶ Treatment approaches focus on eradicating infection and supporting failing organ systems, as well as preventing nosocomial complications.

CASE 31–4.   A patient who had a colectomy 5 days earlier is seen with a blood pressure of 70/40 mm Hg and a temperature of 39°C.

   A. What is your differential diagnosis?
   B. What are your initial treatment steps?

32

Nephrology

▶ ETIOLOGY

What is meant by acid-base balance?

The normal arterial pH is between 7.37 and 7.43. This is the physiologic pH at which cellular function is normal. To maintain this normal pH, an accumulation of any acid must be buffered by a base and vice versa. During daily metabolism, carbon dioxide accumulates (which can generate carbonic acid as it combines with water), and nonvolatile acids such as sulfuric acid are generated from amino acid metabolism. To maintain acid-base balance, the body must excrete this acid. The lungs must properly expire CO_2 and the kidney must excrete hydrogen ions, typically in the form of NH_4^+ and $H_2PO_4^-$. Therefore, the lungs and the kidneys are the principal organs maintaining acid-base balance.

What is an acidemic pH?

An arterial pH less than 7.37 is an acidemic pH and results from a pathologic process that results in acidosis. A metabolic acidosis results from either the accumulation of a nonvolatile acid or the loss of bicarbonate. A respiratory acidosis results from the build-up of CO_2 and an inability of the lungs to expire the CO_2. Causes of metabolic and respiratory acidosis are listed in Table 32–1.

What is an alkalemic pH?

An arterial pH greater than 7.44 is an alkalemic pH and suggests an excessive loss of hydrogen ion or excessive ventilation of CO_2. Causes of an alkalemic pH are listed in Table 32–2.

What is the anion gap?

Calculation of the anion gap is extremely useful in narrowing the differential diagnosis in an acid-base disorder. The anion gap is the difference between the major plasma cation (sodium) and the major

TABLE 32-1

Causes of Metabolic and Respiratory Acidosis

Metabolic (HCO$_3^-$ < 24)	Respiratory (Pco$_2$ > 40)
Elevated Anion Gap	Excess sedation
Lactic acidosis	Extreme obesity
Ketoacidosis	Respiratory muscle weakness
Diabetes	Guillain-Barré syndrome
Starvation	Myasthenia gravis
Toxic ingestions	Periodic paralysis
Salicylates	Hypokalemia or hypophosphatemia
Ethylene glycol	Spinal cord injury
Methanol	Airway obstruction
Toluene	Foreign body
Paraldehyde	Endotracheal tube malposition
	Secretions/vomitus
Normal Anion Gap	Laryngospasm
Renal acidification defects	Disorders of gas exchange
Renal tubular acidosis	Asthma
Renal failure	Pneumonia
Gastrointestinal bicarbonate losses	COPD
Diarrhea	Hemothorax, pneumothorax
Ureterosigmoidostomy	Excess oxygen delivery in CO$_2$-retaining COPD patients

COPD, chronic obstructive pulmonary disease.

measured anions (chloride and bicarbonate). Thus, the anion gap = $Na^+ - (Cl^- + HCO_3^-)$, and the normal anion gap is 12 mEq/L. In the high anion gap acidoses, there is an accumulation of a Na^+-unmeasured anion that accounts for the elevated anion gap. For example, in lactic acidosis, the lactate anion circulates as Na^+lactate$^-$. Review Table 32–1 to note how the presence or absence of an anion gap can help in the differential diagnosis of the pathophysiologic process. The mnemonic MULE PAK can help in remembering the causes of a high anion gap metabolic acidosis: *M*ethanol, *U*remia, *L*actic acidosis, *E*thylene glycol, *P*araldehyde, *A*spirin, *K*etoacidosis.

In an acid-base disorder, how does the body compensate?

In a primary acid-base disorder, there is an attempt to normalize the pH by a variety of compensation mechanisms. In a metabolic acidosis, the appropriate compensating response would be to hyperventilate and expire more CO_2. In a respiratory acidosis, the kidney

TABLE 32-2

Causes of Metabolic and Respiratory Alkalosis

Metabolic (HCO_3^- > 24)	Respiratory (Pco_2 < 40)
Gastrointestinal loss of H+	Hyperventilation
Vomiting	Pulmonary emboli
Gastric suctioning	Pneumonia
Chloride-losing diarrhea	Pulmonary fibrosis
Renal loss of H+	Pulmonary edema
Mineralocorticoid excess	High altitude
Diuretics: loop and thiazide	Psychogenic/anxiety
Bicarbonate excess	Salicylates
Milk-alkali syndrome	Hepatic failure
Blood transfusions containing citrate	Pregnancy
Administration of $NaHCO_3$	Sepsis
Volume depletion	Excess mechanical ventilation
Increases the concentration of plasma	Pain
bicarbonate	

attempts to compensate by reabsorbing bicarbonate and excreting more hydrogen ion. Therefore, in a primary disorder, there is an expected compensation that should occur (Table 32–3).

▶ **EVALUATION**

How do I diagnose an acid-base disorder?

An arterial blood gas and electrolyte panel are necessary. First, examine the pH to determine the primary process as either an acidosis or alkalosis. Next, examine the Pco_2 and HCO_3^- to determine if the primary process is of metabolic or respiratory origin. Check to see if the expected compensation has occurred (see Table 32–3). Then calculate the anion gap. By performing this analysis, you should be able to identify the primary acid-base disorder and whether there has been an appropriate compensation. These steps can help identify the potential differential diagnosis and help in planning therapy. They are summarized in Table 32–4. The Cases at the end of the section illustrate these styles.

Could there be multiple primary disorders mixed together?

Absolutely. Any patient may have more than one primary disorder occurring simultaneously. For example, a patient with a metabolic

TABLE 32–3

Acid-Base Disorders and Expected Compensations

Disorder	Primary Change	Expected Compensation
Metabolic acidosis	$HCO_3^- < 24$	$Pco_2 = 1.5 \times HCO_3^- + 8\ (\pm 2)$ or Pco_2 = last two digits of pH
Metabolic alkalosis	$HCO_3^- > 24$	$Pco_2 = 0.9 \times HCO_3^- + 16\ (\pm 5)$ or Pco_2 = last two digits of pH
Respiratory acidosis	$Pco_2 > 40$	*Acute* HCO_3^- increases 1 mEq/L for every 10 mm Hg increase in Pco_2 *Chronic* HCO_3^- increases 3.5 mEq/L for every 10 mm Hg increase in Pco_2
Respiratory alkalosis	$Pco_2 < 40$	*Acute* HCO_3^- decreases 2 mEq/L for each 10 mm Hg decrease in Pco_2 *Chronic* HCO_3^- decreases 5 mEq/L for each 10 mm Hg decrease in Pco_2

acidosis who does not have the expected respiratory compensation would therefore be suffering from a primary metabolic acidosis superimposed on a primary respiratory acidosis.

Is there another use for the anion gap?

Yes. The anion gap can help determine if there are two metabolic processes occurring simultaneously. For every rise in the anion gap of 1 mEq/L above normal, the serum HCO_3^- should fall by 1 mEq/L. Therefore, the change in the anion gap should equal the change in the serum HCO_3^- from normal. This is referred to as the "delta-delta." So, determining the change in the anion gap above normal, if any, and adding this number to the serum HCO_3^- is important. If

TABLE 32–4

Sequential Approaches to Acid-Base Disorders

Examine the pH for acidemia or alkalemia, and determine if the primary process is metabolic or respiratory in origin.
Determine if the expected compensation has occurred.
Calculate the anion gap.
Determine the "delta/delta" to rule out mixed metabolic processes.

adding the change in the anion gap from normal to the HCO_3^- brings the HCO_3 above 24, there is a concurrent metabolic alkalosis involved. If the value is less than 24, there is a concurrent non-gap acidosis involved (see Cases).

▶ TREATMENT

If the primary disorder is a metabolic acidosis, the underlying cause such as a lactic acidosis or a ketoacidosis should be treated. If the acidosis is from an ingestion, dialysis may be required. If the primary process is a metabolic alkalosis, typically occurring from volume depletion, therapy with intravenous (IV) sodium chloride should be initiated. A primary respiratory acidosis suggests inadequate ventilation, and treatment revolves around improving pulmonary function. Therapy for a primary respiratory alkalosis should be directed at correcting the stimulus leading to hyperventilation.

K E Y   P O I N T S

▶ In an acid-base disturbance, determine the primary disorder and then determine whether the appropriate compensation has been made.

▶ Regardless of the pH, calculate the anion gap to help detect mixed disorders.

▶ In any given patient, it is possible to have two or three mixed primary disorders that would each require therapy.

CASE 32-1. A 43-year-old man is admitted with intractable nausea and vomiting. He is placed on nasogastric suctioning. On the second hospital day, he develops worsening abdominal pain and hypotension. The laboratory tests reveal Na^+ of 140 mmol/L, Cl^- of 98 mmol/L, HCO_3^- of 20 mmol/L, glucose of 150 mg/dL, pH of 7.35, and Pco_2 of 36 mm Hg.

A. What is the primary acid-base disorder?
B. Is the expected compensation occurring?
C. Are there mixed acid-base disorders present?
D. What could explain these acid-base findings?

CASE 32–2. A 28-year-old diabetic man is involved in a motor vehicle accident and sustains chest wall trauma. On arrival he has a blood pressure of 130/80 mm Hg and a respiratory rate of 36 breaths/min. The initial laboratory results are pH of 7.50, P_{CO_2} of 20 mm Hg, Na^+ of 133 mmol/L, Cl^- of 96 mmol/L, HCO_3^- of 14 mmol/L, and glucose of 408 mg/dL.

    A. What is the primary acid-base disorder?
    B. Is the expected compensation occurring?
    C. Are their mixed acid-base disorders present?
    D. What could explain these acid-base findings?

ACUTE RENAL FAILURE

▶ ETIOLOGY

What is acute renal failure (ARF)?

ARF implies a sudden decrease in the function of the kidneys. Reduced renal function usually presents as a rising serum creatinine level and/or oliguria. Serum creatinine levels are usually at a steady state, so a rise in creatinine implies an inability of the kidneys to excrete this and other substances.

What are the causes of ARF?

ARF is caused by reduced perfusion of the kidney (termed *prerenal* causes), an intrinsic renal abnormality affecting either the glomerulus or the renal tubules (termed *renal* causes), or an obstruction beyond the kidney that prevents urine excretion (termed *postrenal* causes). The potential causes of ARF are summarized in Table 32–5.

In hospitalized patients, what are the most likely causes of ARF?

In any hospitalized patient with ARF, a bladder catheter should be placed to allow for accurate assessment of urine output and to ensure that there is no obstruction to urine excretion by the prostate or bladder. In patients with a properly working bladder catheter, the most likely causes of ARF are prerenal or tubular causes. Rarely does ARF present as an acute glomerular lesion or higher acute obstruction. Therefore, hospitalized patients with ARF have usually developed renal perfusion abnormalities or a tubular insult.

TABLE 32–5

Acute Renal Failure

Prerenal Causes	Renal Causes	Postrenal Causes
Intravascular volume depletion	Tubulointerstitial disease	Bilateral ureteral obstruction
Gastrointestinal losses	Pyelonephritis	Kidney stones
Dehydration	Interstitial nephritis	Blood clots
Massive hemorrhage	from drugs	Accidental ligation
Skin losses from fever or burns	Hypercalcemia	Retroperitoneal fibrosis
Extravasation of fluid into	Multiple myeloma	Ureteral
interstitium	Cholesterol embolization	strictures/valves
Impaired cardiac output	Tubular necrosis	Tumor encasement
Congestive heart failure	Ischemic injury	
Myocardial infarction	Aminoglycosides	Bladder obstruction
Pericardial tamponade	Radiocontrast agents	Prostate enlargement
Cardiogenic shock	Chemotherapeutic	Nonfunctional bladder
Peripheral vasodilation	agents	catheter
Sepsis	Rhabdomyolysis	Bladder stones, clots
Vasodilating medications	Glomerular disease	Bladder trauma
Other	Acute glomerulonephritis	Urethral strictures,
Aortic dissection	Malignant hypertension	trauma
Bilateral renal artery dissection,		
embolus		
Hepatorenal syndrome		

▶ **EVALUATION**

How can prerenal ARF be differentiated from ARF due to a tubular insult?

By assessing how the renal tubules are reabsorbing sodium and water, the clinician can usually distinguish between prerenal and tubular causes of ARF. In states of renal hypoperfusion, the kidney attempts to restore its perfusion by avidly reabsorbing salt and water to expand the intravascular volume. With this avid sodium and water resorption, there is less sodium and free water in the urine. Injured renal tubules, however, are incapable of reabsorbing sodium and water fully, and more of these constituents appear in the urine. Therefore, by assessing the urine sodium concentration and calculating the fractional excretion of sodium (FE_{Na}) (Table 32–6), a clinician can determine

TABLE 32–6

Calculation of the Fractional Excretion of Sodium (FE$_{Na}$)

$$FE_{Na}(\%) = \frac{Na\ excreted}{Na\ filtered} \times 100$$

$$= \frac{(U_{Na})\ (V)}{(P_{Na})(GFR)} \times 100$$

$$= \frac{(U_{Na})\ (V)}{(P_{Na}) \left(\dfrac{U_{cr}V}{P_{cr}} \right)} \times 100$$

$$= \frac{(U_{Na})\ (P_{cr})}{(P_{Na})\ (U_{cr})} \times 100$$

Fe$_{Na}$, Fractional exeretion of sodium; U$_{Na}$; urine sodium; U$_{cr}$; urine creatinine; P$_{Na}$, plasma sodium; P$_{cr}$, plasma creatinine; V, urine volume; GFR; glomerular filtration rate.

how filtered sodium is being handled by the kidney. By determining the specific gravity of the urine and the urine osmolality, the clinician can determine whether water is being avidly reabsorbed. These measurements help distinguish between the two most common causes of ARF in hospitalized patients: prerenal and tubular causes (Table 32–7).

Are a 24-hour urine collection and renal ultrasound useful in the evaluation of ARF?

Usually not. A 24-hour urine collection is useful in the assessment of chronic renal failure but not acute renal failure. Because in ARF renal function is changing suddenly, the 24-hour urine results, which change day to day, would not be useful. A renal ultrasound is useful to rule out obstruction that has resulted in hydronephrosis and/or hydroureter. If a bladder catheter is working properly, the likelihood of obstruction's causing ARF is remote. In the evaluation of ARF, renal ultrasound examinations are reserved for more com-

TABLE 32–7

Laboratory Parameters in ARF

Prerenal Causes	Renal Causes	Postrenal Causes
U_{Na} < 40 mEq/L	U_{Na} > 40 mEq/L	U_{Na} > 40 mEq/L
FE_{Na} < 1%	FE_{Na} > 1%	FE_{Na} > 1%
Specific gravity > 1.015	Specific gravity ~ 1.010	Specific gravity 1.010
BUN/Cr > 20:1	BUN/Cr 10–15:1	Urine osmolality < 350
Urine osmolality >	Urinalysis	Urinalysis
500 mOsm/kg	Tubulointerstitial disease	Nondysmorphic RBCs
Urinalysis	Renal tubular cells	Crystals
Minimal cells	Sterile pyuria	Malignant cells
Minimal proteinuria	Eosinophiluria	
	WBC casts	
	Mild to moderate proteinuria	
	Tubular necrosis	
	Renal tubular cells	
	Granular casts	
	Mild to moderate proteinuria	
	Glomerular	
	Dysmorphic RBCs	
	RBC casts	
	Moderate to heavy proteinuria	

FE_{Na}, fractional excretion of sodium; U_{Na}, urine sodium; BUN/Cr, blood urea nitrogen/creatinine ratio; RBC, red blood cell; WBC, white blood cell.

plicated cases in which the etiology remains unclear after initial evaluation.

How does the microscopic evaluation of the urine help in determining the cause of ARF?

In prerenal conditions, the kidney itself is normal but underperfused. Therefore, there should be benign urine microscopy with no evidence of renal cells or casts. In the tubular disorders, urine microscopy is more active with cells and/or casts. In acute tubular necrosis, the urinalysis contains renal tubular cells and granular casts. Tubulointerstitial nephritis may present with a mixture of urinary polymorphonuclear cells (such as neutrophils and eosinophils), renal tubular cells, and possibly white blood cell casts. If the microscopic exam shows few red blood cells but the dipstick shows significant heme pigment, the urine may contain myoglobin or hemoglobin, either of which is a tubular toxin. This may indicate rhabdomyolysis or massive hemolysis as the etiology of the ARF.

▶ TREATMENT

What are the goals of treatment in ARF?

During an acute decline in renal function, fluid and electrolyte management can be difficult. The goals of treatment, therefore, are to avoid fluid imbalances or electrolyte disturbances that may be dangerous.

What are the treatment approaches in ARF?

In any patient with ARF, a bladder catheter should be placed to monitor the urine output accurately. If ARF develops in a patient with a preexisting bladder catheter, the catheter should be flushed to ensure that it is patent and not obstructing urine flow.

If the patient is thought to have prerenal causes for ARF, measures should be taken to improve renal perfusion. Administering crystalloid or colloid solutions would be indicated. A reasonable crystalloid administration would be normal saline as a 250- to 500-mL bolus, which could be repeated in 1 hour. Central venous pressure (CVP) monitoring can help determine the amount of fluid needed to restore normal central volume. If renal perfusion is compromised by depressed cardiac output, the treatment should be directed toward improving cardiac output with inotropic therapy, vasodilatory agents, or diuretics.

If the patient is thought to have intrinsic renal failure, which is usually a tubular defect, a careful review of recently started medications should be performed. If there is a likelihood of allergic interstitial nephritis, the offending medication should be stopped. If tubular necrosis is suspected from a medication, that medication should be stopped.

In patients who develop oliguria during ARF, fluid intake and output should be carefully balanced to avoid fluid overload that could result in pulmonary edema. The oliguria decreases electrolyte excretion, and daily monitoring of electrolytes is indicated.

What is the major electrolyte disturbance in ARF?

Reduced urinary excretion of potassium could lead to hyperkalemia. Hyperkalemia can result in neuromuscular and cardiac conduction abnormalities and lethal arrhythmias. In patients with nonoliguric ARF, urinary losses of potassium may prevent hyperkalemia. In oliguric or anuric ARF, however, hyperkalemia is common. Potassium values should be followed at least daily in patients with ARF, and hyperkalemia should be treated if found.

What is the treatment of hyperkalemia?

As mentioned, hyperkalemia can result in life-threatening cardiac arrhythmias. If the patient demonstrates ventricular ectopy or QRS prolongation attributed to hyperkalemia, the initial treatment is IV calcium gluconate to stabilize cardiac conduction, followed by attempts to shift potassium to the intracellular space and to bind available potassium (Table 32–8). Refractory hyperkalemia in ARF may require urgent dialysis.

What are additional treatment concerns?

In addition to the potential for hyperkalemia and fluid imbalances, the patient with ARF may develop hyperphosphatemia. Dietary phosphate begins accumulating in ARF, so the patient's nutrition should be restricted in phosphorus. In addition, the inability of the kidney to excrete H^+ may result in metabolic acidosis. Adding base in the form of oral or IV sodium bicarbonate may be indicated.

TABLE 32–8

Treatment of Hyperkalemia

Protect and stabilize neuromuscular and cardiac conduction.
    Calcium gluconate 10 mL of a 10% solution IV over 2 minutes. May be repeated at 1 hour.
Shift potassium from the extracellular to intracellular space.
    One 50-mL ampule of D-50-W IV followed by 10 units of regular insulin IV.
    May be repeated in 3 to 4 hours.
    Sodium bicarbonate 1 ampule (44.6 mmol) IV.
Bind the excess potassium.
    Sodium polystyrene sulfonate (Kayexalate) 15 to 30 g in 50 to 100 mL of 20% sorbitol orally
      every 4 to 6 hours.
    If the patient is unable to take orally, give as a retention enema: 50–100 g sodium
      polystyrene sulfonate in 200 mL of 20% sorbitol.
    Can be repeated in 4–6 hours.
If necessary, consider urgent removal of potassium.
    Hemodialysis

K E Y   P O I N T S

▶ In hospitalized patients who develop ARF, the most likely causes are prerenal or tubular insults.

▶ In ARF, the urinalysis and FE_{Na} can help distinguish between prerenal or tubular etiologies.

▶ ARF with oliguria requires careful monitoring of fluid balance and a potassium restriction in both the diet and IV fluids.

CASE 32–3. A 46-year-old man is involved in a motor vehicle accident and sustains multiple fractures and a head injury. He requires mechanical ventilation, operative repair of the fractures, antibiotics, and transfusions. On the eighth hospital day, he develops fever, hypotension, and oliguria. His serum creatinine level rises, suggesting ARF.

    A. What are the possible etiologies of his ARF?
    B. How would you begin your evaluation?
    C. What treatment would you initiate?

ELECTROLYTE DISTURBANCES

SODIUM

▶ **ETIOLOGY**

What causes hypernatremia?

Hypernatremia is caused by lack of or inability to obtain water, by excess sodium in the plasma, or by renal water loss. Inadequate water intake is probably the most common cause, occurring in post-operative or debilitated patients. Reduced thirst can in rare cases result from destruction of the osmoreceptors that regulate thirst; this can occur from tumors or granulomatous involvement, vascular injuries, trauma, inflammation, developmental defects, or degenerative lesions of the hypothalamus. Hypernatremia may also result from hypertonic sodium administration such as sodium bicarbonate or hypertonic saline. Occasionally, inadequate pituitary secretion of antidiuretic hormone (ADH) (central diabetes insipidus) or interference with the kidney's response to ADH (nephrogenic diabetes insipidus) causes inability to concentrate the urine maximally, leading to hypernatremia (Table 32–9).

    Increased renal water loss is seen with the use of diuretics or secondary to an osmotic diuresis that can occur with dextrose, mannitol, high-protein tube feeding, or IV hyperalimentation.

What causes hyponatremia?

Reduced serum sodium concentration usually indicates a hypo-osmolar state or a shift of free water to the extracellular fluid due to hyperglycemia. For every 100 mg/dL rise above the normal glucose concentration of 100 mg/dL, the serum sodium concentration falls 1.6 mEq/L.

TABLE 32–9

Causes of Nephrogenic Diabetes Insipidus

Renal disease: renal failure, amyloidosis, sickle cell disease, light chain disease, Sjögren's
  syndrome, obstructive uropathy, pyelonephritis, acute tubular necrosis, lead nephropathy
Pregnancy
Metabolic: hypokalemia, hypercalcemia
Drug induced: lithium, demeclocycline, amphotericin B, loop diuretics
Osmotic diuresis
Familial

True hypotonic hyponatremia can be categorized by volume status as hypovolemic, euvolemic, or hypervolemic. In hypovolemic hyponatremia, sodium losses exceed volume losses, as occurs in certain renal and gastrointestinal (GI) losses (i.e., thiazide diuretics or diarrhea). With hypervolemic hyponatremia, patients have total body sodium excess with greater excess of body water mainly in the interstitial space, but the effective circulating arterial volume is decreased, thus producing edema with altered systemic hemodynamics. Hyponatremia with normal volume occurs most often from an inappropriate release of ADH with no stimulus for sodium retention or from psychogenic polydipsia. The causes of the syndrome of inappropriate ADH (SIADH) are listed in Table 32–10.

▶ EVALUATION

How do patients with sodium disturbances present?

The clinical signs of chronic hypernatremia include thirst, dehydration, weakness, and neurologic findings, including coma. Acute hypernatremia can cause intracranial hemorrhage and venous sinus thrombosis.

TABLE 32–10

Causes of Syndrome of Inappropriate Antidiuretic Hormone

Pulmonary disease: lung abscess, severe pneumonia, mechanical ventilation with PEEP,
  tuberculosis
Tumor: renal cell, small cell lung carcinoma, leukemia, Hodgkin's disease
CNS disorders: meningitis, encephalitis, tumor, abscesses, subarachnoid hemorrhage,
  cerebrovascular accident
Drugs: carbamazepine, oxytocin, thiazide diuretics, antipsychotics, chlorpropamide, vincristine,
  cyclophosphamide, clofibrate, NSAIDs
Endocrine disorders: primary adrenal failure, hypothyroidism

PEEP, positive end-expiratory pressure; CNS, central nervous system; NSAID, nonsteroidal anti-inflammatory drug.

Symptoms of hyponatremia include confusion, disorientation, nausea, diarrhea, and anorexia due to brain swelling. Seizures or coma may occur with severe or rapidly developing hyponatremia.

What tests help differentiate diagnoses in sodium disturbances?

In hypernatremia, reduced volume of highly concentrated urine suggests impaired water intake. On the other hand, polyuria, defined as urine output exceeding 3 L/day, can reflect water diuresis or solute (osmotic) diuresis. Once osmotic diuresis (urine osmolality >1200 mOsm/day) is excluded, polyuria is due to either diabetes insipidus or primary polydipsia. Accurate diagnosis may require an overnight water deprivation test and the administration of exogenous ADH (vasopressin).

The presence of volume depletion and excess allows for the categorization of hyponatremia. Measurement of urinary sodium is helpful in establishing the route of sodium wasting; urine sodium is greater than 20 mEq/L in renal wasting disorders and less than 10 mEq/L in GI losses. The laboratory features of SIADH include low blood urea nitrogen (BUN), creatinine, and uric acid, as well as urinary sodium greater than 40 mEq/L.

> ▶ **TREATMENT**

How do I treat hypernatremia?

Repair of solute excess or deficit should begin prior to correction of the relative water deficit; then calculate the free water deficit, which is equal to

$$[(serum\ sodium/140) - 1] \times 0.6 \times weight\ in\ kilograms$$

Replacement of the total free water deficit with D-5-W over 36 to 48 hours should not reduce the sodium faster than 0.5 to 1 mEq per hour to avoid cerebral edema. Treatment of diabetes insipidus is correction of the underlying disorder, if possible. Central diabetes insipidus may respond to vasopressin or desmopressin, whereas treatment of nephrogenic diabetes insipidus includes thiazide diuretics and dietary sodium restriction.

How do I treat hyponatremia?

An attempt should be made to treat the underlying disorder. Initial treatment of mild euvolemic hyponatremia is restriction of total water intake. Severe hyponatremia with neurologic symptoms should be treated with hypertonic saline and loop diuretics. Treat hypovolemia with IV normal saline. Management of hypervolemic hyponatremia includes both salt and water restriction along with diuretics at the lowest doses to maintain the patient's comfort. Care should be taken to raise the serum sodium level judiciously (<1 mEq/L per hour) to a final value of not more than 130 mEq/L to avoid central pontine myelinolysis and permanent neurologic damage.

K E Y   P O I N T S

▶ Categorize hyponatremia by volume status.

▶ Treat sodium imbalances according to symptoms.

▶ Correct sodium imbalances no faster than 1 mEq/L per hour.

CASE 32–4. A 50-year-old woman weighing 80 kg has small cell lung cancer with a 1-week history of confusion and fatigue. The laboratory values show a plasma Na^+ of 100 mEq/L, Cl^- of 70 mEq/L, plasma osmolality (P_{osm}) of 205 mOsm/kg, and urinary osmolality of 500 mOsm/kg.

   A. What is the likely cause of this woman's hyponatremia?
   B. How would you correct her plasma sodium?

POTASSIUM

▶ ETIOLOGY

What causes hyperkalemia?

Fictitious hyperkalemia results from hemolysis during blood sample collection or from extreme thrombocytosis or leukocytosis. True hyperkalemia occurs with transcellular shift or release of potassium, excessive intake, or inadequate excretion (Table 32–11).

What causes hypokalemia?

Hypokalemia can be approached in a similar fashion to that of hyperkalemia. The mechanisms responsible include altered transcellular distribution into cells, inadequate intake of potassium, and excessive excretion from either GI or renal routes (Table 32–12).

TABLE 32–11

Causes of Hyperkalemia

Transcellular shift or release into ECF: vigorous exercise, acute metabolic or respiratory acidosis, administration of glucose in a diabetic, or β_2-receptor blockade, α-adrenergic stimulation, acute tumor lysis, rhabdomyolysis, or in vivo hemolysis
Excessive intake: increased dietary intake or salt substitutes, potassium-containing medications
Inadequate excretion: acute or chronic renal failure, hypoaldosteronism, inhibition of renin-angiotensin axis (β-blockers, ACE inhibitors, heparin, NSAIDs), potassium-sparing diuretics (spironolactone, amiloride, triamterene), renal parenchymal diseases with tubulointerstitial damage (partial obstruction, cyclosporine, lithium, sickle cell nephropathy)

ECF, extracellular fluid; ACE, angiotensin-converting enzyme; NSAID, nonsteroidal anti-inflammatory drug.

▶ EVALUATION

How do patients with potassium abnormalities present?

The clinical signs of both hyperkalemia and hypokalemia involve disturbances in cardiac, skeletal muscle, and nerve tissue. Hypokalemia causes impaired GI motility and muscle weakness. Cardiac alterations are less likely but may occur in patients receiving digoxin. If hyperkalemia is severe, paresthesias and weakness of the extremities may occur followed by flaccid paralysis and hypoventilation. The most serious consequences are cardiac arrhythmias.

What evaluation is needed for patients with hypokalemia?

Patients on offending medications (such as non-potassium-sparing diuretics) may not need further evaluation. If excessive potassium loss is suspected, timed urinary potassium measurement may help.

TABLE 32–12

Causes of Hypokalemia

Transcellular shift into cells: β-adrenergic stimulation (in asthma or for inhibition of labor), intravenous glucose in normal individuals or insulin in diabetics, bicarbonate administration, rapidly growing tumor
Inadequate intake: decreased dietary intake results in mild hypokalemia
Excessive excretion: diarrhea, renal losses including non-potassium-sparing diuretics, chronic metabolic acidosis and metabolic alkalosis, primary hyperaldosteronism, secondary hyperaldosteronism (congestive heart failure, cirrhosis, nephritic syndrome, Bartter's syndrome, vomiting), renal tubular disorders (renal tubular acidosis, postobstructive diuresis, multiple myeloma, amphotericin B, hypomagnesemia)

When hypokalemia is due to GI losses, urinary potassium excretion declines to less than 20 mEq/day; by definition, urinary potassium excretion exceeds this rate in renal causes of hypokalemia. In replacement-resistant hypokalemia, serum magnesium must be checked and replaced if low.

What electrocardiographic (ECG) findings suggest a potassium abnormality?

In hyperkalemia, peaked T waves progress to widened QRS complexes and later a sine-wave pattern as serum potassium concentration worsens. Hypokalemia causes flattened T waves, bradycardia, and the appearance of U waves.

▶ TREATMENT

How do I treat hyperkalemia?

For severe hyperkalemia or ECG changes, immediate treatment is necessary to avoid cardiac arrhythmias. Initially, IV calcium gluconate is given to stabilize cardiac membranes (it does not affect the potassium level). Immediately following this, parenteral glucose, insulin, and bicarbonate can be given to shift potassium into cells. Inhaled α-agonists are also effective in shifting potassium into cells. Finally, removal of potassium from the body is accomplished with loop diuretics, cation exchange resins (Kayexalate), and dialysis if necessary.

How do I treat hypokalemia?

For diuretic-induced hypokalemia, potassium chloride should be given, whereas hypokalemia caused by diarrhea and by renal tubular disorders should be treated with alkalinizing potassium salts. Most patients should be treated by oral administration of liquid solutions or tablets. For severe, symptomatic hypokalemia, potassium chloride may be given intravenously, no faster than 10 mEq/hr.

K E Y   P O I N T S

▶ **Think of potassium disorders by mechanism: transcellular shift, intake, and losses.**

▶ **Refractory hypokalemia may be due to coexistent hypomagnesemia.**

▶ **Check an ECG in hyperkalemia and treat according to findings.**

CASE 32–5. A 60-year-old man with chronic kidney disease was placed on an angiotensin-converting enzyme inhibitor along with his regimen of β-blocker to help control his hypertension. A week later he presented to you with weakness and palpitations. His laboratory values revealed a plasma Na^+ of 133 mEq/L, K^+ of 6.9 mEq/L, Cl^- of 101 mEq/L, HCO_3^- of 18 mEq/L, and creatinine of 3.3 mg/dL. An ECG was normal.

   A. What are the likely contributors to this man's hyperkalemia?
   B. How would you treat his hyperkalemia?
   C. If the patient was asymptomatic and there were no ECG changes, would your treatment be different?

CALCIUM

▶ ETIOLOGY

What causes hypercalcemia?

The causes of hypercalcemia are listed in Table 32–13. In ambulatory and young patients, hyperparathyroidism accounts for more than 90% of the cases, whereas among hospitalized and older patients, cancer is the most common cause (65%).

What causes hypocalcemia?

Causes of true hypocalcemia (low ionized calcium) are listed in Table 32–14. Apparent hypocalcemia occurs in states of hypoalbuminemia, because most serum calcium is bound to albumin. Total calcium drops by 0.8 mg/dL for every 1 mg/dL fall in albumin; however, free (ionized) calcium is not affected.

▶ EVALUATION

How do patients with calcium abnormalities present?

The symptoms of hypercalcemia are nonspecific and include fatigue, weakness, anorexia, depression, constipation, and abdominal pain (as in nephrolithiasis and, rarely, pancreatitis). Severe hypercalcemia may cause personality changes and even confusion and coma.

TABLE 32–13

Causes of Hypercalcemia (in order of prevalence)

Primary hyperparathyroidism
Drug induced (thiazide diuretics)
Malignancy
   Osteolytic metastasis (breast cancer)
   PTH-related hormone (lung cancer)
   Direct bone destruction (lymphoma)
Milk-alkali syndrome
Granulomatous disease (TB, sarcoidosis) with increased vitamin D levels
Immobilization
Hyperthyroidism

PTH, parathyroid hormone; TB, tuberculosis.

Acute symptoms of hypocalcemia include tetany, papilledema, and seizures. Dental changes, cataracts, and confusion are features of chronic hypocalcemia. Classic findings of tetany are Trousseau's sign (carpal spasm with blood pressure cuff inflation) and Chvostek's sign (facial twitching with tapping of the cheeks).

What evaluation is needed in patients with calcium derangements?

Available clinical data along with measurement of the serum intact parathyroid hormone (PTH), phosphate, and urinary calcium may help differentiate the many diseases of hypercalcemia. If there is no obvious malignancy and the PTH level is not elevated, check the serum levels of vitamin D.

For hypocalcemia, check albumin, magnesium, phosphate, PTH, vitamin D, and creatinine levels. PTH level is low with primary hypoparathyroidism and hypomagnesemia but elevated with other causes of hypocalcemia.

TABLE 32–14

Causes of Hypocalcemia

Hyperphosphatemia (renal failure, tumor lysis, rhabdomyolysis)
Acute pancreatitis
Hypoparathyroidism
Low magnesium
Vitamin D deficiency (renal failure)
Intravascular complexing with citrate (blood transfusions)

▶ TREATMENT

How do I treat hypercalcemia?

Always treat the underlying cause, if possible. Severe hypercalcemia should be treated with hydration, then furosemide, followed by bisphosphonates and calcitonin, if required. Hemodialysis should be considered in patients who have a serum calcium level higher than 18 mg/dL and neurologic symptoms.

How do I treat hypocalcemia?

Mild hypocalcemia can often be treated by increasing dietary calcium intake. Symptomatic hypocalcemia requires IV replacement with calcium gluconate or even more rapidly with calcium chloride. In patients who are refractory, check the serum magnesium level and replace the magnesium if low. Oral vitamin D and calcium carbonate may be necessary for treatment of hypoparathyroidism.

K E Y   P O I N T S

▶ Hypercalcemia is most likely caused by hyperparathyroidism or malignancy.

▶ If hypocalcemia is refractory, check serum magnesium level and correct as needed.

CASE 32–6. A 45-year-old man with peptic ulcer disease with a baseline creatinine of 1.2 mg/dL is found to have constipation and abdominal pain, with laboratory values showing a plasma Ca^{2+} of 11.7 mg/dL, HCO_3^- of 18 mEq/L, and creatinine of 2.7 mg/dL.

    A. What is the likely cause of this man's lab abnormalities?
    B. How would you treat him?

FLUID STATUS ASSESSMENT AND TREATMENT

What is the role of fluid assessment in surgery?

Fluid status assessment is an important and recurrent task in managing the surgical patient. The goal is to continuously provide optimal intravascular volume and thus avoid shock and maintain end-organ perfusion. Failure to perform a quick and accurate fluid status assessment may result in tissue hypoxia, leading to multiple organ failure and possibly death. Even the untrained person can identify obvious shock, but by then, even appropriate treatment may be too late. It takes careful assessment, training, and experience to identify beginning or minimal volume deficits, correction of which may prevent the shock and organ insults from occurring in the first place. Restated, early shock is difficult to diagnose, but treatment is readily effective; late-stage shock, after organ failure is imminent, is simple to diagnose, but treatment is usually ineffective.

What is the normal distribution of body fluids?

The body is composed mostly (60%) of water that resides in two separate components: intracellular and extracellular (Fig. 32–1). The extracellular fluid either is in the blood stream or lymphatics (intravascular) or bathes the cells (interstitial). Fluid shifts between the compartments are driven by ionic and osmotic gradients. Intracellular fluids have higher concentrations of potassium, magnesium, organic phosphates, and proteins (Fig. 32–2).

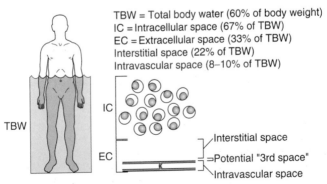

TBW = Total body water (60% of body weight)
IC = Intracellular space (67% of TBW)
EC = Extracellular space (33% of TBW)
Interstitial space (22% of TBW)
Intravascular space (8–10% of TBW)

Interstitial space
Potential "3rd space"
Intravascular space

Figure 32–1. Body fluid compartments: Normal body distribution of water. (From Adams GA, Bresnick S: On Call Surgery, 2nd ed. Philadelphia, WB Saunders, 2001, p 115.)

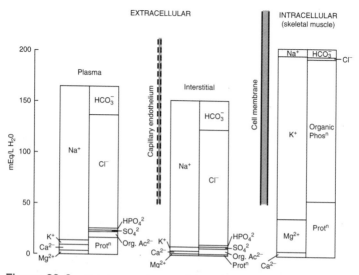

Figure 32–2. Solute constituents (electrolytes and others) of intracellular and extracellular fluid compartments. (From Lyerly HK, Gaynor JW: The Handbook of Surgical Intensive Care, 3rd ed. St. Louis, CV Mosby, 1992, p 404.)

What are body fluid requirements?

For homeostasis, adult surgical patients need about 1500 mL/m² of water per day to compensate for sensible (measurable) fluid losses (urine, feces, drains and tubes) and insensible (not measurable) losses (lungs, skin, open wounds). Fluid losses are increased by fever, tachypnea, vomiting, diarrhea, GI fistulas, large open wounds, and burns (Table 32–15).

How is fluid distribution affected by surgery or trauma?

Following cellular injury, capillary permeability increases and fluid shifts from the intravascular space to the interstitial space. These pathologic fluid shifts are called *third-space losses* and commonly follow surgery or other trauma. The volume of third-space loss is proportional to the cellular insult—it may exceed 10 L in major burns or severe pancreatitis. Because the shift occurs from the intravascular space, the intravascular fluid must be replaced. With resolution of the edema (usually several days after the insult), the third-space fluids are reabsorbed into the circulation.

TABLE 32-15

Daily Fluid and Electrolyte Losses

Losses	H₂O (mL/day)	Na⁺ (mEq/day)	K⁺ (mEq/day)
Sensible Losses			
Urine	800–1500	10–150	50–80
Stool	0–250	0–20	Trace
Sweat	0–100	10–60	0–10
Insensible Losses			
Lungs	250–450	—	—
Skin	250–450	—	—
Total Output	**1300–2750**	**20–230**	**50–90**

What are the clinical signs of fluid overload?

A presumptive diagnosis of fluid overload can be made based on a history of excess fluid intake or previous heart failure and symptoms of dyspnea and orthopnea. Fluid overload leads to tachypnea, jugular venous distention, pitting edema, rales on lung auscultation, and, in adults, an S_3 murmur (dull low-pitched early diastolic, heard best at the cardiac apex with patient in the left lateral decubitus position).

What are the clinical signs of fluid depletion?

Findings of thirst, vomiting, diarrhea, oliguria, and presence of a major burn can predict hypovolemia.

Examination should evaluate for orthostatic vital sign changes, mucous membranes, tearing, skin turgor, capillary refill, and neck veins and include auscultation of the heart and lungs. Hypovolemia results in tachycardia, hypotension, dry mucous membranes, skin tenting, capillary refill greater than 2 seconds, flat neck veins, and, especially in children, an overall ill appearance. Decreased pulse pressure (systolic minus diastolic) may be a sign of acute hypovolemia.

To some extent, the degree of chronic dehydration can be determined from the clinical signs. Thirst with few other clinical signs predicts a 2% body weight water deficit. Severe thirst, dry mouth, and low urine output predicts a 6% deficit. With mental status changes and weakness, assume at least a 7% to 15% deficit.

What is the difference between intravascular fluid changes and total body fluid changes?

Recognize that total body fluid states and intravascular volume states are different.

Some clinical signs (loss of skin turgor; dry axillae, tongue, and mucous membranes; lethargy) denote chronic body fluid depletion. Others result from the autonomic response to acute intravascular volume loss (cool, clammy skin; agitation). Others simply denote inadequate intravascular volume (tachycardia, hypotension, postural changes). A patient does not need to be total-body depleted to be hypovolemic. For example, a patient with severe pancreatitis and third-space sequestration who has been partially fluid resuscitated may be total-body "fluid overloaded" (increased body weight and edema) but still be hypovolemic (inadequate intravascular volume).

How reliable are these clinical signs?

Clinical parameters are helpful in making an initial assessment that a major fluid problem exists, especially in chronic and subacute conditions. In the acute setting, and especially in the intensive care unit (ICU), they are not so helpful. Numerous studies have shown that even the normal-appearing patient can be grossly under-resuscitated, and large volumes can be lost before vital signs change (Table 32–16). The interactions of pulse, blood pressure, flow, and volume are extremely complex, and obvious changes occur only after failure of compensatory mechanisms. Young patients especially may compensate for fluid loss without much change in vital signs until a limit is reached when compensatory mechanisms fail and the patient rapidly decompensates. Elderly patients, especially those taking β-blockers, may not demonstrate a tachycardia in response to hypovolemia.

In the ICU patient, clinical signs of fluid overload (jugular venous distention, crackles on auscultation, and peripheral edema) alone are

TABLE 32–16

Estimated Fluid and Blood Losses*

	Class I	Class II	Class III	Class IV
Blood loss (mL)	<750	750–1500	1500–2000	>2000
Blood loss (% blood volume)	<15	15–30	30–40	>40
Pulse rate (beats/min)	<100	>100	>120	>140
Blood pressure	Normal or increased	Decreased	Decreased	Decreased
Respiratory rate (breaths/min)	14–20	20–30	30–40	>35
Urine output (mL/hr)	>30	20–30	5–15	<5
Central nervous system /mental status	Slightly anxious	Mildly anxious	Anxious and confused	Confused and lethargic
Fluid replacement	Crystalloid	Crystalloid	Crystalloid and blood	Crystalloid and blood

*Based on the initial presentation of the patient (70-kg man).

not reliable indicators of intravascular volume. A thorough assessment of the patient's history (including intake and output data, weight changes, urine output changes), examination (including vital sign changes, breathing pattern, systolic blood pressure variations), and response to fluid bolus may be sufficient, but often an accurate estimate requires more invasive hemodynamic monitoring.

What are the laboratory signs of altered fluid status?

Lab findings of volume status may also be difficult to interpret. A decreased hematocrit may be a sign of blood loss (hypovolemia), but the hematocrit in a rapidly bleeding patient remains normal until equilibration occurs with other body compartments. An increased hematocrit may indicate dehydration (also hypovolemia). Electrolytes may be normal in a patient with hypovolemia from bleeding or isotonic fluid loss. Rising BUN and creatinine levels may indicate poor renal perfusion from hypovolemia but may also represent renal failure from other causes. A rising BUN/creatinine ratio may point toward volume depletion.

Decreasing urine volumes associated with increased color and density may indicate hypovolemia or the acute onset of renal failure. FE_{Na} may help in the differentiation (see section on Acute Renal Failure; see Table 32–6). It is important to obtain an accurate recording of urine output in any patient for whom fluid status is in question. Placement of a urinary catheter (Foley) is a safe and rapid approach to this.

Chest radiography findings of hypervolemia (pleural effusions, septal lines, peribronchial cuffing, redistribution of lung densities) are not reliable indicators in the portable supine films of ICU patients, although vascular pedicle width and cardiothoracic ratio may be. An incidental finding on computed tomography of decreased inferior vena cava diameter may indicate severe hypovolemia.

What other measures can be used to assess fluid status?

When fluid status is not clear from clinical and laboratory parameters, and especially when the patient has not responded appropriately to initial fluid resuscitation, invasive hemodynamic monitoring is indicated. Placement of a CVP catheter is usually the first step, although pulmonary artery catheters give a more accurate measure of left heart filling pressures. However, even both of these measure pressure as a surrogate for volume, and both have been shown to misrepresent volume status in many clinical situations. Changes in cardiac output and systemic venous oxygen saturation may be more sensitive indicators. Other measures of resuscitation—such as thoracic bioelectrical impedance analysis, tissue oxygenation, and gastric tonometry—have not proved reliable enough for widespread clinical use.

The best measure of adequacy of resuscitation may be the physiologic response to a fluid bolus. A rapid IV fluid challenge of

500 or 1000 mL has little risk; if it results in improvement in clinical parameters or cardiac output, fluids clearly are indicated. The response of CVP or pulmonary artery measurements may also be a clue to fluid status: a transient rise with return to near baseline shortly after a fluid bolus indicates that yet more fluids will be well tolerated. Numerous studies have shown that despite fulfilling many of our standard criteria for adequate fluid resuscitation, many patients still have occult hypovolemia and hypoperfusion and that correction of this deficit improves outcome.

What is the role for diuretics in assessment of fluid status?

Although diuretics are sometimes given to patients with decreasing urine output, their use may unknowingly exacerbate a hypovolemic state, precipitating renal failure and shock. Even hypovolemic patients may respond to furosemide with a brisk diuresis, so this response is not helpful in diagnosing the fluid status. Oliguria is not a sign of diuretic deficiency.

What are the options in fluid replacement?

Crystalloids are electrolyte-containing solutions that are available in a wide variety of combinations (Table 32–17). Crystalloids given intravenously into the intravascular compartment equilibrate with the other compartments, such that the patient in shock from blood loss may require three times the volume of crystalloid infusion replacement to maintain normovolemia.

Colloids contain large molecules that do not penetrate membranes and thus remain in the vascular space. Hetastarch, dextran, and albumin are examples. Colloid blood products (e.g., fresh frozen plasma, cryoprecipitate, platelets) have the same effect but are limited in supply, may carry blood-borne diseases, and should be used only to correct a specific coagulation defect.

Blood transfusions are usually given in the form of packed red blood cells. Depending on the urgency, give universal donor (O Rh-negative, which is immediately available), type specific (e.g., A Rh-positive, which is availabe in 15 to 30 minutes), or cross-matched blood that is tested against the patient's serum for the presence of hemolytic antibodies (allow 45 minutes for cross match).

In general, fluids lost are replaced with the same fluids—a rapidly bleeding patient needs red blood cell replacement. Numerous studies have demonstrated no clear benefit of colloids over crystalloids in shock resuscitation. Crystalloids are more easily available and much less expensive; therefore, Ringer's lactate solution and normal saline are the usual fluids of choice.

How do I determine initial fluid orders?

The goal of IV fluid therapy is to maintain normovolemia; deficits should be corrected rapidly without causing fluid overload. Patients

TABLE 32-17

Electrolyte Composition (in mEq/L) of Commercially Available Intravenous Solutions

	Na⁺	Cl⁻	K⁺	HCO₃⁻	Ca²⁺	Osmolality	pH	Calories/L
Crystalloid								
0.9% NaCl (NS)	154	154				292	5	
0.9% NaCl + 5% dextrose (D-5-NS)	154	154				565	5	200
0.45% NaCl (1/2 NS)	77	77				146		
0.45% NaCl + 5% dextrose (D-5-1/2 NS)	77	77				420		200
0.2% NaCl + 5% dextrose (D-5-1/4 NS)	34	34				330		200
D-5-W						274	4	200
D-10-W						548		400
Ringer's lactate	130	109	4	(28)	3	277	6.5	
3% NaCl	513	513				960		
Colloid								
Hetastarch	154	154				310	5.5	
55 Plasma protein factor	145	100	0.25				6–7	

in overt shock should receive volume as rapidly as possible until hemodynamic measures are normal. Aggressive hemodynamic monitoring is indicated in these patients. For more stable patients, deficits should be calculated and then replaced over 24 to 48 hours, beginning by replacing half of the deficit in 6 to 8 hours and then reassessing the patient.

Fluid losses commonly occur in surgical patients and should be corrected prior to induction of anesthesia, which may precipitate shock in a hypovolemic patient.

K E Y   P O I N T S

▶ Significant abnormalities in fluid status can be hidden by apparently normal vital signs until rapid decompensation occurs.

▶ Third-space losses in the surgical patient should be anticipated and aggressively treated.

continued

> ▶ Crystalloids are fluids of choice in the treatment of shock.
>
> ▶ The best measure of fluid status may be the physiologic response to a fluid bolus.

CASE 32–7. A 60-year-old man is being admitted with a 12-hour history of vomiting, crampy abdominal pain, an exam that reveals abdominal distention, hyperactive cavernous bowel sounds, and diffuse tenderness. A plain abdominal film shows multiple loops of distended air-filled small bowel. Electrolytes are normal. He is scheduled to go to the operating room in 4 hours for treatment of his small bowel obstruction.

A. How would you manage his fluids?

CASE 32–8. A 55-year-old woman is now 2 days following colostomy for perforated sigmoid diverticulitis with fecal peritonitis. She received aggressive fluid resuscitation and is 5 kg over admission weight. Her pulse is 108 beats/min and the blood pressure is 110/70 mm Hg. Urine output was 10 mL in the last hour. A recent arterial blood gas showed pH of 7.34, Pco_2 of 38, and Po_2 of 92 on 60% oxygen and 5 cm of positive end-expiratory pressure. Her CVP is 5 (normal = –2 to +6) and pulmonary artery occlusion (wedge) pressure is 10 (normal = 2 to 12).

A. What fluid orders are most appropriate?

33

Surgical Nutrition

Improvements in the care of critically ill and trauma patients have increased the need to evaluate and support surgical patients' nutritional status for prolonged periods of time. Greater numbers of severely injured trauma patients are surviving longer, often with prolonged ventilatory support and intensive care unit (ICU) stays.

The relationship between patients' prehospital nutritional status and complication rates in the perioperative period has long been recognized. Recent data have linked nutritional status and manipulations of nutritional support to preventing immune depression, maintaining the gut barrier to bacteria, and modifying the systemic inflammatory response syndrome (SIRS). Patients with liver or kidney disease, previously not thought to be candidates for surgery, are an increasing percentage of surgical practice. These patients do better in terms of survival, complications, and return to preoperative baseline functioning if their nutritional needs are supported during their hospitalization. Because of this, an understanding of nutritional support needs to be a priority in the care of the surgical patient.

▶ EVALUATION

How do I identify a patient at preoperative risk of protein-calorie malnutrition?

A careful medical and dietary history can identify patients at risk. Patients are at significant risk for an increase in complication rate if they have lost more than 10 pounds or 10% of their body weight in the immediate preoperative period. For example, the elderly are often significantly malnourished without the antecedent weight loss that is often seen in cancer patients. Patients with kidney or liver disease often have specific deficiencies in trace elements, protein, or vitamins that can contribute to poor nutritional status and increase specific complication risks. Patients with gastrointestinal (GI) obstruction, chronic vomiting, or chronic diarrhea may present malnourished, as well as have electrolyte abnormalities that should be addressed before undergoing surgery. A patient can be suffering from protein-calorie malnutrition even in the presence of obesity, and a severe degree of malnutrition can affect the surgical course.

On physical examination, look at the fit of their clothing to assess for recent changes in weight. Skin changes or loss of muscle mass in the temporal region or in the intrinsic muscles of the hand can clue you in to dietary deficiencies. Abnormalities in routine laboratory tests, including complete blood count (CBC), electrolyte panel, liver function tests, clotting tests, albumin, and transferrin, can alert you to occult protein-calorie malnutrition. Many times the patients who are severely malnourished are in urgent or emergent need of surgical intervention and cannot have their nutritional status improved prior to surgery. Elective or semi-elective procedures should be delayed to allow interventions to improve nutritional status if possible.

A list of abnormalities that should alert you to possible malnutrition is contained in Table 33–1. Some of the findings are nonspecific and others reflect a deficiency of a vitamin or trace element that often accompanies protein-calorie malnutrition.

Which patients should receive supplemental nutrition in the hospital?

Any patient that you anticipate will be unable to eat a meal for more than 7 days should be considered for nutritional support.

TABLE 33–1

Features Associated with Patients at Nutritional Risk

History
Recent weight loss of ≥10 lb or 10% body weight
Surgical condition predisposing to ↓ oral intake or ↑ diarrhea
Underlying medical condition (ESRD, cirrhosis, CHF)
Advanced age
Chemotherapy or radiation therapy
Social: Lack of economic or physical support systems in the home

Physical Exam
Skin: dry texture, rash, hyperkeratosis, nail deformities
Mouth: cheilosis, glossitis, mucosal atrophy, poor dentition
Hair: texture, recent loss, loss of pigmentation
Heart: JVD, enlarged heart, gallop
Abdomen: hepatomegaly, ascites, abdominal mass, fistula
Neurologic: peripheral neuropathy, dorsolateral column deficit
Muscular/extremities: temporal, or extremity muscle wasting, pedal edema

Laboratory Tests
CBC: thrombocytopenia, ↓ hematocrit, ↑ MCV, ↓ WBC, ↓ total lymphocyte count (<1000/mm^3)
Electrolyte abnormalities associated with ESRD or chronic GI losses
Liver function tests: transaminases, bilirubin, or alkaline phosphatase, ↑ PT/INR, ↓ albumin
    (normal, 4.5–3.5; moderate malnutrition, 3.5–2.5; severe malnutrition, <2.5 g/dL)

CBC, complete blood count; CHF, congestive heart failure; ESRD, end-stage renal disease; GI, gastrointestinal; JVD, jugular vein distention; MCV, mean corpuscular volume; PT/INR, prothrombin time/International Normalized Ratio; WBC, white blood cell count.

The route of delivery depends on the clinical status of the patient. There is mounting evidence that enteral feeding may in fact help to modify the SIRS response and improve the gut mucosal barrier against bacterial translocation into the blood stream; thus, it is the preferred mode of nutritional support. However, many surgical patients cannot receive nutrition through the GI tract owing to postoperative ileus, enterocutaneous fistulas, severe inflammation within the abdominal cavity, or intolerance of enteral feeding for other reasons. These patients should not be allowed to become malnourished while they await an improvement in GI function and should be started on total parenteral nutrition (TPN) feeds via a central venous catheter. Administration of nutrition via a peripheral line (peripheral parenteral nutrition [PPN]) cannot provide the nutritional support needed for complete nutrition in patients under surgical or traumatic stress, and the formulations are irritating to peripheral veins. PPN is not an optimal method of supplementing nutrition to those patients who are severely malnourished or need complete nutritional support.

How do I know how many calories the patient needs?

The amount of calories needed by a patient can be estimated, calculated, or measured. Estimates of calorie and protein requirements based on the patient's weight and normal levels of stress are a reasonable starting point for most patients. For patients in whom specific stresses are present, the Harris-Benedict formula, based on the body surface area and sex of the patient, with modifications to account for stress and activity factors, may give a more accurate estimation of the caloric needs.

One way to ensure that you are providing enough calories and protein is to measure the nitrogen balance of the patient. The patient remains in negative nitrogen balance as long as the needs are not being met. Normal patients have an obligate negative nitrogen balance following surgery, but this is exacerbated and prolonged by postoperative complications or malnutrition.

The most accurate manner to measure the caloric requirements is to use indirect calorimetry, but this is not available in many centers, and this degree of accuracy in calorie delivery is rarely necessary outside of the research setting.

To measure the relative amounts of carbohydrate and fat used for energy, a respiratory quotient (RQ) can be calculated. An RQ of 1.0 indicates that pure carbohydrate is being oxidized and an RQ of 0.7 results from burning only fat. Manipulation of the relative amount of calories derived from fat can be used in patients in whom severe sepsis and respiratory distress result in CO_2 retention.

Table 33–2 summarizes the commonly used formulas for determining the adequacy of nutritional support.

What are the options for enteral nutrition?

Enteral nutrition can be used to supplement the diets of patients who are able to eat but cannot take in sufficient calories to support their needs or may be used as the sole source of calories and protein. If the patients are well nourished, they will be able to tolerate

---

TABLE 33–2

Caloric Needs of Adults

Surgical and Trauma Patients

Estimated (male or female)
Calories
    25–30 kcal/kg (for weight loss)
    30–35 kcal/kg (for weight maintenance)
    35–40 kcal/kg (for weight gain)
Protein
    0.8–2 g/kg

Calculated: Modified Harris-Benedict formula
Male: $[66.5 + (13.7 \times \text{wt kg}) + (5 \times \text{ht cm}) - (6.7 \times \text{age yr})] \times \text{AF}^* \times \text{IF}^\dagger$
Female: $[66.5 + (13.7 \times \text{wt kg}) + (5 \times \text{ht cm}) - (6.7 \times \text{age yr})] \times \text{AF}^* \times \text{IF}^\dagger$
   *Activity factor (AF)
     Confined to bed   1.2
     Ambulatory   1.3
     Fever factor   1.3
   †Injury factor (IF)
     Surgery   1.1–1.2
     Infection   1.2–1.6
     Trauma   1.1–1.8
     Sepsis   1.4–1.8

Burn Patients

Estimated (male or female)
35–40 kcal/kg + 40 kcal/% body surface area (BSA) burn
Protein 1.5–2.5 g/kg

Calculated (for weight maintenance)
Male: $(25 \text{ kcal} \times \text{preburn wt} \times \text{BMR age factor}^\ddagger) + (40 \text{ kcal} \times \%\text{BSA burn})$
Female: $(22 \text{ kcal} \times \text{preburn wt} \times \text{BMR age factor}^\ddagger) + (40 \text{ kcal} \times \%\text{BSA burn})$
   ‡Basic metabolic rate (BMR) age factor
     20–40 yr   1.00
     40–50 yr   0.95
     50–75 yr   0.90
     > 75 yr   0.80

Measurements
Nitrogen intake = nitrogen intake – nitrogen output
Indirect calorimetry (Weir formula)
   Kcal/min = 3.9 (O_2 consumption) + 1.1 (CO_2 production – 2.2 (urine nitrogen)
Respiratory quotient (RQ)
   Nonprotein RQ = $[CO_2 \text{ production} - 4.8 \text{ (urine nitrogen)}] \div [O_2 \text{ consumption} - 5.9 \text{ (urine nitrogen)}]$

formulas that contain intact proteins. These supplements may be delivered orally, by nasoenteric access, or by direct enteric access, such as feeding jejunostomy or gastrostomy.

Patients with moderate to severe malnutrition or under severe metabolic stress are not able to absorb the nutrients from standard formulas. Special formulas, containing small-molecular-weight polypeptides or individual amino acids, are useful in this subset of patients. They are more expensive, however, and can produce a secretory diarrhea secondary to the high osmolarity; thus, it may take longer to advance the rate to the goal rate. The taste of these elemental formulas is usually not tolerated orally, and direct enteral access is required. As soon as the patient's condition improves, you should consider switching to a standard formula. There are special formulations specific for patients with medical problems, such as hepatic failure or renal failure, that limit the amount of protein and fluid. Likewise, for patients with diabetes there are formulations to help regulate hyperglycemia. Because these medical conditions often do not resolve as the patient's condition improves, the special formula should be maintained until the patient is tolerating the appropriate oral diet.

A sample table of enteral feeding formulations appears in Table 33–3; however, the specific brands of enteral nutrition will vary

---

TABLE 33–3

Enteral Feeding Formulations

Formulation Type	Trade Name
Standard isotonic (1 cal/mL)	Isocal, Ensure, Boost, Osmolite, Nutren 1.0, Resource standard
Standard with fiber (1 cal/mL)	Boost with Fiber, Ensure with Fiber, Ultracal, Nutren 1.0 with Fiber, Jevity
Standard high protein (1 cal/mL)	Boost High Protein, Osmolite HN, Ensure High Protein, Promote, Replete, Impact
Blenderized	Compleat
Calorie dense (1.5 cal/mL)	Boost Plus, Ensure Plus, Nutren 1.5, Resource Plus, Osmolite HN Plus, Pulmocare
Calorie dense (2 cal)	Deliver 2.0, TwoCal HN, Nutren 2.0
Glucose intolerance	Glytrol, Glucerna, Choice DM, Diabetisource
Hepatic	Nutrihep, Hepatic-Aid
Semi-elemental (1 cal/mL) (low albumin, poor absorption)	Peptamen, Criticare HN, Vital HN, Vivonex
Renal insufficiency (predialysis) (1 cal/mL)	Suplena, Renacal
Renal failure (on dialysis) (1 cal/mL)	Magnacal renal, Nepro
Immune enhancing	Immun-Aid, Impact, Stresson Multifibre
Standard pediatric (1 cal/mL)	Kindercal, PediaSure with Fiber
Semi-elemental pediatric (1 cal/mL)	Neocate
Protein module*	Promote, Casec
Carbohydrate module*	Polycose Powder, Moducal
Fat module*	Microlipid
Carbohydrate-fat mixture*	Duocal

*For use in pediatric patients with metabolic abnormalities.

from institution to institution. A formulary can be obtained from the pharmacy to help with administering enteral feeds. Most formulations have the proper ratio of calories from carbohydrates, fats, and proteins to provide a balanced diet. Standard formulas usually contain 1 kcal/mL. Concentrated formulas provide up to 2 kcal/mL for patients who require fluid restriction.

What role do vitamins and trace elements play in nutritional support?

The fat-soluble vitamins A, D, and E participate in wound healing and immune function. Vitamin K, which is stored in the liver, is essential for the production of certain clotting factors and should be supplied weekly in patients on parenteral nutrition. Baseline deficiencies of fat-soluble vitamins are rare, except in patients who have had a prehospitalization weight loss. Water-soluble vitamins such as the B vitamins, vitamin C, niacin, folate, biotin, and pantothenic acid serve as cofactors to many metabolic processes. Only vitamin B_{12} is stored to any extent, so these vitamins should be supplemented in parenteral nutrition. Intravenous multivitamin formulations such as M.V.I.-12 provide sufficient amounts of vitamins in patients unable to take enteric supplements. Trace elements, such as iron, zinc, copper, chromium, selenium, manganese, and molybdenum, play roles in metabolism, immune function, and wound healing and should be supplemented in patients on TPN. Trace elements are available in combination formulas such as Multitrace-5 Concentrate. Iodine is a key component of thyroid function, which is a part of the neuroendocrine response to stress and trauma. Chronically malnourished patients can be iodine deficient, so iodine should be included in TPN formulations. The vitamins and trace elements are included in enteral formulations, but if the patient is not receiving a goal rate of feeding, he or she may not receive sufficient quantities of these essential vitamins or elements.

Are all proteins alike?

Amino acids are the building blocks of proteins. There are 20 amino acids, divided into essential and nonessential amino acids. The essential amino acids cannot be manufactured by the body and thus must be provided in the diet. A lack of any one of the essential amino acids can lead to muscle catabolism and continued negative nitrogen balance in spite of adequate calorie delivery. Certain amino acids participate in metabolic processes that are important for patients under metabolic stress. For example, alanine and glutamine participate in a cycle that prevents the loss of carbon during starvation. Glutamine is thought to have trophic effects on the GI mucosa and may play a role in the maintenance of the mucosal barrier to bacterial translocation. Arginine, a semi-essential amino acid, enhances T-cell activation. Branch-chain amino acids are the preferred fuels for cardiac and skeletal muscle during starvation. Protein formulations in TPN and enteral nutritional formulas are balanced and complete, and rarely do specific amino acids need to be supplemented. The most common exception in practice is the addition of glutamine to enteral formulations for the intestinal trophic effect, as well as potential reduction in the stress response and septic complications in critically ill patients.

Do patients need fat in nutritional supplements?

Fat is a highly efficient way to deliver calories and is a component of all enteral nutritional supplements. Just as there are essential amino acids, there are essential fatty acids that the body cannot make for itself. Patients on TPN typically have lipid infusions three times per week to prevent essential fatty acid deficiency. Because you can deliver higher amounts of calories in less volume (2 kcal/mL), lipids are particularly useful in burn patients, who have extremely high caloric requirements secondary to the burn injury.

▶ TREATMENT

How do I start enteral nutrition?

Access to the GI tract must be established either (1) by nasoenteric tube, with the tip positioned in the first portion of the duodenum, or (2) by direct access via feeding gastrostomy or jejunostomy placed surgically or with the aid of endoscopy or interventional radiology. Direct access is preferred for patients in whom long-term supplementation can be anticipated (>4 weeks).

Standard formulations are usually iso-osmolar and thus can be started at full strength (approximately 40 mL/hr). The rate is then increased according to a schedule over the next few days until the patient has achieved a goal rate that will deliver the estimated or calculated protein and calorie requirements based on the modified Harris-Benedict formula. Hyperosmolar formulas should be started at quarter strength at 40 mL/hr, increased to half strength on day 2 at the same rate, then full strength on day 3 at the same rate. Much of the difficulty encountered in establishing enteral feeding in patients requiring complex or elemental formulations stems from starting at full strength or advancing to full strength too quickly, leading to setbacks and fluid shifts that these more critically ill patients cannot tolerate. Once the patient is tolerating the full-strength feeds at 40 mL/hr, the rate may be increased until reaching goal rate over the next few days.

The head of the bed should be elevated to 30% at all times when infusing enteral feeds to help prevent aspiration. Residual fluid should be checked every 4 hours, and the infusion should be stopped temporarily for residual fluid that exceeds 150 mL. Infusion may be restarted after 2 hours if the residual resolves.

How do I monitor patients with established enteral feeding?

Patients should have standard laboratory parameters checked once a week, including CBC, complete chemistry panel, copper, zinc, magnesium, transferrin, and triglyceride. Continued abnormalities in these values may indicate inadequate supplementation or may alert you to a patient who is not able to absorb standard formulations. These patients may need to be switched to a more elemental feeding formulation for a period. Patients may be intolerant to enteral nutritional supplementation for a variety of reasons. Sudden intolerance of enteral feeding presents as high residuals or back-up of enteral feeding into a nasogastric suction tube and can alert you to an occult intra-abdominal process.

What are the common complications of enteral nutrition?

Nausea, vomiting, and abdominal distention occur in 25% of patients on enteral tube feeds. Aspiration can occur even around a tracheostomy or cuffed endotracheal tube, so it is important to monitor the patient for signs of feeding intolerance. Diarrhea can occur in up to 60% of patients receiving enteral feedings. In evaluating a patient with diarrhea, it is important to rule out other causes such as medications or antibiotics or infectious etiologies, such as *Clostridium difficile* colitis. Diarrhea can also lead to severe fluid shifts and breakdown of the perianal and sacral skin in bedridden patients. The work-up should include imaging studies of the abdomen, because diarrhea is often the first sign of intra-abdominal abscess or fistula formation.

How do I start total parenteral nutrition (TPN)?

Central venous access needs to be established, most commonly through the subclavian vein or internal jugular vein. Once the proper positioning of the catheter is established radiographically, a standard TPN formulation can be started at 40 mL/hour. The standard TPN solution contains 15% to 25% glucose and 8.5% amino acids. A patient-specific goal rate of TPN should be achieved within 72 hours. Electrolyte abnormalities can be adjusted by manipulating the solute concentrations in the TPN, but electrolyte abnormalities in patients on TPN are commonly iatrogenic. Hyperglycemia is common in patients on TPN. Avoid huge changes in the electrolyte concentration or in additives such as insulin, because a miscalculation can result in having to throw away an entire day's worth of TPN at considerable cost and will lead to interruptions in nutrition. Never administer TPN as a fluid bolus to treat deficits in intravascular volume. The high-solute concentration causes an osmotic diuresis and exacerbates the hypovolemia.

How do I monitor patients while they are on TPN?

Patients on TPN need closer monitoring of electrolytes and blood glucose than patients placed on enteral feeding, because the potential for shifts is much greater. Patients often have hyperglycemia with the institution of TPN, and insulin should be administered using a sliding scale. Once the goal rate of TPN is achieved, the amount of insulin usage should be monitored over a 3-day period. If the amount of insulin usage is relatively constant, two thirds of the amount of daily insulin usage can be added to the next day's bag of TPN. Note that this calculation of insulin needs assumes that the patient is not hyperglycemic secondary to other causes such as line sepsis. When a patient has been on TPN for a longer period without problems or changes in the composition of the formula, standard labs may be checked once a week, including CBC, complete chemistry panel, copper, zinc, magnesium, transferrin, and triglyceride. The monitoring of patients on TPN must include monitoring for the common complications of TPN. These are mainly associated with the central venous catheter.

What are the complications of TPN?

Complications occur in 5% to 8% of patients receiving TPN, and the overall mortality is 0.2%. Complications during line placement include pneumothorax, hemothorax, and arterial puncture. Air embolus can occur when a line is being placed, when it becomes accidentally disconnected, or when it is removed. Life-threatening sepsis is the most serious complication associated with TPN, and meticulous care of the catheter and maintenance of a dedicated TPN port can reduce the incidence of this complication. When a line infection is suspected, the catheter should be replaced, preferably with a new stick at a different site. Exchange over a wire is acceptable in cases where blood cultures are negative but infection is suspected. Hyperglycemia that suddenly worsens or appears in a patient who has previously been stable can signal a potential line infection. This can occur even in the absence of the other common presenting features of fever, erythema, tenderness, or pus around the insertion site and should prompt a work-up or a line change. A flow chart for the management of line infection appears in Figure 33–1.

Patients on TPN can have severe iatrogenic electrolyte abnormalities and other metabolic derangements such as hyperosmolar nonketosis coma, metabolic acidosis, and liver function test abnormalities consistent with cholestasis. Meticulous attention to fluid status, insulin needs, and major and minor electrolyte levels is critical, particularly at the institution of TPN. Patients on prolonged TPN may experience deficiencies in vitamins and trace elements if they are not checked on a periodic basis.

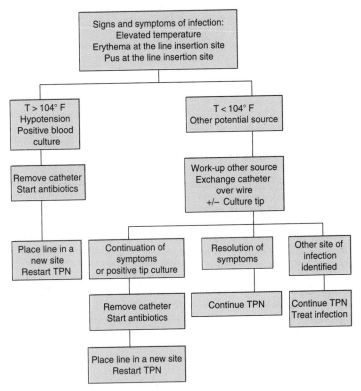

Figure 33–1. Algorithm for the management of line infections associated with total parenteral nutrition (TPN) administration.

What are immune-enhancing diets?

Malnourishment or catabolism caused by trauma, sepsis, or surgical stressors can lead to impairment of immune function. The effect can be the result of an overall deficiency in caloric intake or deficiencies in specific components of the diet such as trace elements, vitamins, omega-3 fatty acids, or specific amino acids that enhance the integrity of the gut barrier to bacterial translocation. Practically all forms of immunity may be affected by deficiencies in one or more of these nutrients. Animal and human studies have demonstrated that adding the deficient nutrient back to the diet can restore immune function and resistance to infection. Vitamins C and E and zinc are the most studied micronutrients that affect immune function, but omega-3 fatty acids, selenium, copper, and vitamins B_6 and B_{12} have also been found to affect the immune system in experimental models.

There are many formulations that have what are considered optimal immune-enhancing combinations of proteins, calories, and micronutrients. There are some preliminary studies that demonstrate that these formulations can produce measurable differences in parameters of immune function when compared with standard complete nutrition formulations, but the impact on the outcomes of critically ill surgical patients as measured by decreased length of stay and decreased morbidity and mortality is not yet fully understood.

K E Y P O I N T S

▶ Nutritional support is a high priority for all surgical patients. It supports many of the functions that determine the complexity of the perioperative course and the eventual outcome, such as wound healing and immune function.

▶ Although enteral nutritional support is the preferred route of supplementation, it is common for the surgical or trauma patient to have conditions that preclude its use.

▶ Modern formulations of enteral and parenteral nutrition can allow you to lessen the impact of underlying medical conditions on the perioperative course.

▶ There is compelling evidence to suggest that we can manipulate nutritional parameters to improve patient outcomes and reduce perioperative complications.

CASE 33–1. A 20-year-old man is an unrestrained passenger in a motor vehicle accident. His injuries include a lumbar spine injury with a near-complete cord transection at L1–2, multiple rib fractures on the left side, a splenic rupture requiring exploratory laparotomy and splenectomy, and a grade 2 liver laceration that was able to be controlled without resection. He had a massive fluid resuscitation in the trauma bay and the operating room. He returns to the ICU intubated and sedated. His admission weight is 74 kg and his height is 6 ft, 2 in (188 cm).

A. What are his estimated caloric needs and the calculated caloric requirements?
B. What are his daily protein requirements?
C. What would be the best route of nutrition and when should you start feeding?

CASE 33–2.

A 68-year-old man presents to your office with progressive dysphagia. He has lost 40 lb in the last 3 months. He had a mid-esophageal adenocarcinoma identified by his gastroenterologist, who was unable to pass the endoscope distal to the tumor in the mid-esophagus. His work-up reveals that tumor is encasing the left pulmonary artery and left main stem bronchus. The medical oncologist would like to try neoadjuvant therapy to see if the tumor can be shrunk to the point that a resection can be considered.

  A. What are his options for nutritional access?

  B. How do you assess the degree of malnutrition in this patient?

Two months later he has completed his neoadjuvant therapy with what appears to be a complete response to the therapy by computed tomographic scan and you are considering resection. He has gained only 10 lb because of debilitating nausea and diarrhea secondary to his chemotherapy.

  C. How will you handle his nutrition perioperatively?

34

Surgical Oncology

The field of surgical oncology is broad and spans many of the chapters in this text. Specific cancers of the gastrointestinal tract, the lung, or the thyroid gland, for example, are addressed in those chapters. This chapter focuses on general principles and on melanoma and sarcoma.

GENERAL PRINCIPLES

What is cancer?

In a general sense, the term *cancer* describes any abnormal outgrowth of cells that no longer follow normal developmental pathways of clonal expansion and differentiation. This may include proliferation of an immature cell type, lack of inhibition due to geographic boundaries, or abnormal clonal immortality.

What is Surgical Oncology?

Surgical Oncology is part of the medical armamentarium against cancer, which also includes Medical Oncology and Radiation Oncology and many ancillary services. The goal of any cancer treatment is the cooperative approach to screening, diagnosis, staging, humane treatment, and follow-up of a variety of neoplastic diseases. Not all cancers are amenable to surgical treatment, but some rely heavily on surgical extirpation for disease control or cure. Up to 55% of cancer patients have a surgical approach to their disease.

Cancer surgery is based on the principle that control of the primary site of tumor growth can diminish the chance of subsequent distal spread.

What are the principles of the surgical treatment of cancer?

The surgical approach to cancer follows some basic rules to minimize the chance of local or distant recurrence.

Excise the entire tumor when possible.
  Do not leave neoplastic tissue behind if at all possible. Make the incision large enough to facilitate removal of the mass. Excise an

appropriate margin of "normal" tissue surrounding the tumor. The extent of this margin is based on the type of tumor and other functional and cosmetic factors.

Avoid spilling tumor cells back into the body.
It is best to avoid any tissue planes that contain tumor. Avoid cutting across the tumor, protect the wound edges, and change gloves and instruments after contamination with tumor cells. Cytotoxic solutions have been used to wash the operative site, but many of these have offered no advantage.

Avoid vascular spread.
Manipulation of the tumor during resection greatly increases the chance of hematogenous spread. Limit handling of the mass ("no-touch" technique). Identify outgoing vasculature and perform early ligation of these vessels.

What are tumor markers?

Tumor markers are molecules measurable in the serum that are associated with the presence or recurrence of a specific tumor type. The specificity and sensitivity for each marker vary. Although the presence of a measurable marker has greatly facilitated the diagnosis of many tumors, most are not reasonable as screening tests. A list of the more common markers is listed in Table 34–1.

MELANOMA

▶ ETIOLOGY

What is melanoma?

Melanoma results from malignant transformation of melanin-producing cells. Melanocytes are of neural crest origin and are present throughout the body, especially in the skin, mucous membranes, eyes, upper esophagus, and meninges.

Melanoma is most commonly associated with presentation in the skin, though it can occur anywhere that melanocytes are present. It accounts for 4% to 5% of all skin cancers. Although not common, it occurs in young patients and is second only to leukemia in killing cancer patients 15 to 34 years of age.

What are the risk factors for development of melanoma?

Risk factors involved in the development of melanoma include the following:

TABLE 34-1

Common Tumor Markers

Marker	Associated Tumor Types	Associated Nonmalignant Conditions
α-Fetoprotein	Hepatocellular, testicular	Hepatitis, cirrhosis, pregnancy, IBD
β-Human chorionic gonadotropin	Trophoblastic tumors, testicular	Pregnancy
CA 15–3	Breast	Hepatitis, cirrhosis, benign breast disease
CA 19–9	Colorectal, pancreatic, stomach	Hepatitis, cirrhosis, sclerosing cholangitis, other cholestatic disease
CA 50	Colorectal, pancreatic, stomach	Pancreatitis, cirrhosis, sclerosing cholangitis, ulcerative colitis
CA 125	Ovarian, gynecologic tumors	Pancreatitis, jaundice, pregnancy, menstruation, endometriosis, PID, renal insufficiency
CA 242	Colorectal, pancreatic, stomach	Pancreatitis, cirrhosis, sclerosing cholangitis, ulcerative colitis
Carcinoembryonic antigen	Colorectal, pancreatic, breast, lung, stomach	Hepatitis, cirrhosis, hyperbilirubinemia, peptic ulcer, pancreatitis, IBD, renal insufficiency, COPD
erb B-2	Breast, ovarian, stomach	—
Prostate-specific antigen	Prostatic	Benign prostatic hypertrophy, prostatic massage or biopsy

COPD, chronic obstructive pulmonary disease; IBD, inflammatory bowel disease; PID, pelvic inflammatory disease.

Several sunburns in early life
Celtic heritage
Dysplastic nevus syndrome
Xeroderma pigmentosa
Family history of melanoma

The only identified preventable risk factor is sun exposure, and it is important to recommend the use of sunblock to patients at risk.

▶ **EVALUATION**

How is melanoma identified?

Melanoma on the skin usually presents as a new skin lesion or as a change in an existing mole. Changes might include growth, change in color, irregularity or the borders, or ulceration. Lesions may also bleed. Changes that should be considered important are abbreviated by the acronym ABCDE:

A: Asymmetry
B: Border irregularity

C: Change in color
D: Diameter exceeding 6 mm
E: Elevation from the skin

What are the histologic variants of melanoma?

Four histopathologic variants are identified: (1) lentigo maligna; (2) superficial spreading; (3) acral lentiginous; and (4) nodular. All spread in a horizontal fashion except the nodular variant.

Lentigo Maligna Melanoma. This variant is found in sun-exposed regions of the skin, especially the face, and is characterized by presentation in the sixth through eighth decades of life. This lesion tends to be thin and has a relatively good prognosis. A lesion may typically arise from a brown macular lesion called a Hutchinson's freckle.

Superficial Spreading Melanoma. This is the most common histologic variant. It tends to grow radially (horizontally) for a time before it grows vertically into the skin.

Acral Lentiginous Melanoma. This lesion is associated with the palms, soles, and nails. It has a poor prognosis.

Nodular Melanoma. This lesion does not grow radially; rather, vertical growth predominates. The margin tends to be more linear and uniform.

What are the prognostic features of melanoma?

The extent of spread is the most important prognostic feature. This includes both measurement of the vertical penetration of the tumor and assessment of lymphatic spread. The American Joint Committee on Cancer (AJCC) uses a staging system as listed in Table 34–2. This is based on a system developed by Breslow. A corollary system, developed earlier by Clark, is based on the depth of invasion relative to normal skin structures. Lesions of less than 0.76 mm are considered *thin* lesions; lesions of 0.76 to 4.0 mm are considered *intermediate* lesions; and lesions deeper than 4.0 mm are *thick* lesions. The

TABLE 34–2

Staging System for Melanoma

Stage	Thickness	Description
I	<1.5 mm	Localized
II	>1.5 mm	Localized
III	Any	Only 1 involved regional node basin, or 1–4 nodes in-transit
IV	Any	Advanced regional metastases or any distant metastasis

From Sabiston DC, Lyerly HK: Textbook of Surgery: The Biological Basis of Modern Surgical Practice, 15th ed. Philadelphia, WB Saunders, 1997, p. 521.

TABLE 34–3

Melanoma Mortality Rates Based on Lesion Penetration

Depth of Penetration (mm)	10-Year Mortality (%)
1	10–20
3	45
6	70

prognosis worsens with the depth of the lesion. The 10-year mortality based on penetration is shown in Table 34–3.

Other factors that affect outcome include age at presentation, whether the lesion is ulcerated, sex, race, site of presentation, and histologic characteristics.

How are initial lesions handled?

The most important first step is accurate diagnosis and staging. Any suspicious lesion should be evaluated with a full-thickness, excisional biopsy if possible. In cosmetically sensitive areas, an incisional biopsy may be taken that does not include the entire lesion as long as it obtains a full-thickness sample. There is no difference in outcome for these patients as long as the lesion is accurately staged and subsequently completely removed.

Careful examination of regional lymph node beds is an important part of the initial evaluation. Look for any enlarged or firm nodes.

▶ TREATMENT

How is the surgical site handled after the diagnosis of melanoma is made?

The surgical site should be handled with a wider, local excision of the site, with 2-cm margins. Margins of 1 cm may be used safely for lesions of 1-mm depth or less.

How are lymph node beds evaluated?

Lymphatic beds with clinically palpable nodes require exploration and biopsy. There has been much recent discussion on how to evaluate clinically negative lymph node beds. Some investigators believe that in cases of intermediate-thickness primary lesions, these lymph node beds should be evaluated by elective lymph node dissection (ELND). Because most thin lesions are unlikely to spread and most thick lesions have already manifested distant spread, neither of these groups benefit from ELND.

In the setting of clinically negative lymph node beds, most surgeons would start with lymphoscintigraphy to look for primary nodal drainage sites, then excise the "hot" node (sentinel lymph node biopsy).

How does melanoma recur?

When melanoma recurs, it does so in the following pattern:

Local: 16%
Regional lymph nodes: 60%
Distant: 24%

Distant spread is thought to occur hematogenously. Approximately 20% to 30% of patients with intermediate-thickness melanoma have recurrent disease within 5 years.

How is recurrent melanoma treated?

With any evidence of recurrence, the cancer should be restaged, and further treatment depends on the extent of the documented spread. Local recurrence, without lymphatic or distant spread, is treated with surgical excision. Margins wider than 2 cm are usually encouraged. If regional lymph nodes are affected without evidence of distant metastatic disease, a lymph node dissection of the affected bed is performed. This can greatly increase survival.

Distant metastatic spread is treated with systemic chemotherapy. Conventional cytotoxic regimens have only 20% to 40% response rates, however, and are considered palliative. The biologic modifier interferon-α2b has been used with reasonable success, with prolongation of time to relapse from 0.98 years to 1.7 years and prolongation of overall survival from 2.8 to 3.8 years in high-risk groups. With interferon-α2b treatment, overall 5-year survival has increased from 36% to 47%.

K E Y   P O I N T S

▶ The only controllable risk factor for the development of melanoma is sun exposure.

▶ The key to diagnosis is a high suspicion and observation of existing skin lesions.

▶ Prognosis is based on the depth of skin invasion and lymph node spread.

▶ Surgical management is used in control of the primary lesion and for regional lymph node spread.

CASE 34–1. A 48-year-old woman admits to several sunburns in her youth as a swim instructor. She presents with a 3-mm purplish-brown spot on her left shoulder. She states that it used to be much smaller and that she has recently noted some bleeding from the site.

A. How would you diagnose this lesion?
B. What other examination is important?
C. What radiographic study may be necessary?
D. How would you treat a 0.72-mm-deep lesion?

SARCOMA

▶ ETIOLOGY

What are sarcomas?

Sarcomas are rare tumors arising from cells of connective tissue origin. They encompass a wide variety of tumor types, as listed in Table 34–4. Sarcomas make up 1% of adult neoplasms and 15% of pediatric malignancies. One half of these tumors occur on the extremities. The three most common histologic subtypes in adults are liposarcoma, malignant fibrous histiocytoma, and leiomyosarcoma.

What factors predispose to sarcoma development?

Many predisposing factors have been associated with the development of sarcoma, but none are strong links. These include genetic disorders such as neurofibromatosis, retinoblastoma, Gardner's

TABLE 34–4

Distribution of Sarcoma Histologic Subtypes

Subtype	Distribution (%)
Liposarcoma	22
Leiomyosarcoma	19
Malignant fibrous histiocytoma	17
Fibrosarcoma	10
Synovial sarcoma	7
Malignant peripheral nerve sheath tumor	5
Embryonal rhabdomyosarcoma	4
Other*	16

*Other subtypes include Ewing's sarcoma, myxoid chondrosarcoma, and myxoid liposarcoma.

syndrome, or Li-Fraumeni syndrome; a history of radiation or chemical exposure; trauma; and a history of lymphedema. Genetic translocations and point mutations have been associated with sarcoma development as well, most specifically the loss of tumor suppressor genes *P53* and/or *RB1*.

▶ **EVALUATION**

How do sarcomas present?

Patients with sarcoma usually present with a firm mass; one third of the masses cause pain. If the mass is not readily palpable, such as a mass in the retroperitoneum, it may grow to great size before diagnosis.

How is the diagnosis confirmed?

Once a mass is identified as suspicious for sarcoma, definitive tissue diagnosis is required. The technique for biopsy is an important consideration. The sample needed for analysis needs to be of sufficient size to allow delineation of tissue architecture as well as cellular identification, so often a fine-needle aspiration is inadequate. A larger biopsy approach is favored, such as core-needle biopsy or incisional biopsy. The other important consideration is the orientation of any surgical incision used to obtain the biopsy. The incised tissue will be removed en bloc during the definitive surgical procedure if the diagnosis is confirmed. The biopsy incision should be oriented in a direction that minimizes tissue and functional loss of the limb or body site in question.

How are sarcomas staged?

Once diagnosis is confirmed, the tumor is staged with respect to the grade of the tumor (based on the biopsy specimen), the size of the initial mass (usually based on magnetic resonance imaging scan), and the extent of spread. Lymph node spread is discovered in less than 3% of sarcomas. Extremity sarcomas tend to spread hematogenously to the lungs, and visceral sarcomas tend to spread to the liver. In low-grade extremity lesions, a chest radiograph is sufficient to detect metastatic spread, but high-grade lesions require computed tomographic scanning of the chest and abdomen.

What are the important prognostic factors in staging sarcoma?

The grade of the tumor is determined by histology of the biopsy specimen. The degree of mitotic activity, cellularity, presence of necrosis, and stromal content all are important. In general, division of the grades into two groups (low grade and high grade) is sufficient for prognostication. Low-grade lesions have a less than 15% chance of metastasis, versus a greater than 50% chance seen with high-grade lesions.

The size of the original tumor is important because tumors greater than 5 cm have a greater chance of metastasis, but this prognostic factor is not as important as histologic grade.

The AJCC system for sarcoma grading is listed in Table 34–5.

▶ TREATMENT

How are sarcomas treated?

The main therapy for soft tissue sarcomas is surgical excision. Goals of surgical resection include complete resection of the mass, preferably with 2- to 3-cm margins, and maximal preservation of

---

TABLE 34–5

AJCC TNM Staging System for Soft Tissue Sarcomas

Primary Tumor (T)

TX	Primary tumor cannot be assessed
T0	No evidence of primary tumor
T1	Tumor 5 cm or less in greatest dimension
	T1a superficial tumor
	T1b deep tumor
T2	Tumor more than 5 cm in greatest dimension
	T2a superficial tumor
	T2b deep tumor

Note: Superficial tumor is located exclusively above the superficial fascia without invasion of the fascia; deep tumor is located either exclusively beneath the superficial fascia, superficial to the fascia with invasion of or through the fascia, or both superficial yet beneath the fascia. Retroperitoneal, mediastinal, and pelvic sarcomas are classified as deep tumors.

Regional Lymph Nodes (N)

NX	Regional lymph nodes cannot be assessed
N0	No regional lymph node metastasis
N1*	Regional lymph node metastasis

Note: Presence of positive nodes (N1) is considered Stage IV.

Distant Metastasis (M)

MX	Distant metastasis cannot be assessed
M0	No distant metastasis
M1	Distant metastasis

Stage Grouping

Stage I	T1a, 1b, 2a, 2b	N0	M0	G1–2	G1	Low
Stage II	T1a, 1b, 2a	N0	M0	G3–4	G2–3	High
Stage III	T2b	N0	M0	G3–4	G2–3	High
Stage IV	Any T	N1	M0	Any G	Any G	High or Low
	Any T	N0	M1	Any G	Any G	High or Low

Used with the permission of the American Joint Committee on Cancer (AJCC), Chicago, Illinois. The original source for this material is the *AJCC Cancer Staging Manual, Sixth Edition* (2002) published by Springer-Verlag New York, www.springer-ny.com.

limb or body region function. If meticulous dissection is performed, nearby neurovascular bundles can be spared.

Adjuvant therapy can include radiation therapy such as external-beam radiation or brachytherapy. Chemotherapy has not been shown to be efficacious.

How is recurrence treated?

Despite adequate resection and adjuvant therapy, as many as one third of these tumors recur. The mean time to recurrence is 18 months.

Patients with confirmed recurrence are restaged and the site of recurrence is re-excised. Metastatic disease is excised as it occurs. In as many as 50% of patients with pulmonary metastasis from an extremity sarcoma, that site may be the only site of spread. Those who are candidates for thoracotomy may have a 20% to 30% 3-year survival rate after resection of pulmonary metastases.

Despite recent trials of high-dose systemic cytotoxic chemotherapy, patients with unresectable pulmonary or extrapulmonary metastatic disease have a uniformly poor prognosis.

K E Y   P O I N T S

▶ Sarcoma is a rare tumor of the connective tissue.

▶ Diagnosis is made by a biopsy of sufficient size to assess tissue architecture.

▶ Prognostic factors include histologic grade, tumor size, and the extent of spread throughout the body.

▶ The major treatment modality is surgery, with adjuvant radiation therapy.

CASE 34–2. A 34-year-old man presents with a 10-cm mass on his right thigh. This has been slowly growing for more than a year. It now bothers him when he walks. On physical examination, a $10 \times 7 \times 5$-cm mass is noted, fixed to the underlying tissue on the medial aspect of his thigh. Distal motor and sensory exam is normal. Distal pulses are symmetrical.

    A. How would you diagnose this mass?
    B. What considerations are important in choosing a biopsy technique?
    C. Once the diagnosis is made, how is a sarcoma staged?
    D. How is a high-grade sarcoma of this size treated?

35

Trauma

TRAUMA ASSESSMENT

What is the significance of injury management in the field of medicine?

Injury is the most common cause of death up to the age of 40 years and the third leading cause of death overall. For ages 1 to 34 years, more lives are lost from injury than all other causes combined. For people aged 15 to 24 years, 80% of deaths are injury related. Many more patients are injured and survive, accounting for about 2.5 million hospital admissions and 37 million emergency department visits per year in the United States.

Whereas more than half of deaths due to injury occur at the site of injury, most injured patients do not have life-threatening injuries. But for the few patients who do have immediately life-threatening injuries, the speed and efficiency of care determine survival. The first hour, the so-called golden hour, during which more than half of hospital deaths due to injury are said to occur, belies the true window of opportunity for correct management, which may be only a few minutes in some patients or days in others. Any physician can perform a primary assessment and initiate treatment of the injured patient. However, a well-prepared, organized, and orchestrated trauma team in a dedicated trauma system has been shown to significantly decrease complications and deaths.

What are the major causes of death following injury?

Motor vehicles and firearms account for most deaths due to injury in the United States. More than one third of deaths are intentional (suicide and homicide). Early deaths are usually from severe brain injury (40%) or massive hemorrhage into the chest or abdomen (30%).

What are the initial steps in assessment of the injured patient?

The American College of Surgeons Committee on Trauma has fostered and disseminated a standard of care for injured patients called Advanced Trauma Life Support (ATLS). ATLS is accepted and used in evaluation and resuscitation in the United States and abroad. This protocol recognizes that the most immediately life-threatening problems must be diagnosed and treated first (primary survey) and that a more thorough evaluation (secondary survey) should be completed when the patient is stabilized. The most immediate problems are Airway, Breathing, Circulation, and neurologic Disability. This is known as the ABCDs. Oxygen supply to vital organs cannot be maintained without ventilation and distribution of blood.

Trauma management is unique in requiring that separate goals be attained immediately and simultaneously, including restoring organ perfusion, diagnosing all significant injuries, and beginning definitive therapy.

What are the basics of airway control in trauma?

First the airway should be assessed for patency. If a patient can talk normally, the airway is patent. If not, the airway should be rapidly assessed for obstruction. If a clear and reliable airway cannot be established or if the patient has major alterations in level of consciousness (Glasgow Coma Scale score ≤8) or a major burn or inhalation injury, the priority is to establish an airway by orotracheal intubation using rapid-sequence induction. Airway problems not severe enough to require immediate intubation still require frequent reevaluation. Injuries leading to hematoma or swelling in the neck may cause sudden airway obstruction, making later intubation impossible. Though intubation attempts can sometimes cause complications, a much more serious problem results from delaying an intubation until the airway is lost. Rarely, rapid and safe intubation is not possible and a surgical airway is required. A cricothyroidotomy is performed by making a short transverse incision over the cricothyroid membrane.

All injured patients should be assumed to have a cervical spine fracture until this can be reliably excluded. Until such clearance is possible, it is important to maintain cervical spine precautions—stabilization collars should be left in place, and during intubation or other movement, one person should be assigned the task of maintaining spinal alignment.

What are the basics of breathing assessment in trauma?

Breathing is assessed by listening for good breath sounds on both sides. In intubated patients, correct tube position and ventilation should be confirmed by measurement of end-tidal CO_2. Absence of breath sounds on the left may be due to intubation of the right main stem bronchus. Absence of breath sounds, especially if associated with deviation of the trachea to the opposite side, may also be due to tension pneumothorax, which should be immediately treated by pleural decompression with a needle or chest tube. Other injuries that should be diagnosed during the primary survey include flail chest, massive hemothorax, and open pneumothorax. Supplemental oxygen should be given until it is clearly unnecessary.

What are the initial steps in assessment and resuscitation of circulation?

Circulation is assessed by feeling for a peripheral pulse, looking for skin perfusion, and evaluating level of consciousness. A strong radial pulse, warm and pink skin, and normal mentation are reassuring signs. Conversely, a patient with only a weak or thready carotid pulse, ashen or gray skin, and confusion is clearly in shock. Shock in the injured patient is assumed to be caused by bleeding until proven otherwise (see Table 35–5). A patient in shock requires immediate volume resuscitation and simultaneous evaluation for the source of bleeding. External bleeding should be diagnosed and controlled by direct pressure during the primary survey. Scalp lacerations are a commonly underestimated cause of major blood loss, and this bleeding should be controlled immediately—suturing of arterial vessels is sometimes required.

Internal and thus occult causes of bleeding and shock in injured patients must be suspected and diagnosed. Massive hemothorax diagnosed by physical exam or chest radiograph should be treated by a large-bore chest tube (36 French*) and may require thoracotomy if bleeding persists (>200 mL/hr). Abdominal bleeding in the unstable patient is best diagnosed by focused abdominal sonography for trauma (FAST) ultrasound in the trauma room and treated by immediate laparotomy. Major bleeding may result from pelvic fractures, especially when there is posterior element disruption. Pelvic bleeding may be slowed by stabilizing the pelvis, even by tying a bed sheet around it, but is definitively treated in most centers by angiographic embolization. Major blood loss can occur from long bone fractures, especially if multiple; adequate splinting limits blood loss by limiting fracture movement.

Nonbleeding causes of shock include tension pneumothorax, treated by chest tube; pericardial tamponade, treated by pericardial decompression and subsequent thoracotomy; and spinal shock from cervical spinal cord injury, treated by fluid replacement and pressors. Because the initial response to head injury with intracranial bleeding is hypertension and bradycardia (Cushing's reflex), shock should not be attributed to head injury. Shock from head injury does occur, but only after irreversible brain stem herniation causes loss of all vasoregulatory function.

An injured patient who has any evidence of circulatory compromise should have at least two large-bore intravenous catheters placed and infusion begun with warm crystalloid (Ringer's lactate or

---

*French size is the circumference of the tube in millimeters.

normal saline). Patients in shock from bleeding should immediately receive universal donor (O negative) packed red blood cells.

Why should neurologic disability be assessed during the primary survey?

Approximately half of prehospital and in-hospital trauma deaths result from head injury. For patients with space-occupying lesions (epidural and subdural hematomas), time to surgical decompression is a critical determinant of outcome. A rapid neurologic examination should be performed as part of the primary survey. At the least, level of consciousness should be noted—optimally, assessment should include the Glasgow Coma Scale score (see Table 35–11). Patients often deteriorate after arrival or may require sedation and paralysis, obscuring later neurologic exams. Most treatable intracranial injuries produce a deterioration of mental status; detection of changes in status requires that an initial baseline has been recorded and repeat examinations are performed.

What are the elements of the secondary survey of injured patients?

The secondary survey is a history and physical examination focused on detecting all injuries and including frequent reassessment of vital functions. History obtained should include allergies, medications, and prior medical and surgical problems. Be listening also for other important details related to the trauma that may help predict potential specific areas of injury. Examination includes a head-to-toe visual and tactile evaluation of the entire body.

The head and neck area is examined for scalp and facial lacerations and underlying injuries. Eyes are checked for visual acuity, pupillary response, range of movement, and bleeding. Palpation of bony prominences reveals most facial fractures. Detection of midface fractures may require placing a gloved finger in the mouth and attempting to move the central incisors. Basilar skull fractures may present only with bruising around the eyes ("raccoon's eyes") or behind the ears (Battle's sign) or with hemotympanum or cerebrospinal fluid (CSF) leak. Cervical immobilization is maintained until instability can be excluded clinically or radiologically.

A careful visual assessment of the thorax is important to detect paradoxical movement or splinting. The chest should be palpated carefully for tenderness, crepitus, or rib instability. This is usually done first by compressing the sternum toward the spine and then by medial compression of both hemithoraces with the examiner's hands on each side of the chest.

A thorough but gentle abdominal exam must be performed. A seat belt mark should increase concern about abdominal, especially intestinal, injury. Recognize that significant blood loss can be hidden within a minimally tender abdomen. Persistent or increasing peritoneal signs or unexplained shock remain clear indications for abdominal exploration.

The pelvic ring is assessed by applying pressure at the symphysis pubis and rocking the pelvis at the anterior iliac spines. The perineum, genitalia, and rectum must be assessed to exclude lacerations, hematomas, and open fracture.

Every extremity bone must be palpated and every joint ranged to avoid missing fractures. Pulses and circulatory status are checked to exclude vascular injuries.

A thorough neurologic exam includes Glasgow Coma Scale scoring (see Table 35-11) and checking for sensation and motor strength in all extremities.

More detailed discussions of region-specific injuries are contained in subsequent sections.

What are standard adjuncts to the examination of the injured patient?

Nasogastric Tube. Gastric distention is common in the injured, especially children, and should be prevented by placement of a gastric tube. This is usually placed nasally, but in a patient with possible basilar skull or maxillofacial fracture it should be placed orally to avoid the unusual but reported complication of the nasogastric tube's entering the brain through a cribriform plate fracture. Untreated gastric dilation may cause hypotension, bradycardia, and vomiting with aspiration.

Foley Catheter. Catheterization of the bladder provides for frequent urinary output measurements to assess perfusion and an immediate urine sample to check for hematuria. Before the catheter is placed, a perineal and rectal exam must always be done to look for blood at the urethral meatus, for perineal hematoma, or for a high or not palpable prostate, which may indicate a urethral injury.

Chest and Pelvis Radiographs. Breath sounds may be present even with major pneumothoraces or hemothoraces, and some thoracic injuries (e.g., aortic tear [wide mediastinum], esophageal or bronchial injury [pneumomediastinum]) cannot be diagnosed by physical exam alone. Pelvic fractures may be missed on exam and are a frequent cause of occult blood loss. Therefore, standard radiologic studies in major blunt trauma include chest and pelvis plain films.

Ultrasound and Computed Tomography. Rapidly and accurately diagnosing abdominal injuries remains an enigma. FAST is reliable in detecting peritoneal blood. Computed tomography (CT) is accurate in diagnosing most abdominal injuries and is obtained in stable patients with a questionable abdominal examination.

What is the tertiary survey?

Injuries may be missed on the initial evaluation. Patients may be distracted by other injuries, intoxicated, or rushed directly to the operating room. A complete trauma assessment must include a history and physical exam after these problems have resolved. This tertiary survey is usually completed the morning after admission.

What are some common pitfalls in assessment of the injured patient?

Optimum resuscitation of the severely injured patient remains a challenge even for the experienced trauma team. Some pitfalls are preventable, including failure to treat the life-threatening problems first (such as the obtunded patient who develops respiratory arrest during the CT procedure) and failure to appreciate the magnitude of insult (such as the elderly man with multiple rib fractures who is sent home, then develops pneumonia and respiratory failure). There is inherent conflict in providing fail-safe care (never missing an injury) and cost-effective care (avoiding unnecessary tests). This conflict can lead to errors both ways. Finally, indefensible errors result from failure to do a complete examination (such as missed additional stab wounds from failure to look at the back).

Some particular injuries are missed because their diagnosis remains difficult. The physician must remain wary of these particular problems. A chest radiograph may reveal an obvious wide mediastinum or obscured hemidiaphragm heralding, respectively, aortic or diaphragmatic disruption, but more commonly the findings are subtle. Blunt injuries to the carotid arteries must be suspected to order the duplex ultrasound needed for the diagnosis. Despite the relative accuracy of abdominal CT, intestinal and pancreatic injuries remain difficult to diagnose. Optimum care requires a high index of suspicion and a willingness to repeat the CT scan or operate based on clinical concern.

K E Y   P O I N T S

▶ Assessment of the trauma patient should follow an orderly script, addressing first the life-threatening problems: Airway, Breathing, Circulation, and neurologic Disability.

▶ In severe trauma, to obtain optimum outcome, evaluation, and treatment, diagnosis and resuscitation must proceed rapidly and simultaneously with an organized plan.

▶ Common pitfalls in trauma assessment should be known and anticipated.

CASE 35–1. A young man presents to the emergency department shortly after a motorcycle accident. His pulse is 130 beats/min and his blood pressure is 88/50 mm Hg. He is conversant but disoriented and confused. He has dyspnea, tenderness, crepitus, and absent breath sounds on the left side and moderate diffuse abdominal and pelvic pain and tenderness.

A. Outline, in order, the steps you would take to evaluate and treat this patient.
B. List five injuries that must be suspected in all patients with major blunt injury because their diagnosis remains difficult.

CASE 35–2. A 17-year-old boy presents to the trauma room with a stab wounds to the left anterior chest and to the left upper abdomen. Initial primary survey is normal with pulse of 92 beats/min and blood pressure of 120/80 mm Hg. The vital signs slowly deteriorate. A chest radiograph reveals a small left hemothorax. A chest tube is placed, and 250 mL of blood is drained without improvement in vital signs.

A. What should be the next steps in evaluation and treatment?

ABDOMINAL TRAUMA

What causes abdominal trauma?

The abdomen is the third most commonly injured body region, following the head and extremities. Abdominal trauma is a source of significant morbidity and mortality, with both penetrating and blunt mechanisms of injury. Penetrating injuries are more straightforward in both their presentation and work-up compared with blunt trauma. Blunt trauma often occurs in association with other multisystem injuries. Therefore, diagnostic approaches to abdominal trauma differ according to the mechanism of injury.

BLUNT TRAUMA

▶ ETIOLOGY

What is the etiology of blunt abdominal trauma?

Blunt trauma is the most common mechanism of injury, with motor vehicle accidents accounting for approximately 75% of all blunt injuries to the abdomen. Injury is produced by compression of the abdominal contents against the vertebral column or rib cage, by increase in intra-abdominal pressure with rupture of a hollow-viscus organ or injury to a solid organ, or by rapid deceleration leading to shearing or tearing of the structures and/or their vascular pedicles.

▶ EVALUATION

How is blunt abdominal trauma diagnosed?

Physical examination remains the single most important tool for determining the need for laparotomy versus further diagnostic work-up. In a hemodynamically stable patient who is awake and alert, physical examination of the abdomen should be reliable. However, the presence of central nervous system injury (either closed head injury or spinal cord injury), intoxication (drugs or alcohol), or distracting injuries (long bone and/or pelvic fractures) can render the physical examination unreliable in the blunt trauma victim. In addition, the need for sedation, intubation, respiratory support, or operative intervention for extra-abdominal injuries (head injury, orthopedic fractures) also limits the utility of the physical examination. Hence, the trauma surgeon may need to rely on the multiple diagnostic modalities available. The major diagnostic modalities beyond physical examination include diagnostic peritoneal lavage (DPL), CT of the abdomen (CTA), ultrasonography, and diagnostic laparoscopy (DL).

What is a diagnostic peritoneal lavage (DPL)?

DPL was first introduced by Root and colleagues in 1965 as a method for intraperitoneal evaluation following severe blunt trauma. This technique is useful primarily for diagnosing hemoperitoneum, but it is also helpful in the presence of hollow-viscus injury with enteric contamination. DPL can be performed using closed percutaneous, open, or semi-open techniques. Patients must have a nasogastric tube and Foley catheter placed for gastric and bladder decompression prior to any of these approaches.

The open technique uses a longitudinal incision in the periumbilical area (above the umbilicus in the case of a pelvic fracture or pregnancy, otherwise below) down to the peritoneum, which is visualized and incised for direct insertion of the dialysis catheter in the direction of the pelvis.

The percutaneous approach employs the Seldinger technique. The skin is incised, and a 21-gauge needle is inserted intra-abdominally through which a wire is placed. A dilator is then placed over the wire, and finally the catheter is inserted.

With the semi-open technique, the skin and/or fascia is incised and the catheter is blindly advanced into the peritoneal cavity. Following insertion, aspiration is attempted. If more than 10 mL of gross blood or any intestinal contents are aspirated, the test is considered grossly positive. If not, 1000 mL (15 mL/kg in children) of warm crystalloid is infused through the catheter, allowed to mix with the intra-abdominal contents, and drained via gravity.

What is considered a positive DPL?

Results constituting a positive DPL are listed in Table 35–1.

What are the advantages and disadvantages associated with DPL?

DPL is the most sensitive method for detecting intraperitoneal blood. However, it cannot specify the exact source of bleeding, and only about 30 mL of blood is needed to produce a microscopically positive lavage. As a result, as many as 15% of patients with a positive DPL undergo a nontherapeutic laparotomy. In fact, prior to the introduction of selective nonoperative management of solid-organ injuries, it was thought that practically every damaged spleen

TABLE 35–1

Criteria for Positive DPL Following Blunt Abdominal Trauma

Immediate Aspirate (grossly positive)	
Blood	> 10 mL
Abdominal fluid	Enteric contents
Lavage fluid through chest tube or Foley	
*Lavage Fluid (microscopically positive)**	
Red blood cells	> 100,000/mm^3
White blood cells	> 500/mm^3
Amylase	> Serum
Alkaline phosphatase	> 3 IU/L
Enteric contents	Vegetable matter, bile

*Instillation of 1 L of crystalloid and withdrawal of at least 250 mL to ensure mixing and sampling of the entire abdominal cavity.

DPL, diagnostic peritoneal lavage.

required removal and every liver injury required hemostasis and drainage. It has become apparent that a significant number of these procedures were nontherapeutic; that is, at exploration, the spleen and/or liver was no longer bleeding. Accordingly, the role of DPL has been redefined, and it is used primarily for rapid screening in the hemodynamically unstable patient and evaluation for hollow-viscus injuries.

Diaphragmatic injuries and injuries to the retroperitoneal structures can often be missed by DPL. The only absolute contraindication to DPL is an obvious need for exploratory celiotomy. Previous celiotomy with resultant adhesions can make DPL difficult and is considered a relative contraindication.

What is CT of the abdomen (CTA)?

The technique for CTA has become fairly standardized. Beginning at the lower chest, 1- to 2-cm cuts are taken down through the pelvis. Both nonenhanced scans and contrast-enhanced scans may be performed. Nonenhanced studies demonstrate intra-parenchymal hematomas that can be missed on contrast CTs. Oral contrast delineates the location and integrity of the upper gastro-intestinal tract. Intravenous contrast is given to define organ injury, to evaluate vascular supply, and occasionally to demonstrate active bleeding.

What are the advantages and disadvantages of CTA?

CTA can be quite helpful in the evaluation of blunt trauma and seems to be gradually replacing DPL as the routine method for screening for blunt abdominal trauma. In fact, CTA is fast becoming the workhorse for the evaluation of blunt abdominal trauma. It provides a window into the patient and allows us to "see" the injuries. Specific advantages of CTA include its noninvasive nature and its ability to (1) specify the site of injury; (2) better localize the source of intraperitoneal fluid; (3) grade solid-organ injuries; (4) evaluate associated injuries (vertebral and pelvic fractures); and (5) delineate the retroperitoneum, helping to define injuries to the pancreas, duodenum, and genitourinary tract.

However, there are several inherent disadvantages of CTA. It requires transporting the patient to a site outside the immediate resuscitation room (i.e., radiology department) and takes time to perform. It also requires additional personnel to perform and interpret the scan, with greater associated costs. Consequently, CTA should be performed only in the hemodynamically normal and stable patient. In addition, CTA is limited in the diagnosis and detection of diaphragmatic, pancreatic (50% missed early), and bowel injuries.

As discussed earlier, there has been a recent push toward the nonoperative management of solid-organ injuries. As a result, CTA has assumed increasing importance because it allows us to see the severity of organ damage. In fact, CTA provides the opportunity of observing patients with a limited liver or splenic injury, decreasing the number of nontherapeutic laparotomies and reevaluating known organ injury later in the patient's course (either as an inpatient or as an outpatient).

Is there a role for abdominal ultrasound?

Although abdominal ultrasonography has been used extensively in Europe and Japan for more than a decade to evaluate patients with blunt abdominal trauma, it has only recently gained popularity in the United States. Ultrasonography can be performed by the trauma surgeon in the resuscitation room during the initial evaluation. The subphrenic spaces, subhepatic space, paracolic gutters, pelvis, and pericardium are examined for the presence of fluid. Ultrasonography provides similar information as DPL. Specific advantages of ultrasonography include its (1) relatively low cost; (2) ability to quickly detect intraperitoneal fluid; (3) noninvasiveness; (4) portability; and (5) repeatability. Disadvantages include reliance on operator dependability, missed bowel and pancreatic injuries, and a relatively low specificity for individual organ injury. In addition, ultrasonography is technically limited by obesity, subcutaneous emphysema, and bowel distention with air.

How has the advent of diagnostic laparoscopy (DL) affected the diagnosis and/or treatment of abdominal trauma?

DL has been used with increasing frequency among trauma patients. Because of its relatively low sensitivity for hollow-viscus injury, DL has been used primarily for detection of peritoneal penetration. Once injury is identified, a formal laparotomy is performed. It is unclear whether DL has a significant impact on the evaluation of blunt abdominal trauma. Although DL does not visualize the retroperitoneum well, it does allow evaluation of the diaphragm. Another significant problem is its limited evaluation of the extent and depth of both liver and splenic injuries. In addition, the invasiveness of DL carries the risk of trocar injury, gas embolization, and tension pneumothorax.

Does angiography or magnetic resonance (MR) imaging play a role in the acute trauma setting?

Other diagnostic modalities can be used to evaluate the patient with blunt abdominal trauma. Although angiography has been used as a screening tool in the past, it is no longer practical in this regard. However, it has certain specific applications in which it is both diagnostic and potentially therapeutic (such as angioembolization). Angiography may be helpful in the patient with evidence of ongoing blood loss but without a readily identifiable source of hemorrhage (retroperitoneal hematoma without pelvic fracture). The other primary role for angiography is in the setting of a pelvic fracture, where it is used to identify and embolize pelvic arterial bleeding.

Magnetic resonance (MR) imaging is valuable for evaluating abdominal pathology; however, it is not practical in the multiply injured trauma patient.

Is there a difference between hemodynamically unstable and stable patients in terms of their diagnostic work-up?

Until now, the focus of the discussion has been on the hemodynamically stable patient. In the case of the unstable patient, however, the most important determination the trauma surgeon must make is whether the patient is exsanguinating into the abdominal cavity. There are only four places to lose enough blood to produce instability: (1) external environment, (2) chest, (3) retroperitoneum, and (4) abdomen. In addition, estimates of blood loss should be assigned to individual injuries. A general guideline is shown in Table 35–2. By quantitating blood loss from associated injuries, one can evaluate the hemodynamically unstable patient more efficiently, because diagnostic modalities for evaluating the hemodynamically unstable patient are limited. With ongoing blood loss, varying degrees of shock ensue (Table 35–3).

CTA is too time-consuming for assessment of an unstable patient, requiring transport to the radiology department and performance of the scan. DL is also limited because of the need for special equipment, the inability to rapidly assess the abdominal cavity, and the potential for the pneumoperitoneum to compromise an already tenuous hemodynamic status. Thus, for the hemodynamically unstable patient, either DPL or ultrasonography should be performed in the resuscitation room to definitively rule out intraperitoneal hemorrhage as the source of the patient's instability prior to further diagnostic work-up.

TABLE 35–2	
Estimated Blood Loss	
Injury Description	**Blood Loss (Units)***
Facial fractures	1
Humerus fracture	1
Multiple rib fractures	1–2
Pelvic rami fractures	1–2
Tibia fracture	1–2
Femur fracture	2
Sacroiliac disruption	2–10

*Add 1 to 2 units for open fractures.

TABLE 35–3

Shock States

Degree	Blood Volume Lost (%)	Signs and Symptoms
Mild	<20	Delayed capillary refill, thirst
Moderate	20–40	Tachycardia, restlessness
Severe	>40	Hypotension, altered mental status

Do the criteria for a positive DPL change in the setting of hemodynamic instability?

Because the main concern is whether there is significant intraperitoneal hemorrhage, DPL is an ideal procedure. In this case, however, only a grossly positive lavage (aspiration of >10 mL of blood) should be considered diagnostic. Hemodynamic instability is unlikely to be present based on a microscopically positive DPL. Therefore, in the unstable patient, a grossly positive DPL is a rapid indicator of significant intra-abdominal hemorrhage.

Is there a simplified approach to the patient with blunt abdominal trauma?

For the hemodynamically stable patient (Fig. 35–1), primary survey, including assessment of the ABCDs, must be performed, followed by a thorough physical examination and plain radiographs of the chest and pelvis. Further diagnostic evaluation is necessary for patients with equivocal findings on examination. CTA provides information regarding both solid organs and retroperitoneal structures. If there is significant solid-organ injury with hemoperitoneum, evidence of hollow-viscus injury, or hemoperitoneum in the absence of solid-organ injury, the patient should undergo exploratory laparotomy. For those with less significant solid-organ injury and minimal hemoperitoneum, observation in an intensive care setting (intensive care unit [ICU] or postanesthesia care) is possible. If free fluid is the only finding, DPL should be done to rule out hollow-viscus injury.

As with the hemodynamically stable patient, in the unstable patient (Fig. 35–2), primary survey including the ABCDs must be performed, followed by a thorough physical examination and plain radiographs of the chest and pelvis; plain films of the chest and pelvis rule out major intrathoracic and retroperitoneal hemorrhage. In the absence of a pelvic fracture, the likelihood of a retroperitoneal hemorrhage is low. After plain films, either a DPL or ultrasonography is performed. If the DPL is grossly negative for blood, other causes for shock must be considered.

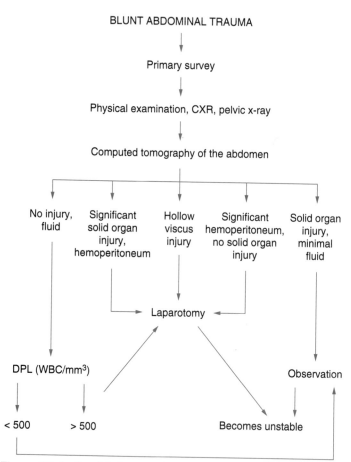

Figure 35–1. Simplified approach for evaluation of the hemodynamically stable patient following blunt abdominal trauma. CXR, chest radiograph; DPL, diagnostic peritoneal lavage; WBC, white blood cell.

PENETRATING TRAUMA

▶ **ETIOLOGY**

What is the etiology of penetrating abdominal trauma?

Stab and gunshot wounds constitute the majority of penetrating injuries to the abdomen. Significant intra-abdominal injury is associated with 66% of stab wounds and 80% of gunshot wounds.

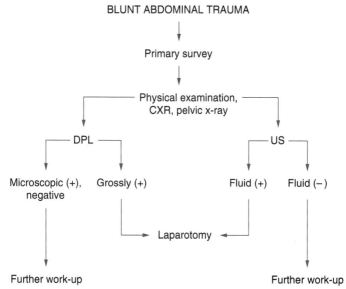

BLUNT ABDOMINAL TRAUMA

Primary survey

Physical examination,
CXR, pelvic x-ray

DPL

Microscopic (+),
negative

Grossly (+)

US

Fluid (+)   Fluid (−)

Laparotomy

Further work-up

Further work-up

Figure 35–2. Simplified approach for evaluation of the hemodynamically unstable patient following blunt abdominal trauma. CXR, chest radiograph; DPL, diagnostic peritoneal lavage; US, ultrasonography.

Consequently, any wound from the nipple line to the gluteal crease has the potential for peritoneal or retroperitoneal injury.

▶ EVALUATION

How is penetrating abdominal trauma managed?

Any penetrating abdominal wound associated with either hemodynamic instability or clear signs of peritoneal irritation on physical examination of the abdomen requires urgent exploratory celiotomy. In the stable patient with equivocal abdominal findings, however, there are five basic approaches: (1) observation, (2) local wound exploration, (3) DPL, (4) DL, and (5) CTA.

What is a local wound exploration?

Local wound exploration is employed for the evaluation of stab wounds. After the site of penetration is sterilely prepped and draped, the stab wound and surrounding tissues are anesthetized. The wound is then extended both proximally and distally so that it is approximately three times its original length to allow adequate exploration. The tract is then carefully followed with subsequent identification of the anterior and posterior fascia and the peritoneum if the wound extends to these levels. If these structures cannot be adequately visualized, another diagnostic modality should be used.

Does the location of the stab wound influence patient management?

Anterior wounds (ventral to the midaxillary lines and from the sub-costal region to the inguinal ligament) and flank wounds (between the anterior and posterior axillary lines) can be locally explored. If the posterior fascia is clearly intact, the patient can be discharged. If the anterior fascia is violated and peritoneal penetration cannot be assessed, further diagnostic work-up should be performed. This can be helpful in reducing the rate of negative laparotomies and missed injuries.

Posterior stab wounds are difficult to assess because of the extremely thick groups of paraspinal muscles. In such patients, observation with serial abdominal examinations is often adequate. In addition, triple-contrast CT scans can be performed with oral, intravenous, and rectal contrast for both posterior stab wounds and flank wounds in which local exploration was not possible.

The concern with lower thoracic wounds is that there can be diaphragmatic penetration with subsequent intra-abdominal injury. Both DPL and DL can be used in this situation.

A problem with DPL has been establishing a red blood cell (RBC) count that is appropriate for injury. Various centers have reported positive values ranging from as low as $>10,000/mm^3$ RBC to $>50,000/mm^3$ RBC to as high as $>100,000/mm^3$ RBC. In addition, as mentioned previously, DPL frequently misses hollow-viscus injuries in the acute setting.

What is the role of abdominal ultrasonography in penetrating trauma?

The best role for ultrasonography in the setting of penetrating abdominal trauma is in the assessment of the pericardium and cardiac injury. It is more cost-effective than performance of a pericardial window, and the results may influence the incision or order of exploration. Nevertheless, ultrasonography remains of questionable value in evaluating penetrating abdominal trauma, and more clinical trials are necessary to further define its role in this setting.

Does the management of penetrating abdominal trauma secondary to gunshot wounds differ from trauma secondary to stab wounds?

The diagnostic evaluation of patients with gunshot wounds and equivocal abdominal findings is essentially the same as that for stab wounds. However, given the fact that gunshot wounds have a greater likelihood of producing injury and a higher degree of injury, physical examination tends to be less equivocal in the presence of peritoneal penetration. In fact, in patients with clear peritoneal irritation, the only immediate blood work that is necessary is a type and cross match.

DL plays a similar role in the evaluation of gunshot wounds; however, a low threshold for laparotomy should be maintained because intestinal injuries can be missed. As with stab wounds, DPL should be used with caution because of conflicting criteria concerning positive results (see earlier).

What is the treatment for specific organ injuries?

Splenic injury is usually the result of blunt trauma. In hemodynamically stable patients with lower-grade injuries (Table 35–4) and without CT evidence of pseudoaneurysm or extravasation, observation with serial hematocrit determinations followed by repeat CTA is acceptable. In the latter situation, angiography with embolization should be performed. In the hemodynamically unstable patient, urgent celiotomy should be performed and may consist of hemostatic control, splenorrhaphy, partial splenectomy, or, most likely, splenectomy.

Similar to splenic injury, liver injury is usually the result of blunt trauma. Again, hemodynamically stable patients with lower-grade injuries (Table 35–5) and without CT evidence of pseudoaneurysm or extravasation can be usually be managed with observation and

TABLE 35-4

Spleen Injury Scale: American Association for the Surgery of Trauma

Grade	Type of Injury	Injury Description
I	Hematoma	Subcapsular, nonexpanding, <10% surface area
	Laceration	Capsular tear, nonbleeding, <1 cm parenchymal depth
II	Hematoma	Subcapsular, nonexpanding, 10–50% surface area; intraparenchymal, nonexpanding, <5 cm in diameter
	Laceration	Capsular tear, active bleeding; 1–3 cm parenchymal depth that does not involve a trabecular vessel
III	Hematoma	Subcapsular, >50% surface area or expanding; ruptured subcapsular hematoma with active bleeding; intraparenchymal hematoma >5 cm or expanding
	Laceration	>3 cm parenchymal depth or involving trabecular vessels
IV	Hematoma	Ruptured intraparenchymal hematoma with active bleeding
	Laceration	Involves segmental or hilar vessels producing major devascularization (>25% of spleen)
V	Laceration	Completely shattered spleen
	Vascular	Hilar vascular injury that devascularizes spleen

TABLE 35–5

Liver Injury Scale: American Association for the Surgery of Trauma

Grade	Type of Injury	Injury Description
I	Hematoma	Subcapsular, nonexpanding, <10% surface area
	Laceration	Capsular tear, nonbleeding, <1 cm parenchymal depth
II	Hematoma	Subcapsular, nonexpanding, 10–50% surface area; intraparenchymal, nonexpanding, <10 cm in diameter
	Laceration	Capsular tear, active bleeding; 1–3 cm parenchymal depth, <10 cm in length
III	Hematoma	Subcapsular, >50% surface area or expanding; ruptured subcapsular hematoma with active bleeding; intraparenchymal hematoma >10 cm or expanding
	Laceration	>3 cm parenchymal depth
IV	Hematoma	Ruptured intraparenchymal hematoma with active bleeding
	Laceration	Parenchymal disruption involving 25–75% of hepatic lobe or 1–3 Couinaud's segments within a single lobe
V	Laceration	Parenchymal disruption involving >75% of hepatic lobe or >3 Couinaud's segments within a single lobe
	Vascular	Juxtahepatic venous injuries (retrohepatic vena cava, central major hepatic veins)
VI	Vascular	Hepatic avulsion

serial hematocrits followed by repeat CTA. However, observation entails admission to an ICU with continuous hemodynamic monitoring and repeated examinations by the responsible physician. Operative management consists of simple repair with or without drainage, suture ligation of bleeding vessels, débridement of devitalized tissue, or packing (temporary packing with laparotomy pads.

Small bowel injuries require either primary repair or resection with anastomosis. Similar to small bowel injuries, colonic injuries can be treated with either primary repair or resection and anastomosis. However, there are certain situations in which a colostomy should be performed. Management of duodenal injuries differs from management of the rest of the small bowel. These injuries tend to be more hazardous, with an increased likelihood of breakdown of the repair. Nevertheless, most can be managed with primary repair. However, extensive injuries may require resection, patching, afferent and efferent tubes, or pyloric exclusion.

What is the importance of missed injuries?

The importance of a meticulous evaluation of all patients presenting with abdominal trauma regardless of the etiology cannot be stressed enough. In a busy trauma center, it is easy to overlook minor details as multiple patients arrive at the same time. It is the role of the trauma surgeon to ensure that nothing is missed. A missed injury can be catastrophic, leading to prolonged hospital/ICU stays, intra-abdominal sepsis and/or hemorrhage, and frequently death.

K E Y   P O I N T S

▶ Physical examination is the single most important tool for determining the need for laparotomy versus further diagnostic work-up.

▶ Hemodynamic instability in the resuscitation room is secondary to intra-abdominal hemorrhage until proven otherwise.

▶ Multiple diagnostic modalities exist for the evaluation of blunt abdominal trauma, especially in the presence of coexisting orthopedic fractures, closed head injuries, and substance abuse.

▶ Missed injuries can be catastrophic—all patients presenting with abdominal trauma regardless of the etiology must be completely evaluated.

CASE 35–3. A 28-year-old man is an unrestrained driver in a motor vehicle crash. He is awake and alert with stable vital signs. He complains of left upper quadrant tenderness but has no signs of peritonitis.

   A. What is the next step in management of this patient?
   B. If the patient had altered mental status secondary to a closed head injury or substance abuse, would this alter the management?
   C. If the patient's vital signs were unstable, would this alter the management?

CASE 35–4. An 18-year-old man sustains a knife stab wound to the anterior abdominal wall. He is awake and alert with stable vital signs and no complaints of abdominal pain.

   A. What is the next step in management of this patient?
   B. If the patient's vital signs were unstable or he complained of diffuse abdominal tenderness, would this alter the management?

OTHER TRAUMA

THERMAL INJURIES

Burns are a major health problem in the United States, with approximately 2.5 million people seeking treatment each year, resulting in 150,000 hospitalizations and 6000 fatalities. Morbidity is highest in the very young and very old. Factors determining burn mortality include size and depth of injury, age, comorbidities, and presence of inhalation injury.

▶ ETIOLOGY

What causes different kinds of burns?

Thermal burns most commonly occur as the result of contact with a hot object, exposure to flame, or scalding with hot liquids. Exposure to intense cold can also result in tissue injury or death. Chemical burns occur as the result of contact with caustic substances (usually acids or alkalis).

How are burns classified?

Tissue damage or destruction as the result of thermal or chemical insult results in a burn. Traditionally, burns have been classified as first through fourth degree, but a more useful distinction is partial thickness or full thickness (Table 35–6).

▶ EVALUATION

How are burn victims evaluated?

As in any injured patient, it is necessary to follow the ABCDs of resuscitation. Burn patients often have other injuries, and these need to be addressed. A complete history and physical exam are mandatory. Burns disrupt temperature autoregulation and fluid homeostasis. Patients should be kept warm and in clean, dry dressings until they reach the definitive care center. If there is any question of patency or inhalation injury, the airway should be secured with endotracheal intubation. Large-bore vascular access should be established. All lines should be securely sewn in place (tape does not stick to burned tissue). A nasogastric tube and Foley catheter should be placed.

What steps are involved in the initial resuscitation?

Following assessment and management of the airway and breathing, lactated Ringer's solution should be started at a rate based on

TABLE 35-6

Characterization of Burns

Burn Depth	Structures Involved	Appearance/Exam	Treatment Required
Superficial partial thickness	Epidermis and superficial dermis	Reddened/blistered, painful, blanches with pressure	Débridement of all blisters and dead tissue dressings as indicated
Deep partial thickness	Epidermis and most of dermis	Red with sloughing epidermis, usually wet, painful, may not blanch with pressure	Débridement (may require tangential excision); coverage with grafts or dressings to minimize conversion to full thickness
Full thickness	Full thickness of skin and variable underlying tissues	White, red, or charred; dry, insensate	Early excision and grafting

the size of the patient adjusted for the size of the burn. Multiple formulas exist to calculate resuscitation requirements (see Table 35–6), but a good starting point is 2 mL/kg/% burn. One half of this volume should be infused over the first 8 hours following injury, with the remaining half being divided over the ensuing 16 hours. The "clock" starts at the time of injury, not at the time that resuscitation is instituted. Delay in resuscitation of even 1 or 2 hours dramatically increases fluid requirements and mortality. Fluid rate should be adjusted to maintain a urine output of 1 mL/kg/hr.

What is involved in the initial wound management?

Prior to reaching the definitive care center, burn wounds should be dressed in clean, dry dressings. Wet dressings may contribute to heat loss and promote bacterial growth. Topical antimicrobials probably accomplish nothing in the first 24 to 36 hours and may make the depth of injury difficult for the definitive caregiver to assess.

If wounds are full thickness and circumferential around an extremity or the trunk, circulation or breathing may be compromised. In this case, escharotomy may be required. This is performed with electrocautery at the bedside. Anesthesia is generally not needed because burned tissue is insensate.

Chemical burns require extensive irrigation (30 to 60 minutes of spray and scrub; soaking in a tub may actually extend the injury to unaffected areas). The chemical should be washed off the patient and onto the floor. Dry chemicals or chemical-soaked clothing should be removed prior to irrigation. Neutralization of acids with base or vice versa should be avoided.

How are inhalation injuries evaluated?

Inhalation injury results from chemical insult to the trachea, bronchi, and lungs occasioned by breathing the products of combustion. Direct thermal injury to the lungs is rare. Inhalation injury should be suspected in any patient with a history of a flame or chemical burn in an enclosed space. Other findings suggestive of the diagnosis are singed nasal or facial hair, carbonaceous sputum, burns to the central face, or an elevated carboxyhemoglobin level. The diagnosis should be confirmed with bronchoscopic evaluation.

Endotracheal intubation should be performed early in patients with inhalation injuries because swelling during resuscitation may result in sudden loss of airway and may make intubation extremely difficult.

How are electrical injuries evaluated?

Electrical injuries fall into two categories: The more common are *low-voltage conduction injuries* (<500 V) that result in local skin burns at the entrance and exit sites. Deep tissue injury may result from tissue heating as the current flows along the path of least resistance. *High-voltage injuries* also have local and deep tissue effects, but there is generally a component of flash injury as well. This results from the heat produced when the electricity arcs from the conductor to ground. High-voltage injuries are commonly associated with cardiac, renal, neurologic, and ophthalmic problems. In either setting, a thorough examination is warranted, and compartment syndrome or nerve compression must be addressed with formal fasciotomies if indicated. Carpal tunnel and tarsal tunnel canal releases are also commonly required. Extensive tissue necrosis may be present in deep tissues with apparently normal overlying structures.

▶ **TREATMENT**

What is the initial surgical management of thermal injuries?

Surgical care of burn wounds is directed first toward removal of nonviable tissue. This is accomplished with early excision to the level of living tissue and coverage of the wound, either permanently with autograft or temporarily with allograft. Infected burn wounds are generally managed with initial excision and temporary coverage, with subsequent autografting after the wound bed shows signs of healing. After coverage has been achieved, function becomes the major focus. Releases of scar contractures and aggressive therapy are directed toward maximizing the ability of the patients to move and function as best they can. Cosmetic concerns are generally addressed after these issues are resolved.

What grafting techniques are used?

Skin grafts are generally classified as *full thickness*, in which a piece of skin is excised to the level of subcutaneous fat and then used to cover an open area; or *partial thickness*, in which epidermis along with some dermal elements are tangentially excised and used to cover areas that have no skin elements present. Both techniques are commonly used, and both have advantages and disadvantages. Full-thickness donor sites require coverage or closure and cannot be reharvested. Partial-thickness skin is cosmetically inferior, especially when meshing is required to expand coverage; it tends to contract more, and scarring is more pronounced. However, donor sites may be harvested multiple times at relatively short intervals.

In situations where little donor site is available, techniques such as the use of cultured epithelium or widely meshed autograft may be employed.

What are the infectious risks?

The skin is the primary defense against infection. Burn patients are at high risk of sepsis and death as a result of loss of skin integrity. Invasive procedures and vascular access devices compound this problem. Prophylactic broad-spectrum antibiotic coverage with subsequent conversion to directed therapy is warranted in these patients. Assiduous attention to cleanliness and débridement of nonvital tissues on an ongoing basis is also mandatory. Often the use of topical antiseptic agents such as Dakin solution, mafenide (Sulfamylon) solution, or silver nitrate can be helpful. Routine use of silver sulfadiazine over grafts is generally contraindicated because it has been shown to inhibit epithelialization.

What are the rehabilitation steps following thermal injury?

Initial rehabilitation is geared toward maximizing function and range of motion and inhibiting scar formation. Aggressive active and passive exercises are mandatory. The best way to deal with scar contraction is prevention through aggressive therapy. Adjuncts to exercise include pressure garments and splinting. Surgery may be required to release scars that interfere with function.

K E Y   P O I N T S

▶ Thermal injuries are a common cause of death and serious disability in the United States.

▶ Morbidity is determined by depth and extent of injury, age, prior medical diseases, and association with other injuries, especially smoke inhalation.

continued

▶ Survival from major burns requires effective emergency management of the *airway*, by early intubation; *breathing*, by early institution of oxygen; *circulation*, by early, aggressive fluid resuscitation; and *prevention of infection*, by early burn débridement and coverage.

▶ Successful rehabilitation from major burn injury requires long-term planned coordination of multiple disciplines, including burn surgery, physical and occupational therapy, and social and psychological services.

CASE 35–5. A 55-year-old alcoholic man sustains 50% partial- and full-thickness burns after his cigarette set his bed on fire in a small apartment. The firemen initially had trouble finding the patient in the room because of thick smoke. On arrival, the patient is somewhat drowsy but complaining of pain. His vital signs are normal and he is phonating normally.

    A. Outline a treatment plan.

CHEST INJURY

What are the incidence and mortality of thoracic trauma?

Thoracic injuries account for 20% to 25% of deaths due to trauma. Approximately 16,000 deaths per year in the United States are attributable to chest trauma. The overall mortality from thoracic trauma is estimated at approximately 10%. However, certain intrathoracic organ injuries carry a large mortality. For example, mortality from cardiac and thoracic vascular injuries can exceed 60% depending on the type of injury.

Although many injuries to the chest can be devastating, 80% to 85% of the patients with thoracic trauma can be managed with tube thoracostomy and observation. Less than 10% of blunt chest injuries and only about 15% to 30% of penetrating chest injuries require thoracotomy. Approximately 10% of penetrating chest injuries injure the heart. Of the patients with penetrating thoracic injuries, 20% have associated injuries to the diaphragm and abdominal viscera.

Approximately 66% of patients with blunt trauma sustain chest injury. Pulmonary contusion is the most common lung injury and accounts for 30% to 75% of these injuries.

Chest injuries encompass a wide spectrum of injuries ranging from simple thoracic wall trauma to devastating cardiac, pulmonary, and esophageal injuries. The clinical presentation of thoracic injuries can vary from total absence of symptoms to profound shock and patients arriving in extremis. Hypoxia, hypercarbia, and acidosis often result from thoracic injuries. Immediate deaths are usually due to major cardiac or thoracic aortic injury.

What are the most immediate life-threatening chest injuries?

The most immediate life-threatening injuries causing early deaths are cardiac tamponade, aortic disruption, and continued intrathoracic hemorrhage. Later deaths are due to respiratory complications, infection, multisystem organ failure, and, rarely, unrecognized injuries. Other immediately life-threatening injuries that should be identified during the primary survey include tension pneumothorax, massive hemothorax, open pneumothorax, and flail chest. Perforation of the esophagus or the tracheobronchial tree, diaphragmatic rupture, and myocardial or pulmonary contusion are examples of other potentially fatal injuries that should be identified during the secondary survey and treated. Lethal thoracic injuries are listed in Table 35–7.

What is the pathophysiology and treatment of tension pneumothorax?

Tension pneumothorax is accumulation of air in the pleural space secondary to a valve mechanism created by the egress of air from the injured pulmonary parenchyma. This results in a progressive increase in tension in the injured hemithorax, causing displacement of the mediastinum toward the uninjured side. Displacement of the

---

TABLE 35–7

Lethal Thoracic Injuries

Simple pneumothorax
Hemothorax
Pulmonary contusion
Tracheobronchial tree injuries
Blunt cardiac injuries
Traumatic aortic disruption
Traumatic diaphragmatic injuries
Mediastinal traversing wounds

mediastinum with twisting of the superior and inferior venae cavae in their axes causing subsequent decrease in venous return, cardiac filling, and cardiac output results in hypotension and potential cardiac arrest. Presentation is similar to that of cardiac tamponade, with distention of jugular veins. Exam may reveal absent breath sounds on the affected side and tracheal deviation.

Treatment consists of decompression of the affected hemithorax temporarily via needle thoracostomy inserted in the second intercostal space at the midclavicular line followed by immediate chest tube insertion. Decompression of a tension pneumothorax usually results in immediate resolution of symptoms.

What is hemothorax and how it is diagnosed and treated?

Hemothorax is defined as the presence of free blood within a pleural cavity from either blunt or penetrating injury. Frequently, it coexists with pneumothorax. Symptoms range from minimal to severe respiratory and circulatory compromise depending on the amount of blood loss. Symptomatic patients usually complain of chest pain and dyspnea. Diminished breath sounds with dullness to percussion help distinguish this entity from pneumothorax. This is a clinical diagnosis. In the stable patient, a definitive diagnosis is made with chest radiography, although a small amount of hemothorax may be evident only by CT scan and may be missed in the initial chest radiograph. It is critical to remember that a pleural effusion in trauma patients is a hemothorax until proven otherwise. Larger collections of blood require evacuation via tube thoracostomy. Bleeding exceeding 1000 to 1500 mL of blood or hemodynamic instability is an indication for an emergency thoracotomy. Inadequately drained hemothorax or clotted hemothorax should be further evaluated with a chest CT scan and may require thoracoscopy for evacuation.

What are the indications for the use of tube thoracostomy?

Tube thoracostomy (chest tube placement) is required in a large number of the patients with chest injury. Frequently it is the sole intervention required for the treatment of pneumothorax. Chest tubes are placed under local anesthesia to evacuate air or blood from the pleural space.

Indications for placement of tube thoracostomy include simple pneumothorax, tension pneumothorax, and hemothorax. Other patients who may benefit from prophylactic tube thoracostomy are selected patients with suspected severe lung injury, especially those requiring air or ground transfer; individuals undergoing general anesthesia for other injuries; or patients requiring positive pressure ventilation who have suspected lung injury.

The procedure can easily be performed at the bedside. The insertion site is usually the nipple level anterior to the midaxillary line. An incision is made and carried through skin and subcutaneous structures sharply. The chest cavity is entered bluntly in the fifth intercostal space, above the rib to avoid injury to the neurovascular bundle and the lung. Trocars should never be used, since 15% of the population has some type of pleural adhesions that may result in parenchymal lung injury. Iatrogenic injuries to the pulmonary parenchyma result in significant hemorrhage because the lung is a low-pressure high-flow system. Chest tubes of at least 36-French or larger are used in adults to evacuate hemothorax. Smaller tubes can be used to drain simple pneumothorax. Sterile collecting systems are available and allow safe autotransfusion of the evacuated blood.

What is the diagnosis and treatment of flail chest?

Flail chest is defined as double fractures in three of more adjacent ribs. It can be diagnosed clinically and radiographically. A flail segment due to separation of sternum from the costochondral joints or adjacent broken ribs is known as a *central flail chest*. The diagnosis is made clinically and not radiographically because costochondral cartilages are not visualized on films. The flail segment moves independently and paradoxically during the respiratory cycle. Negative pressure generated in inspiration by the descent of the diaphragm and expansion of the chest wall leads to inward movement of the flail segment. In contrast, expiration generating positive intrathoracic pressure pushes the segment outward, unlike the remaining part of the chest wall. Although this movement is rather dramatic, the underlying pulmonary contusion is the main determinant of the final outcome.

Respiratory support, aggressive pulmonary toilet, and pain management are the mainstays of treatment. The need for intubation is determined in each case. Respiratory compromise is evidenced by fatigue and progressively deteriorating lung mechanics. The results of arterial blood gases usually indicate the need for endotracheal intubation. Selective intubation and application of positive end-expiratory pressure provides internal chest wall stabilization. The use of thoracic epidural analgesia provides excellent pain control and eliminates the need for endotracheal intubation in a large number of these patients.

What are the indications for emergency department thoracotomy?

Emergency department thoracotomy is indicated for patients arriving in cardiopulmonary arrest secondary to penetrating wounds to the chest, particularly penetrating cardiac injuries. It is most successful in patients with short transport times and witnessed arrest or objectively measured physiologic parameters such as pupillary response, spontaneous respiration, presence of a carotid pulse, or extremity movement.

The chest is approached via a left anterolateral thoracotomy through the fifth intercostal space. The incision is extended from the xiphisternal junction just below the nipple toward the axilla to the anterior border of the latissimus dorsi in a curvilinear fashion. Once the thoracic cavity is entered, the pericardium is opened longitudinally anterior to the phrenic nerve. This allows evacuation of the pericardial blood causing tamponade, open cardiac massage, and repair of penetrating cardiac injuries. Subsequently the left lung is retracted anteriorly to visualize and cross clamp the descending aorta. By this maneuver all remaining blood volume is redistributed to the head and heart while control of distal hemorrhage is achieved. In some patients, direct control of exsanguinating intrathoracic hemorrhage can also be obtained.

Success rates are lower in patients who have penetrating abdominal injuries. Similarly, this procedure is rarely indicated in blunt trauma because of attendant low survival rates and poor neurologic outcomes; therefore, it should be reserved for patients who arrive in the emergency department with measurable vital signs and suffer witnessed cardiac arrest. Survival rates range from approximately 1.5% for blunt trauma to 15% to 20% for penetrating cardiac injuries.

What is a transmediastinal wound?

Transmediastinal wounds are defined as injuries that involve an ipsilateral hemithoracic cavity and mediastinum or both hemithoracic cavities and mediastinum. They are generally caused by missile injury. The thoracic cavity should be conceptualized as three separate cavities contained within the thorax: the two pleural cavities containing the ipsilateral lung and hilar structures, and the mediastinum containing the heart, thoracic great vessels, major airways, esophagus, and thymus. Mediastinal traversing gunshot wounds pose a great challenge in their diagnosis and management. The presence of multiple vital structures in this anatomic area makes the diagnostic work-up and treatment challenging.

Generally, patients presenting with unrelenting hypotension and/or cardiopulmonary arrest require emergency thoracotomy or median sternotomy as life-saving measures. Patients who present with hemodynamic stability should undergo a detailed systematic diagnostic work-up to exclude cardiac, great vessel, tracheal, and esophageal injuries. Following the primary and secondary surveys, a plain chest radiograph is essential to rule out the presence of hemothorax or pneumothorax. FAST performed in the emergency department is essential for the diagnosis of hemopericardium. In recent years a CT scan of the chest has been used to delineate missile tracks, thus guiding further diagnostic work-up. The thoracic aorta and great vessels are usually evaluated with angiography.

Esophageal injuries are the most difficult to detect. Esophagoscopy and/or esophagography should be used in all patients with suspected injury. Bronchoscopy is used to investigate the trachea and proximal airways.

What is the mechanism and treatment of pulmonary contusion?

Pulmonary contusions are the result of direct blunt trauma to the chest. Less frequently they are due to shock waves produced by explosions or high-velocity missiles. Clinical presentation may range from the asymptomatic patient to a patient with severe respiratory distress requiring ventilatory support. The chest radiograph may be normal initially but usually reveals a well-localized opacification. CT scan of the chest is helpful in establishing the diagnosis as well as excluding other associated intrathoracic injuries such as thoracic aortic injury. Treatment is symptomatic and consists mainly of aggressive pulmonary toilet, respiratory support as needed, and pain control. Antibiotics are not indicated unless the presence of infection has been established. Judicious fluid management is of utmost importance because the injured lung is susceptible to fluid underload and overload.

What is the mortality of thoracic aortic injuries and how can they be diagnosed?

Penetrating injuries to the thoracic aorta are highly lethal—most patients die instantly. Approximately 85% of the patients with blunt injuries die within minutes from the injury. In the group of patients that survive to arrive at the hospital, approximately 1% die per hour for the first 48 hours. The primary mechanism of injury is rapid deceleration of the body resulting in rupture of the aorta at the points of fixation, namely the aortic root and descending aorta distal to the ligamentum arteriosum.

Establishing a diagnosis may not be easy in patients with occult injuries; therefore, a high index of suspicion is essential. Only one third of the patients are symptomatic, having dyspnea, chest and back pain, and absence of pulses in the lower extremities. Occasionally higher blood pressure in the upper extremities compared to the lower is present. Widened mediastinum, loss of contour of the aortic knob, left apical cap, left pleural effusion, loss of the aortopulmonary window, depression of the left main stem bronchus and displacement of trachea, and nasogastric tube displacement to the right are some of the indirect indicators of aortic injury that can be seen in a plain chest radiograph. However, 25% of the patients with injuries have a normal chest radiograph on admission. Table 35–8 lists the radiographic findings consistent with aortic disruption.

Helical CT scan of the chest is an excellent tool for evaluation of the thoracic aorta and mediastinum, and it has become the most

TABLE 35–8

Findings in Plain Chest Radiograph Indicating Thoracic Aortic Injury

Widened mediastinum (>8 cm)
Loss of contour of the aortic knob
Left apical cap
Left pleural effusion
Loss of aortopulmonary window
Rightward deviation of a properly placed nasogastric tube
Displacement of the trachea
Depression of the left main stem bronchus
Sternal, clavicular, first rib, or multiple rib fractures

commonly used imaging study for the diagnosis of this particular injury. Transesophageal echocardiography has also been proven helpful as a diagnostic tool in some trauma centers. Aortography remains the gold standard for diagnosis. Once the diagnosis is established, maintaining systolic blood pressure is essential to avoid rupture of a contained hematoma until surgical control can be obtained. A left posterolateral thoracotomy provides the best exposure for surgical repair. The use of a prosthetic graft is almost always necessary and can be achieved with or without the use of cardiopulmonary bypass.

What is the importance of diaphragmatic injuries?

Diaphragmatic injuries are frequently associated with other severe injuries. In the absence of diligent investigation they may remain undetected, resulting in serious delayed complications such as traumatic diaphragmatic hernia with visceral strangulation and necrosis. Blunt ruptures of the diaphragm occur in less than 10% of the patients sustaining severe blunt trauma, most commonly on the left. In penetrating trauma, thoracoabdominal injuries located below the nipple line pose a significant risk for diaphragmatic injury. In the presence of diaphragmatic injury, approximately 80% to 90% of patients have significant associated intra-abdominal injuries.

Patients can be asymptomatic or demonstrate nonspecific physical findings. Specific symptoms may be due to associated injuries. Imaging studies such as CT scanning are nonspecific. Approximately 25% of the patients may have a normal chest radiograph. Obscured diaphragmatic border, irregular contour, associated hemothorax or pneumothorax, elevated hemidiaphragm, a nasogastric tube noted in the left hemithoracic cavity, and air mass or air-fluid level above the diaphragm are indirect indicators of diaphragmatic injury. DPL is nonspecific for the diagnosis of this particular type of injury. DL or thoracoscopy may be necessary in asymptomatic patients with suspected diaphragmatic injury to establish the diagnosis

What is the incidence of esophageal injuries, and how are they diagnosed and treated?

Traumatic esophageal injuries are rare, accounting for less than 1% of all intrathoracic injuries. They represent one of the most challenging injuries due to the complexity of their diagnosis and treatment. It is estimated that a busy urban trauma center treats approximately three to five patients with penetrating esophageal injuries a year. Blunt esophageal trauma is extremely rare, with an estimated incidence of 0.001%. Approximately 30% of all esophageal injuries are intrathoracic. Because of the esophagus' protected location, esophageal injuries are rarely isolated. An average of two associated injuries is usually found in these patients.

Thoracic esophageal injuries are notoriously silent. They should be suspected with the presence of pneumomediastinum or hematemesis in the absence of gastric or duodenal injury. On rare occasions the diagnosis can be made when gastric contents and food particles are evacuated from the left chest following tube thoracostomy.

Rigid esophagoscopy in combination with esophagography can establish the diagnosis in 90% of the cases. Occasionally the diagnosis can be made intraoperatively. Because the thoracic esophagus is mostly a right-sided organ, most injuries are approached via a right posterolateral thoracotomy; however, lower thoracic esophageal injuries can be approached through a left posterolateral thoracotomy. Approximately 80% of all esophageal injuries can be repaired primarily, 3% to 4% require resection and diversion, and approximately 11% can be treated by drainage alone. Esophageal injuries carry a significant mortality rate, ranging from 15% for penetrating trauma to 10% for blunt trauma. Mortality rates triple in patients undergoing surgery with delays longer than 24 hours.

What is the incidence and prognosis of cardiac injuries, and how are they evaluated?

Cardiac injuries are among the most lethal organ injuries. Cardiac injuries represent 10% of all penetrating chest injuries. Many patients are dead at the scene or arrive at trauma centers in extremis. Diagnostic investigations are undertaken in patients who present in relatively stable condition and in whom the diagnosis is not certain. In most cases an immediate thoracotomy or median sternotomy is necessary.

Cardiac tamponade occurs commonly in patients sustaining penetrating injuries, but it can also occur with blunt trauma. Even a small amount of blood can significantly restrict cardiac activity and interfere with cardiac filling. Cardiac tamponade is immediately life-threatening. Frequently the diagnosis is difficult. The classic diagnostic Beck's triad, consisting of venous pressure elevation as evidenced by jugular venous distention, hypotension, and muffled heart tones, is present in only 10% of the patients. Pulsus paradoxus, defined as a decrease in systolic blood pressure of more than 10 mm Hg during spontaneous inspiration, is another sign of cardiac tamponade.

Chest radiography may be helpful in 30% to 50% of the cases, mainly by depicting an enlarged cardiac silhouette, pneumopericardium, or enlarged upper mediastinum, although often there is little opportunity to obtain a chest radiograph. Echocardiography is a valuable tool to detect hemopericardium as part of the FAST exam.

Pericardiocentesis is of limited value in large trauma centers. If the diagnosis of cardiac injury is in doubt, a subxiphoid pericardial window can be performed; if positive, it is then followed by median sternotomy and cardiac repair.

Overall survival is 10% to 15%, with 30% to 35% survival in patients who survive long enough to arrive at the hospital. Survival rates of 10% to 15% for gunshot wounds and 60% to 65% for stab wounds are achieved in highly experienced trauma centers. Blunt cardiac rupture is extremely rare, accounting for 0.5% of all blunt trauma hospital admissions. Although patients are often asymptomatic, clinical presentation may range from cardiac arrhythmias to cardiogenic shock. Diagnosis is established by obtaining serial troponin levels and electrocardiograms. Patients with positive findings may require additional investigation with a formal echocardiogram.

What other injuries can be seen in chest trauma?

Tracheobronchial injuries can also occur in chest trauma, and they are frequently lethal. The trachea is in close contact with the esophagus and surrounded by vital structures. Injuries to these other mediastinal structures are common and often fatal. A substantial number of these injuries are recognized only after death. The reported incidence varies from 0.2% to 8%. Extensive mediastinal emphysema is the dominant sign on plain chest radiography or chest CT scan. Flexible bronchoscopy is the procedure of choice for the diagnosis. Treatment can be conservative in minimal or sealed injuries. Larger injuries require surgical treatment, usually through a right thoracotomy.

Several large thoracic vessels can also be injured in penetrating or blunt chest trauma. Penetrating trauma causes approximately 90% of the thoracic vascular injuries, whereas blunt trauma is the most common cause of thoracic aortic injuries. Injuries to the innominate; subclavian and proximal carotid injuries; and brachiocephalic, subclavian, internal jugular vein and superior vena cava trauma can also occur. All these injuries pose various diagnostic and therapeutic challenges.

K E Y   P O I N T S

▶ Primary and secondary surveys are indispensable tools in the assessment of all trauma patients.

▶ When the patient's condition allows, diagnostic adjuncts are invaluable.

▶ In the presence of hemodynamic instability or peritoneal signs, an operation is almost always indicated.

CASE 35–6. A 22-year-old man is brought to the hospital after suffering a single stab wound 2 cm below his left nipple. He is fully awake, alert, and oriented; his heart rate is 127 beats/min, his respiratory rate is 42 breaths/min, and his blood pressure is 90/42 mm Hg. Breath sounds are significantly decreased in the left chest.

    A. List all the procedures that his initial assessment should include.

    B. List all the possible injuries that need to be addressed.

    C. Describe the treatment plan once the initial assessment is completed.

CASE 35–7. A 46-year-old man is brought to the emergency department following a motor vehicle crash. He complains of severe chest pain and shortness of breath. His Glasgow Coma Scale score is 15, his heart rate is 113 beats/min, his blood pressure is 164/48 mm Hg, and the respiratory rate is 37 breaths/min. His primary survey is otherwise unremarkable. His secondary survey reveals severe tenderness in the left anterior chest with a flail segment.

    A. What are the life-threatening injuries that must be immediately addressed?

    B. What should the diagnosis and management of the fail chest include?

MAXILLOFACIAL INJURIES

▶ **ETIOLOGY**

What causes maxillofacial injuries?

Maxillofacial injuries encompass both soft and hard tissue trauma. Facial fractures are most commonly due to motor vehicle accidents (automobile, motorcycle, pedestrian), altercations, sport injuries, falls, and gunshot wounds. Open fractures require urgent treatment, but closed fractures also benefit from early treatment, which results in improved functional and aesthetic outcomes.

▶ **EVALUATION**

How do I start my work-up in the emergency department?

Patients with facial trauma frequently have other injuries, and a full trauma team evaluation is warranted. The ATLS protocol is implemented and the initial ABCs of resuscitation are followed. Airway obstruction due to hematoma and active bleeding may necessitate endotracheal intubation and/or emergent cricoidectomy/tracheostomy. Aspiration of blood, saliva, and gastric contents frequently accompanies maxillofacial injuries and can be prevented by intubation. Bleeding from head and neck lacerations is brisk. If the laceration appears minor, the bleeding is frequently overlooked during the initial trauma evaluation and resuscitation period. The accumulated blood loss from head and neck lacerations, especially from the scalp, can quickly be great enough to require transfusion. Blind clamping to control bleeding is not recommended, especially in the face and neck regions, because of the relatively superficial location of important nerves. Bleeding can usually be controlled with direct compression until direct surgical control is performed.

What are the physical exam findings?

The initial management of maxillofacial injuries begins with a thorough history (when possible) and physical examination. The mechanism and time interval from the injury, loss of consciousness, and vision and occlusion changes are important points to address. The patient's medical history may provide details that influence the type or timing of treatment.

   The physical examination is done in an orderly manner from calvarium, ears, forehead, nose, orbit-zygoma, maxilla, mandible, chin, and oral cavity. Lacerations, abrasions, and contusions are noted at each site. Signs of facial fractures include facial asymmetry, bony step-offs, decreased or double vision, malocclusion, and diminished facial nerve or trigeminal nerve function. Other signs include airway obstruction, soft tissue crepitus, intraoral lacerations, and nasopharyngeal bleeding.

The locations and depths of lacerations are documented in each facial subunit. A sensory and motor nerve exam of the face is imperative and should be done before local anesthesia is administered. The supraorbital, infraorbital, and mental divisions of the trigeminal nerve should be assessed for sensation. Facial expression should be compared for symmetry. Thin, bloody fluid coming from the nose or ears should raise the possibility of CSF leak and basilar skull fracture.

All scalp and facial bone surfaces are palpated. During the oral cavity exam, the maxillary and mandibular dentition are palpated, noting intraoral lacerations and broken, avulsed, or loose teeth. The dental arches should be assessed for lateral or anteroposterior movement. Dentures and nonfixed bridgework may be removed to permit accurate evaluation. The excursion and occlusion of the jaws are noted, and deviation on movement is observed. The patient's subjective sensation of malocclusion is an important clue to the presence of a mandibular or maxillary fracture. Intranasal examination permits identification of hematoma or septal deviation-fracture.

Extraocular movement, pupillary response, and visual acuity are assessed. The combination of a palpebral and conjunctival hematoma represents an orbital fracture until excluded by radiographic confirmation. Formal ophthalmologic consultation is necessary if an orbit fracture is present to rule out corneal, scleral, lens, retinal, optic nerve, and other injuries.

What types of imaging studies are necessary?

Injuries of the brain frequently accompany facial fractures. Axial CT radiographs of the brain are done to diagnose intracranial bleeding or other injury, and the facial fracture pattern is identified. When necessary, true coronal plane CT images are later obtained to fully evaluate the orbital floor. A three-dimensional CT reconstruction of the face and calvarium provides a clear picture of the fracture locations and bone fragment relationships. Cervical spine radiographs are done to diagnose bone or ligament injury prior neck movement and removal of the cervical collar.

▶ TREATMENT

How do I treat facial lacerations?

Lacerations require high-pressure irrigation and layered suture repair. Tetanus prophylaxis and toxoid are administered as necessary.

A careful sensory and motor exam is performed for documentation of loss of nerve and muscle function prior to injection of local anesthesia and wound closure. Road tattoo and gross foreign body contamination are débrided. Deep wounds may have a facial nerve laceration in which repair is necessary. Alignment of anatomic landmarks at the laceration site ensures the best repair. For example, the vermilion border must be reapproximated accurately during lip laceration repair, and the gray line/ciliary margin must be aligned during eyelid laceration repair.

When do I treat facial fractures operatively?

In general, displaced facial bone fractures need reduction because the functional and aesthetic tolerance for bony misalignment is low. Facial bone asymmetry is readily visible due to the superficial location of bones under the skin. Malunion occurs when the fracture is not reduced appropriately, which presents a more technically difficult refracture/reposition operation for correction. Moreover, facial bone fractures heal rapidly secondary to the robust blood supply in the head and neck region and thus are easiest to repair soon after injury.

For multisystem trauma patients, facial fracture treatment can progress in the absence of significant increased intracranial pressure. Altered mental status, including coma, need not exclude the treatment of a facial injury. In consultation with the neurosurgery team, intracranial pressure can be monitored, a prognosis determined from the CT scan, and the decision made about when to perform facial fracture repair. Patients with isolated facial fractures can undergo repair as soon as logistically feasible. In general, fractures are repaired from peripheral to central. This algorithm is particularly relevant for panfacial fracture repairs, in which bilateral frontal, zygomatic, maxillary, mandibular, and NOE fractures may be present in various combinations. Successful repair reestablishes both proper facial anterior projection and width through realignment of the facial vertical and horizontal buttresses.

What are the types of facial fractures and how are they treated?

Nose

Nasal bone fractures are quite common. Adequate reduction can usually be done acutely in the office or emergency department with local anesthesia and sedation. However, optimal reduction for more displaced fractures is best obtained in the operating room with its inherent better lighting, instrumentation, and anesthesia. Closed reduction is performed by both external pressure and internal pressure through the nares. A dorsal nasal splint is used for 5 to 7 days to hold the reduction. Septoplasty is performed when the septum is fractured and deviated. A septal splint and nasal packing are placed postoperatively to hold reduction, control bleeding, and prevent hematoma formation. The packing is removed after 24 to 72 hours.

Mandible

Mandible fractures cause malocclusion, most commonly an anterior open bite secondary to premature contact of the molars. With body and parasymphyseal fractures, an intraoral laceration is commonly present between the teeth in the alveolar ridge at the fracture site. Loose teeth with roots in the fracture line may need extraction. Numbness commonly occurs in the inferior alveolar nerve distribution if a fracture occurs in the body through the canal. Pain in the temporomandibular joint region occurs with subcondylar fractures, and tenderness is present directly over all facial bone fracture sites.

Orbit-Zygoma

Orbit fractures can occur in the rims, roof, or floor and thus involve components of several facial bones. The exact fracture pattern must be determined with CT imaging to plan incision locations. An isolated orbital floor blow-out fracture causes orbit contents (fat and extraocular muscles) to herniate into the maxillary sinus. If the inferior oblique muscle is entrapped, globe excursion will be limited and diplopia will result. Enophthalmos occurs after the initial edema resolves and the globe has inferior and posterior displacement. Floor blow-out fractures generally require repair when the size is greater than 1 cm^2 to prevent late enophthalmos. Orbital roof fractures commonly cause exophthalmos due to displacement of the globe anteriorly. Floor, roof, and medial wall blow-out fractures are treated with bone grafts by most craniofacial surgeons. However, some surgeons also use synthetic implants, including meshed-metal plates.

Zygoma

Tetrapod fractures of the zygoma denote fractures at the lateral and inferior orbital rims, lateral zygomaticomaxillary buttress, and zygomatic arch. These fractures displace the zygomatic complex (malar eminence) posteriorly and inferiorly. Three-point rigid fixation is necessary to prevent relapse; thus, plate fixation at the lateral and inferior rims and at the buttress is performed for adequate stabilization. The zygomatic arch is plated when its fracture(s) remain displaced after reduction of the zygomatic complex.

Le Fort

There are three types of Le Fort fractures, and each can be unilateral or bilateral. Le Fort I fractures occur through the medial and lateral maxillary buttresses (Fig. 35–3). Le Fort II fractures denote naso-maxillary separation from the facial skeleton (Fig. 35–4). Le Fort III fractures represent craniofacial disjunction, in which the maxilla and zygoma are separated from the cranial base as a single unit (Fig. 35–5). With panfacial fractures (generally defined as five or more fractures), combinations of Le Fort fractures (e.g., Le Fort I and III) can occur on the same side.

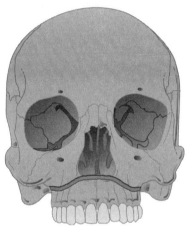

Figure 35–3. Le Fort I fracture pattern. The zygomaticomaxillary and nasomaxillary buttresses are fractured.

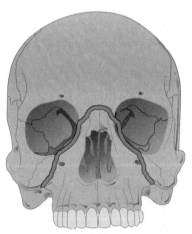

Figure 35–4. Le Fort II fracture pattern. Nasomaxillary separation from the facial skeleton occurs.

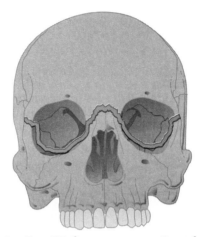

Figure 35–5. Le Fort III fracture pattern. Craniofacial disjunction occurs, in which the nasomaxillary (Le Fort II) segment and zygoma are separated from the cranial base.

Nasal-Orbital-Ethmoid

Nasal-orbital-ethmoid (NOE) fracture refers to fractures of the nasal bones and medial orbital wall. They result in lateral displacement of the medial canthus with subsequent telecanthus on the ipsilateral side. NOE fractures are approached with combinations of incisions that include direct approaches through lacerations immediately above the NOE fracture, lower eyelid incisions, and a coronal incision. In older patients, a gull-wing forehead incision is occasionally used.

Frontal Sinus

Careful evaluation for possible anterior and posterior frontal sinus wall fractures is important in patients with forehead trauma and other facial fractures. If the posterior wall is fractured, a risk of dural tear with CSF leak and frontal lobe contusion is present. The posterior wall is removed, the mucosa is stripped, and the duct and sinus are obliterated using bone, fat, or dermis grafts (cranialization). The anterior wall fracture fragments are reduced and plated. Late mucoceles can develop if the mucosa is not stripped completely or the duct is not obliterated. The mucoceles can become infected and erode into the intracranial space, resulting in lethal meningitis. Isolated anterior wall fractures require bone reduction, but mucosal stripping is necessary only when the fractures are extensive or the duct is fractured.

What is mandibular-maxillary fixation (MMF) and when is it used?

Repair of Le Fort and mandible fractures begins with establishment of mandibular-maxillary (also called "intermaxillary") fixation (MMF). The teeth of the upper and lower jaws are ligated to arch bars, which are then ligated to each other. Wear facets are matched on the teeth to guide the occlusion into its preinjury pattern during MMF. This provides stability to the fracture fragments and maintains the correct dental relationships. Loose or severely carious teeth in the fracture line are extracted to promote proper fracture healing. Oral hygiene is maintained with frequent mouthwashes with antibiotic and peroxide solutions.

MMF treatment length is variable and depends on the type and pattern of fractures. When tension bands and rigid plates are placed across isolated mandible fractures, MMF can be released at the conclusion of surgery in the operating room. Elastic band guidance is still commonly used thereafter to retrain the masticatory musculature. In the case of mandibular subcondylar fractures, MMF is kept in place 2 to 6 weeks, depending on the compliance and overall health of the patient. Restrictions include a soft diet, no chewing, no contact sports, and no altercations. Young, compliant patients can heal within 2 weeks. Older and more debilitated patients require more time to achieve adequate bony healing such that their jaw fracture reductions will be maintained after the MMF is discontinued.

What are the surgical incisions used to approach the fractures?

The calvarium, orbits, and jaws are accessed through several incisions, performed alone or in combination, depending on the fracture location(s). The incisions are coronal scalp, lateral brow or lateral upper blepharoplasty, transcutaneous subciliary or transconjunctival lower eyelid with or without lateral canthotomy, and intraoral maxillary or mandibular vestibule (Fig. 35–6). An external Risdon incision in the upper neck and can also be used to approach the mandible, but an obvious scar is present and the marginal mandibular branch of the facial nerve is at risk for injury. Lacerations over fracture sites can also be reopened and used for bony approaches. This is commonly useful for repairing NOE fractures.

What hardware is used for repair of facial fractures?

Rigid plate and screw fixation has been the standard of care for facial fracture treatment for the last 10 to 20 years. These systems range in screw size from 1.0 to 1.3 mm for orbital rims, 1.5 to 2.0 mm for zygoma or maxillary fractures, and 2.0 to 2.4 mm for mandibular fractures. However, during the last 5 years,

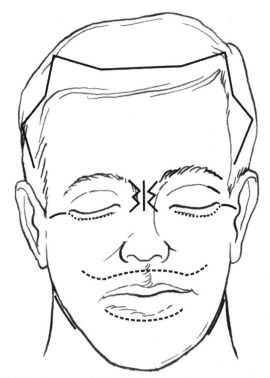

Figure 35–6. Incisions *(dashed lines)* used to approach the facial skeleton.

resorbable palate and screw systems have become available. The resorbable systems are currently not as rigid as the metal (titanium alloy) systems, and thus loss of bone reduction is possible. They are used mostly in children and in orbital rim locations on adults.

What are the important aspects of postoperative care?

Patients are hospitalized overnight for uncomplicated open reduction internal fixations. Intravenous pain medication, sedation, fluids, and antibiotics are administered. The patient's head is elevated on two or three pillows, and cool packs are placed to reduce swelling. Corticosteroids are frequently given both during surgery and immediately thereafter for 1 or 2 days to reduce facial edema. Antibiotics are given 1 to 5 days postoperatively to reduce infection rates. Plain facial radiographs are obtained in the immediate postoperative period for evaluation of the fracture reduction and hardware location.

K E Y   P O I N T S

▶ Follow the ABCs of resuscitation.

▶ Control bleeding, protect the cervical spine, and rule out fracture with radiographs.

▶ Complete maxillofacial bone imaging includes CT of the face with axial 3-mm and coronal 2-mm cuts.

▶ Irrigate and débride wounds and make suture repairs as necessary.

▶ Undertake operative fracture repair early

CASE 35–8. A 22-year-old man is ejected from an automobile in a roll-over accident. He has a brief (<30-second) loss of consciousness at the scene. On presentation to the emergency department, he has a blood pressure of 100/60 mm Hg, heart rate of 100 beats/min, and Glasgow Coma Scale score of 15. He complains of blurred vision, a numb left cheek, and epistaxis.

A. What are your initial diagnoses?
B. What findings will you look for on physical exam?
C. How will you determine the extent of his injuries?
D. What will be your operative plan?

CASE 35–9. A 45-year-old intoxicated man is struck in the face during an altercation and presents to the emergency department. He has no loss of consciousness, blood pressure of 110/60 mm Hg, and heart rate of 90 beats/min. He complains of pain and swelling along the right side of his face. He cannot close his mouth and is bleeding intraorally.

A. What is(are) the most likely facial fracture(s)?
B. What findings will you look for on physical exam?
C. How will you determine the extent of his injuries?
D. What will be your operative plan?

FRACTURES

▶ ETIOLOGY

What is a fracture?

In general terms, a fracture occurs as a result of a traumatic event and is defined as a break in the continuity of a bone. Fractures may occur from a variety of different mechanisms ranging from a simple break with minimal soft tissue damage to a highly comminuted fracture with a limb-threatening soft tissue injury. Fractures may be either open or closed and can be further classified based on fracture pattern, displacement, and location within a given bone.

One of the more difficult objectives for medical students and interns on an orthopedic rotation is to accurately describe radiographs of a fracture to a senior colleague. We have developed a simple mnemonic *(PLASTER OF PARIS)* to allow clinical clerks to organize their analysis effectively (Table 35–9).

What are the different types of fracture patterns?

Fracture patterns occur in response to various types of loading. A *transverse fracture* pattern occurs when the bone fails in tension

---

TABLE 35–9

Mnemonic for Fracture Description*

P lane of fracture (transverse/oblique/spiral)
L ocation (which bone/where in bone)
A rticular surface involvement (including growth plate injuries)
S imple vs. comminuted
T ype of fracture (classification system)
E xtent of fracture (complete/greenstick)
R eason (traumatic/pathologic/stress)

O pen vs. closed
F oreign bodies

Dis**P** lacement (translation)
A ngulation
R otation
I mpaction (periarticular spaces)
S hortening (diaphyseal spaces)

*The first section *(PLASTER)* allows a general overview of the fracture, whereas the second *(OF)* describes the soft tissue injury as seen on the radiographs. The final section *(PARIS)* describes the position of the different fracture fragments.

and the major fracture line runs perpendicular to the long axis of the bone. *Oblique fractures* occur under conditions of compression, and the major fracture line runs at some angle less than perpendicular to the long axis when viewed in one plane but appears transverse in a plane 90 degrees from the first. A *butterfly fragment* occurs when bending loads are applied and the bone fails in tension on one side and compression on the other side. *Spiral fractures* occur under conditions of torsion, and the fracture line appears oblique in both the anteroposterior and lateral planes. *Comminuted fractures* occur when the bone fails as a result of a high-energy mechanism under a variety of different loading conditions. In comminuted fractures there are at least three major fragments and two fracture lines (Fig. 35-7).

How are fractures classified with respect to location within the bone?

Long bones may be divided into different regions, including diaphyseal, metaphyseal, and epiphyseal (Fig. 35-8). Fractures in these anatomic regions have their own specific characteristics that impact management. For example, diaphyseal fractures occur through thick cortical bone with a small cross-sectional diameter, whereas metaphyseal fractures occur through cancellous bone with a much larger cross-sectional diameter. Epiphyseal fractures are frequently intra-articular and include fracture fragments with articular cartilage.

How are fractures involving the growth plate of long bones classified?

Pediatric physeal fractures are characterized using the Salter-Harris classification. The physis (growth plate) is a unique cartilaginous structure that is frequently weaker than bone in torsion, shear, and bending, which predisposes the child to injury in this location. Fractures involving the physis may interfere with the blood supply, resulting in growth arrest.

Salter-Harris type I fractures are transphyseal separations. These fractures typically have an excellent prognosis, although complete or partial growth arrest may occur if they are displaced.

Salter-Harris type II fractures occur through the metaphysis and the physis. The metaphyseal fragment is known as the *Thurston-Holland fragment* and is usually associated with an intact periosteal hinge. These fractures have an excellent prognosis unless displaced, which may result in partial or complete growth arrest.

Salter-Harris type III fractures are transphyseal; they exit the epiphysis, resulting in intra-articular displacement. These fractures require anatomic reduction without violation of the

Type A   Simple fractures
Type B   Wedge fractures
Type C   Complex fractures

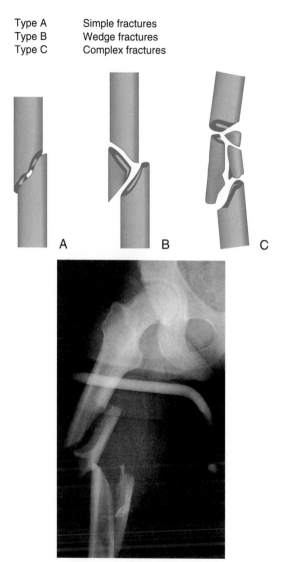

Figure 35–7. Comminuted fractures. *A,* Type A, simple fractures. *B,* Type B, wedge fractures. *C,* Type C, complex fractures. *Lower,* In comminuted fractures, there are at least three major fragments and two fracture lines. (*A* to *C,* From Rüedi TP, Murphy WM [eds]: AO Principles of Fracture Management. Davos, Switzerland, AO Publishing, 2000, p 52.)

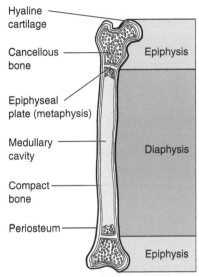

Figure 35–8. Bone regions. Long bones may be divided into different regions, including diaphyseal, metaphyseal, and epiphyseal.

physis. Prognosis for these fractures is guarded because partial growth arrest and deformity are not uncommon.

Salter-Harris type IV fractures are physeal fractures that traverse the metaphysis and the epiphysis. Anatomic reduction without violation of the physis is essential. Prognosis is guarded because partial growth arrest resulting in angular deformity is common.

Salter-Harris type V fractures are crush injuries to the physis and are difficult to diagnose on initial radiographs. Prognosis is poor because growth arrest and partial physeal closure commonly result (Fig. 35–9).

How are fractures classified in terms of displacement?

Fracture fragment position should be described in complete detail, including displacement (translation), angulation, rotation, and length (Fig. 35–10). These descriptive terms have important implications in both the acute setting and the healed fracture when defining residual deformity or malunion.

Displacement is defined as translation of the distal fragment in relation to the proximal fragment in either a medial or lateral direction. Translation can also occur in the sagittal plane in an anterior or posterior direction. Angulation describes the direction in which the apex of the angulation points. There are two types of coronal plane angulation. In varus angulation the apex points away from the mid-

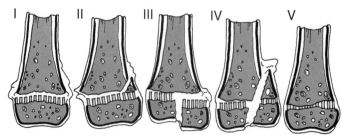

Figure 35–9. Salter-Harris fractures. Salter-Harris type fractures are traumatic injuries to the pediatric physis. In displaced epiphyseal fractures, prognosis is guarded because of the potential for partial physeal closure and growth arrest. (Redrawn from Salter RB, Harris WR: Injuries involving the epiphyseal plate. J Bone Joint Surg 1963;45A:587.)

line, whereas in valgus angulation the apex points toward the midline. Angulation can also occur in the sagittal plane and is described as either apex anterior or apex posterior. The rotation of a fracture is described as either internal or external, depending on the position of the distal fragment relative to the proximal fragment along the long axis of a bone. Length refers to shortening or distraction of the fracture fragments.

How are fractures formally classified?

There are many classification schemes currently used to categorize fractures. There are classification systems specific for a particular

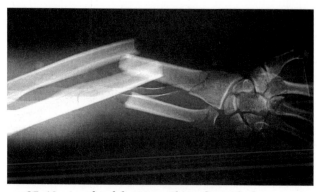

Figure 35–10. Angulated fractures. This radiograph shows a comminuted both-bones forearm fracture. The distal fractures are essentially undisplaced. In the mid-shaft area, both the radius and ulna are shortened and 100% displaced in an ulnar direction. The fracture is angulated approximately 30 degrees, apex radial. Angulation can also occur in the sagittal plane (lateral radiograph) and is described as either apex anterior or apex posterior. Rotation is difficult to assess.

anatomic site or injury, such as the Schatzker classification of tibial plateau fractures or the Winquist-Hansen classification of femoral shaft fractures. These are usually named for the surgeon who devised the classification. There are many examples of this method throughout the orthopedic literature. There are two classification methodologies that employ an alphanumeric system and are based on fracture severity, bone location, and segment. The AO/ASIF (AO/Association for the Study of Internal Fixation) system and the OTA (Orthopaedic Trauma Association) system were developed to standardize the classification of fractures (see Table 35–9).

What is an open fracture and how are open fractures classified?

An *open fracture* refers to an osseous disruption that results in a break in the skin and soft tissue with direct communication to the fracture and its hematoma. Any wound occurring on the same limb as a fracture must be evaluated as an open fracture until proven otherwise. The soft tissue injury in an open fracture has important consequences to consider. The wound is exposed to the outside environment and can be contaminated. Crushing, stripping, and devascularization results in soft tissue compromise and increased susceptibility to infection. Fracture healing may be compromised. Destruction or loss of the soft tissue envelope may affect the method of treatment and ultimately the functional outcome in fracture management.

▶ EVALUATION

How are patients with fractures evaluated?

After the initial resuscitation and stabilization of a trauma or multiply injured patient, a pertinent history and systematic examination of the patient should be undertaken. The entire spine, pelvis, and all extremities should be inspected and examined. Potential spine and pelvic injuries should be assessed. Lateral cervical spine and anteroposterior pelvic radiographs should be obtained in the trauma patient. One should also consider a lateral radiograph of the thoracolumbar spine in the initial assessment of the patient. CT scanning and/or MR imaging should be considered to further delineate injury to the spine if plain radiographs or physical examination are suspicious for bony or neurologic injury.

Extremity injuries should be identified. The skin and soft tissue damage to the extremity should be assessed. The neurovascular status of the injured limb should be assessed and an angiogram obtained if vascular injury is suspected. Anteroposterior and lateral radiographs of the extremity should be obtained as indicated by physical examination, injury pattern, and patient complaints. The joint above and below an apparent limb injury should be included in the radiographic assessment. Provisional reduction of the fracture should be considered, particularly if the skin or soft tissues are compromised by the fracture deformity. Dislocations of joints should be reduced if possible without undue force. The extremity should be splinted to prevent further soft tissue damage and hemorrhage prior to transport to the operating room. Wound hemorrhage should be addressed with direct pressure rather than tourniquets or clamps.

▶ TREATMENT

What are the principles of fracture management?

Fracture management begins with a complete history and physical examination. One should determine the condition of the soft tissue and whether the injury is open or closed. Neurovascular status is assessed. Radiographs and advanced imaging studies are reviewed and a determination is made whether the fracture will require operative or nonoperative treatment. The timing of surgery is also an important consideration, with early intervention indicated in the following cases: (1) femoral or pelvic fractures that carry a high risk of pulmonary complications such as fat embolus syndrome or adult respiratory distress syndrome; (2) open fractures; (3) fractures associated with vascular injury that requires repair; (4) fractures associated with active or impending compartment syndrome, such as a tibia fracture; (5) unstable cervical or thoracolumbar spine fracture/dislocation with incomplete or worsening neurologic deficits; and (6) multiply injured patients that are hemodynamically stable.

Many nonoperative and surgical treatment options are available for the care of fractures. Although many general principles apply, the specific treatment of a fracture varies widely depending on surgeon experience and training as well as on patient demands and expectations.

Following the initial assessment of a fracture, reduction can be carried out by one of two methods. *Closed-reduction techniques* require traction and a reversal of the forces that produced the injury. Splints are initially employed to maintain alignment of the fracture and allow for swelling without vascular compromise. *Open reduction* requires surgical intervention and placement of internal fixation devices to stabilize the fracture. As a general rule, closed reduction techniques are used initially to manage fracture deformity to protect the soft tissue envelope from further damage until the definitive treatment can be performed. Closed techniques can also be employed in simple low-energy fractures in which satisfactory alignment can be restored and maintained until complete healing occurs or in patients who are not candidates for operative treatment because of systemic or local factors.

How are open fractures treated?

Open wounds in the setting of a fracture should not be explored in the emergency department if operative intervention is planned. These wounds should not be irrigated or probed in the emergency department because this may further contaminate the tissues. Only obvious foreign bodies that are easily accessible—not bone fragments—should be removed. These wounds should be covered with a sterile saline–soaked gauze pad. Tetanus prophylaxis should be given in the emergency department, and parenteral antibiotics should be initiated.

Open fractures constitute an orthopedic emergency, and the patient should undergo a formal irrigation and débridement before fracture stabilization. Intervention within 8 hours of an open fracture may result in a lower incidence of wound infection and osteomyelitis. The principles of an adequate irrigation and débridement cannot be overstated. The open wound should be extended proximally and distally to fully examine the zone of injury. Meticulous débridement should be performed, starting with the skin and progressing to the muscle. All devitalized tissues should be removed. Small and completely detached bone fragments that serve no structural purpose may be removed. One should avoid creating large skin flaps, which may further devitalize already compromised tissues. Neurovascular structures and tendons should be preserved. The fracture surfaces should be exposed and débrided. Pulsatile low-pressure or gravity-flow lavage irrigation should be performed using at least 4 L of normal saline with or without antibiotics solution. Traumatic wounds should not be closed. Serial débridements may be performed every 48 hours as necessary until the wounds are clean.

Fracture stabilization is generally performed at the time of the initial débridement. In open fractures with extensive soft tissue injury, stabilization of the fracture with internal or external fixation provides protection of the soft tissue envelope, access to the wounds for dressing changes, and stability of the fracture for mobilization of the patient.

Wound coverage following open fractures should be performed when there is no further evidence of necrosis or contamination. Ideally this is accomplished within the first week of injury. There are three methods for providing definitive wound coverage: delayed primary wound closure, split-thickness skin graft, and rotational or free muscle flap. The type of coverage depends on the severity of the original injury and its location on the extremity.

Bone grafting should be considered for segmental or significant bony defects. Iliac crest bone grafting is the gold standard. The timing of the bone graft is controversial, with some surgeons advocating the grafting at the time of definitive wound coverage and others waiting until the soft tissues have completely healed, which usually takes 6 weeks.

What are the principles of open reduction and internal fixation?

The operative treatment of fractures requires a thorough knowledge of the anatomy and various surgical approaches to the injury site. A complete understanding of the various fixation devices is necessary, and one should employ sound biomechanical principles when performing open reduction and internal fixation. The choice to proceed with open reduction and internal fixation depends on having a stable soft tissue envelope that will tolerate the surgical trauma and recognizing fractures that will heal with a better functional outcome treated operatively versus nonoperatively. Open reduction and internal fixation are useful for intra-articular fractures in which anatomic reduction and early mobilization have been shown to be beneficial. Operative treatment is also considered in fractures that would heal with a clinically significant deformity resulting in a functional impairment. Rarely are fractures treated surgically simply to promote or accelerate the healing process. Finally, early operative intervention is recommended in the patient with multiple trauma to mobilize the patient and minimize the risks associated with prolonged bed rest and recumbency.

The Swiss Association for the Study of Internal Fixation, known as the AO, pioneered the techniques of internal fixation. The evolution of the AO principles of internal fixation included four doctrines (Table 35–10), which were expected to improve the results of fracture treatment.

TABLE 35–10

AO Principles of Internal Fixation

1. Anatomic reduction of the fracture fragments, particularly in joint fractures
2. Stable internal fixation designed to fulfill the local biomechanical demands
3. Preservation of the blood supply to the bone fragments and the soft tissue by means of atraumatic surgical technique
4. Early, active pain-free mobilization of muscles and joints adjacent to the fracture, preventing the development of fracture disease

From Müller ME, Allgöwer M, Schneider R, Willenenner H: Manual of Internal Fixation. Techniques Recommended by the AO-ASIF Group., 3rd ed. revised 1995. Berlin, Springer Verlag, p. 2.

KEY POINTS

▶ Bony fractures occur in a wide variety of patterns depending on the magnitude and direction of the force applied at the time of injury.

continued

▶ A complete description of the fracture is required to determine management: plane of fracture, exact location, angulation and displacement, simple or comminuted, closed or open, and if open, the degree of associated soft tissue injury.

▶ Orthopedic trauma emergencies include open fractures, dislocations, fractures associated with compartment syndrome or vascular compromise, and unstable spinal fractures associated with incomplete or worsening neurologic deficits.

▶ Major blood loss may be associated with fractures, especially pelvic fractures with posterior element disruption and femoral fractures.

CASE 35–10. A 54-year-old woman had a fall on her outstretched hand (FOOSH) after tripping in her home. She complains of a deformed, painful right wrist. Examination reveals an obvious "dinner fork" deformity of her wrist with pain to gentle palpation. The skin is contused but intact. She has a normal neurovascular examination with the exception of paresthesia in the distribution of the median nerve. The patient has good pulses and capillary refill. See the plain radiographs on the facing page.

A. Outline a treatment plan the orthopedic consultant is likely to choose.

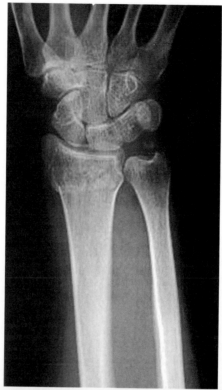

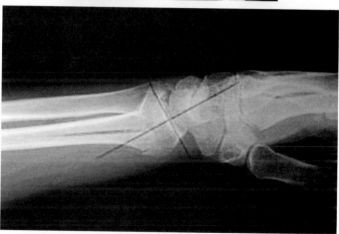

Case 35–10

CASE 35–11. A 76-year-old woman had a fall while
walking to the bathroom. She has mild dementia, congestive
heart failure, and hypertension. She complains of pain in her
right hip. Examination reveals a shortened, externally rotated
leg. She has pain to any motion in her hip joint. The skin in
contused but intact. She has a normal neurologic
examination. The internal medicine service has seen the
patient and believes that she is in acceptable medical
condition to undergo anesthesia.

A. Outline a treatment plan the orthopedic consultant is likely to
   choose.

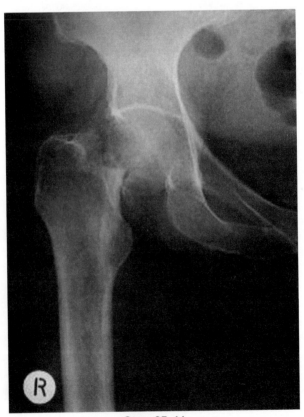

Case 35–11

continued

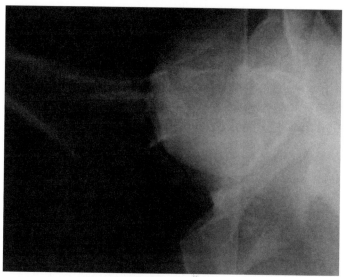

Case 35–11 *continued*

CASE 35–12. A 19-year-old motorcyclist was hit by a truck, sustaining multiple injuries that include a crush injury to the left shin. Examination reveals an obvious deformity of the lower leg with a deep laceration of the mid-shin and crushed and bruised skin extending from mid-shin to the foot. The patient has sensation and movement in the toes, but the foot is cool, pale, and pulseless. Plain radiographs (see the following page) reveal simple tibia and fibula fractures with angulation and displacement.

  A. Outline a treatment plan the orthopedic consultant is likely to choose.

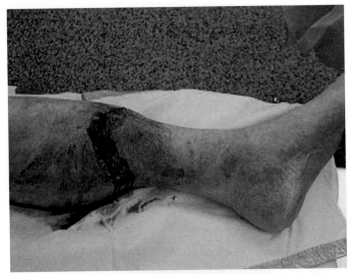

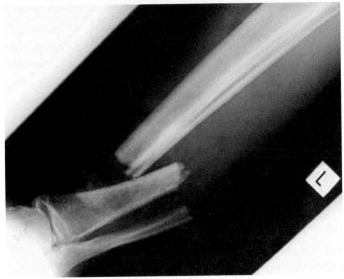

Case 35–12

HEAD AND CERVICAL SPINE INJURY

▶ ETIOLOGY

How common is head injury?

Each year in the United States, 1 million patients with head injuries are treated and discharged from hospital emergency departments and another 230,000 are admitted. Brain injury is present in half of trauma deaths, and alcohol or drug use is found in about half of these deaths.

Motor vehicle accidents are the most common cause, especially in young adults and teenagers.

What is the mortality of head injury?

The majority of head injuries (80%) are mild, and these patients generally do well in the long run, but about half have some post-concussive symptom 6 weeks after injury. Of those with moderate injuries, only 60% make a good recovery, while 7% remain vegetative or die. Severe head injury has an even more dismal prognosis and accounts about one third of trauma deaths.

What are the consequences of gunshot wounds to the head?

Penetrating head injury is increasing in frequency and now accounts for about 15% of deaths due to head injury. The intracranial entrance of bullets and associated bone fragments causes shock waves and cavitation injuries that result in a wide path of destruction. The tissue destruction is associated with a consumptive coagulopathy and vasospasm, which further increase the injury. Mortality exceeds 60%; of survivors, 10% are vegetative or severely disabled. In patients with some hope of survival, surgery may be undertaken to débride necrotic tissue and close the dura.

Where do spinal cord injuries usually occur?

In the United States about 10,000 people per year sustain spinal cord injuries. Cervical injuries are the most devastating and unfortunately also the most common (55%). The C5 vertebra is the most common fractured. Other injuries in the thoracic (30%) and lumbar (15%) locations result in less disability.

▶ **EVALUATION**

How is neurologic status best evaluated?

The level of alertness should be noted on patient arrival and the Glasgow Coma Scale score (Table 35–11) recorded. This remains the best clinical evaluation of injury severity and ultimate prognosis. Though the Glasgow Coma Scale score, along with findings on CT scan, can be helpful in predicting outcome, only very good and very bad outcomes can be predicted with any degree of confidence, especially in children.

What trauma patients need a head CT scan?

Trauma patients with documented loss of consciousness and any sustained neurologic impairment need CT scanning immediately. The same applies to patients with persistent amnesia for the event or suspected skull fractures and any patient with definite or suspected neurologic deterioration. Age older than 40 years implies a higher risk of severe injury and hence imparts an even greater need for expeditious CT scan.

TABLE 35–11

Glasgow Coma Scale[*]

Variable	Points
Eye Opening (E)	
Spontaneous	4
To speech	3
To pain	2
None	1
Motor Response (M)	
Obeys commands	6
Localizes pain	5
Withdraws from pain	4
Abnormal flexion	3
Abnormal extension	2
None	1
Verbal Response (V)	
Oriented	5
Confused conversation	4
Inappropriate words	3
Incomprehensible sounds	2
None	1

[*]Glasgow Coma Scale scoring = E + M + V points.

How does one make the diagnosis of basilar skull fracture?

The only evidence for basilar skull (base of skull) fracture may be found by examination of the external auditory canal and tympanic membrane for bleeding secondary to disruption of that bony canal or membrane. These fractures may also present with bruising around the eyes ("raccoon's eyes") or behind the ears (Battle's sign). Leakage of CSF denotes significant skull injury. This leak usually stops spontaneously but may require elevation of the head of the bed, CSF drainage, or, rarely, surgical intervention.

Which patients with blunt trauma need cervical spine radiographs?

All patients with major blunt trauma, especially those with head or facial injuries, should be assumed to have cervical spine injuries until proven otherwise. These patients must be treated with cervical spine immobilization until instability has been excluded either clinically or radiologically. Patients who are fully awake, are not intoxicated, have no distracting pain, have no tenderness in the cervical spine, and are able to rotate, flex, and extend the head without pain may be cleared clinically and do not require cervical spine radiographs. Otherwise, patients must be cleared radiologically; a fine-cut CT scan with coronal and sagittal reconstructions is the study least likely to miss a fracture or dislocation.

How does one know which vertebral fractures are stable?

All cervical spine fractures should be assumed to be unstable and evaluated by a neurosurgeon. In patients with tenderness over the posterior neck but *no* fractures on CT scan, flexion-extension radiographs may confirm stability of the cervical spine (i.e., no ligamentous injury). However, in patients with fractures, the movement necessary to obtain these images may result in spinal cord injury. Neurologic deficit or radiographically demonstrated fracture are contraindications for flexion-extension films.

What is the difference between epidural and subdural hematomas?

It is helpful to distinguish mass lesions, which often require immediate surgical evacuation, from diffuse lesions, for which protection of secondary brain injury by nonsurgical means is the only therapeutic option (Table 35–12). Mass lesions include subdural, epidural, and intracranial hematomas. Hemorrhagic lesions also include traumatic subarachnoid hemorrhage, which is not in itself an actual mass lesion.

TABLE 35–12

Categories of Head Injury

Category	Description
Focal	Epidural hematoma
	Subdural hematoma
	Subarachnoid hemorrhage
	Intraparenchymal contusions and hematomas
	Penetrating injuries
Nonfocal	Mild concussion
	Major concussion
	Diffuse axonal injury

Acute subdural hematomas are the most commonly seen mass lesions. They occur as a result of a deceleration injury, in which the brain actually continues to move a few millimeters in the direction of the head-motion vector. This takes place when the skull comes to a sudden stop against a static object, such as a dashboard or windshield. The negative pressure on the side opposite the impact causes bridging veins to tear, thereby causing a hematoma. This negative pressure also causes severe cortical and subcortical damage and consequent swelling. Associated parenchymal bleeding and contusion are common and often determine a poor outcome even if the hematoma is small, and even after it is decompressed.

Epidural hematomas occur most commonly when the middle meningeal artery is lacerated by a temporal skull fracture due to a direct blow. But they can also be seen at other sites on the skull. The clinical course sometimes includes a period of lucidity immediately after the injury, followed by deterioration to coma as the hematoma expands. This lucid interval is found in a minority of patients. Epidural hematomas affect only 3% of patients with major head injury. Without craniotomy, these patients usually deteriorate rapidly and die. Because the parenchymal brain injury is often minimal, if timely surgical decompression is accomplished, they may rapidly recover normal neurologic function.

What is the significance of diffuse axonal injury (DAI)?

Diffuse axonal injury (DAI) is generally a widespread brain injury that occurs when shear forces injure or transect long axons of cerebral neurons. Some transected neurons degenerate, but others that are only stretched may heal if conditions remain optimal. These conditions include adequate cerebral flow and oxygenation. The initial CT scan may be unimpressive, though DAI may coexist with mass lesions, especially subdural and parenchymal hematomas. When there are enough transected pathways, significant permanent deficits result.

What are the clinical signs of increasing intracranial pressure (ICP)?

Deterioration of mental status, vomiting, and hypertension with bradycardia or tachycardia may be indicative of increased intracranial pressure (ICP). The skull contains about 80% brain, 10% blood, and 10% CSF. When brain swelling occurs, the cerebrum enlarges and fluids are displaced from the intracranial compartment. Thereafter, compliance decreases and ICP rises rapidly. As the ipsilateral uncus of the medial temporal lobe swells and compresses the pupilloconstrictor (exterior) fibers of the peripheral 3rd cranial nerve, pupillary dilation occurs. In actuality these 3rd cranial nerve fibers are usually compressed between the posterior cerebral and superior cerebellar arteries (review circle of Willis anatomy) as the swelling uncus pushes one of these against the other. In this manner, an enlarging focal hematoma or diffuse brain swelling eventually causes transtentorial herniation, loss of brain stem function, and death.

Which patients need ICP monitoring?

ICP monitoring is recommended for all patients with severe head injury (Glasgow Coma Scale score 3 to 8) and abnormal CT. It is also recommended for patients with severe head injury and age older than 40 years, systolic blood pressure less than 90 mm Hg, or clinical signs of elevated ICP (Table 35–13). The goal of ICP monitoring is to identify and treat pressure peaks and therefore consistently preserve cerebral blood flow. Normal ICP is less than 15 mm Hg, and treatment is instituted for pressures higher than 20 mm Hg. Treatment options are many (Table 35–14).

TABLE 35–13
Brain Trauma Foundation Guidelines for the Management of Severe Head Injury

1. First priority for head injured patient is complete and rapid physiologic resuscitation.
2. No specific treatment should be directed at intracranial hypertension in the absence of signs of transtentorial herniation or neurologic deterioration.
3. When signs of transtentorial herniation or neurologic deterioration not attributable to extracranial explanations are present, the physician should assume that intracranial hypertension is present and treat it aggressively with
    a. Hyperventilation
    b. Mannitol, but only under conditions of adequate volume replacement.
4. The mean arterial pressure should be maintained above 90 mm Hg throughout the patient's course (to maintain a cerebral perfusion pressure of >70)

continued

Table 35-13. Brain Trauma Foundation Guidelines for the Management of Severe Head Injury *continued*

5. Intracranial pressure (ICP) monitoring is appropriate in patients with severe head injury (Glasgow Coma Scale score 3–8)
   and
   An abnormal CT scan of the head (i.e., hematomas, contusions, edema, compressed basal cisterna)
   or
   A normal CT and age >40 years
   Motor posturing
   Systolic blood pressure <90 mm Hg
6. ICP treatment should be initiated at an upper threshold of 20–25 mm Hg and corroborated by frequent clinical examinations and cerebral perfusion pressure data.
7. Cerebral perfusion should be maintained at a minimum of 70 mm Hg.
8. Hyperventilation
   a. Prolonged hyperventilation (Pco_2 <25) should be avoided.
   b. Prophylactic hyperventilation (Pco_2 <35) should be avoided for the first 24 hours if possible.
   c. Hyperventilation therapy may be necessary for brief periods when there is a sudden ICP rise and/or acute neurologic deterioration.
9. Mannitol is used for control of raised ICP in boluses of 1 g/kg body weight. Euvolemia should be maintained by adequate fluid replacement. A Foley catheter is essential in these patients.
10. High-dose barbiturate therapy may be considered in hemodynamically stable, salvageable severe head injury patients with refractory intracranial hypertension.
11. Nutrition: 140% of resting metabolic expenditure (100% if paralyzed) using enteral or parenteral formulas containing at least 15% of proteins is replaced by the 7th day after injury.
12. Seizures: prophylactic use of phenytoin, carbamazepine, or phenobarbital is not recommended for preventing late post-traumatic seizures. Anticonvulsants may be used to prevent early post-traumatic seizures in patients at high risk.

How is cerebral blood flow (CBF) measured?

In the laboratory setting, cerebral perfusion has been measured using radioisotope uptake, thermodilution, transcranial Doppler, jugular venous oxygen saturation, direct measurement of brain Po_2, and other techniques.

However, at the bedside, cerebral blood flow and oxygenation are not easily quantified, although techniques and instrumentation for these are in clinical trials. Cerebral perfusion pressure (CPP) is currently used as a surrogate measure. CPP is calculated by subtracting the intracranial pressure (ICP) from the systemic mean arterial pressure (MAP) (CPP = MAP − ICP). Most recommend maintaining a CPP higher than 70 when possible. A range of devices may be used to measure ICP. Intraventricular catheters offer the advantage of access to withdraw CSF, which facilitates the lowering of ICP.

TABLE 35-14

Options for Treatment of Severe Head Injury
Maintain normal intravascular volume
Vasopressors to maintain CPP >70 (phenylephrine, epinephrine, dopamine)
CSF drainage
Mannitol
Sedation and paralysis
Beta-blockers to control hypertension
Barbiturate coma
Maintain $Pao_2 > 80$
Correct coagulopathy
Moderate hypothermia, avoid fever
Elevate head of bed
Minimal hyperventilation
Hypertonic saline
Insulin to control hyperglycemia (possible option)
Maintain normal serum sodium and magnesium levels
Bifrontal craniotomy
Enteral nutritional support

CPP, cerebral perfusion pressure; CSF, cerebrospinal fluid.

When is a patient "brain dead?"

Brain death indicates the cessation of brain function and indicates the inability to maintain life without continuation of life support. The presence of brain death indicates that further care is clearly futile, is a legal requirement for transplantation donation, and is a legally sufficient reason to withdraw clinical care (i.e., the patient is declared dead).

To make the determination of brain death, a neurologic exam must reveal absence of motor response to deep central pain and absent brain stem function. For absent brain stem function, there must be the following:

1. No pupillary, corneal, or gag reflexes
2. No oculocephalic or oculovestibular reflexes
3. No spontaneous breathing (i.e., an apnea test with no breathing despite hypercapnia)

Oculocephalic ("doll's eye test") and oculovestibular (cold caloric) tests evaluate the 3rd, 6th, 8th cranial nerves and nuclei and the ascending brain stem pathways. They consist of the following:

Doll's eye test—rapidly rotate the head from side to side. In a normal test (in a live patient) the eyes remain "looking" at a fixed external point.
Cold caloric test—ice water is infused onto the tympanic membrane. In a normal test for a comatose patient (not brain

dead), the eyes drift toward the stimulus, then a cortical response directs the eyes back to midline, resulting in nystagmus.

The determination of brain death also requires the absence of other possible causes of coma, such as temperature higher than 32.2°C, drugs, shock, or anoxia, and should not immediately follow cardiac resuscitation.

▶ TREATMENT

What are basics of management of major head injury?

Because nothing can be done to reverse the initial brain injury, treatment is focused on preventing any secondary injury, foremost by maintaining good cerebral perfusion. As is always the case, airway, breathing, circulation, and neurologic disability remain priorities. Because systemic hypotension is associated with double the mortality in head injury, the first goal is to maintain normal blood pressure and oxygenation. Also critical is the need for immediate decompression of focal hematomas that may rapidly enlarge and cause brain herniation.

Current recommendations for optimum management of severe traumatic brain injury are outlined in a consensus document from the Brain Trauma Foundation (see Table 35–13). Common sense and clinical studies support additional treatments, including elevation of the head of the bed to decrease cerebral edema through the augmentation of venous drainage and maintenance of normal serum glucose, sodium, magnesium, clotting factors, temperature, and nutrition.

There are now good scientific data and consensus that some therapies are not beneficial, including prophylactic hyperventilation and steroids. Prophylactic hyperventilation to reduce ICP was previously popular, but subsequent studies demonstrated that the resulting cerebral vasoconstriction often causes cerebral ischemia. Moreover, the beneficial effects lasted only 24 hours. Currently patients are maintained on mild hyperventilation (Pco_2, 35); hyperventilation is then increased only in response to brief peaks in ICP.

Unproven but potentially beneficial treatments are sometimes used in patients for whom outcome appears dismal. Barbiturate-induced coma may provide some cerebral protection but may be detrimental if cerebral blood flow is compromised by hypotension. Mild hypothermia is thought to provide some protection to the brain but may result in its own complications, and a recent large study of this treatment failed to show any substantially significant benefit in outcome.

How are skull fractures treated?

Skull fractures indicate of major energy transfer and potential for underlying injury, including associated arterial injuries (epidural bleed) or dural sinus tears. Patients with skull fractures should, at the least, be admitted to the hospital for observation. The diagnosis is usually made by CT scan in the emergency department.

Depressed skull fractures are generally repaired, especially if there is a CSF leak, an impingement of brain, or a cosmetic deformity. A laceration over a depressed fracture is an indication for expeditious surgical repair and antibiotic coverage.

A basilar fracture is a relative contraindication for antibiotics. This is because the basilar fracture is in direct contact with the patient's sinus mucosa, to which he or she is already acclimated. Antibiotics will likely change those flora to species to which the patient is less acclimated. On the other hand, immunization against the common basilar fracture–associated meningitides is a commonly offered option.

What is the initial care of a patient with spinal cord injury?

Immediate treatment of spinal cord injury includes stabilization and steroid treatment. Immobilization initially may be with hard cervical collar and log roll precautions but may require traction, special orthoses, or surgical fusion. Though the effectiveness of steroids remains controversial, their use has become the standard of care, and methylprednisolone should be started within 3 hours of injury with a 30 mg/kg bolus followed by 5.4 mg/kg/hr for 23 hours. The exact level of sensory and motor deficit for each side should be clearly documented. Patients with deteriorating function may require further immediate evaluation and may require urgent cord decompression.

K E Y   P O I N T S

▶ Maintain oxygen and cerebral perfusion by attention to ABCDs.

▶ Provide immediate diagnosis and evacuation of mass lesions.

▶ Pay attention to details in ICU support especially to maintain CPP and avoid secondary brain injury.

CASE 35–13. An unhelmeted motorcyclist is hit by a car and arrives in the emergency department in coma and shock.

continued

CASE 35–13. *continued*

A. Outline the immediate priorities in management.
B. What are the most important initial steps to provide optimum neurologic outcome?

Following chest tube placement to treat a tension pneumothorax and splenectomy for abdominal hemorrhage, a CT of the head demonstrated frontal contusions but did not show any hematomas or midline shift. The patient remains obtunded with a Glasgow Coma Scale score of 5. Toxicology screen is negative. The patient is taken to the ICU.

C. Outline the optimum subsequent management of this patient with head injury.
D. Should this patient have an ICP monitor placed?
E. What measures should be taken if the ICP abruptly rises ?

UROLOGIC INJURY

▶ ETIOLOGY

What are the usual causes of urologic trauma?

Each of the four main components of the urologic system (kidney, ureter, bladder, and urethra) display different patterns of injury due to their relative positions within the body and degree of protection by surrounding bony and muscular structures. Blunt mechanisms such as falls and motor vehicle crashes produce 80% to 90% of all urologic injuries, with penetrating truncal trauma by missiles, knives, and other piercing agents accounting for the remaining 10% to 20%. An additional, although much smaller, proportion of injuries occurs iatrogenically during abdominal or pelvic surgery.

The kidney is the most frequently injured urologic organ, involved in up to 90% of cases of truncal trauma. Damage to the ureter, although rare, is most often due to penetrating injuries to the flank or back, with 90% of these resulting from a gunshot wound. Bladder injuries are largely caused by blunt forces such as falls, vehicular crashes, and direct pelvic-crushing forces and have been associated with a pelvic fracture in up to 89% of cases. Urethral disruptions also most commonly result from blunt forces and are seen almost exclusively in men. The greater length of the male urethra in comparison to the much shorter and protected female urethra accounts for this sex discrepancy. Fractures of the anterior elements of the pelvic ring (the superior and inferior pubic rami) are a well-described risk factor for injuries to the urethra.

How are urologic injuries classified?

Injury to each of the four segments of the urologic system (kidney, ureter, bladder, and urethra) can be classified by the application of a standardized Urologic Injury Scale (Table 35–15). Grading of urologic injury by this method requires the use of various modalities, including radiologic imaging procedures such as CT, intravenous pyelography (IVP), arteriography, and direct organ inspection at the time of emergency surgery. The size of associated hematoma,

TABLE 35-15	
Urologic Injury Scale	
Grade* and Type	**Injury Description[†]**
Renal Injury	
I Contusion	Microscopic or gross hematuria; urologic studies normal
Hematoma	Subcapsular, nonexpanding without parenchymal laceration
II Hematoma	Nonexpanding perirenal hematoma confined to the renal retroperitoneum
Laceration	<1 cm parenchymal depth of renal cortex without urinary extravasation
III Laceration	>1 cm parenchymal depth of renal cortex without collecting system rupture or urinary extravasation
IV Laceration	Parenchymal laceration extending through the renal cortex, medulla, and collecting system
Vascular	Main renal artery or vein injury with contained hemorrhage
V Laceration	Completely shattered kidney
Vascular	Avulsion of renal hilum that devascularizes the kidney
Ureter Injury	
I Hematoma	Contusion or hematoma without devascularization
II Hematoma	≤50% transaction
III Laceration	>50% transaction
IV Laceration	Complete transaction with 2-cm devascularization
V Laceration	Avulsion of renal hilum that devascularizes the kidney
Bladder Injury	
I Hematoma	Contusion, intramural hematoma
Laceration	Partial thickness
II Laceration	Extraperitoneal bladder wall laceration ≤2 cm
III Laceration	Extraperitoneal (>2 cm) or intraperitoneal (2 cm) bladder wall lacerations
IV Laceration	Intraperitoneal bladder wall lacerations >2 cm
V Laceration	Intraperitoneal or extraperitoneal bladder wall laceration extending into bladder neck or ureteral orifice (trigone)

continued

Table 35–15. Urologic Injury Scale *continued*		
Grade* and Type	**Injury Description†**
Urethral Injury	
I Contusion	Blood at urethral meatus; urethrography normal
II Stretch injury	Elongation of urethra without extravasation on urethrography
III Partial disruption	Extravasation of urethrographic contrast medium at injury site, with contrast visualized in the bladder
IV Complete disruption	Extravasation of urethrographic contrast medium at injury site, without visualization in the bladder; <2 cm of urethral disruption
V Complete disruption	Complete transaction with >2 cm urethral separation, or extension into the prostate or vagina

*Advance one grade for multiple injuries to the same organ.
†Based on the most accurate assessment at autopsy, laparotomy, or radiologic study.
From Moore EE, Shackford SR, Pachter HL, et al: Organ injury scaling: Spleen, liver, and kidney. J Trauma 1989;29:1664.

the length and depth of organ laceration, and the presence of major vascular disruptions (such as to the renal arteries) all are features that can be quantified and therefore used to grade injuries to these organs, allowing the clinician to establish therapeutic priorities and estimate prognosis.

▶ EVALUATION

What is hematuria, how is it measured, and why is it important?

Hematuria, or the presence of blood in the urine, may be described as either gross (visible to the naked eye) or microscopic (detected only under magnification or by dipstick techniques) and is one of the hallmarks of urologic injury. Hematuria is associated with an injury incidence rate of the urologic tract of up to 94%. Studies have determined that the widely available dipstick urine tests, which quantify hematuria on a linear scale from "negative" to "3+," are for all practical purposes as sensitive as microscopic urinalysis, which determines the number of erythrocytes per high-power field. Unfortunately, there exists only a poor correlation between the degree of hematuria and the severity of the injury. Many relatively innocuous and self-limiting kidney injuries present rather dramatically with gross hematuria, whereas other, more potentially serious injuries can present with no blood in the urine at all or are associated with only minute amounts that are seen only microscopically. Indeed, hematuria is notoriously absent in several specific types of urologic injury: up to 40% of renal pedicle vascular disruptions and 70% of injuries to the ureter present with a normal urinalysis.

Despite these apparent inconsistencies, the value of determining the presence of hematuria lies in its high sensitivity for injury to the various urologic organs. Thus, the presence of hematuria after truncal trauma mandates further investigations in most patients to rule out significant injuries. The nature and complexity of such investigative maneuvers depend to a large degree on the clinician's index of suspicion for major injury, which should be based on the injury mechanism as well as on the physical examination of the patient. In general, microscopic hematuria mandates further investigation if it is associated with significant flank or back pain, tenderness or hematoma, or hemodynamic instability or shock.

Which diagnostic techniques are available to assess urologic system injury?

The choice of test largely depends on the portion of the urologic system that is suspected of harboring an injury. *Plain film radiographs* of the abdomen and pelvis are not sensitive enough to demonstrate specific urologic injuries, although they are excellent tools for diagnosing fractures of the lower spine and of the pelvis, which are commonly associated with injuries of the adjacent kidney, bladder, or urethra.

Excretory urography, or IVP, is a widely available test that may demonstrate major parenchymal injuries to the kidney or may suggest renal arterial inflow disruption or congenital absence. The IVP may be performed "on table" during emergency surgical exploration of the abdomen to more completely stage renal or ureteral injuries or to establish the presence of a functioning contralateral kidney if a nephrectomy is being contemplated. A useful variant of this technique that may elucidate a ureteral or bladder injury intraoperatively involves the administration of rapidly excreted *intravenous dyes* such as methylene blue or indigo carmine. Brightly colored urine usually leaks out from small bladder or ureteral injuries and stains the surrounding tissues, thus directing the surgeon's eyes to the area in question.

CT scan is the most sensitive and specific tool for determining the presence and nature of renal injuries, although it is more time-consuming and should not be performed on unstable patients. It allows for the preoperative staging of the injured kidney (see Table 35–15), a crucial element in the decision to embark on nonoperative management of these injuries.

Retrograde contrast cystography not only remains the most reliable method with which to diagnose bladder rupture but also can distinguish between the intraperitoneal and extraperitoneal varieties and therefore determines the appropriate management of these injuries.

Contrast retrograde urethrography (*RUG*) must be performed in any patient with a potential urethral disruption and should always precede the insertion of an indwelling Foley bladder catheter in these patients.

Finally, formal *renal angiography* is useful in cases of suspected renal vascular pedicle injury that cannot be fully delineated on the CT scan.

What should be ruled out prior to insertion of a Foley catheter into the bladder of a male trauma victim?

The potential for a urethral injury should be entertained, and if high, further investigated. Blind insertion of an indwelling bladder catheter may further disrupt a partial urethral tear, making subsequent repair and healing much more difficult. Therefore, any patient with a suspected urethral disruption must first be studied with RUG to image the full length of the urethra and rule out such injuries. The study consists of an oblique plain radiograph of the pelvis that is taken during slow injection of 15 to 20 mL of iodinated water-soluble contrast into the male urethral meatus via a soft latex catheter carefully inserted 1 to 2 cm into the urethral bulb.

What signs and symptoms should raise a suspicion for urologic trauma after a blunt mechanism of injury?

Gross hematuria should always initiate further investigation to rule out a major urologic injury. The nature of the investigation depends on which portion of the urinary tract is under suspicion from the patient's history and physical findings on examination. When hematuria is microscopic, a history of shock (systolic blood pressure lower than 90 mm Hg in the adult) requires urologic imaging to rule out hemorrhage from a kidney injury. Flank ecchymosis or tenderness, associated lower thoracic or upper lumbar vertebral fractures, and lower rib fractures are relative indications for additional studies to rule out kidney laceration, hematomas, and vascular disruptions, although the diagnostic yield in these cases is low. Blood at the urethral meatus, as well as a nonpalpable prostate, a scrotal hematoma, or an inability to void spontaneously, are common signs in men with traumatic urethral disruptions. Suprapubic or lower abdominal pain and tenderness, especially if associated with a pelvic fracture, may indicate laceration or rupture of the underlying bladder and should be investigated with contrast cystography.

What signs on the physical exam should raise a suspicion for urologic injury after a penetrating mechanism of injury?

All stab, shotgun, and gunshot wounds of the anterior abdomen, back, flank, and groin have the potential to injure any of the various components of the urologic system. Clearly, patients in shock should be explored without delay to control exsanguinating hemorrhage. Bullets known or thought to have violated the peritoneal cavity almost always produce injuries that require surgical control, so these patients merit prompt exploration as well. Injuries with trajectories tangential to the trunk or those suspected of causing only isolated renal injury may be staged radiographically, assuming the patient remains hemodynamically normal and has no other indication for immediate surgical exploration. In any case, the presence of peritonitis in the victim of penetrating truncal trauma merits prompt abdominal exploration.

What organ-specific injuries are commonly seen in patients with urologic trauma?

The kidney is the organ most commonly injured by both blunt and penetrating mechanisms. In blunt truncal trauma, renal injury is sustained in up to 94% of cases, although a relatively small proportion of these are considered life threatening. The spectrum of injury can vary from the usually self-limited minor renal contusions and shallow lacerations, to deeper and more complex parenchymal disruptions, to exsanguinating injuries of the vascular pedicle that require emergency operative control and repair or even nephrectomy.

The ureter is well protected from blunt forces by the musculature of the retroperitoneum and the adjacent spine, although it is quite vulnerable to direct injury from missiles and knives. Additionally, blast forces from bullets passing through adjacent tissue may produce ureteral devascularization and delayed necrosis leading to perforation or stricture. Unless diagnosed intraoperatively, a ureteral disruption presents in a delayed fashion as a urinoma, which is a free intraperitoneal collection of urine that may be noted as a flank mass producing abdominal pain, tenderness, and fever.

The bladder may sustain lacerations from sharp spicules of fractured pelvic bones, most commonly the pubic rami. Also, the bladder may rupture directly into the peritoneal cavity or, more commonly, into the retroperitoneal spaces from a sudden increase in the intravesical pressure as a result of a direct blow or deceleration.

The urethra in the male is vulnerable to disruption over its posterior segments as a result of a straddle injury or from direct avulsion from the bladder base in severe pelvic blunt trauma. Fractures of the anterior elements of the pelvis can also disrupt the anterior segments of the urethra in the male and should alert the clinician to this possibility any time a patient sustaining blunt pelvic injury cannot void spontaneously, has blood at the urethral meatus, has a nonpalpable or "high-riding" prostate on digital rectal exam, or develops a scrotoperineal hematoma. In women, urethral injuries are rare due to the urethra's much shorter length but can still occur in association with severe open pelvic fractures involving the anterior bony elements.

> **TREATMENT**

What are the initial priorities in patients with suspected urologic injuries?

A significant proportion of early morbidity and mortality in victims of trauma results from a rather small collection of injuries, most of which can be diagnosed and controlled in the first few minutes of care. Examples include upper airway obstruction (from either oropharyngeal or tracheal injuries, or due to occlusion by foreign bodies or the tongue), tension pneumothorax, severe pulmonary contusion, exsanguinating disruption of major blood vessels, solid organs, or long bones, and cerebral or spinal cord injuries causing potentially irreversible brain damage or loss of peripheral vascular tone (i.e., neurogenic shock).

The principles of trauma resuscitation allow for a rapid evaluation and control of these usually lethal injuries and always take precedence over the management of any specific organ trauma. This approach involves diagnosing and securing the compromised airway, ensuring effective breathing (i.e., optimizing oxygenation and CO_2 exchange), evaluating the circulation (i.e., diagnosing shock and controlling hemorrhage while replenishing lost intravascular volume), assessing neurologic disability, and ensuring full *exposure* of the patient to allow a complete head-to-toe, front-to-back physical examination. Once these basic areas have been evaluated and major life-threatening problems controlled or ruled out, specific injuries to the urologic system may proceed as part of the secondary survey of the patient.

How is blunt injury to the kidney best managed?

A patient presenting in shock with evidence of renal injury by virtue of gross hematuria is best served by immediate exploratory celiotomy for evaluation and control of the bleeding kidney, assuming the absence of any other extra-abdominal injuries that could account for the hemodynamic instability. However, an average of only 10% of patients presenting with blunt renal trauma ultimately require operative control and repair of their kidney injuries, despite the frequently dramatic degree of hematuria with which these patients arrive to the emergency department. Accordingly, a significant majority of blunt renal trauma can be successfully managed nonoperatively once the appropriate urologic imaging and staging procedures are complete. Safe and effective implementation of this nonsurgical approach obviously requires that the patient remain hemodynamically normal as well as lack any other indications for emergency surgical exploration. Close monitoring of the patient's vital physiologic parameters, such as blood pressure, heart rate, and urine output, and frequent abdominal re-examinations are mandatory elements of the nonoperative management approach, because any significant changes in these signs and symptoms may signal the presence of ongoing bleeding or peritonitis—which is best treated surgically. For this reason, any patient with a major renal injury who is a candidate for nonoperative management is best served by close monitoring in an ICU until the clinician is certain that hemorrhage has not recurred.

An absolute indication for operative exploration of a renal injury is evidence of continued or recurrent bleeding from the kidney producing hemodynamic instability or ongoing transfusion or fluid requirements. Prolonged urine extravasation from the collecting system that does not diminish after a period of observation is a relative indication for surgery. A CT scan demonstrating a nonfunctioning kidney usually indicates either renal pedicle vascular thrombosis or avulsion.

In the stable patient in whom ongoing bleeding is unlikely, these injuries are best left alone, since surgical intervention to repair renal vascular injuries has not been show to improve the renal salvage rate and often results in nephrectomy.

How are injuries to the bladder best managed?

Blunt bladder disruptions are approached selectively, because the type of rupture (intraperitoneal vs. extraperitoneal) dictates the therapeutic approach, consisting of either immediate surgical intervention or nonoperative management.

An intraperitoneal bladder rupture is usually diagnosed during exploratory surgery or, more commonly, at the time of contrast cystography, when the free-flowing, radiopaque contrast can be seen on the abdominal radiograph delineating loops of intestine or adjacent to the liver or spleen. This type of injury is customarily repaired surgically so as to prevent continued urine leakage and peritonitis, although a small percentage of cases may respond to simple decompression via the indwelling bladder catheter if the disruption is not too large.

Conversely, an extraperitoneal bladder rupture is distinguished by a much more limited extravasation of contrast and urine, which is effectively contained by the adjacent intact peritoneum and retrovesical tissues. A 2-week period of bladder decompression followed by contrast cystography to document healing is all that is required in these patients, assuming the absence of associated pelvic or intra-abdominal injuries mandating surgical control.

Finally, bladder trauma caused by penetrating mechanisms such as knives or bullets is almost universally surgically repaired at the time of abdominal exploration for other injuries.

K E Y   P O I N T S

▶ The urologic system is composed of several different organs; injury to each is characterized by a particular pattern of injury and requires a specific diagnostic and therapeutic approach.

▶ Hematuria is the hallmark of urologic injury, although a complete history and physical examination are mandatory to determine the severity of the injury and the need for further diagnostic and therapeutic maneuvers.

▶ Hematuria associated with flank tenderness and shock often indicates the need for immediate surgical exploration of the kidney to rule out and control exsanguinating injury.

▶ Pelvic fractures are frequently associated with injuries to the bladder, especially in patients presenting with gross hematuria.

▶ Urethral trauma should always be ruled out in a man sustaining pelvic or perineal trauma prior to insertion of an indwelling bladder catheter.

▶ Most kidney injuries in stable patients and most extraperitoneal bladder ruptures may be managed nonoperatively with excellent results.

CASE 35–14. A 41-year-old woman falls 7 m from a balcony onto a concrete sidewalk. She is alert and complains of back and abdominal pain. Despite receiving a rapid infusion of 1500 mL of intravenous crystalloid, her blood pressure remains low at 90 /64 mm Hg and her pulse rate elevated at 128 beat/min. On examination you note tenderness in the left upper quadrant of the abdomen and over the left flank. Her pelvis is nontender and shows no signs of instability. Insertion of a Foley bladder catheter returns grossly bloody urine.

  A. What are your immediate priorities?
  B. What type of urologic system injury do you suspect?
  C. What associated nonurologic system injuries may also be
     present?

CASE 35–15. A 23-year-old man sustains a crush injury to the pelvis when he strikes a telephone pole while riding his motorcycle. On arrival to your emergency department, he complains of severe pain in the suprapubic and inguinal regions and refuses to flex his hips, because of pain. His vital signs are normal. A chest radiograph is normal, but the anteroposterior view of the pelvis shows pubic symphysis separation and fractures of both pubic rami on the right with moderate displacement.

    A. What segments of the urologic system are at risk for injury?
    B. How would the findings of scrotal hematoma direct your approach in this case?
    C. When would you insert a Foley bladder catheter in this patient?

CASE 35–16. A 35-year-old woman is assaulted with a lead pipe, sustaining several blows to her back and flank. She complains of severe pain in these areas, although her vital signs are normal. Her urinalysis is grossly free of blood but shows 10 to 20 red blood cells per high-power field on microscopic analysis. Radiographs of her thoracic and lumbar spine are normal, as is a radiograph of her chest.

    A. Describe your differential diagnosis for her microscopic hematuria.
    B. What further investigations are indicated?

VASCULAR INJURY

▶ ETIOLOGY

What is a vascular injury?

All forms of trauma (blunt, penetrating, burn) disrupt blood vessels, but these are often unnamed small branches or capillaries in the subcutaneous tissue or muscle. On trauma services a "vascular injury" refers to damage to a major named artery or vein in the neck, thorax, abdomen, or extremity. Because most major named vessels lie adjacent to other named vessels, structures, or viscera, combined injuries are common and complicate the care of the vascular injury.

What causes a vascular injury?

All injuries related to trauma are secondary to the transfer of kinetic energy ($KE = \frac{1}{2} mv^2$, where m = mass and v = velocity) during the incident. This kinetic energy associated with a motor vehicle crash (blunt trauma) is usually transmitted to the victim by mechanisms of deceleration or compression, each of which can cause vascular injuries. For example, a sudden deceleration of the victim against a shoulder harness restraint may cause a stretching injury to the carotid artery in the neck. Disruption of the intima (the inner lining of the artery) with or without injury to the media may lead to impaired arterial flow, emboli to the brain, or complete thrombosis of the carotid artery. In such a patient, neurologic sequelae rather than overt bleeding would result from the vascular injury. Compression of the mid-aspect of the popliteal artery by a posterior dislocation of the knee sustained in a motor vehicle crash or fall might also lead to an intimal injury with secondary thrombosis. In this patient, signs of ischemia in the leg and foot would then occur.

With penetrating trauma caused by knives or low-velocity missiles from civilian handguns (muzzle kinetic energy of a missile from a .357 Magnum handgun = 535 ft-lb), vascular injuries are caused by cutting or laceration from the object. If a critical organ such as the brain or heart or a major blood vessel is injured by a low-velocity missile, death may result even though impact kinetic energy is low.

What are the types of vascular injuries?

In general, these include nonperforating injury of the wall only, perforation of the wall, transection of the vessel, and spasm of the vessel. When all the subtypes of these major categories are included (Table 35–16), a large number of clinical presentations are possible.

TABLE 35–16

Types of Vascular Injuries

Nonperforating injury of the wall
   Subintimal or intramural hematoma
   Intimal flap with or without occlusion of the vessel
Perforating injury of the wall
   With hemorrhage or early traumatic false aneurysm
   With or without arteriovenous fistula
Transection of the vessel
Spasm of the vessel

▶ EVALUATION

What are "hard" signs of a vascular injury?

"Hard," or overt, signs of a vascular injury include bleeding, pulsatile (arterial) or nonpulsatile (venous) hematoma, a palpable thrill/audible bruit characteristic of an arteriovenous fistula, or one or more of the six "Ps" of arterial occlusion (*p*ulselessness, *p*allor, *p*aresthesias, *p*ain, *p*aralysis, *p*oikilothermia). A laceration of a vessel most commonly leads to hard signs such as bleeding, hematoma, or an arteriovenous fistula. Either penetrating or blunt injury can cause transection of a vessel or an intimal injury with secondary thrombosis and lead to the six Ps. The type of hard sign that results from a vascular injury is related to the size of the patient, the direction of the injury (especially for missile wounds), the location of the injury, and the kinetic energy transferred. For example, a gunshot wound to the brachial artery in a thin patient often results in external bleeding because there is little soft tissue to tamponade the injury. An obese patient with an oblique track of a missile through large muscles adjacent to a penetrating wound to the brachial artery would more likely present with a pulsatile or expanding hematoma. Any patient who arrives in the emergency department with measurable vital signs after sustaining a gunshot wound of the infrarenal abdominal aorta or inferior vena cava is likely to have extensive retroperitoneal tamponade (pulsatile or nonpulsatile hematoma) rather than free bleeding.

What are "soft" signs of a vascular injury?

"Soft," or subtle, signs of a vascular injury include history of external bleeding at the scene or in transit to the hospital, proximity of wound or blunt injury to a vessel, a small nonpulsatile hematoma, or a neurologic defect in a nerve adjacent to a named vessel. A patient with a laceration of a peripheral artery or vein may bleed enough at the scene to cause hypovolemic shock. Vasoconstriction is a normal physiologic response in such a patient and may cause cessation of external bleeding until resuscitation occurs in the emergency department. The absence of current external bleeding does not, therefore, rule out a vascular injury. In patients with only proximity of a penetrating injury to a peripheral artery and no other symptoms or signs, 3% to 18% will be found to have some type of abnormality on an arteriogram. Approximately 90% to 95% of these injuries are minor wall abnormalities that do not affect flow and can be managed without operation (see later).

What are the signs of peripheral vascular injury on physical examination?

Signs of peripheral vascular injury include bleeding, a hematoma, a thrill or bruit, or diminished or absent pulses.

Either pulsatile or nonpulsatile bleeding observed on inspection of an extremity is suggestive of a major vascular injury but is not pathognomonic. This is because small vessels in the injured skin or muscle can bleed at a significant rate in normotensive individuals. Bleeding from such vessels, however, does not occur at the rate of or with the force associated with hemorrhage from a major named vessel.

A hematoma in an extremity may represent an injury to underlying soft tissue, a fracture of the underlying bone, or injury to a major artery or vein. Hematomas related to contusions, fractures, or venous injuries are nonpulsatile and do not expand significantly when observed in the emergency department. Those caused by fractures of underlying bone are usually diffuse and are often associated with deformity of the extremity and bony crepitus on examination. Hematomas overlying injuries to major named arteries are obviously pulsatile and continue to expand when observed.

An arteriovenous fistula in an extremity is diagnosed by palpation of a thrill (feels like a continuous vibration) and auscultation of a bruit (continuous murmur). The thrill and bruit disappear when the site of the fistula is compressed by the examiner.

A major injury to an artery in an extremity is always suggested by a *diminished or absent pulse* at the wrist or ankle and pallor or delayed capillary refill in the fingernails or toenails.

Other signs of arterial occlusion previously listed (paresthesias, pain, paralysis, poikilothermia) occur when there has been a delay in diagnosis and neuromuscular damage has occurred. Any diminished or absent pulse distal to a fracture or dislocation in an extremity should be reassessed after the fracture is realigned or the dislocation is reduced.

What are the signs of vascular injury in the trunk?

A patient with an injury to a major named vessel in the superior mediastinum (great vessels) may present in one of several ways. Such patients may be asymptomatic (intima/media injury only); may have a mediastinal or extrapleural hematoma on a chest radiograph (tamponade or perforation); may be hypotensive and have a hematoma on a chest radiograph (inadequate tamponade); or may have profound hypotension on admission (bleeding into pleural cavity).

A patient with an injury to a major named vessel in the abdomen may present in one of several ways. Almost all patients with such an injury have a period of hypotension in the field or on arrival in the emergency department.

Those with injuries to veins that are tamponaded by the retroperitoneum (i.e., inferior vena cava, renal vein, iliac vein) or base of the mesentery (superior mesenteric vein) may become normotensive with the infusion of crystalloids in the emergency department and remain so until the hematoma is opened in the operating room.

Those with injuries to abdominal arteries often have profound hypotension in the field, have only a transient improvement in blood pressure after the infusion of crystalloids, and develop abdominal distention if an emergency operation is delayed.

If a major injury to a common or external iliac artery has occurred, the ipsilateral pulse in the femoral artery may be diminished or absent.

Which diagnostic test based on an extension of the physical exam may be helpful in the diagnosis of a peripheral arterial injury?

In patients who are hypothermic or hypotensive and have peripheral vasoconstriction, it may be difficult to determine if a peripheral arterial pulse is diminished as compared to the opposite extremity. The same is often true in patients with significant exogenous obesity. It may be helpful to measure an ankle/brachial index (ABI) or brachial/brachial index (BBI) (ABI or BBI = systolic blood pressure in injured lower or upper extremity distal to site of injury divided by systolic blood pressure in uninjured upper extremity). This can be performed using a hand-held Doppler device to auscultate the systolic pressures and is known as an arterial pressure index. A ratio of 0.9 or less has been verified in a limited number of clinical studies as strongly suggestive of an arterial injury in an extremity and should be followed by more advanced diagnostic tests.

Is duplex ultrasound helpful as a diagnostic test in a patient with a possible peripheral arterial injury?

Ultrasound is defined as sound waves exceeding 20,000 cycles/sec and is outside the range of human hearing. For clinical purposes, medical ultrasound devices exceed 1 million cycles/sec. A diagnostic duplex ultrasound probe emitting 7.5 million cycles/sec can be placed over a peripheral artery to determine the appearance of the wall and lumen (real-time brightness or B-mode image) and the flow in the vessel (pulsed-wave Doppler image). The performance and interpretation of diagnostic duplex ultrasound require special training, but the accuracy in detecting peripheral arterial injuries has exceeded 95% in several studies.

What is the role of arteriography, CT angiography, and MR angiography in diagnosing a cervical, truncal, or peripheral arterial injury?

Arteriography refers to the injection of a radiopaque (shows as white on radiograph or CT film) contrast agent into a vessel that may be injured and a simultaneous radiograph, CT, or MR image. It is used to rule in or rule out an arterial injury when physical examination is

TABLE 35–17
Possible Abnormalities on an Arteriogram
Extravasation of dye from vessel   Hematoma containing dye adjacent to vessel injury (early traumatic false aneurysm)   Irregularity of wall with intact flow   Obstruction or severe narrowing   Area of spasm with intact flow

equivocal or cannot be performed. In difficult anatomic areas, an arteriogram may be used to precisely localize the site of a known arterial injury. An arterial injury is present if any of the abnormalities listed in Table 35–17 are noted on the arteriogram. Although venography is rarely indicated in trauma patients, the same findings would be suggestive of a venous injury.

Digital-contrast arteriography uses less contrast than with a routine arteriogram, and blood vessels appear as a dark color. CT and MR arteriography are expensive but have an emerging role in evaluating cervical and mediastinal vessels in patients with blunt trauma.

▶ TREATMENT

Can injuries to major vessels be treated nonoperatively?

In hemodynamically stable patients with nonperforating injuries of the wall or spasm of the vessel and intact distal flow of the contrast agent on an arteriogram, nonoperative management is acceptable because experience has shown that many of these injuries heal spontaneously.

Can injuries to major vessels be treated with endovascular procedures?

An endovascular procedure is defined as the percutaneous insertion of an expandable stent or stent graft under fluoroscopy to treat a lesion of the arterial wall. In patients with atherosclerotic arterial lesions, endovascular stents have been used to treat narrowed areas, and stent grafts to treat infrarenal abdominal aortic aneurysms. On trauma services in hemodynamically stable patients, endovascular procedures have been limited to the treatment of arterial lesions in areas that are difficult to expose (high internal carotid artery, subclavian artery) or when the standard operation may be too risky for the multiply injured patient (stent graft for contained rupture of the descending thoracic aorta). Data on long-term complications and patency of such grafts are unavailable at this time.

What is the treatment in the emergency department for patients with bleeding from a vascular injury?

In patients with active bleeding from the face or neck, manual or gauze pad pressure of the site should be performed at the same time as the airway is assessed. When there is bleeding into the airway or obstruction by a cervical hematoma, either endotracheal intubation or a cricothyroidotomy is performed. Patients with thoracic or abdominal vascular injuries and active bleeding are moved directly to the operating room for simultaneous resuscitation with intravenous fluids and blood and operative control. Significant bleeding from a vascular injury in an extremity is controlled by pressure to the site, compression on a proximal pressure point (i.e., brachial artery in antecubital area, femoral artery in groin), or the application of a temporary proximal tourniquet as the patient is moved to the operating room.

What are the basic principles of vascular repair in the operating room?

Wide preparation and draping around the site of the vascular injury are necessary to allow for extensions of the original incision. When active bleeding is occurring from an injury in the proximal extremity and a tourniquet cannot be placed, direct pressure is maintained on the site as the incision is made in line with the underlying vessel. Vascular clamp control of the vessel proximal and distal to the area of hemorrhage is then performed, and the magnitude of the injury is assessed. Options for management of vascular injuries are described in Table 35–18. After a complex arterial repair in an upper or lower extremity, it is often worthwhile for the surgeon to perform an intraoperative arteriogram to assess the status of suture lines and distal flow. All vascular repairs must be covered by healthy soft tissue to avoid desiccation of the vessel and later breakdown of the repair. When repair of an obstructed artery in an extremity is delayed, ischemic edema and a reperfusion injury may occur in the muscle compartments of the forearm or leg before and after restoration of arterial inflow. Extensive muscle edema

---

TABLE 35–18

Options for Management of Vascular Injuries

Suture repair of perforation or laceration (i.e., arteriorrhaphy or venorrhaphy)

Borrowed vein or synthetic patch repair of perforation or laceration (i.e., patch arterioplasty or venoplasty)

Resection of injured segment and reapproximation of the open ends (i.e., end-to-end anastomosis)

Resection of injured segment and insertion of a substitute vascular conduit (i.e., interposition autogenous vein or synthetic graft)

(intracompartmental pressure >30 to 35 mm Hg) is relieved by longitudinal incisions through the overlying skin, subcutaneous tissue, and enveloping fascia.

What are the complications of arterial repairs?

Early postoperative complications include bleeding from the suture line, distal embolism of clot, thrombosis of the repair, and a missed distal compartment syndrome. Later postoperative complications include stricturing at the site of the repair, thrombosis, infection at the site of the repair with leakage of blood, and an aortogastrointestinal fistula (thoracic or abdominal aorta).

K E Y   P O I N T S

▶ Patients with active external bleeding need direct compression and early operation.

▶ Patients with active internal bleeding need an emergency thoracotomy or laparotomy.

▶ Patients without active bleeding are assessed by physical examination, duplex ultrasound, and/or some form of arteriography with a contrast agent.

CASE 35–17. A 20-year-old man sustained a gunshot wound to the upper left arm and has a nonpulsatile local hematoma with an intact radial pulse at the wrist and a normal BBI.

    A. What are possible causes of the hematoma?
    B. Does the patient need any diagnostic tests?
    C. Does the patient need an emergency operation?

CASE 35–18. A 40-year-old man suffered an open fracture-dislocation of the left knee in a motorcycle crash and has a cool, pulseless left foot.

    A. Which artery is likely to be injured?
    B. Does the patient need any diagnostic tests?
    C. What treatment would you suggest?

36

Vascular Disease

AORTIC VASCULAR DISEASE

▶ ETIOLOGY

What are common causes of thoracic and abdominal aortic aneurysms?

Most aortic aneurysms are caused by atherosclerosis or aortic wall degeneration. A common underlying defect is vessel wall weakness secondary to loss of elastin and collagen. Risk factors for aortic aneurysms include hypertension, smoking, chronic obstructive pulmonary disease (COPD), male gender, and advanced age.

What is the definition of an aortic aneurysm?

Aneurysm of the aorta is enlargement of the aortic diameter by 150% compared to the normal aorta.

What are aortic dissections?

Aortic dissections are separations of the aortic wall due to an intimal tear and disease in the tunica media. A true and a false lumen are formed, and a re-entry tear may also occur. Etiologies include hypertension, trauma, and connective tissue disorders (Marfan's syndrome), and cystic medial necrosis. Usual symptoms include abrupt onset of severe chest pain radiating to the back. The patient describes the pain as "tearing." It may result in cardiac tamponade, aortic insufficiency, and aortic branch occlusion or shearing leading to multiple symptoms. Classification of aortic dissections helps organize treatment plans. Stanford type A dissections involve the ascending aorta, whereas Stanford type B dissections involve the descending aorta distal to the left subclavian artery. All type A dissections need operative repair due to the risk of pericardial tamponade.

What is aortic occlusive disease, and what are its common etiologies?

Aortic occlusive disease is significant atherosclerosis of the aorta with calcification of the aortic wall. It results in aortic narrowing of major aortic branch vessels, including celiac, superior mesenteric, renal, inferior mesenteric, and common iliac arteries. There is usually no aneurysm formation. Risk factors are those similar to atherosclerosis.

▶ EVALUATION

What are important questions in the history to ask the patient with aortic disease?

In addition to a careful history and physical exam, symptoms of back pain, postprandial pain, and impotence are important to ask about. Suspect severe aortoiliac occlusive disease (Leriche's syndrome) in men with hip and buttock claudication and impotence. Most aortic aneurysms are asymptomatic and are discovered during routine abdominal exam by the primary care physician. Asking if the patient has had any family member diagnosed with an aortic aneurysm is important and may help direct the exam.

What findings on physical exam should be noted?

The aorta bifurcates usually at the level of the umbilicus. Careful palpation of the abdomen between the xiphoid and umbilicus is important in aortic evaluation. A pulsatile mass indicates an aneurysm. A tender pulsatile mass or back pain on palpation should be immediately reported since it may reflect a weakening aortic wall and pending rupture. Auscultation of the abdomen may help detect renal or iliac artery bruits.

What radiographic imaging helps?

In a stable patient diagnosed with aortic aneurysm, abdominal ultrasound and/or abdominal CT scans can be ordered to help diagnose and measure the aneurysm diameter. Magnetic resonance (MR) imaging is also a suitable option to help follow the aneurysm, especially in those patients with renal failure. Aortograms are useful to evaluate aortic main branch vessels but not to measure the aortic diameter since they provide visualization only of the lumen.

What other organ systems should also be evaluated?

All patients should undergo a full evaluation of their other comorbidities, including cardiac, pulmonary, renal, and nervous systems.

What is the relationship between aortic diameter and risk of rupture?

Small aneurysms (<5 cm) have a risk of rupture at 4% per year. Aneurysms that are 5 cm have a 10% risk of yearly rupture. Aneurysms greater than 7 cm have a 30% yearly risk for rupture. Thus, all aortic aneurysms greater than 5 cm should be considered for repair.

How is aortic occlusive disease treated?

Once the diagnosis of aortoiliac disease is confirmed by imaging, these patients benefit from aortic femoral bypass with prosthetic graft. Isolated, small iliac occlusions can also be treated with iliac angioplasty and stenting with favorable results. In either case, preservation of the internal iliac artery flow is important to protect against further impotence and colonic ischemia.

What are the proper ways to treat abdominal aortic aneurysms?

Most aneurysms can be repaired on an elective basis. Standard open repairs require either a midline incision and formal exploratory laparotomy or left upper quadrant transverse incision for a retroperitoneal approach. Either approach can be used. Retroperitoneal approaches limit third-space fluid losses, decrease postoperative pain, and are convenient in patients who have had previous abdominal explorations. In either case, aortic control is obtained below the renal arteries by a large clamp. Distal control is either on the distal aorta or iliac arteries bilaterally. The aneurysm is opened and the contents (thrombus) are removed. A prosthetic graft (aortic tube or aortoiliac) material is then sewn to the healthy proximal aortic stump and distally to the iliac arteries. The old aneurysm wall is then used to cover the synthetic graft material to prevent a possible late erosion of the graft into the bowel.

What is the present state of endovascular treatment of aortic aneurysms?

Endovascular treatment of some infrarenal aortic aneurysms is an option. Presently, there are two U.S. Food and Drug Administration–approved devices for transluminal placement of an endoprosthesis in aneurysms via femoral artery access. The patient's aortic anatomy must be suitable for the device selected, including small aortic neck diameter (<28 mm), long aortic neck (usually >10 mm below the renal arteries), and large iliac arteries. This procedure can be performed with minimal blood loss since it entails bilateral femoral cutdowns to place the sheaths that will provide access for device deployment.

What are the signs of aortic aneurysm rupture and how do we treat it?

Patients usually have abdominal pain, a pulsatile mass, and hypotension. The pulsatile mass is usually left of midline and above the umbilicus. Once the diagnosis is confirmed by history and physical exam, resuscitation is started, and these patients must be rushed to the operating room to control the aorta and repair the aneurysm with graft placement. Risk factors for rupture include large aortic diameter, hypertension, COPD, and recent rapid expansion. Thirty-three percent of all aortic aneurysms larger than 5 cm will rupture in 5 years.

What are the indications for aortic aneurysm repair?

The indications for aortic aneurysm repair include whether the patient is experiencing symptoms, as discussed earlier, has an aortic diameter greater than 5 cm, or shows an aortic diameter growth greater than 5 mm over a 1-year period.

What is the operative mortality for aneurysm repairs?

In elective repair, the operative mortality is 4%. When the aortic aneurysm has ruptured, the operative mortality is greater than 50%. The most common cause of postoperative death following aortic aneurysm repair is myocardial infarction.

What are the potential operative complications?

Potential operative complications include atheroembolism, acute renal failure, ureteral injury, cardiac complications, hemorrhage, stroke, and colonic ischemia. Colonic ischemia usually occurs if the inferior mesenteric artery is sacrificed during surgery and presents in the first week postoperatively. Signs include heme-positive stool or bright red blood per rectum. Diagnosis is confirmed by sigmoidoscopy or colonoscopy.

K E Y   P O I N T S

▶ Good history and physical exam are important in treating aortic disease.

▶ Symptomatic cases must be treated and evaluated immediately.

▶ Work-up for aortic disease requires complete radiographic imaging.

▶ Treatment options range from complex operative repairs to endovascular approaches based on patient choice, anatomy, and overall health.

CASE 36–1. A 75-year-old man with a history of coronary artery disease, hypertension, and a pulsatile mass presents to the emergency department with a 2-hour history of back pain radiating down his left groin. The patient has a blood pressure of 120/80 mm Hg and a heart rate of 75 beats/min. He denies chest pain or shortness of breath.

    A. How do you evaluate this patient?
    B. What is your differential diagnosis?
    C. What tests or studies would you order?
    D. What are the treatment options?
    E. What would you do differently if he was hypotensive and in shock?

CAROTID VASCULAR DISEASE

▶ ETIOLOGY

What are common causes of carotid dissections?

Carotid dissections are usually spontaneous, rare events. They may present as Horner's syndrome, sudden onset of temporal headache with neurologic deficit, or cranial nerve compression. Usual etiologies include hypertension or trauma to the cervical region. Duplex ultrasound or MR imaging can confirm the diagnosis. Asymptomatic dissections can usually be followed with anticoagulation, blood pressure control, and follow-up imaging.

What are common causes of carotid occlusive disease?

Carotid occlusive disease is usually caused by atherosclerosis. Plaques are localized to a small segment of the carotid bifurcation extending up the first portion of the proximal internal carotid artery. Other causes include fibromuscular dysplasia or radiation arteritis.

What are the risk factors of carotid vascular disease?

Risk factors include tobacco use, hypertension, elevated cholesterol levels, and diabetes.

What is the usual etiology of the neurologic symptoms?

Acute neurologic events secondary to carotid vascular disease usually result from either decreased blood flow (high-grade carotid stenosis) or embolization of plaque or thrombus from the carotid plaques.

What is the common etiology of recurrent carotid artery disease?

After successful carotid endarterectomy, recurrent early stenosis is caused by intimal proliferation of smooth muscle cells. Late recurrence is almost always recurrent atherosclerosis.

▶ EVALUATION

What are important questions in the history to ask the patient with carotid disease?

In addition to a complete history and physical exam, the history must focus on any acute or chronic neurologic findings. Patients must be evaluated for symptoms of visual changes, hemispheric symptoms (motor and sensory), speech disturbance/aphasia, or dizziness. Syncope, ataxia, or vertigo usually result from vertebral basilar insufficiency and require evaluation of bilateral vertebral arteries.

What findings on physical exam should be noted?

It is important to document blood pressure in both arms. Each patient should have the carotid, superficial temporal, and subclavian arteries palpated and the differences reported. The neck should be auscultated for bruits, which may indicate carotid stenosis.

What is the definition of amaurosis fugax, transient ischemic attack, and stroke?

Amaurosis fugax is an episode of temporary monocular blindness. It is reported as a "curtain coming down" in the visual field and is seen with microemboli from the ipsilateral carotid bifurcation to the retina.

Transient ischemic attacks (TIAs) are focal neurologic deficits with resolution of all symptoms within 24 hours.

A *stroke* or *cerebrovascular accident* is an acute, focal neurologic deficit with incomplete recovery.

Remember that hemispheric symptoms are contralateral to the lesion; that is, a left hemispheric TIA results in right arm weakness and aphasia and is due to a left carotid plaque. The opposite is true for right hemispheric TIAs.

What radiographic imaging helps?

Usually a high-quality carotid ultrasound/duplex is all that is needed. It provides the general location of the lesion and the degree of stenosis based on velocity profiles. Elevated velocities and duplex imaging correlate well with the degree of stenosis. Other tests used after ultrasound are MR imaging, oculoplethysmography, and cerebral arteriograms. Angiograms are usually reserved for recurrent lesions or those in which carotid stenting is a consideration. Degree of stenosis can also be calculated from angiogram measurements when taking the ratio of the disease-free internal carotid artery diameter and the stenosed artery diameter.

What other organ systems should also be evaluated?

All patients should undergo full neurologic and cardiac evaluation preoperatively and postoperatively.

What are the indications for carotid endarterectomy?

The indications for carotid endarterectomy include the following:

Asymptomatic, internal carotid artery stenosis >70%
TIA with >50% internal carotid stenosis
Cerebrovascular accident with substantial neurologic recovery
   and >50% stenosis

▶ TREATMENT

When do you treat asymptomatic carotid artery disease?

Most prospective studies have reported that asymptomatic carotid lesions with greater than 70% stenosis should be electively treated by carotid endarterectomy. Prospective, randomized trials have shown that carotid endarterectomy results in a significant decrease in risk of stroke and/or death compared with medical therapy.

How do you prepare the patient for carotid surgery?

Patients should have a complete evaluation by an anesthesia team prior to operation. In the operating room, the patient should have two intravenous lines and an arterial line. Usually general anesthesia is preferred, but regional anesthesia is a suitable option for certain patients. During the operation, patients may require pressors to increase the blood pressure and vasodilators to control hypertension.

What important cervical structures do you identify during carotid surgery?

After making a cervical incision over the sternocleidomastoid muscle, important structures to identify are the platysma muscle, internal jugular vein, facial vein, common carotid artery, internal carotid artery, superior thyroid artery, ansa cervicalis, vagus nerve, and hypoglossal nerve (cranial nerve XII).

How do you perform a carotid endarterectomy?

Once the major anatomic structures are identified and the vessels are carefully dissected and controlled to prevent embolization, the patient is systemically heparinized. Once the patient is heparinized fully, the internal carotid artery, common carotid artery, and external carotid artery are sequentially clamped. An arteriotomy is created from the common carotid artery extending through the plaque to the internal carotid artery. A temporary shunt is usually inserted to carry blood flow to the brain while the carotid artery is clamped. The endarterectomy involves complete removal of the diseased intima and atherosclerotic carotid plaque from the carotid bifurcation. Care is taken to ensure a smooth-flow surface without intimal flaps or dissections. Once the endarterectomy is complete, the arteriotomy is closed either primarily or with a patch to enlarge the lumen.

How do you monitor the patient in the postoperative period?

Once the operation is complete, the patient is neurologically evaluated in the operating room. The patient is then moved to a monitored setting where close monitoring of neurologic function and blood pressure is started. Periods of severe hypertension and hypotension are to be aggressively treated to ensure a good, safe recovery. Continue the patient on aspirin, and check the incision for hematomas.

What other options are available to treat carotid disease?

Recently, certain carotid lesions have been treated with angioplasty and stenting, especially recurrent lesions in patients with scarring or radiation of the neck. Although this procedure is becoming increasingly common in certain investigational centers, the procedure has not gained widespread acceptance. Distal protection devices to prevent embolic strokes during the procedure are still being developed. At present, a formal, prospective, multicenter study is being organized to help determine the role of this procedure.

What are common complications after carotid surgery?

Complications following carotid endarterectomy are unusual, with combined stroke/death rates of 0% to 2% for asymptomatic lesions and 1% to 4% for symptomatic lesions. Potential complications include myocardial ischemia, stroke, bleeding, and cranial nerve injury (vagus, hypoglossal, marginal mandibular nerve, and superior laryngeal nerve).

What is the treatment for an occluded carotid artery?

There is no treatment. Totally occluded carotid arteries are not surgically explored. There is no role for thrombectomy or endarterectomy.

K E Y　　　P O I N T S

▶ Good history and physical exam are important in treating carotid vascular disease.

▶ Work-up usually requires auscultation of the neck for bruits and duplex ultrasound to determine the degree of stenosis.

▶ Carotid endarterectomy is the standard of care for asymptomatic and symptomatic high-grade carotid stenoses.

▶ Carotid stenting is an investigational procedure that is currently being evaluated with clinical trials.

▶ The effectiveness of carotid stenting compared with carotid endarterectomy is not yet known.

CASE 36–2. A 77-year-old woman was noted to have a left carotid bruit on routine physical exam at her physician's office. She is referred to you for further evaluation.

    A. What is important in her history?
    B. What tests would you order?
    C. What are the treatment options based on?

CASE 36–3. An 82-year-old patient just underwent successful left carotid endarterectomy for an asymptomatic high-grade lesion 4 hours earlier and now cannot move his right arm or leg.

    A. How do you evaluate the patient?
    B. What do you order?
    C. What do you do?

DEEP VENOUS THROMBOSIS

▶ ETIOLOGY

What are the risk factors for deep venous thrombosis (DVT)?

Risk factors include age older than 40 years, immobilization, previous DVT or pulmonary embolism, malignancy, obesity, prolonged operation, trauma, pelvic or hip operation, varicose veins, recent myocardial infarction, congestive heart failure, stroke, air travel, and pregnancy. Hemostatic risk factors that also contribute to the formation of DVTs include functional and quantitative abnormalities in proteins C and S, antithrombin III deficiency, antiphospholipid antibodies, lupus anticoagulant, myeloproliferative disorders, factor V Leiden mutation, prothrombin 20210A, and hyperhomocystinemia.

Why are surgical patients at increased risk for developing DVTs?

After most surgeries, patients are immobile or inactive. This is especially true for orthopedic patients. There are also reports of DVT with hip replacement surgery owing to direct vascular damage to major veins from retraction and manipulation of the veins. Furthermore, tissue damage from all types of surgery leads to increased activated serum coagulation factors, not just at the local surgical site, but systemically.

What is Virchow's triad?

Virchow's triad is a set of factors that promote venous thrombosis: hemostasis, wall damage, and hypercoagulability. Hemostasis may be a result of prolonged bedrest, paralysis, or varicose veins. Wall damage may result from trauma, including both accidental and iatrogenic, secondary to hip surgeries. Hypercoagulability can result from increased tissue factors after surgery, the presence of activating factors with cancer, or the decrease in coagulation inhibitors as in inherited antithrombin III deficiency and dysfunctional activated protein C.

How are venous thrombi different from arterial thrombi?

Venous thrombi are redder, are less compact, and contain red blood cells in a fibrin matrix. Arterial thrombi contain more platelet aggregates, which gives them a whiter appearance.

What is a potential severe consequence of DVT?

The most feared complication is pulmonary embolism. In more than 90% of the cases of pulmonary embolism, the embolus is believed to originate from the deep veins of the legs.

What is post-thrombotic, or postphlebitic, syndrome?

This is thought to result from valve damage in the veins secondary to DVT. Long-term consequences include pain, swelling, skin changes (stasis dermatitis), dermatosclerosis, and stasis ulceration. A significant number of patients with DVT eventually develop this condition, although the extent and location of DVT are not predictive. Persistent obstruction of the deep veins is highly associated with the post-thrombotic syndrome. Deep venous reflux can develop in venous segments not initially involved with DVT, especially with more proximal chronic venous obstruction. This can be treated with graduated compression stockings.

▶ EVALUATION

How significant is the physical examination in detecting DVT?

Physical examination, although important, is insensitive in detecting DVT. Nearly 80% of deep venous thrombi are not detectable by physical examination. If present, reported symptoms in patients with DVT may include calf swelling, lower extremity tenderness, fever, and a positive Homans' sign.

What characterizes a positive Homans' sign?

Calf pain with dorsiflexion of the foot at the ankle joint indicates a positive Homans' sign.

What is phlegmasia cerulea dolens?

Phlegmasia cerulea dolens is unilateral swelling, pain, and cyanosis of the leg due to massive occlusion of the iliofemoral vein, which may progress to venous gangrene. Patients often have a history of DVTs and superficial thrombophlebitis.

What are the different radiographic modalities used to detect DVT?

Ultrasonic duplex scanning is the test of choice for detecting DVT. It consists of B-mode gray scale imaging and Doppler flow analysis. Possible findings include visualization of the thrombus as an echogenic filling defect within the vein, inability to compress the vein, or detection of an abnormal flow pattern. Partial obstruction, for example, changes the normal phasic flow into a continuous flow pattern. Venography has previously been the gold standard, but it has declined in use because it is invasive and requires the injection of contrast medium.

▶ TREATMENT

What are the major methods of prevention of DVT?

There are both pharmacologic and mechanical methods used to prevent DVT. Mechanical methods include support stockings, sequential compression boots, and early ambulation. Compression stockings have been shown to be as effective as low-dose heparin in patients who have had abdominal surgery. Together these mechanical prophylactic methods decrease the rate of DVT by 50% to 65%, and unlike pharmacologic methods, pose virtually no risk of bleeding.

What are some of the major pharmacologic agents used to treat DVT?

In many studies, it is accepted that the use of unfractionated heparin decreases the risk of DVT by 50% to 70%. The problem with unfractionated heparin is that it requires subcutaneous injections or intravenous dosing. In addition, it requires monitoring in the form of partial thromboplastin times. Warfarin is another useful drug for treating DVT, and it can be given orally. However, its anticoagulation effect as measured by the International Normalized Ratio (INR) (prothrombin time) usually does not reach therapeutic values until 3 or 4 days after the initiation of therapy. To bridge this gap, heparin is usually given to patients until the warfarin becomes therapeutic. Low-molecular-weight heparin (LMWH) is considered a third form of prophylaxis and has been found to be more effective than unfractionated heparin, dextran, and warfarin in patients undergoing elective hip surgery. Aspirin has also been used successfully in total joint surgery. LMWH has the widest application and a beneficial risk/benefit profile for postoperative DVT prophylaxis.

What are some of the complications of anticoagulants?

The most common complication is abnormal bleeding. This can be problematic because localized bleeding can result in a hematoma that may be susceptible to infection. This would be catastrophic for prosthetic graft or joint replacement procedures. Heparin has been noted in some cases to cause thrombocytopenia. Warfarin has been associated with skin necrosis, but this occurs only in patients with protein C or S deficiencies who are given warfarin without adequate anticoagulation from unfractionated heparin or LMWH.

What is the indication for thrombolytics in the management of DVT?

Thrombolysis may be indicated for cases of iliofemoral DVT, in the hope of preventing the results of long-term occlusion such as valvular incompetence and chronic venous insufficiency. To date, no objective data confirm this theoretical advantage.

What is the treatment regimen, if any, for a pregnant patient with DVT?

Heparin therapy is preferred because it does not cross the placenta. Warfarin is teratogenic and can cause fetal or neonatal hemorrhage. A standard dosing of heparin is a 5000-unit bolus followed by a 5- to 10-day continuous infusion. It can be continued throughout pregnancy until the start of labor. After delivery of the baby, warfarin is administered for at least 6 weeks or until there is a 3-month total of anticoagulation. LMWHs are attractive because they have a lower incidence of thrombocytopenia and less risk of hemorrhage and can have a once-a-day dosing schedule owing to greater bioavailability than unfractionated heparin.

CASE 36–4. A 32-year-old woman complains of left leg pain and swelling 3 days after undergoing an uncomplicated laparoscopic appendectomy.

A. How do you evaluate the patient?
B. What tests do you order?
C. What are this patient's risk factors?
D. What are your treatment options?

PERIPHERAL VASCULAR DISEASE

▶ ETIOLOGY

What are the important causes of peripheral arterial obliteration?

Atherosclerosis is the underlying cause in most patients. Thromboangiitis obliterans, or Buerger's disease, although more common in the Middle East and the Far East, is a rare cause of peripheral ischemia in the United States. Pathologically, it is a chronic inflammatory process involving the neurovascular bundle of the medium and small vessels of the hands and feet leading to arterial and venous thrombosis and fibrosis. Buerger's disease typically occurs in the 3rd and 4th decades of life in individuals with heavy tobacco usage. Cessation of tobacco usage can effectively halt the progress of Buerger's disease. Vasculitis, popliteal artery entrapment, and cystic adventitial disease of the popliteal artery are other rare causes of peripheral vascular disease.

What are the risk factors?

The incidence and progression of atherosclerosis are clearly accelerated in the presence of diabetes mellitus, hypertension, hyperlipidemia, lipoprotein abnormalities, homocystinemia, and tobacco usage. Male gender and advanced age are also risk factors for peripheral vascular disease.

What is claudication?

Claudication, derived from the Latin verb meaning "to limp," is a form of functional ischemia; that is, blood flow is normal in the resting limb but cannot be increased in response to exercise. The patients manifest extremity pain, usually in the calf, which is reproducibly precipitated by exercise and promptly relieved by rest.

Claudication pain usually presents as an ache or cramp or severe fatigue in some cases.

What is critical limb ischemia?

Critical limb ischemia is a result of reduction of blood flow in the extremity to a level below that required for normal resting tissue metabolism. It manifests as either recurring, ischemic rest pain that usually is a severe, burning pain located at the metatarsal heads or chronic, painful (unless diabetic neuropathy is present), nonhealing ulceration or gangrene of the foot or toes. Ischemic rest pain typically occurs at night and frequently awakens the patient from sleep. The pain is exacerbated by elevation and relieved by a dependent position. Many patients find relief of their pain by sleeping with the extremity dangling over the side of the bed.

What are the two types of gangrene?

The two types are wet gangrene and dry gangrene. Wet gangrene is infected and presents as a poorly demarcated, erythematous, foul-smelling, vesicular, or draining lesion. Dry gangrene is aseptic and presents as a sharply demarcated, black-brown, dry, and often odorless lesion.

What is the natural history of claudicants?

Three fourths of nondiabetic claudicants remain stable or show some improvement 2 to 5 years after onset of symptoms. Only 5% to 7% need amputation of the extremity. Patients who continue to use tobacco and or who have diabetes mellitus fare worse than those who do not have these coexistent risk factors.

What is the natural history of patients with ischemic rest pain or necrosis?

Ischemic rest pain or necrosis is a limb-threatening condition. Without surgical intervention, 100% of patients with ischemic rest pain or necrosis would lose the affected limb.

▶ EVALUATION

What is the simplest test used to evaluate patients for arterial occlusive disease?

The ankle-brachial index (ABI) is defined as the systolic blood pressure of the ankle divided by that of the arm. This test is easily performed at the bedside with a hand-held Doppler unit. An ABI of less than 0.95 is considered to be abnormal. Claudicants usually have an ABI in the range of 0.5 to 0.9. Patients with ischemic rest pain have an ABI in the range of 0.2 to 0.5. Patients who present with tissue necrosis usually have an ABI of less than 0.3. The presence of arterial medial calcification that is common in patients with diabetes mellitus can cause a false elevation of the ABI. In patients with significant claudication who have a minimally decreased ABI, exercise testing can be used to increase the sensitivity of Doppler-derived segmental pressure. Exercise causes vasodilation, but the stenosis prevents sufficient blood flow to the distal extremity to maintain local blood pressure.

What are the three major studies of the noninvasive vascular laboratory?

Arterial study in the vascular laboratory evaluates Doppler waveform analysis to detect loss of the normal triphasic pattern in diseased arterial system, plethysmography to detect reduction in extremity volume changes with systole, and duplex ultrasound to detect jets and turbulence caused by stenosis.

What are other studies used in the evaluation of patients with peripheral vascular disease?

Arteriograms can show the anatomic lesion and are usually performed only after a decision for operative or angioplastic intervention has been made. With the digital subtraction technique, angiography can be performed with a small amount of dye load. A critical arterial stenosis is a lesion that has more than 50% diameter reduction (or >75% reduction in the cross-sectional area) based on arteriographic criteria. MR angiography with gadolinium and carbon dioxide angiography are study modalities that are especially useful in patients with renal insufficiency.

▶ TREATMENT

What are the indications for medical treatment?

Medical treatment is indicated in most patients with claudication. Walking exercise regimen, smoking cessation, weight reduction, diabetic control, hypertension control, hyperlipidemia control, and antiplatelet therapy are the foundations of medical treatment. Walking exercise therapy is the most effective treatment of claudication. Current opinion indicates that walking exercise allows muscles to be more efficient at extracting oxygen from the blood. Multiple studies have documented a mean increase of 179% in initial claudication distance and a mean increase of 122% in maximal walking distance. Homocystinemia can be treated with vitamin B supplementation; however, the effect of vitamin B supplementation on the progression of atherosclerosis is not yet proven. Rheologic agents such as pentoxifylline have been shown to have some benefits in clinical improvement of patients with claudication symptoms. Cilostazol, a cyclic adenosine monophosphate phosphodiesterase inhibitor, has recently been shown to be of benefit in improving walking distance in patients with claudication.

What are the indications for operative intervention?

Critical limb ischemia is a clear indication for arterial reconstruction because of its poor outcome if left untreated. Claudication imposing an unacceptable alteration in patients' lifestyle, preventing them from participating in a treatment program (e.g., post–coronary artery bypass exercising program), or precluding them from gainful employment is also an indication for operative intervention.

What are the different options of surgical revascularization?

A successful bypass requires optimal inflow as well as outflow. Bypass procedures can be performed with autogenous vein or prosthetic (expanded polytetrafluoroethylene [ePTFE]) grafts. Patency rate is superior for autogenous vein grafts compared to prosthetic grafts, especially with infrapopliteal bypasses. The primary 5-year patency rate is reported to be 65% to 80% for infrainguinal bypasses with greater saphenous vein graft and 59% for all femoropopliteal bypasses performed with ePTFE. Infrapopliteal bypass using ePTFE has a dismal patency rate of 22% at 3 years.

Autogenous vein grafts can be used in a reversed or in situ manner with valve lysis. The superiority of one approach over the other has not been documented in randomized clinical trials.

What is the role for endovascular interventions in the management of chronic lower extremity ischemia?

For the symptomatic, short, focal stenoses of the aorta or iliac arteries, percutaneous transluminal angioplasty (PTA) is a viable treatment option. Stent placement should be considered for lesions that are recurrent or occluded and for postangioplasty dissection or residual stenosis. PTA is also appropriate for short (<2 cm) focal stenoses in the superficial femoral or popliteal arteries. Routine stent placement in the femoropopliteal segment has not been shown to extend long-term patency rates; therefore, it should be considered only for extensive or flow-limiting postangioplasty dissection. Infrapopliteal angioplasty should be considered only for the rare patient with a short, focal tibial artery stenosis, limb-threatening ischemia, and contraindications to operation.

KEY POINTS

▶ Atherosclerosis is the predominant cause of peripheral arterial occlusive disease.

▶ ABI is an easy test that can be done at the bedside to evaluate patients with arterial occlusive disease.

▶ Claudicants have a benign natural history; therefore, surgical intervention is not indicated in all patients with claudication.

▶ Surgical intervention is indicated in patients with critical limb ischemia or those with claudication that imposes an unacceptable alteration in their lifestyle or precludes them from gainful employment.

CASE 36–5. A 60-year-old man presented to the emergency department with pain and nonhealing ulcers of the left foot.

    A. How do you evaluate this patient?
    B. What studies would you order?
    C. What are your treatment options?

VASCULAR ACCESS FOR HEMODIALYSIS

What is hemodialysis?

Hemodialysis is the process by which fluid, electrolytes, and metabolites are removed from the blood by equilibration against an appropriate solution from which the blood is separated by a semipermeable membrane. Patients without adequate renal function cannot survive without hemodialysis, peritoneal dialysis, or renal transplantation.

What is required for successful hemodialysis?

Blood flows of at least 250 mL/min are needed to achieve satisfactory dialysis in the average adult. In addition, blood returning to the patient must be separated from blood being withdrawn so that it will not be removed and dialyzed a second time (recirculation). Access systems must be sufficiently durable to permit satisfactory blood flows three times per week, 4 or 5 hours each time. Unmodified peripheral vessels are not capable of meeting these requirements.

What access systems are available?

There are three basic types of vascular access for hemodialysis: autologous arteriovenous fistulas, arteriovenous grafts, and dual-lumen central venous catheters. Each has its own advantages and disadvantages. See the summary in Table 36–1.

What is an autologous arteriovenous fistula?

If the cephalic vein at the wrist is anastomosed to the adjacent radial artery, the vein will gradually dilate and thicken. The names Brescia and Cimino are usually associated with these autologous fistulas; they described the procedure in 1966. After 6 or 8 weeks,

TABLE 36–1

Summary of Vascular Access Systems for Hemodialysis

Type	Availability	Longevity
Central venous catheters		
Uncuffed	Immediate*	Weeks/months
Cuffed	Immediate	Months
Arteriovenous grafts	7–10 days	1–2 years
Autologous arteriovenous fistula	Minimum 6 weeks	Indefinite

*Lowest risk

if the fistula develops successfully, the vein will be easily visible throughout the forearm. Because of turbulent flow there is a palpable thrill and audible bruit. The vein can then be cannulated with two 15-gauge needles, one for outflow and one for return, placed far enough apart to prevent recirculation. Blood flows in excess of 250 mL/min are routinely obtained. These fistulas are remarkably durable. Ninety percent of those that are working 1 year after creation are still working 2 or 3 years later.

One of the disadvantages of an autologous fistula is that it cannot be used for 6 or 8 weeks. Ideally, if the need for dialysis is anticipated, these fistulas can be created weeks or months in advance. Unlike prosthetic grafts, which deteriorate over time, autologous fistulas generally improve the longer they are in place. If dialysis is needed before an autologous fistula is ready for use, a dual-lumen central venous catheter can be inserted. The patient can then undergo venovenous dialysis for several additional weeks or months while the native fistula matures.

When are arteriovenous grafts appropriate?

If the patient does not have suitable forearm vessels to permit creation of a native fistula, or if such a fistula has failed, vascular access can be obtained by placement of a prosthetic graft between a suitable artery and a suitable vein. The artery must be capable of delivering blood flows of at least 300 to 400 mL/min. The vein must provide low-pressure outflow. The grafts are usually PTFE or modified bovine arterial heterografts (specifically processed carotid arteries from cows). The usual configurations are straight forearm (radial artery at the wrist to an antecubital vein), loop forearm (brachial artery at the antecubital, passing distally, then looping back to an antecubital vein), or straight upper arm (distal brachial artery to proximal brachial/distal axillary vein). Grafts are rarely placed in the lower extremities because of a high rate of complications. The grafts are passed through subcutaneous tunnels that are superficial enough to allow them to be easily felt. They are usually also visible. The grafts should not be punctured before they have had time to become incorporated into the subcutaneous tissues, usually 10 to 14 days. Premature use can lead to bleeding into the subcutaneous tunnel, causing hematoma formation and possible thrombosis or infection. If a prosthetic graft becomes infected, it must be removed.

Advantages of arteriovenous grafts are that they can be created in essentially all patients, even those with poor peripheral vessels. They can be used much earlier than native fistulas and can be placed in a variety of locations. The 6-mm, 7-mm, or 8-mm conduits are usually used, making needle placement relatively easy.

If flow is too great, the patient may experience distal ischemia ("steal" syndrome). If this is severe, the graft may need to be ligated. The greatest disadvantage of prosthetic grafts is their lack of durability. They typically develop a stenosis at or near the venous anastomosis, probably related to turbulent flow from size and compliance differences between the graft and the vein. As stenosis increases, resistance increases, flow decreases, and eventually thrombosis occurs. Less than 75% of grafts are patent at 1 year, less than 60% at 18 months, and essentially none at 2 years. Frequently it is possible to declot thrombosed grafts and revise the venous anastomosis by endarterectomy and patch angioplasty. After one or two revisions, however, most thrombosed grafts must be abandoned and a new access established using other vessels at a different location.

After antecubital veins become unusable, it is necessary to place grafts in the upper arm, using the distal axillary/proximal brachial veins. Eventually, if the patient lives long enough, all venous access sites may be used up. The patient must then switch to peritoneal dialysis, be managed as long as possible with central venous catheters, receive a transplant, or die. Every access must therefore be planned to make optimal use of the patient's peripheral veins. Hence the rule for graft placement: "Stay as peripheral as possible for as long as possible."

Because of the vital importance of peripheral veins in the long-term management of hemodialysis patients, it follows that *everything possible should be done to preserve all forearm veins in all patients with established or potential chronic renal insufficiency* (e.g., patients with diabetes, collagen vascular disease, chronic pyelonephritis, hypertension, polycystic kidney disease). All doctors, nurses, and other health care workers should be taught the importance of not injuring forearm veins in such patients. Always draw blood samples or start intravenous infusions using veins distal to the wrist or in the neck or in the lower extremities.

When are central venous catheters used?

Large-bore, dual-lumen central venous catheters permit venovenous dialysis. Because of the large size of the central vessels (superior vena cava, right atrium), blood flows in excess of 300 mL/min can be easily obtained. The lumen used to withdraw blood and deliver it to the dialysis machine is 1.5 to 2.0 cm above (peripheral to) the lumen used to return blood from the machine. This, plus a high rate of flow in the vessels, prevents recirculation. Recirculation occurs when returning blood is commingled with the blood being withdrawn, thus returning to it to the machine and dialyzing it a second time. This decreases the efficiency of dialysis per unit time, and, unless the duration of treatment is increased, the patient will be underdialyzed.

There are two types of central venous dialysis catheters: uncuffed and cuffed. Uncuffed catheters are simply semirigid double-lumen plastic tubes approximately 4 mm in diameter and 13 to 15 cm in length with proximal and distal openings as described earlier. They can be placed at the bedside using the Seldinger technique. The vein is located with an 18-gauge needle and a guidewire passed. A dilator is then passed over the guidewire, followed by the dialysis catheter itself. Uncuffed catheters are typically placed in the femoral or internal jugular veins. *Dialysis catheters should* never *be placed in the subclavian veins. Cannulation of subclavian veins by these large-bore catheters frequently leads to stenosis and thrombosis, rendering the ipsilateral extremity unusable for future access procedures.*

The advantage of uncuffed catheters is that they can be used immediately and can be placed at the bedside, when the patient is too sick to be safely transported to the operating room or if an operating room is not available in a timely fashion. The disadvantage is that, because they pass through the skin and tend to move in and out a few millimeters, they usually become infected after 2 to 3 weeks.

Cuffed catheters were developed to decrease or delay the incidence of infection. A cuff of soft, rough plastic cloth is attached to the catheter 19 to 20 cm from the tip. After accessing the internal jugular vein, a small incision is made on the upper chest, and the catheter is passed subcutaneously so that the cuff is buried 2 to 7 cm from the exit site. Over the next few days the cuff "scars" into the subcutaneous tissues. This prevents the catheter from moving back and forth in the tunnel. This is thought to reduce the incidence of infection. Cuffed catheters are softer than uncuffed ones and may be less traumatic to the central vessels. On the other hand, they are larger ($\leq 3 \times 6$ mm in cross-sectional diameter) and therefore require a larger puncture site in the vein.

Initially it was hoped that tunneled cuffed catheters would provide permanent access for patients on chronic hemodialysis. That has not proven to be case because, unlike fistulas and grafts, they are not completely subcutaneous and have only intermittent rather than continuous flow. They therefore remain prone to infection and thrombosis. They are, however, more durable than uncuffed catheters, typically providing satisfactory access for weeks or months—and occasionally for as long as a year. They can be used immediately on insertion. They are currently used to provide dialysis on a short- or medium-term basis, allowing time for a native fistula to mature, for a prosthetic graft to heal into place, for a determination to be made as to whether the patient's renal failure is acute or chronic, or for the patient to decide between hemodialysis and peritoneal dialysis.

In addition to the risks of thrombosis and infection, placement of these catheters is fraught with all the usual hazards of central venous catheter insertion, magnified by the size of the dilators and catheters involved. Serious and even fatal complications have occurred.

▶ EVALUATION

The optimal type of hemodialysis access to be established for any given patient depends on three factors: the type of renal failure (acute or chronic), the length of time before the access must be available for use, and the adequacy of the patient's forearm vessels.

What would the history determine?

The history should determine whether the renal failure is potentially reversible. Patients suffering from acute tubular necrosis or toxic or obstructive nephropathy may recover renal function within 6 to 8 weeks. Establishment of a fistula or a graft is not necessary in such patients. They would be best served by insertion of a tunneled cuffed central venous dialysis catheter. The catheter would be available for immediate use and would be likely to provide satisfactory access for 2 to 3 months, allowing adequate time for renal function to return. If, on the other hand, renal failure is thought to be irreversible, some type of subcutaneous access, such as a fistula or a graft, should be placed.

The history should also ascertain how soon the access system must be available for use. If the patient is acutely uremic and in congestive failure or severe electrolyte imbalance, immediate dialysis is indicated, and a venovenous catheter should be inserted. If the patient is gravely ill, an uncuffed catheter placed at the bedside into a femoral vein is the access of choice. If, on the other hand, the patient will not need to start dialysis for several months, an autologous fistula would be indicated (these only improve with time). Conversely, grafts deteriorate with time and should not be placed unless they will be needed within 2 to 3 weeks.

What should the physical examination focus on?

Physical examination focuses primarily on assessing the status of the patient's forearm veins and radial pulses. The key question is whether the vessels are adequate for creation of an autologous fistula between the distal radial artery and the cephalic vein at the wrist. This procedure (Brescia, Cimino, or Brescia-Cimino fistula) is the vascular access of choice for hemodialysis and should be attempted whenever suitable vessels are available. Theoretically an Allen test should be performed to assess the status of the ulnar artery and palmar arch. In practice this is rarely necessary or helpful. The fistula involves an end-of-vein to side-of-artery anastomosis that should preserve flow into the distal artery; clinically significant ischemia of the hand is rarely if ever seen following this procedure. Moreover, because these patients require some type of arteriovenous fistula or graft to maintain life, it may be necessary to compromise and assume some risk of distal ischemia to provide the type of access that is essential to their continuing survival.

If forearm vessels are not suitable for an autologous fistula, the antecubital space should be examined to see if there is a vein large enough to provide venous outflow for an arteriovenous graft. Even if no veins are apparent, this area should be explored surgically to look for vessels that may be deep and not readily detectable on physical examination. Occasionally ultrasound is used to map the size and course of upper extremity veins to aid in the planning of vascular access procedures.

In matching the access to the patient, what should I keep in mind when considering an access approach?

Keep in mind the following:

Type of renal failure (acute vs. chronic)
Presence and quality of vessels
When dialysis will be necessary

How do I decide which approach to take?

The following principles apply when choosing between access approaches:

Use an autologous fistula, if at all possible
Use a cuffed internal jugular catheter if dialysis is needed before
    the fistula has matured
Use a prosthetic arteriovenous graft if
    Autologous fistula is not possible
    Dialysis is imminent (7 to 10 days)
Use an uncuffed catheter if dialysis is needed in less than 7 to 10
    days

    Application of these principles leads to the following recommendations:

1. A seriously ill patient should have an uncuffed catheter placed into a femoral vein at the bedside.
2. A patient with potentially reversible renal failure should have a tunneled cuffed catheter placed.
3. Fistulas and grafts should not be placed until it is clear that renal function will not return.
4. If the patient has suitable forearm vessels, an autologous fistula at the wrist is always the access of choice for chronic hemodialysis. Ideally this procedure should be done 2 to 3 months before it will be needed, allowing time for maturation.
5. If dialysis must be instituted before the fistula has matured, a tunneled cuffed catheter should be placed and used until the fistula is mature.

    If the patient will not require dialysis for several weeks or months, and if he or she does not have suitable vessels for an autologous fistula, nothing should be done. Arteriovenous grafts should be placed no more than 10 to 14 days before they will be needed. This is sufficient time for them to become incorporated into the subcutaneous tissues. Unlike autologous fistulas, prosthetic grafts do not improve with time—they only deteriorate.

K E Y   P O I N T S

▶ Vascular access is essential for survival of patients with end-stage renal disease who require hemodialysis.

▶ There is no perfect access system: all eventually fail. Each access must therefore be planned to make optimal use of the patient's peripheral vessels.

▶ *Never place a dialysis catheter into a subclavian vein; use this route only if neither internal jugular vein can be cannulated.*

▶ Autologous fistulas are more durable and have fewer complications than prosthetic arteriovenous grafts.

▶ Autologous fistulas improve with time; prosthetic grafts deteriorate.

▶ Preserve all forearm veins in all patients with potential or established chronic renal insufficiency (e.g., diabetes, collagen vascular disease, chronic pyelonephritis, hypertension).

▶ Plan ahead. Create autologous fistulas early, as soon as dialysis seems likely (these systems only improve with time).

CASE 36–6. A 22-year-old man presents with acute renal failure secondary to gentamicin toxicity. Laboratory studies include blood urea nitrogen (BUN) of 200 mg/dL, creatinine of 20 mg/dL, and potassium of 6.5 mg/dL. He has strong radial pulses and excellent cephalic veins at the wrist bilaterally.

    A. What access procedure do you recommend? Why?

CASE 36–7. A 22-year-old man presents with fatigue and shortness of breath. His laboratory studies include a BUN of 200 mg/dL, creatinine of 20 mg/dL, and potassium of 6.5 mg/dL. An ultrasound shows small kidneys, and a biopsy shows end-stage renal disease, not otherwise specified. He has strong radial pulses and excellent cephalic veins at the wrist bilaterally.

    A. What access procedure or procedures do you recommend? Why?

CASE 36–8. A 74-year-old woman has insulin-dependent diabetes mellitus. Six months earlier her BUN was 20 mg/dL and her creatinine was 2.0 mg/dL. Now her BUN is 4.0 mg/dL and her creatinine is 4.5 mg/dL. She has excellent forearm vessels.

A. What access procedure do you recommend? Why?

CASE 36–9. Assume that the same patient as in Case 36–8 has poor forearm vessels.

A. What access procedure do you recommend? Why?

Case Answers

► **ABDOMINAL MASS**

3–1, A. Learning objective: *The prior melanoma history is very important, but don't eliminate other causes of abdominal mass.*[AU1] The history is an important tool in the evaluation of abdominal masses. Determine the chronicity and any symptoms associated with the mass.

3–1, B. Learning objective: *A thorough physical exam is important. Do not forget a complete exam of lymph nodal beds.* A full exam of the mass is warranted. Define the size, shape, mobility, and any tenderness. The history of melanoma increases the concern that the mass is a recurrence of her tumor. Look for other sites of possible recurrence.

3–1, C. Learning objective: *All labs and studies are indicated by the suspected diagnosis.* In a patient with suspected recurrence of melanoma, appropriate studies might include CBC, alkaline phosphatase, and thoracic, abdominal, and pelvic CT scanning.

3–1, D. Learning objective: *The ultimate goal to evaluation of abdominal masses is diagnosis.* Tissue diagnosis of a solid mass is the most important end point. In the case of potential recurrence of melanoma, an FNA or incisional biopsy is necessary.

3–2, A. Learning objective: *History often holds the key to diagnosis.* The rapid onset associated with weight-lifting holds the key that tissue stress may be the etiology of this mass.

3–2, B. Learning objective: *Physical examination can further narrow the differential diagnosis.* The mass is palpable, tender, and nonreducible. The mass may be localized to the abdominal wall, though this may be difficult to discern. A thorough physical exam reveals that he is otherwise healthy and in good shape.

3–2, C. Learning objective: *Keep an open mind.* Although the likely diagnosis is a hernia, there are a number of other etiologies that may cause these symptoms, such as an abdominal wall tumor (lipoma or sarcoma) with acute rupture or bleed into the tumor mass, an abscess, and a spontaneous hemorrhage into the subcutaneous tissues.

3–2, D. Learning objective: *Use laboratory and radiographic studies to confirm your suspected diagnosis.* In this patient, specific laboratory tests may not be helpful. A CT scan through the region will give structural information.

3–2, E. Learning objective: *Once again the history is key.* Knowing that the patient is anticoagulated will direct your diagnosis toward a spontaneous bleed. Check the patient's hematocrit and coagulation status. A CT scan with IV contrast may show if there is any active extravasation in this mass. Treatment plans depend on the coagulation status and whether there is evidence of ongoing bleeding. Simple correction of an abnormal INR may be all that is necessary. Ligation of an actively bleeding blood vessel may also be required.

▶ ABDOMINAL PAIN/DISTENTION

4–1, A. Learning objective: *Recognize that a number of etiologies may lead to abdominal distention in the elderly patient.* There are several possibilities causing abdominal distention in this patient. The patient may have a mechanical large bowel obstruction due to a stricture from diverticulitis. Other causes of large bowel obstruction would include volvulus or carcinoma. He also could have a small bowel obstruction secondary to adhesions from his past surgery, a hernia, or neoplasm. The distention could also be due to an ileus secondary to acute diverticulitis, pericolonic abscess, or other intra-abdominal inflammatory foci. You should also consider intestinal ischemia in the diagnosis.

4–1, B. Learning objective: *Describe physical findings and other tests that help differentiate between ileus and mechanical bowel obstruction.* Inspect and palpate the abdomen to assess for masses or regions of tenderness. Listen for bowel sounds and decide whether they are decreased, as in ileus, or resemble rushes and tinkles, as in obstruction. Perform a rectal exam and feel for rectal or pelvic masses and check for occult blood to evaluate for malignancies. Check CBC to evaluate for signs of acute infection (ileus) or chronic anemia (chronic gastrointestinal blood loss with malignancy). Order a KUB and decide whether the picture is most consistent with ileus, small bowel obstruction, or large bowel obstruction (see Table 4–2). Perform sigmoidoscopy to screen the rectosigmoid for obstructing masses. Consider barium enema if large bowel obstruction is still a concern; however, CT may be helpful to better characterize the nature and location of bowel obstruction. Check for inflammatory masses or abscesses that could be causing ileus. If intestinal ischemia is considered, perform visceral angiography.

4–2, A. Learning objective: *Recognize that intestinal obstruction can present with atypical signs and symptoms.* With the patient's significant past surgical history, she is certainly at risk for adhesive disease with resultant small bowel obstruction. The findings of diarrhea, dull percussion note, localized distention, and decreased bowel sounds may seem atypical for obstruction. Distention from intestinal obstruction typically results in tympany on abdominal percussion. Nevertheless, as the dilated loops of bowel become filled with fluid, the percussion note may become dull. Similarly, bowel sounds may decrease with progressive obstruction. The patient's localized abdominal distention could be due to a fixed closed-loop obstruction. Diarrhea may be more prominent than obstipation with partial bowel obstruction. Finally, even the KUB may be misleading since fluid-filled loops of bowel may be invisible on plain radiographs.

4–2, B. Learning objective: *Recognize that solid-organ enlargement or neoplastic processes can cause abdominal distention.* Although the patient describes a rather acute course for this process, it may have been present for a longer period. Therefore, an ovarian tumor or other intra-abdominal mass is a distinct possibility.

4–2, C. Learning objective: *Understand which imaging tests have the greatest yield in patients with abdominal distention.* A KUB may be diagnostic of small or large bowel obstruction and should be the first imaging study obtained. Nevertheless, nonspecific findings may be seen and in the case of solid-organ distention of the abdomen, the films will be normal. Therefore, CT would be the test of choice to differentiate bowel obstruction from intra-abdominal mass.

▶ **ACUTE ABDOMEN**

5–1, A. Learning objective: *Abdominal pain has a wide differential diagnosis.* To narrow the diagnosis, take a careful history, followed by a complete physical examination. The lack of fever is somewhat helpful in ruling out an inflammatory cause of the pain, but this is not reliable because nearly a third of patients with appendicitis have no elevation of their temperature. More data must be collected to narrow the differential further. Although this patient most likely has a perforated ulcer, other diagnoses to entertain include biliary obstruction/colic, pancreatitis, hepatitis, appendicitis, colitis, and gastroenteritis.

5–1, B. Learning objective: *Pain syndromes can change over time.* Abdominal pain is not a static symptom—it will develop, intensify, and resolve over time. Appendicitis and bowel perforation are good examples. As the disease process develops, inflammation increases, or fluid spilling from a perforation may cause irritation to a wider region of the peritoneum and cause a change in symptoms. When a patient is hospitalized, make it a point to perform frequent "serial exams" to look for changes in the abdominal pain.

5–1, C. Learning objective: *Further studies are directed by the differential diagnosis.* Apart from some standard initial tests (CBC, UA, upright chest radiograph), the further work-up is dictated by clinical suspicion. Following a complete history and physical examination, the differential diagnosis should be pared down to a handful of causes. Order studies that differentiate between the remaining things on this list. This patient may also need an amylase, lipase, liver function tests, and a three-way radiographic examination of the abdomen.

5–1, D. Learning objective: *Therapy and diagnosis can coexist.* Following your examination, while the patient is undergoing diagnostic testing, pain can be treated. Patients with derangements in their vital signs (tachycardia, hypotension) need rapid intervention, such as fluid resuscitation, and invasive monitoring of their intravascular volume status.

5–2, A. Learning objective: *The likely unifying diagnosis is diabetic ketoacidosis (DKA).* This would explain the acidosis, abdominal pain and the elevated blood glucose. DKA is one of many medical conditions that can mimic surgical acute abdominal pain. Others include myocardial infarction, pneumonia, sickle cell crisis, acute intermittent porphyria, familial Mediterranean fever, and urinary tract infection.

5–2, B. Learning objective: *Medical problems can coexist with surgical problems.* Remember that DKA is a symptom of lack of diabetic control, and when a patient presents in DKA, that a source of the problem must be sought. Noncompliance is a likely suspect, but infections also cause loss of insulin responsiveness. In the presence of abdominal pain, you must rule out an intra-abdominal infection such as appendicitis as a cause for the DKA.

5–2, C. Learning objective: *Try to optimize the patient for the operating room.* To prepare a patient for the operating room, recognize that the patient who is already is being physiologically stressed by the disease is about to get physiologically stressed by the application of anesthesia, blood loss, and surgical resection. Most anesthetic agents contribute to hypotension, so be sure to have adequate IV access and attempt to fluid-resuscitate the patient. Have blood available if deemed necessary. Further invasive monitoring such as a Foley catheter, central venous access, or pulse oximetry may be necessary. In this diabetic patient, an attempt to control the glucose levels should be made, but this may not be possible until the pathology has been corrected. Those patients with infections may need parenteral antibiotics.

5–3, A. Learning objective: *The history is consistent with a ruptured abdominal aortic aneurysm.* The history alone is sufficient to suspect this diagnosis, and the patient may be too unstable for further work-up. Although other causes of abdominal pain are possible, there are some etiologies that are devastating if ignored, and action must be taken without delay.

5–3, B. Learning objective: *If the patient is unstable, therapeutic considerations outweigh diagnostic ones.* This patient is critically ill. He needs fluid resuscitation and a trip to the operating room to correct his problem. Often, a surgeon has to act on very limited information.

5–3, C. Learning objective: *Early operation is the key to this patient's survival.* The only way a patient with a ruptured abdominal aortic aneurysm can survive is with early control of the hemorrhage and repair of the aorta. There are few instances when this sort of speed to the operating room is necessary, but it is vitally important that you learn when this action is warranted.

▶ BREAST MASS

6–1, A. Learning objective: *Recognize the components of a complete initial evaluation for breast mass.* Part of the initial work-up of a palpable breast mass is to take a history that helps with risk stratification. This includes taking an accurate breast cancer history for her family members, particularly first-degree relatives. You need to know if she has had any previous mammograms or biopsies of the breast and, if so, what were the results. This information helps you refine your index of suspicion for malignancy.

6–1, B. Learning objective: *Recognize the features on physical exam that make potential malignancy more likely.* She has several features of her mass that are worrisome for potential malignancy, such as ill-defined border and overlying skin changes. With one or more of these features present in the initial evaluation, you would want to proceed to biopsy immediately without getting a mammogram first. The choice of biopsy (either FNA or core biopsy) depends on the capabilities in your clinic; however, some tissue diagnosis is warranted as a component of her initial evaluation.

6–1, C. Learning objective: *A comprehensive history is important in the evaluation of breast masses.* The patient gave a history of new onset of vertigo and multiple falls. Although she was not able to identify any specific trauma to the involved breast, it was most likely a traumatic injury to the breast because it resolved so rapidly. She was sent for further evaluation by a neurologist and was found to have benign positional vertigo secondary to a middle ear condition that resolved spontaneously over the next several months.

6–1, D. Learning objective: *Needle biopsies can yield false-negative results due to sampling error.* A patient such as this with several worrisome features on physical exam needs to be evaluated very carefully and completely. A positive needle biopsy at the initial evaluation may allow you to proceed with definitive therapy such as mastectomy or lumpectomy with axillary dissection in one stage. A negative needle biopsy of a persistent worrisome lump should prompt an open surgical biopsy. The sensitivity of FNA for a palpable mass is between 70% and 88%, probably due to sampling error.

Patients with a negative FNA, a lump with benign features on physical exam, and a low-risk history should be offered a biopsy or close follow-up. However, if there is anything in the history that indicates high risk or if the lesion has malignant features, an open biopsy should be done.

6–1, E. Learning objective: *Each breast mass needs to be evaluated individually.* The rounded mass as described is an example of the type of mass that most surgeons are comfortable following without biopsy, particularly in young patients. It is small, with benign features on mammogram, and has been present for a number of years without change. Had this been the first mammogram on which the breast mass was noted, and it was nonpalpable as this one was, an ultrasound-guided FNA or a mammographically guided core or open biopsy would be appropriate. Close follow-up can be done with a reliable patient with a low-risk lesion. The patient should be seen and examined again in 3 to 6 months. She should be encouraged to do monthly self-exams and counseled to return to the clinic immediately if there are any changes that she notes in either lesion before the next scheduled visit.

6–2, A. Learning objective: *Recognize that the diagnostic work-up needs to be tailored to each clinical scenario.* Mammography is not as sensitive in patients younger than 40 years of age owing to the greater density of the breast tissue. She was recently lactating and therefore most likely has very dense breast tissue and will likely not tolerate the mammogram due to discomfort. Patients still produce milk for several months after ceasing to nurse, so she is still at risk for mass lesions related to her milk ducts. Ultrasound is the best tolerated study and will most likely yield useful information. In her case the lesion was found to be solid with irregular borders and complex internal echoes, with some shadowing indicating internal calcifications. This makes it a high-risk lesion on sonogram.

6–2, B. Learning objective: *Recognize that painful lesions are not always benign.* Breast cancers most commonly present as painless masses unless the disease is advanced. Only about 11% of breast cancers present as painful breast masses. However, the presence of pain in this patient is not in any way reassuring when there are multiple features on clinical exam and ultrasound that are worrisome. An FNA was done in the clinic that day, revealing mammary carcinoma.

▶ **CHANGES IN BOWEL HABITS**

7–1, A. Learning objective: *Understand the presentation of a colon cancer.* The presentation of constipation and decreasing stool caliber in a patient older than 40 years of age must be considered cancer until proven otherwise.

7–1, B. Learning objective: *Understand what history is important to obtain from patients in whom colon cancer is suspected.* The suspicion of colon cancer is reinforced with a history of occasional blood in the stool or weight loss in the last year.

7–1, C. Learning objective: *Understand what studies are important to obtain from patients in whom colon cancer is suspected.* After a complete history and physical examination (including a rectal examination), consider anoscopy if a mass is palpable. A CBC should be obtained.

7–1, D. Learning objective: *Understand that the colon must be visualized in some way to confirm the suspected diagnosis.* Arrange for the patient to return in a few days, after the results of the CBC are available. Prior to the follow-up visit, arrange for a bowel prep so that the patient may be studied with sigmoidoscopy. If a sigmoidoscopy is negative, a complete colonoscopy or barium enema should be performed.

▶ FREE INTRAPERITONEAL AIR

8–1, A. Learning objective: *Understand the findings of peritonitis.* This patient has classic findings of peritonitis, and this constitutes a surgical emergency. The sudden onset of abdominal pain that increases in severity should raise the suspicion of a bowel perforation.

8–1, B. Learning objective: *Understand the work-up of suspected bowel perforation.* The initial clinical work-up should include a CBC, urinalysis, and upright chest radiograph.

8–1, C. Learning objective: *Understand that peritonitis is a surgical emergency and requires operative intervention.* Regardless of the results of the laboratory and radiographic studies, this patient needs an exploratory laparotomy. Notify the operating room and begin fluid resuscitation.

▶ GI BLEEDING

9–1, A. Learning objective: *First considerations should be to support the patient's vital functions, such as airway, breathing, blood pressure, and volume status.* Endotracheal intubation should be obtained if there are airway or ventilation concerns. IV access should be always be established. Two large-bore IVs are necessary.

9–1, B. Learning objective: *Although the first thought is that the patient is bleeding from varices, such a patient has many potential sources of bleeding, such as a peptic ulcer or a Mallory-Weiss tear.* Endoscopy is indicated to obtain a diagnosis.

9–1, C. Learning objective: *The goal of therapy is to first stop the hemorrhage.* Then, and only then, deal with long-term treatment issues.

9–2, A. Learning objective: *This patient could have any of the causes of GI bleeding mentioned. However, evaluation for cancer is mandatory because this is a likely cause of the hemorrhage.* A thorough diagnostic work-up is indicated, which may include esophagogastroduodenoscopy, colonoscopy, or barium enema.

▶ HEMOPTYSIS

10–1, A. Learning objective: *Know the common sites of hemoptysis.* The bronchial arteries are the source of bleeding in most chronic parenchymal lung infections and lung tumors.

10–1, B. Learning objective: *Bronchiopulmonary artery embolization is a useful treatment option for patients with massive hemoptysis.* Embolization is used for patients who have multiple sites of bleeding or bilateral disease, for nonsurgical patients, or as a temporizing measure for patients who are awaiting surgery.

10–1, C. Learning objective: *Know the common causes of hemoptysis.* Causes of hemoptysis include pneumonia, carcinoma, pulmonary hypertension, coagulopathy, and bronchitis. In adults, the most common cause of hemoptysis is bronchitis.

▶ INGUINAL/SCROTAL SWELLING

11–1, A. Learning objective: *Recognize the difference in clinical presentation and physical examination findings of inguinal hernia and hydrocele in a child.* Indirect inguinal hernia and hydrocele are the two most likely diagnoses. If the mass reduces into the abdomen, it is an inguinal hernia. If it does not reduce, it is either an incarcerated hernia or a communicating hydrocele. These can usually be differentiated by careful palpation of the spermatic cord in the groin to evaluate for the presence of bowel protruding through the internal ring into the scrotum (hernia) versus no palpable inguinal component as in a hydrocele.

11–1, B. Learning objective: *Provide a rational treatment plan for reducible and irreducible inguinal/scrotal swellings.* If the mass reduces easily, the hernia can be scheduled for elective repair at a convenient time. If the mass reduces with difficulty, the hernia should be repaired the next day. If the mass does not reduce and you can confidently exclude a hydrocele, the patient should be taken immediately for surgical exploration.

11–2, A. Learning objective: *Recognize that acute scrotal swelling can be due to a variety of causes, which are usually age related.* The differential in this patient includes acute epididymitis, testicular torsion, torsion of the appendix testis, testicular neoplasm, and testicular hematoma. He is a bit older than most patients presenting with acute torsion, but the diagnosis must still be considered. The trauma may or may not be related to the pain and swelling; minor trauma can result in bleeding in a preexisting testicular mass. The history of urinary symptoms may make epididymitis more likely.

11–2, B. Learning objective: *Describe physical examination findings and other tests that help differentiate various causes of scrotal swelling.* In testicular torsion, the testicle may be oriented more horizontally, may be pulled up high in the scrotum, and may have an anteriorly located epididymis. Late in the course, with extensive scrotal swelling, these findings may be obscured. Epididymitis may be associated with urinary symptoms or pyuria and can often be differentiated on exam by the tender, indurated epididymis that is palpated posterior to the testicle. Males younger than 20 years of age rarely get epididymitis. With the patient supine, careful lifting up of the scrotum off the exam table will alleviate some of the pain with epididymitis and will not affect or worsen the pain with torsion. A blue dot sign with transillumination of the scrotum is suggestive of torsion of the appendix testis. A testicular neoplasm is usually a nontender, hard mass palpable within the testicle. It can be tender, however, if associated with even minor trauma. Tests that may be helpful to better differentiate these conditions are ultrasound and color Doppler flow studies.

11–2, C. Learning objective: *Recognize which conditions require prompt surgical exploration.* The only condition that needs immediate surgery is testicular torsion. Doppler flow studies may suggest this diagnosis; however, there are reported false-negative examinations. Exploration is warranted if the condition cannot be ruled out.

11–3, A. Learning objective: *State historical factors that may predispose a patient to inguinal hernias and perform a systematic exam of the groin.* A patient should be examined in both the standing and supine positions. Direct observation and palpation of the groin and the inguinal canal via trans-scrotal invagination is important. Chronic straining with cough (smoking, chronic obstructive pulmonary disease, asthma), urination (prostatic enlargement), or constipation (bowel cancer) can predispose to the development of direct inguinal hernias. This is important because these risk factors may need to be addressed prior to repair of the hernia. Examples are prostatectomy for benign prostatic hypertrophy or colonoscopy to rule out a colon lesion.

11–3, B. Learning objective: *Understand the various types of groin hernias.* A femoral hernia bulges below the inguinal ligament, although it may extend above it to some degree. Femoral hernias are most common in females and have a high propensity to incarcerate. Indirect inguinal hernias are congenital remnants of the processus vaginalis and may be felt to protrude on the tip of your examining finger while invaginating the scrotal skin. Direct inguinal hernias bulge directly through the floor of the inguinal canal (more medial) and may be felt more on the volar side of your index finger. The bottom line is that they really can't be accurately differentiated on physical exam and should not be documented as one or the other. Both are repaired through similar groin incisions.

► **JAUNDICE**

12–1, A. Learning objective: *Understand what symptoms are important in evaluating jaundice.* History taking should include questions regarding symptoms, quality and character of pain, gastrointestinal bleeding, fever, and any history of alcohol use or liver disease.

12–1, B. Learning objective: *Understand what laboratory studies are important in evaluating jaundice.* Initial laboratory studies should include a complete liver panel, CBC, and abdominal ultrasound.

12–1, C. Learning objective: *Understand the management steps for obstructive jaundice.* The patient should receive intravenous fluids, antiemetics, analgesics, and broad-spectrum antibiotics. If abdominal ultrasound reveals biliary dilation, an ERCP must be performed expeditiously with diagnostic and therapeutic intent.

► **LEG PAIN, ULCERATION, OR SWELLING**

13–1, A. Learning objective: *An important question to ask patients with claudication is a present smoking history.* Smoking is a major risk factor for peripheral vascular disease. All patients should be encouraged to start a smoking cessation program immediately because clinical results are poor if smoking continues.

13–1, B. Learning objective: *Know the differential diagnosis of leg pain.* The differential includes trauma, muscle cramps, electrolyte deficiencies (e.g., hypokalemia and hypocalcemia), compression of the neurospinal canal, deep tumors/masses, deep venous thrombosis, compartment syndrome, acute ischemia, and, most likely in this case, peripheral vascular disease.

13–1, C. Learning objective: *The most important test to document claudication is an ankle-brachial index.* This noninvasive test helps quantify the decrease in blood flow to the extremity and can help determine the level of occlusions.

13–1, D. Learning objective: *Know the initial treatment plans for claudication.* After review of the history, physical, and ankle-brachial indexes, the patient should be first encouraged to start programs for smoking cessation and graded exercise.

▶ LYMPHADENOPATHY

14–1, A. Learning objective: *Atypical presentations of common diseases are more likely than rare diseases.* The differential diagnosis includes infectious mononucleosis, resolving pharyngitis, lipoma, bronchial cleft cyst, sarcoid, Hodgkin's disease, non-Hodgkin's lymphoma, scrofula, and toxoplasmosis. In a young healthy patient with no other symptoms or signs, a solitary cervical node is usually due to an infectious etiology such as Epstein-Barr virus mononucleosis or pharyngitis. A single large node can actually be a cluster of small nodes that delineate themselves as they regress.

14–1, B. Learning objective: *Order the appropriate tests for a young patient.* Initial testing should include a complete blood count, Monospot, and chest radiograph.

14–1, C. Learning objective: *Plan an appropriate follow-up for cervical lymphadenopathy.* If the CBC and Monospot are normal, call the patient and assess how she feels. The Monospot is negative in 10% of patients with mononucleosis. If she still feels ill, redo the Monospot, review HIV risk factors, and consider an HIV test. If she is feeling better, have her return in 2 to 4 weeks to assess that the node is resolving. Consider PPD test if indicated.

14–2, A. Learning objective: *Always consider malignancy in an older patient.* In an older patient the risk of malignancy is higher and both tobacco and alcohol increase the risk of head and neck malignancy. Unlike the first patient, this differential should stress malignancy until proven otherwise.

14–2, B. Learning objective: *Select appropriate biopsy to exclude malignancy.* In a patient in whom malignancy is strongly suspected, laboratory studies are rarely indicated. Fine-needle aspiration biopsy is the preferred method for diagnosis because excisional biopsy may cause contamination of tissue planes.

▶ MENTAL STATUS CHANGES

15–1, A. Learning objective: *Acute mental status changes require emergent evaluation and treatment.* The cause of this patient's mental status change is initially indeterminate and must be considered life-threatening until a cause is determined and treated. Patients are not usually discharged from the recovery room until awake and alert, so this lethargic state may be a deterioration. Instituting nasal oxygen is indicated unless the patient has chronic obstructive lung disease with CO_2 retention. However, this patient must be examined on an urgent basis. All possible causes of lethargy must be considered, but immediate action should be taken to exclude hypoglycemia (by giving glucose) and narcotic overdose (by giving naloxone [Narcan]).

15–2, A. Learning objective: *Acute alcohol withdrawal is common several days after stopping alcohol intake and may have a wide variety of presentations.* Acute alcohol withdrawal can present with decreased mentation and hallucinations. Be mindful that the patient may not admit to alcoholism, and these symptoms can occur without documentation of alcohol intake.

15–2, B. Learning objective: *Rule out other reversible causes of mental status change before assuming a diagnosis.* All of the common causes of this patient's confusional state should be excluded before arriving at a definitive diagnosis. That said, alcohol withdrawal seems highly likely, and steps should be taken to begin treatment for this disorder, including vigorous fluid replacement and beginning sedation with a benzodiazepine. Deterioration should be expected, and the patient should be moved to an environment where he can receive ongoing nursing surveillance. Once other diagnoses have been excluded, sedation should be increased as needed to ensure that he will not be a danger to himself or others until the delirium resolves.

▶ **NAUSEA AND VOMITING**

16–1, A. Learning objective: *Obtaining a complete surgical history is important.* This man is otherwise healthy, and of greatest significance, he has never had an intra-abdominal procedure performed. In the setting of an unequivocal small bowel obstruction, this is an indication for an exploratory laparotomy.

16–1, B. Learning objective: *Be familiar with the differential diagnosis of small bowel obstruction.* The patient has some obstructive lesion referable to the mid or distal ileum. This condition could be caused by a tumor, inflammatory bowel disease, Meckel's diverticulum, internal hernia, or other inflammatory disease nearby (such as acute appendicitis).

16–1, C. Learning objective: *Any patient presenting with a small bowel obstruction that cannot be attributed to postoperative adhesions requires prompt abdominal exploration.* Prior to induction of anesthesia, the patient requires fluid and electrolyte replacement.

16–2, A. Learning objective: *The etiology of his small bowel obstruction is most likely secondary to adhesions from his prior operation.* A long midline scar has a higher incidence of being associated with obstruction than smaller incisions. In addition, any physician caring for a patient with a history of prior splenectomy and an acute illness must also be cognizant of the possibility of postsplenectomy sepsis.

16–2, B. Learning objective: *Treatment options depend on the prior history of abdominal surgery and whether the obstruction is partial or complete.* Most surgeons would be willing to treat a stable patient with a partial obstruction and normal laboratory values in a nonoperative manner, including fluid and electrolyte resuscitation, no oral intake, and nasogastric decompression. This approach may continue for 24 to 48 hours or until the resolution of symptoms. It is effective in the majority of cases. Common indications for exploration include a complete obstruction or the development of fever, leukocytosis, tachycardia, or increasing abdominal pain or tenderness, all of which may signify bowel ischemia or perforation.

▶ NECK MASS

17–1, A. Learning objective: *Cervical lymphadenopathy in the adult is malignant until proven otherwise.* The two most common cancers are metastatic squamous cell carcinoma and lymphoma. Fine-needle aspiration of the lymph node is safe and highly diagnostic. A complete head and neck examination with panendoscopy should be done.

17–1, B. Learning objective: *The most likely diagnosis is metastatic squamous cell carcinoma of the head and neck.* Patients at risk have a longstanding history of smoking and alcohol intake. The history of dysphagia and the location of the node raise the suspicion of a pharyngeal or esophageal carcinoma.

17–1, C. Learning objective: *An FNA rather than an open lymph node biopsy should be done in this case.* Open cervical lymph node biopsy in metastatic squamous cell carcinoma has been shown to be detrimental and associated with an increase in the risk of local recurrence.

17–2, A. Learning objective: *Check for risk factors for thyroid cancer.* Most thyroid masses occur in women, but the risk of cancer in a thyroid mass is higher in men. A history of low-dose irradiation in childhood is associated with an increased risk of well-differentiated cancer. Family history is important in thyroid cancer.

17–2, B. Learning objective: *A fine-needle aspiration is indicated and is the most effective way to establish the diagnosis.*

An attempt should be made to diagnose or exclude malignancy prior to considering operation.

17–2, C. Learning objective: *If the FNA is inadequate, then repeat aspiration can be performed.* Radionuclide scanning or ultrasound may be helpful in this situation. If the nodule is "hot" or hyperfunctioning, then it is most likely benign and can be observed. If the sample is indeterminate, then it is suggestive of a follicular neoplasm and surgical resection is indicated.

▶ NIPPLE DISCHARGE

18–1, A. Learning objective: *A focused history and physical examination will help guide your treatment.* Certainly bilateral discharge and irritation of the skin in other areas of the body will lend some credibility to her theory that this is an irritation. However, if the irritation is limited to a single nipple, then you need to examine her and rule out Paget's disease of the breast. If after careful examination of both breasts you can identify bloody discharge (particularly unilateral), further work-up is warranted. Her preconceived idea that her physician is being alarmist is an important bit of the history as well. It is important to listen to patients, and you should guide your therapy by what they report as objective findings. You should not let your therapy be guided by their level of concern, whether it is below the level that you feel is appropriate or well above (i.e., the "worried well" patient). A disparity in the patient's level of concern and yours is common in any disease entity but can be particularly marked in diseases of the breast where the emotional undertones are so prominent.

18–1, B. Learning objective: *The patient should be informed that although the majority of the lesions identified in the work-up of bloody discharge are benign, we cannot be sure without tissue.* A minimal amount of tissue necessary to make a diagnosis is removed at the biopsy, with attention to cosmetic result. Document having discussed education about the potential diagnoses, the risks involved in delay of diagnosis in terms of staging, and metastases if an early malignancy is present. Most patients just need to hear and process the information and will respond reasonably. Rarely does a patient continue to refuse a biopsy of a suspicious lesion. Documentation of your discussion in these cases is critical, including a signed statement by the patients saying that they understand the risks involved and are refusing treatment against medical advice.

18–1, C. Learning objective: *Intraductal papilloma is benign disease.* There is some association of intraductal papilloma with future degeneration to DCIS or invasive cancer, so her continued compliance with breast cancer screening including self-exam, mammography, and annual examination by her primary physician or gynecologist should be encouraged. Patients who have had a duct exploration, like patients who have had other types of biopsy for benign breast disease, inevitably scar in the biopsy cavity. A new baseline mammogram 6 months after the biopsy will show the radiographic appearance of the scar after wound healing and scar remodeling have occurred. Patients can then return to a normal yearly schedule of mammographic follow-up.

18–2, A. Learning objective: *There are a variety of medications that can contribute to nipple discharge by affecting the level of circulating prolactin.* Although birth control pills are the obvious medication associated with changes in hormonal levels (particularly in this age group), some other medications would not immediately raise a red flag as being associated. Another important part of the history is stratification risk factors for breast cancer. This can increase or decrease your index of suspicion but also can provide information as to why the patient appears so anxious.

18–2, B. Learning objective: *The character of the breast discharge is fairly benign.* If she is bothered by the discharge, the first step is to stop all medications that may be contributing to the problem. There are many women who produce at least a small amount of fluid even without any secondary cause. It is not pathologic and does not require treatment. Only those patients with persistent, spontaneous discharge that stains clothing on a regular basis require treatment. If the discharge is nonspontaneous, simple reassurance and education about the factors associated with worrisome discharge will suffice.

> ▶ **POSTOPERATIVE BLEEDING**

19–1, A. Learning objective: *Determine if the patient is hemodynamically stable. Then proceed with a further history and physical exam.* She has normal vital signs and is alert and mentating normally. Now complete your physical examination. Remember to remove the surgical dressing and examine the incision and surrounding tissues. Also check for the presence and briskness of distal pulses. Review her history to determine if she has any preexistent conditions that put her at increased risk for bleeding. Send a stat CBC and type and screen to evaluate her hematocrit and prepare for blood transfusion if it becomes necessary.

19–1, B. Learning objective: *Understand the steps of evaluation of a bleeding patient.* This is most likely a case of localized hemorrhage from a blood vessel at the operative site. Ensure that the patient is NPO, and begin intravenous fluid resuscitation. If review of her history reveals a coagulopathic state, begin appropriate therapy. The most prudent plan is to return to the operating room for exploration and ligation of all bleeding vessels. A young and otherwise healthy patient should tolerate this level of hemorrhage. If bleeding is controlled promptly, blood product transfusion will not likely be needed. Although a consensus value has not been reached in this population, most surgeons would feel comfortable allowing her hematocrit to drift below 20% before considering blood transfusion.

▶ POSTOPERATIVE FEVER

20–1, A. Learning objective: *Know the causes of fever in the first postoperative 24 hours.* The differential diagnosis should include atelectasis, wound infection, and fever associated with perforated appendicitis.

20–1, B. Learning objective: *A physical exam must be performed even though it is often unrevealing.* Examine the patient, checking for diminished breath sounds, wound infection, and presence of peritonitis.

▶ SHOCK

21–1, A. Learning objective: *Understand the pathophysiology of the key shock syndromes.* The patient most likely has hypovolemic shock. The pathophysiology is reduction in blood volume from bleeding leading to decreased left ventricular end-diastolic pressure (filling pressure), decreased left ventricular end-diastolic volume (preload), decreased stroke volume, decreased cardiac output despite increased heart rate, decreased oxygen delivery, decreased oxygen consumption despite increased extraction, and development of oxygen-debt shock.

21–1, B. Learning objective: *Use physical exam and laboratory to recognize shock.* This young trauma patient has hypotension, which is one sign of shock. The patient also likely has tachycardia, decreased peripheral pulses, altered mental status, and cool and clammy skin. If urine output is measured, it is likely he will produce less than 0.5 mL/kg/hr. Blood gases likely show a metabolic acidosis, and the serum lactate typically is elevated.

21–1, C. Learning objective: *Provide initial management of shock.* The first priorities are the ABCs. Thus, you must address airway (A) and breathing (B) first. Management of circulation (C) requires a rapid infusion of 1000 mL of crystalloid solution. This may be repeated. If there is no response to 2000 mL of crystalloid, then the patient will require rapid infusion of packed cells—not cross-matched, if necessary. This trauma patient will likely need to go to the operating room for definitive control of bleeding.

21–2, A. Learning objective: *Understand the pathophysiology of the key shock syndromes.* The patient appears to have an intra-abdominal surgical infection, such as ruptured appendicitis or diverticulitis, and most likely has septic shock. The complex pathophysiology includes decreased intravascular volume from fluid losses into the abdomen and fluid leaks into the interstitium, decreased blood volume, decreased left ventricular filling pressures, decreased left ventricular end-diastolic volume, and thus decreased stroke volume. The stroke volume may also be decreased because of circulating myocardial depressant factors associated with systemic infection, which lead to decreased contractility and increased left ventricular end-systolic volume. The decreased stroke volume leads to decreased cardiac output, despite a compensatory increase in heart rate. Decreased cardiac output leads to decreased oxygen delivery. Because there is loss of vasoregulation, there is a decrease in maximal extraction, and the patient is unable to compensate for decreased delivery with increased extraction. Thus, the oxygen consumption falls at a time when oxygen demand is increased from inflammation and fever. The result is oxygen-debt shock.

21–2, B. Learning objective: *Provide initial management of shock.* The approach to managing this patient with septic shock starts with the ABCs. After ensuring adequate airway and breathing, resuscitate the patient with up to 2000 mL of crystalloid. The patient requires definitive operative management of his surgical intra-abdominal problems. The patient may require transfusion, inotropes, or vasopressors both intraoperatively and postoperatively. Placement of a pulmonary artery catheter helps titrate therapy to optimize volume and contractility support.

▶ SHORTNESS OF BREATH

22–1, A. Learning objective: *Recognize life-threatening causes of dyspnea.* The initial objective is to recognize and treat reversible causes of life-threatening shortness of breath. These include acute airway obstruction, pneumothorax, pulmonary embolus, myocardial infarction, congestive heart failure, cardiac tamponade, severe hypoxia, and respiratory failure.

22–1, B. Learning objective: *Learn the initial treatment for patients with dyspnea.* Always begin with the ABCs. Make sure the patient has an adequate and maintainable airway; confirm air movement and circulation. Add supplemental oxygen, apply hemodynamic monitoring, and continually reassess the patient as further work-up continues.

22–1, C. Learning objective: *Identify signs of impending respiratory failure.* Respiratory failure can present with worsening oxygenation or worsening ventilation, often both. As the patients' condition worsens, their respiratory rate may increase or decrease. Their work of breathing may increase or decrease as they become more fatigued. The patient's Sao_2 often falls despite increasing amounts of oxygen. The patient's mental status may decline as $Paco_2$ increases and Pao_2 decreases. It may transition from lucidity to agitation and finally stupor.

▶ URINE OUTPUT CHANGES

23–1, A. Learning objective: *Recognize that simple mechanical causes for an apparent change in a patient's status should be excluded prior to beginning an extensive work-up.* After trauma and surgery, patients most likely have an intravascular deficit. The urine output may dwindle over a course of several hours. A plugged bladder catheter is the most likely cause of abrupt urine volume changes. This can easily be excluded and treated with catheter irrigation. However, hypovolemia from continued bleeding from the liver or other undiagnosed source or myoglobinemia from the fracture site must be considered.

23–1, B. Learning objective: *Recognize the urgency of treatment of oliguria.* This patient must be seen urgently by a physician. Vital signs that are reported to you as "stable" may include a persistent tachycardia, and even normal vital signs may be present with marked under-resuscitation.

23–1, C. Learning objective: *Be able to treat the causes of oliguria.* A fluid bolus should be given. Catheter patency should be confirmed. The patient should be assessed for volume status and, if clearly hypovolemic, should be rapidly resuscitated with more crystalloid and possibly blood transfusion. If the fluid status is unclear, a more objective and invasive measurement may be indicated (central venous pressure or pulmonary artery catheter). Myoglobinuria must be excluded, and this likely requires cutting the cast to examine the leg and measuring compartment pressures. The cause for the oliguria is confirmed when results of urine and serum electrolytes and myoglobin are reviewed.

23–2, A. Learning objective: *Know the differential of polyuria.* This volume of urine output is most likely from diabetes insipidus. Polyuria several days after operation or trauma may result from physiologic resorption of third-space fluids, but the changes are rarely this dramatic.

23–2, B. Learning objective: *Be able to distinguish the causes of polyuria.* Urine and serum samples should be sent for electrolytes and osmolarity, which will demonstrate a high serum sodium and osmolarity and low values for the urine.

23–2, C. Learning objective: *Be able to treat diabetes insipidus.* The first priority is to restore intravascular volume with crystalloid. Treatment is with intravenous vasopressin.

► WOUND PROBLEMS

24–1, A. Learning objective: *Know what factors are important in decreasing the risk of wound infection.* (1) Administer intravenous antibiotics before skin incision. Since gram-negative and anaerobic bacteria cause most infections following colorectal surgery, antibiotic prophylaxis should be directed to cover those organisms. (2) Do not shave the surgical site unless it is immediately before the operation, and preferably do it with a clipper. (3) Prep the skin with antiseptic solution. (4) Pay attention to minimizing tissue injury and avoidance of wound contact with the lumen of the colon. (5) Avoid hypothermia and hypotension, and minimize blood loss.

24–1, B. Learning objective: *Recognize the signs and symptoms of an acute wound infection.* These are signs of a wound infection and the incision should be opened and drained. Check the fascial integrity to determine if this is a superficial or deep wound infection. Antibiotics are usually not necessary unless there is associated cellulitis. Wound cultures are usually not obtained since they do not alter the treatment.

24–1, C. Learning objective: *Recognize the signs of a late wound complication.* This is a description of a sinus tract. The tract should be probed to determine if there is residual suture material. Removal of the foreign object leads to the closure of the sinus tract.

24–2, A. Learning objective: *Understand the management of an acute wound.* The wound should be examined, bleeding controlled, and extent and depth of injury assessed. If the wound is deep and muscles and tendons are involved, then it may be prudent to take the patient to the operating room for repair. If the wound is superficial, then it could be anesthetized with local anesthetic and washed and prepped with antiseptic solution. All foreign objects should be removed and nonviable tissue excised, and the wound can be closed primarily. The patient should receive tetanus immunization or booster if the last tetanus shot was given more than 10 years ago.

24–2, B. Learning objective: *Recognize the importance of the timing of wound closure.* Open wounds that are more than 6 to 8 hours old are contaminated and have a higher chance of developing an infection if closed primarily. These wounds are best handled by topical wound care and healing by secondary intention.

► INGUINAL AND ABDOMINAL WALL HERNIAS

25–1, A. Learning objective: *Be able to generate a list of possible diagnoses in a male patient with a unilateral, tender groin mass.* Possibilities include inguinal hernia, lymphadenopathy, lipoma, hydrocele, varicocele, sebaceous cyst, hidradenitis, and epididymitis. The fact that the mass is reducible strongly favors the diagnosis of an inguinal hernia.

25–1, B. Learning objective: *Be able to logically and comprehensively plan a diagnostic evaluation to reach a definitive diagnosis.* No other diagnostic studies are necessary. If the hernia cannot be reduced, then operative intervention is required in a timely manner.

25–1, C. Learning objective: *Know the different types of hernia repairs available and the best type of repair for each case.* Given that this patient has a unilateral hernia that has not been operated on before, the best approach should be open technique. The type of repair should include a prosthetic mesh for the best long-term results.

25–2, A. Learning objective: *Be able to clinically identify a bowel obstruction and an incarcerated incisional hernia.* Have a wide differential for the cause of pain in this patient, including an incisional hernia and intra-abdominal adhesions. Do not forget to examine for groin hernias.

25–2, B. Learning objective: *Identify patients that require prompt resuscitation and surgical intervention.* This patient has a clinical bowel obstruction with dehydration and possible bowel ischemia. A nasogastric tube should be placed for decompression, lab values should be obtained, and intravenous fluids should be administered judiciously.

25–2, C. Learning objective: *Recognize that operation is required.* This patient demonstrates a bowel obstruction with possible bowel ischemia. After aggressive resuscitation, early operative intervention is required to prevent further ischemia to the bowel. An operative approach should include not only repairing the fascial defect but also assessing the viability of the incarcerated bowel. If irreversible ischemia has occurred, then bowel resection may be required.

▶ **BREAST DISEASE**

26–1, A. Learning objective: *Understand the options for workup of a nonpalpable lesion of the beast.* Mammography allows surgeons to diagnose and treat malignancies of the breast before they are palpable. A breast mass must be at least 1 cm in diameter to be consistently palpable. By the time it is palpable, the lesion has most likely been present for 1 to 5 years. There is potential for spread even at this early stage. Mammographically guided needle localized breast biopsy is a good option for those lesions that are visible on mammogram but not yet palpable. Occasionally a lesion is seen on mammogram, but in only one projection. Adequate localization with mammography requires that the lesion be visible in two fields. If the lesion can be visualized with ultrasound, it is an excellent alternative for localization.

26–1, B. Learning objective: *Understand the patterns of risk associated with the diagnosis of an in situ cancer.* This patient has a prior history of DCIS in the contralateral breast. The presence of DCIS increases the risk of future development of breast cancer in the ipsilateral breast. The risk of recurrence of DCIS or cancer can be minimized with radiation treatment of the remaining breast after margin-negative wide excision. Her newly detected lesion is in the contralateral breast, which makes it a less important component in risk stratification; however, this does not exclude the possibility that this lesion represents a cancer. Tissue confirmation should proceed. Had her original diagnosis been LCIS, the risk of developing a cancer is increased in the contralateral breast as much as in the ipsilateral breast. In this sense, LCIS is thought to be an indicator of a global or genetic propensity toward the development of breast cancer.

26–1, C. Learning objective: *Recognize the criteria that determine surgical options in breast cancer treatment.* The patient has a <1-cm primary lesion that makes her an excellent candidate for breast conservative treatment consisting of wide local excision with axillary node sampling or sentinel node biopsy. She has had breast irradiation in the past and will be able to make an informed decision, knowing how well she tolerates radiation. Because of her diabetes and peripheral vascular disease, she most likely is not a good candidate for breast reconstruction with a TRAM flap but may be able to have subpectoral implant reconstruction. The emotional impact of a diagnosis of cancer or precancer in patients is considerable. Many patients in her position opt for bilateral mastectomy to reduce the stress and fear associated with the increased risk.

26–1, D. Learning objective: *Recognize that there is a limit to the dose of radiation that can be delivered to any given anatomic site.* If her prior radiation had been to the same breast in which she had a newly discovered breast cancer, her surgical options would be confined to mastectomy because she would not be able to receive another full course of radiation postoperatively. The same considerations regarding the possibility of reconstruction would apply as in 26–1, C. The argument for bilateral mastectomy would be less strong because she would have demonstrated significantly increased risk in only one breast.

26–2, A. Learning objective: *Recognize the features of inflammatory breast carcinoma.* This presentation is typical for patients with inflammatory breast cancer. It is an extremely fast growing and aggressive form of breast cancer that is often widely spread at the time of presentation. It is not uncommon for there to be some improvement of appearance with antibiotic treatment, but the mass lesion continues to grow, distinguishing it from mastitis and breast abscess, the two most common diagnoses that are confused with inflammatory breast cancer. Rapid initiation of chemotherapy in combination with radiation is the mainstay of treatment, with surgery having little role in therapy.

26–2, B. Learning objective: *Understand how to quickly provide the diagnostic information needed to start medical therapy of inflammatory breast cancer.* The objective in inflammatory breast cancer is rapid progression to medical therapy. The role of the surgeon in the initial evaluation of this disease is to provide the amount of tissue needed to definitively establish the diagnosis. Fine-needle aspiration does not consistently provide tissue sufficient to provide a profile of histologic markers to aid in the planning of specific courses of chemotherapy. An incisional biopsy of the breast leaves behind a wound in the middle of a tumor that can bleed and will not heal well. If there are easily accessible and clearly involved nodes, an open lymph node biopsy under local anesthetic is a good alternative. I prefer to perform a core-needle biopsy on the main tumor mass to avoid the possibility of a false-negative biopsy of an inflammatory node. The diagnostic histologic finding is lymphatic dermal involvement, which can be established by skin-punch biopsy; however, inflammatory breast cancer is more of a clinical than histologic diagnosis, often making the punch biopsy unnecessary.

26–2, C. Learning objective: *Patients with abnormalities in staging laboratories require further evaluation.* The patient had elevated liver transaminases on the screening lab tests. The purpose of the initial lab studies is to identify those patients who need more extensive evaluation. In this case, a CT scan of the chest and abdomen revealed three lesions in the base of the right lung and one in the liver that likely represented metastases.

▶ PULMONOLOGY

27–1, A. Learning objective: *Peak flow measurement can assess the severity of the attack and also be used to monitor the effectiveness of treatments.* The patient's physical exam and history suggest that she is in moderate distress and may be worsening. The physical exam, however, is a poor gauge of the severity of an asthma exacerbation. A peak expiratory flow rate gives you a baseline estimate of the severity of her airflow obstruction. This can be used to measure the effectiveness of therapy and give a more objective measure of any future changes in the patient's clinical status. Methylprednisolone (Solu-Medrol) and intubation are not indicated at this time because the patient is alert, giving a history, and has yet to receive any other therapy for her exacerbation. Asking her about triggers is also important, but accurately assessing her clinical status and stabilizing her condition should take priority.

27–2, A. Learning objective: *Know what is important in assessing operative risk in an asthmatic patient.* No pulmonary function tests are needed. There are two important considerations when evaluating this patient for elective surgery, the first being the patient's current clinical status and the degree of her airflow obstruction. This patient has normal PEFR and has required minimal therapy for her asthma. Preoperative spirometry and ABG are unlikely to add information to what has already been elicited. The second consideration is the type of surgery that the patient is going to have. Thoracic and high abdominal procedures carry a much greater risk of postoperative pulmonary complications than lower extremity procedures and require extra vigilance. This patient can be cleared to have her hip replacement, and her pulmonary function should be followed throughout the perioperative period with repeated chest examination and PEFR.

27–3, A. Learning objective: *Know when to delay surgery for asthma control.* Several factors play into the appropriate steps to take in this case. First is the patient who is in the midst of an exacerbation with worsening of her already moderate asthma. Though urgent surgery is not contraindicated in this case, the patient's elective hernia repair is not an urgent procedure and the patient has the time to have her asthma symptoms stabilized prior to her procedure. Finally, the mid-abdominal location of the hernia increases the risk for postoperative pulmonary complications and adds another reason to medically maximize the patient's asthma before repairing her hernia.

27–4, A. Learning objective: *Influenza is a dangerous disease in patients with COPD.* Give influenza vaccine. The flu can severely affect patients with COPD, as can pneumonias caused by *Streptococcus pneumoniae*, *Pseudomonas*, or *Haemophilus influenzae*. His pneumococcal vaccination is already up to date. As an adult who is 65 years of age or older and who received his first vaccination before the age of 65, he should have a one-time revaccination if more than 5 years have passed. *H. influenzae* vaccination is given to infants and at this time is not recommended for adults. A *Pseudomonas* vaccination is not currently available.

27–5, A. Learning objective: *Understand the etiologies of COPD.* Order α_1-antitrypsin concentration. Signs and symptoms of COPD in such a young patient are worrisome as a secondary cause of COPD. α_1-Antitrypsin is a likely possibility, given that there was no other history that suggested another cause of COPD.

27–6, A. Learning objective: *Understand the adverse reactions associated with treatment for COPD.* Order a theophylline level. This man is exhibiting the first symptoms of theophylline toxicity. Hyperthyroidism, hypoglycemia, and acute coronary syndromes can demonstrate some of these symptoms but do not fit the clinical picture as well as an elevated serum theophylline level does.

27–7, A. Learning objective: *Understand some of the atypical presentations of lung cancer.* Pancoast's syndrome is most typical for shoulder/arm pain with brachial plexus neuropathies. Horner's syndrome consists of anhidrosis, miosis, and ptosis. Pancoast's syndrome, like this case, can encompass symptoms of Horner's syndrome. SVC syndrome occurs when venous return from the head and upper extremities is blocked by tumor or thrombosis effects on the SVC. The symptoms of SVC syndrome are headache, facial edema, and plethora. Cerebellar ataxia's main symptom is a gait disturbance.

27–8, A. Learning objective: *Know the staging of lung cancer.* This woman had a postobstructive pneumonia in her presentation of lung cancer. Her abdominal pain, elevated AST, and anemia suggest metastatic disease probably of the liver. Metastatic disease defines stage IV.

27–9, A. Learning objective: *Understand the pathophysiology of paraneoplastic syndromes.* This patient is demonstrating the signs and symptoms of Cushing's disease. This is a paraneoplastic syndrome characteristic of the neuroendocrine-active small cell carcinomas.

27–10, A. Learning objective: *Understand the treatment of community-acquired pneumonia.* This patient has uncomplicated community-acquired pneumonia. The most likely pathogens are *Streptococcus pneumoniae*, *Mycoplasma pneumoniae*, *Chlamydia pneumoniae*, and *Haemophilus influenzae*. These can be adequately covered by a macrolide alone. The patient also has discomfort from his symptoms, so a cough suppressant and antipyretic will give him symptomatic relief. The other regimens are for patients with more severe cases of pneumonia or risk factors for drug-resistant or more virulent pathogens.

27–11, A. Learning objective: *Understand the treatment of nosocomial pneumonia.* This patient has a nosocomial pneumonia and a clinical picture suggestive of an aspiration pneumonia. The nasopharynx of hospitalized patients becomes colonized with gram-negative bacteria and these patients are at increased risk for gram-negative infections. They are also at risk for anaerobic infections from aspirated secretions. Given this patient's already tenuous clinical status and her pneumonia, she should receive an antibiotic with broad-spectrum coverage, such as piperacillin/tazobactam. This can be changed to a narrower-spectrum antibiotic once sputum or blood cultures elicit a likely pathogen.

27–12, A. Learning objective: *Understand that failure of pneumonia treatment warrants further work-up.* This patient has a history that is suspicious for a postobstructive pneumonia caused by an endobronchial malignancy. Antibiotic therapy will not be efficacious if this is true. The patient needs a diagnosis and clearance of any obstruction before therapy for the pneumonia will work.

Given the central nature of the infiltrate, the patient would be best served by a bronchoscopy. This test can directly visualize gross abnormalities of the airways, biopsy any suspicious lesions for diagnostic purposes, and provide diagnostic material for tailoring antibiotic therapy.

27–13, A. Learning objective: *Understand the priorities in treating patients with respiratory distress.* The most important first step in therapy of this patient's oxygenation failure is to improve her oxygenation. This can be accomplished by increasing the delivered Fio_2 with oxygen therapy through a nasal cannula or face mask. Diuresis may ultimately improve the patient's condition but takes time.

27–14, A. Learning objective: *Recognize the signs of severe hypoxia associated with hypoventilation.* The patient is hypoventilating from the narcotic and sedative medications she received earlier. This has resulted in a pure respiratory acidosis and obtundation. Correcting the ventilatory failure by replacing the bellows function of the lung with bag-mask ventilation should reverse the obtundation and help prevent any aspiration events. Giving the antidotes can be done after bag-mask ventilation is begun. Intubating the patient should be the next step if bag-mask ventilation and antidote administration do not arouse the patient promptly. Care should be taken to monitor the patient closely afterward because the antidotal medications have a half-life that is shorter than the medications she received and she may have a recurrence of her ventilatory failure.

27–15, A. Learning objective: *Understand the risk factors involved in extubation.* Do not extubate this patient in the OR, and explain your concerns. This patient has multiple known risk factors for postoperative respiratory failure including advanced age, emergent surgery, abdominal aorta repair, and general anesthesia. He may have more risk factors that you are unaware of such as underlying pulmonary disease or tobacco use history. His risk for postoperative respiratory failure is high and should prevent you from extubating him in the operating room or on arrival to the ICU. In this early postoperative period it is impossible to judge whether the patient will be dependent on mechanical ventilation and/or require a tracheostomy. He deserves early postoperative monitoring and a full evaluation of his mental status, respiratory reserve, and upper airway prior to any attempted extubation.

27–16, A. Learning objective: *Recognize the signs and symptoms of pulmonary embolism.* This patient's history is classic for pulmonary embolus. She has two of the three risk factors from Virchow's triad: hypercoagulability (oral contraceptive use) and stasis (a long plane flight). Given the high clinical suspicion for PE and that she has no contraindications to anticoagulation, heparin should be begun immediately, and then her diagnostic work-up should be completed. Given her high clinical probability of PE, either a CT angiogram or $\dot{V}/\dot{Q}$ scan would be an appropriate initial diagnostic test. An echocardiogram would be useful if the patient proves to have a PE because her history suggests she may have some right ventricular dysfunction and be a candidate for thrombolytic therapy.

27–17, A. Learning objective: *Know the steps of treatment for severely symptomatic pulmonary embolism. Consider thrombolytic therapy.* Thrombolytic therapy for PE is a controversial topic. Most experts would now agree that patients with no contraindications to thrombolysis who have right ventricular dysfunction and hemodynamic compromise as this patient has should receive systemic thrombolysis. There is no consensus on what to do with patients with similar degrees of clot burden and right ventricular dysfunction but without signs of hemodynamic compromise. Patients without signs of right ventricular dysfunction should not receive thrombolysis. This patient has somewhere between a 5% and 20% risk of death based on the severity of her PE and as such should be in an ICU for intensive monitoring.

27–18, A. Learning objective: *Understand the risks of anticoagulation therapy and other therapeutic options that are available.* The treatment of choice for DVT is anticoagulation. This patient, however, has a contraindication to anticoagulation because he currently has significant gastrointestinal bleeding that requires transfusion therapy. An interventional radiologist should be called to place an inferior vena cava filter.

> ▶ **ENDOCRINE SURGERY**

28–1, A. Learning objective: *Evaluation starts with a good history and physical exam.* This patient has an incidentaloma. The work-up includes a good history and physical examination. Specific historical points include description of his hypertension, any history of other medical problems, any history of electrolyte abnormalities, or symptoms of palpitations, sweating, or flushing. A family history of endocrine neoplasia should be sought. If there are history or physical exam findings that indicate that the mass may be functional, appropriate specific laboratory studies should be ordered.

28–1, B. Learning objective: *Know the indications for surgery of an adrenal incidentaloma.* The indications for surgery are hyperfunction and size >6 cm. This mass is 5 cm and does not strictly meet the criteria for removal based on size alone. However, in the absence of evidence of function, this patient should be screened in the near future with another CT scan to watch for signs of growth.

28–2, A. Learning objective: *History and physical examination are the first step.* This patient should be queried for symptoms of hyperfunction of the thyroid (palpitations, heat intolerance, nervousness). In addition, other causes of neck masses should be sought (smoking history, recent upper respiratory infection symptoms, trauma).

28–2, B. Learning objective: *Know the initial work-up of a solitary thyroid nodule.* Initial work-up of a thyroid nodule includes thyroid function tests and fine-needle aspiration.

28–2, C. Learning objective: *The primary treatment of thyroid cancer is surgery.* Well-differentiated thyroid cancers can spread by local extension, and clinically suspicious lymph nodes need to be removed with the thyroid.

▶ **GASTROINTESTINAL SURGERY**

29–1, A. Learning objective: *Rule out other causes of right lower quadrant pain.* In women, especially those of childbearing age, always consider the possibility of gynecologic disease mimicking appendicitis. Thus, ask about the dates of last menstrual period (LMP) because right lower quadrant pain at mid cycle could be due to ovulation. Also inquire about recent bouts of vomiting or diarrhea.

29–1, B. Learning objective: *Define the characteristics of the pain.* Discern what the character of the pain is (i.e., sharp, crampy, intermittent, constant). Has the pain changed in character since its onset? Ask about migration of the pain (i.e., from the umbilicus to the right lower quadrant).

29–1, C. Learning objective: *Know that the differential diagnosis for appendicitis is extensive.* In addition to acute appendicitis, consider gynecologic conditions (ovulation, tubo-ovarian abscess, ovarian torsion, ectopic pregnancy), renal conditions (renal colic, urinary tract infection), gastrointestinal conditions (inflammatory bowel disease, irritable bowel syndrome, gastroenteritis), and other causes of abdominal pain (pancreatitis, peptic ulcer disease).

29–1, D. Learning objective: *Know the standard approach for evaluation of a patient with suspected appendicitis.* Obtain a CBC, urinalysis, and amylase to help narrow down the differential diagnosis.

29–1, E. Learning objective: *Know when diagnostic imaging is helpful in the diagnosis of appendicitis.* In a woman with equivocal signs and symptoms of appendicitis, a pelvic ultrasound may be helpful. It is also faster and cheaper than CT scanning and does not subject the patient to unnecessary radiation. Interpretation of the ultrasound is highly dependent on the operator.

29–2, A. Learning objective: *Use the history to narrow the differential diagnosis.* Ask if the pain has always been at its current position or if it shifted during the development of the disease. Also ask if the diarrhea preceded the abdominal pain, or vice versa. Discern the nature of the diarrhea. Has the patient had similar episodes of these symptoms? Has anyone with whom he is in contact been ill?

29–2, B. Learning objective: *Laboratory tests are indicated to narrow the differential diagnosis and also to indicate the severity of the illness.* Because the patient appears quite ill, obtain a full laboratory assessment including CBC, urinalysis, amylase, and metabolic panel.

29–2, C. Learning objective: *Recognize the signs and symptoms of perforated appendicitis.* The patient has signs of peritonitis on physical examination. The history and exam are consistent with perforated appendicitis, or appendiceal abscess.

29–2, D. Learning objective: *Understand the urgency to operate on this patient.* With the diagnosis of peritonitis, this patient needs an exploratory laparotomy regardless of the etiology. Additional tests and consultations are not going to change the clinical course or the need to operate. No further studies are necessary.

29–3, A. Learning objective: *Understand the approach to anal complaints.* The proper exam of this patient includes inspection and palpation of the perianal region, digital exam of the rectum, and anoscopy. In women, a vaginal exam is also necessary to rule out involvement of this organ in the disease process.

29–3, B. Learning objective: *Fifty percent of perirectal abscesses can result in a fistula-in-ano.* A patient who has recently undergone drainage of a perirectal abscess must be followed for the possibility of subsequent development of a fistula-in-ano. Such a fistula presents as an opening in the area of the prior abscess. Gentle digital pressure on the anal sphincter, before and after anoscopy, may produce a purulent discharge at the external fistula opening or in the anal canal at the origin of the fistula.

29–3, C. Learning objective: *Understand the options for treating fistula-in-ano.* A patient with a fistula-in-ano must be treated surgically. Antibiotics have no role in this disease unless there is evidence of cellulitis. Superficial fistulas may be opened and marsupialized. More complex or deeper fistulas may need treatment with seton placement.

29–4, A. Learning objective: *Know the initial evaluation of a patient presenting with suspected biliary pathology.* The history should include characterization of the pain, what brings it on, and what alleviates it. A history of jaundice or shaking chills with fever may be suggestive of obstruction of the biliary tree. If the patient is asymptomatic at the time of the exam, the only study necessary would be an ultrasound of the right upper quadrant. If the patient has persistent symptoms, additional testing might include laboratory studies such as LFTs, CBC, and serum amylase.

29–4, B. Learning objective: *Know the treatment options for cholecystitis.* For most patients without contraindications for surgery, an elective cholecystectomy should be recommended. This may be done laparoscopically or in an open fashion. Rarely, oral agents that dissolve cholesterol stones may be recommended, but these have limited value.

29–5, A. Learning objective: *Know the differential diagnosis of severe abdominal pain.* There are many things that cause severe abdominal pain. In those patients with known cholelithiasis, biliary disease is primary on the list and may include biliary colic, acute cholecystitis, choledocholithiasis with ductal occlusion, ascending cholangitis, and gallstone pancreatitis. Nonbiliary causes of severe abdominal pain are covered in depth in Chapter 4 and may include appendicitis, peptic ulcer disease, gastroenteritis, colitis, diverticulitis, and pyelonephritis.

29–5, B. Learning objective: *Initial evaluation is aimed at eliciting a diagnosis.* Because biliary disease is suspected, initial laboratory studies should include LFTs, CBC, and serum amylase. A urinalysis is also helpful in ruling out urinary pathology. A three-way abdominal series may be obtained to look for bowel obstruction or free air under the diaphragm. The initial imaging study of the biliary tract should include a right upper quadrant ultrasound.

29–5, C. Learning objective: *Know the initial treatment of pancreatitis.* Patients with pancreatitis should be hospitalized. Pain is treated liberally. Because these patients "third-space" a significant amount of fluid, aggressive fluid resuscitation is begun. Place a Foley catheter in those patients in whom the fluid status is in question. Determine the severity of the pancreatitis by applying Ranson's criteria (Table 29–13). Correct electrolyte abnormalities. The patient is placed at bowel rest with fluid hydration, nasogastric suction, and NPO. Antibiotics are rarely necessary.

29–5, D. Learning objective: *Know the optimum timing of surgical treatment.* The treatment for patients with gallstone pancreatitis is cholecystectomy. If gallstones have not been documented, ultrasound is warranted. While the patient is in acute distress, conservative treatment is necessary as outlined in 29–5, C. Most surgeons do not wait for normalization of an elevated amylase before surgery, because this does not correlate well with symptoms. Rather, surgery is safe when the patient no longer has abdominal pain. Surgery is indicated during the acute hospitalization or soon thereafter because 50% of patients have a relapse of symptoms within 6 months. Those patients who do not improve on conservative therapy must be evaluated further to rule out necrotizing pancreatitis or common bile duct obstruction.

29–6, A. Learning objective: *Know that retained common bile duct stones can complicate cholecystectomy.* The likely cause of her symptoms is retention of stones in the common bile duct following cholecystectomy. Arbitrarily, if the stones are found within 2 years of surgery, they are classified as retained, or "secondary," common bile duct stones. Other causes of these symptoms include obstruction of the common bile duct by some other process (stricture or extrinsic mass) or acute hepatitis. In the immediate postoperative period following a cholecystectomy, these symptoms may represent a bile leak or abscess.

29–6, B. Learning objective: *Know the initial work-up for jaundice associated with pain.* Initial work-up includes documentation of the stones. This is usually done by right upper quadrant ultrasound. The study may not show the stones in the common bile duct directly but may show evidence of the stones as dilation of the intrahepatic and extrahepatic bile ducts. CT scan may also be useful in this setting. Laboratory studies should include LFTs, CBC, and serum amylase.

29–6, C. Learning objective: *Know the treatment algorithm for retained common bile duct stones.* Many stones pass on their own. The patient would be treated symptomatically with pain management and careful monitoring of the serum bilirubin as it fell. Patients are hospitalized and kept NPO. Antibiotics are usually started. In those patients with persistent symptoms, an ERCP should be arranged. ERCP gives direct imaging of the bile duct and can be used to either drain the bile duct by stenting or remove the stone.

29–7, A. Learning objective: *Know the symptoms of ascending cholangitis.* These symptom changes are worrisome for ascending cholangitis. This can occur in patients with complete bile duct occlusion despite antibiotics. The constellation of symptoms of fever, right upper quadrant pain, and jaundice is termed *Charcot's triad;* the addition of hypotension and mental status changes make up *Reynold's pentad.* Ascending cholangitis is a manifestation of undrained pus in the biliary tree. It carries a high mortality if untreated.

29–7, B. Learning objective: *Know the treatment of ascending cholangitis.* Ascending cholangitis is a surgical urgency. The infected bile needs to be drained. There are three primary approaches: ERCP with placement of a stent, THC with placement of a transhepatic drain, or emergency surgery with CBDE. These patients are sick and require parenteral, broad-spectrum antibiotics and treatment of their hypotension with fluids and, often, pressors. Transfer to the ICU is often warranted.

29–8, A. Learning objective: *This patient has painless jaundice and should be assumed to have a neoplasm until proven otherwise.* After a complete history and physical, laboratory studies should include CBC, LFTs, and serum amylase. The initial imaging study should be a CT scan.

29–8, B. Learning objective: *Ductal anatomy should be defined.* An ERCP can give information as to the anatomy of the biliary ductal system, and brushings and washings of the duct may lead to tissue diagnosis. Definitive tissue diagnosis is not required prior to operative therapy. Preoperative staging may include a pancreatic-protocol CT scan or magnetic resonance cholangiopancreatography.

29–8, C. Learning objective: *Know the surgical treatment options for bile duct tumors.* If the tumor appears resectable by imaging studies, and if, during the staging work-up, no evidence of metastasis is discovered, an attempt at resection may be planned. The type of surgery is predicated by the location of the mass. A distal mass, near the pancreatic head may be treated with pancreaticoduodenectomy (Whipple procedure). More proximal lesions may be treated with excision of the affected bile duct with adequate margins and reconnection of the bile duct to the intestine by choledochojejunostomy or hepaticojejunostomy. With evidence of metastatic disease or in settings of unresectable tumors, the surgical treatment becomes palliative. The bile is diverted by choledochojejunostomy. Usually, stents placed by ERCP can reopen the bile duct without the need for surgery. There are chemotherapeutic options, but none are associated with long-term survival.

29–9, A. Learning objective: *Generate a list of possible diagnoses in the setting of abdominal pain and emesis.* The diagnostic possibilities should include nonsurgical causes of ileus such as gastroenteritis, nephrolithiasis, uremia/electrolyte imbalance, and side effects of medications such as opiates, anticholinergics, antihistamines, and tricyclic antidepressants. Surgical diagnoses to be considered should include biliary colic, diverticulitis, peptic ulcer disease, hernia, and bowel obstruction.

29–9, B. Learning objective: *Design an appropriate work-up for a patient with suspected bowel obstruction.* Laboratory tests such as a CBC, electrolytes and LFTs, and a urinalysis should help differentiate the entities discussed in 29–9, A. Plain films of the abdomen can help distinguish between a generalized ileus and a specific obstruction of the small or large bowel and may also help to characterize a bowel obstruction as complete or incomplete.

29–10, A. Learning objective: *Recognize the signs and symptoms that determine operative versus nonoperative management of bowel obstruction.* The lack of resolution of the bowel obstruction after 48 to 72 hours of conservative therapy would prompt many surgeons to consider exploratory laparotomy. If the patient develops signs of perforation and/or strangulation, such as localized tenderness, fever, elevated white blood cell count, or metabolic acidosis, operative management is certainly indicated. If follow-up abdominal radiographs show an increased number of dilated bowel loops and air-fluid levels, exploration should be considered. A complete obstruction identified by a small bowel follow-through or CT is also an indication to operate.

29–10, B. Learning objective: *Outline the appropriate postoperative management of a bowel obstruction patient.* When return of bowel function is slow, one must first consider a persistent or recurrent obstruction and manage that entity appropriately. A small bowel follow-through with barium most accurately distinguishes a postoperative ileus from a persistent obstruction. In this patient, a prolonged ileus is most likely, in which case bowel rest should be continued. The patient has had no oral intake for more than 7 days and should receive parenteral nutrition while awaiting adequate gastrointestinal function.

29–11, A. Learning objective: *History taking should focus on separating simple versus complicated diverticular disease and ruling out other causes of lower gastrointestinal obstruction like carcinoma.* One should ask about prior attacks, the nature of obstructive symptoms, any lower GI bleeding, and any history of chronic urinary tract infections or pneumaturia/fecaluria. History should include risk factors for colon cancer, including family history, weight loss, and change in stool habits.

29–11, B. Learning objective: *Initial laboratory and radiographic tests should include CBC with differential, urinalysis, and CT scan.* An abdominal radiograph is not necessary if a CT scan will be done.

29–11, C. Learning objective: *Initial treatment should focus on resuscitating this patient with intravenous fluids and the administration of broad-spectrum antibiotics.* This patient is obviously in significant distress. Because he has localized peritonitis, an immediate operation may be premature. If the CT scan shows a localized intra-abdominal collection, he may be candidate for CT-guided drainage. If a drain can be placed, he could be treated conservatively with bowel rest, IV fluids, and broad-spectrum antibiotics. If he improves over the next 24 to 48 hours, he can likely avoid a two-stage operation and undergo elective resection and primary anastomosis in 6 to 8 weeks.

29–11, D. Learning objective: *Patients may fail conservative management, despite appropriate measures.* Worsening leukocytosis, increasing abdominal pain, and systemic toxicity may be signs that a patient is failing. Patients who do not improve, or who worsen, over a 24- to 48-hour period will likely need an operation. The safest operation to perform in these circumstances is a two-stage Hartmann procedure.

29–12, A. Learning objective: *Recognize the distinct radiologic features of achalasia.* A bird-beak deformity with megaesophagus is pathognomonic for achalasia. His symptoms are characteristic of the disorder. Many patients who are nervous and in high-stress situations have worsening of the symptoms, but the etiology is thought to be a primary motility disorder.

29–12, B. Learning objective: *Understand the nonsurgical options and how they affect subsequent surgery.* Medical therapy for achalasia, although effective, is only a temporary solution, with most patients becoming symptomatic after a short period. It consists of either bougie dilation to disrupt the spasm of the LES or injection with botulinum (Botox) toxin to paralyze the LES. Either one is a viable option until surgery can be performed. The high rate of permanent success associated with surgical treatment with Heller myotomy makes this the preferred treatment. A single treatment with the bougie or injection does not adversely affect the ability to perform surgery. I prefer to wait after botulinum injections until the patient is beginning to experience symptoms again because I monitor the length of the myotomy with intraoperative endoscopy and may do an inadequate myotomy if the LES is still paralyzed. Repeated bougie treatment or botulinum injections can lead to scar formation at the gastroesophageal junction that increases the difficulty and risks of a Heller myotomy and should not be done in patients who are reasonable surgical patients.

29–13, A. Learning objective: *Recognize the symptoms and physical signs of GI cancers.* The patient's pain pattern could result from several different types of intra-abdominal diseases, including diverticulitis, neoplasia, or cholelithiasis. The change in stool caliber and the occult fecal blood make the first two diagnoses more likely. The history of recent weight loss, in association with the other symptoms, should cause you to suspect colorectal cancer.

29–13, B. Learning objective: *Understand the approach to diagnosing GI cancers and cancer staging.* In addition to standard laboratory studies, you should obtain a CEA on this patient. You would also want to undertake a sigmoidoscopy and colonoscopy with biopsy of any mass encountered. A chest radiograph should also be obtained to assess the patient from pulmonary metastases.

29–13, C. Learning objective: *Know the preferred treatment of GI cancers.* If the biopsy reveals cancer, your next steps depend on the location of the tumor. A patient with rectal cancer should undergo CT scanning of the abdomen and pelvis and rectal ultrasound for clinical staging. Preoperative or "neoadjuvant" therapy with radiation and chemotherapy is an option in many patients, and this must be discussed at a joint conference with radiation oncologists, surgical oncologists, and medical oncologists. Preoperative imaging in patients with colon cancer is unnecessary because the surgeon can assess the liver for metastatic disease at the time of exploration and the nodal status is determined from the surgical specimen.

29–14, A. Learning objective: *Recognize the symptoms and physical signs of GI cancers.* A patient with this constellation of signs and symptoms is likely to have pancreatic cancer. Cancer of the distal common bile duct and carcinoma of the ampulla of Vater should also be considered. It is possible that the patient has an obstruction of the common bile duct due to stones, acute chole-cystitis, or chronic pancreatitis, but the weight loss makes cancer the primary diagnosis in the differential.

29–14, B. Learning objective: *Understand the approach to diag-nosing GI cancers and cancer staging.* In addition to standard laboratory examination, you will want to obtain a CA 19-9 level. An ultrasound of the biliary tree and the pancreas will identify masses and evidence of obstruction. UGI endoscopy, ERCP, and abdomi-nal CT scan are also important in preoperative staging. In particu-lar, endoscopic ultrasound of periampullary tumors with biopsy of prominent juxtaduodenal nodes is gaining favor. A chest radio-graph should be performed to rule out pulmonary metastasis.

29–14, C. Learning objective: *Know the preferred treatment of GI cancers.* Patients with cancer of the mid to proximal common bile duct (CBD) can be treated with resection of the gallbladder and most of the CBD, provided that an adequate tumor-free margin can be obtained at the distal CBD. However, most of these lesions are in the distal duct, and along with tumors of the ampulla of Vater, require pancreaticoduodenectomy (Whipple procedure) for any chance of curative resection.

29–15, A. Learning objective: *Recognize the symptoms of IBD.* Although infectious colitis and irritable bowel syndrome are possi-ble considerations in this patient, the chronicity and episodic nature of her symptoms should make you suspicious for a diagnosis of Crohn's disease.

29–15, B. Learning objective: *Understand the steps of evalua-tion for IBD.* With Crohn's disease as the working diagnosis, pay special attention on physical examination to any evidence of peri-anal, abdominal, or extraintestinal manifestations of the disease, such as fistulas, point tenderness, masses, skin lesions, and/or joint abnormalities. Laboratory tests should include CBC, LFTs, and a metabolic screening panel. The colon should be evaluated by either colonoscopy or contrast enema. Colonoscopy has the advan-tage of the availability of biopsy to differentiate Crohn's colitis from mucosal ulcerative colitis in those patients with disease limited to the colon. The upper GI tract should be assessed by GI radio-graphic series, including small bowel follow-through. Upper GI endoscopy can also be useful.

29–16, A. Learning objective: *Understand the risk of colorectal cancer associated with longstanding mucosal ulcerative coli-tis.* In any patient with a history of stool habit changes, the diag-nosis of colon cancer should come to mind (see Chapter 7). This concern should be heightened in a patient with longstanding mucosal ulcerative colitis, especially if the disease was diagnosed at an early age, because the risk of colorectal malignancy increases significantly after 10 years of symptoms. A history of appetite and weight loss makes colon cancer the likely diagnosis until proven otherwise.

29–16, B. Learning objective: *Know the work-up for suspected colon cancer.* After a thorough history and physical examination, including rectal exam and testing for occult blood in the stool, obtain a CBC. Proctosigmoidoscopy should be performed, as well as either complete colonoscopy (preferred) or contrast enema. If a colon mass is detected, biopsy is warranted and additional laboratory studies should include LFTs and CEA.

29–17, A. Learning objective: *Liver tumors may present with nonspecific complaints.* The primary concern in this patient with hepatitis B, weight loss, malaise, and abdominal pain is that he has primary liver cancer. Alternative possibilities include other types of abdominal malignancy and acute-on-chronic hepatitis.

29–17, B. Learning objective: *Understand the initial imaging studies necessary.* Abdominal ultrasound and CT scan of the abdomen are appropriate imaging tests for this patient. CT scan, however, provides more detailed information of a possible HCC lesion and has better resolution than ultrasound.

29–17, C. Learning objective: *Surgical options can cure, but other options are available in nonsurgical candidates.* Surgical resection and orthotopic liver transplantation offer the only chance for cure. Partial hepatic resection (either anatomic or nonanatomic) can be carried out in patients with adequate hepatic reserve. If hepatic reserve is inadequate, liver transplantation can be considered in those without extrahepatic disease, small tumors, and minimal intrahepatic spread.

29–18, A. Learning objective: *Understand the differential diagnosis of an incidentally found liver mass.* The differential diagnosis of a 2-cm lesion found incidentally in this patient is hemangioma, hepatic adenoma, focal nodular hyperplasia, primary liver cancer, metastatic cancer, and bacterial abscess. However, bacterial abscess, primary liver cancer, and metastatic cancer are unlikely in this patient given her history, physical findings, and laboratory tests. With her history of oral contraceptive use, hepatic adenoma is more likely than the other benign tumors in the differential diagnosis.

29–18, B. Learning objective: *Understand the treatment options.* This lesion most likely represents a benign tumor of the liver. Laparoscopic cholecystectomy should be performed with intraoperative inspection of the lesion. If there is any doubt that this lesion is a malignancy, a wedge resection and biopsy should be performed.

29–19, A. Learning objective: *Understand the differential diagnosis of multiple liver lesions.* These multiple lesions in the liver in this patient represent hepatic bacterial abscesses. Although rare, hepatic bacterial abscesses may be a result of perforated appendicitis. Patients present with high fever, sweats, marked leukocytosis, and elevated LFTs.

29–19, B. Learning objective: *Small abscesses may be treated with antibiotics; large abscesses require drainage.* This patient should be adequately fluid resuscitated, placed on IV antibiotics, and have his primary infection treated with appendectomy or percutaneous drainage of his right lower quadrant abscess followed by interval appendectomy. His multiple hepatic abscesses may be adequately treated with IV antibiotics; however, if his clinical status fails to resolve, he may need percutaneous drainage of large abscesses not improving on IV antibiotics.

29–20, A. Learning objective: *Know the key historical points in the evaluation of pancreatitis.* Although this patient gives a good history for chronic pancreatitis, it is important to rule out pancreatic cancer. Despite his history of alcohol abuse, be aware that choledocholithiasis can also cause chronic pancreatitis. Thus, it is important to find out if this patient has gallstones or a history of cholecystectomy. Also inquire whether the patient has had episodes of jaundice, glucose intolerance, or steatorrhea. Has his appetite changed? Does he smoke? Is there a family history of GI tumors?

29–20, B. Learning objective: *There are many causes of recurrent upper abdominal pain.* The leading diagnosis is chronic pancreatitis. Other causes of chronic, relapsing pain include gallbladder disease, peptic ulcer disease, pancreatic cancer, and cancer of other areas of the GI and biliary tracts.

29–20, C. Learning objective: *A thorough physical examination is important in this patient.* Look for signs of malnutrition, jaundice, or abdominal mass. Check for occult blood in his stool. In addition to standard laboratory studies such as CBC and LFTs, an ultrasound of the abdomen can be useful. Abdominal CT scan and upper GI endoscopy may be indicated based on the results of the prior studies. ERCP or MR imaging may be used to define pancreatic ductal anatomy.

29–21, A. Learning objective: *Abdominal pain in the absence of other stated signs or symptoms is a general, nonspecific complaint.* Thus, you need to elicit pertinent information from the patient to develop a working diagnosis and direct your evaluation. For example, this patient's epigastric pain could be due to esophagitis, gastritis, ulcer disease, cholecystitis, pancreatitis, or GI cancer. To develop a reasonable differential diagnosis, you would want to know if this patient has had symptoms of nausea or vomiting, hematemesis, bright red blood per rectum, or melena. You would want to ask if he has had documented prior GI disease, abdominal surgery, or other significant medical problems. Does he take any medications? Has anyone in his family had GI disease or cancer? Has he noticed any weakness or fatigability?

29–21, B. Learning objective: *Weight loss is a worrisome complaint.* Although it is certainly possible that this patient's stated weight loss is due to reduced food intake, you should be concerned about the presence of GI cancer. Your evaluation would commence with routine blood studies, a urinalysis, and a serum amylase and lipase determination. If these studies are normal, your next step should probably be a plain film of the abdomen and ultrasound of the pancreaticobiliary system. If this evaluation is not revealing, you would next want to obtain an esophagogastroduodenoscopy (EGD). A CT scan of the abdomen could be done if the EGD does not establish a diagnosis.

29–21, C. Learning objective: *Patients with gastric ulceration need to undergo routine surveillance endoscopy to assess the healing process.* At the first session, a biopsy of the ulcer must be obtained to rule out an ulcerated gastric cancer. This step would be especially important in the patient with a history of weight loss. Gastric cancer must be strongly suspected in all patients with nonhealing gastric ulcers; therefore, biopsy is recommended of all persistent ulcers noted on follow-up. Resection of a nonhealing gastric ulcer is indicated even if repeated biopsy does not demonstrate malignancy. Any patient with ulcer disease should be tested for *Helicobacter pylori* and treated if the test result is positive.

▶ **HEMATOLOGY**

30–1, A. Learning objective: *In a trauma patient, always assume that the etiology of hypotension is volume loss.* This patient has two possible causes of hypotension. His lack of mobility and sensation suggest a thoracic spine injury, which would contribute to "spinal shock," and he has an open tibial-fibular fracture that has bled an unknown volume at the scene of the accident. He may also have other internal injuries that contribute to his intravascular volume deficit ("hemorrhagic shock"). In a trauma patient, always assume that hypotension is (at least partially) due to blood loss. The treatment is intravascular expansion with crystalloid or blood products.

30–1, B. Learning objective: *Know the options for treating early hypotension during the trauma resuscitation.* The initial resuscitation of this patient should consist of the rapid administration of 2 L of normal saline or lactated Ringer's solution. Subsequent treatment with blood products depends on the patient's response to the initial fluid bolus and on the results of initial laboratory tests.

30–1, C. Learning objective: *Laboratory studies guide the diagnosis and therapy.* In this patient, be concerned about significant blood loss from multiple injuries. It is necessary for him to go to the operating room for repair of his leg fracture; thus, it is important to obtain a baseline hematocrit and hemoglobin. A metabolic panel is helpful to the anesthesiologist in safely administering anesthesia. Some trauma surgeons would obtain a platelet count and coagulation studies at the time of presentation of a massive trauma victim, but this may not be routinely necessary in an otherwise healthy individual.

30–2, A. Learning objective: *Always suspect other sources of blood loss in massive trauma victims.* The leading cause of hypotension is still blood loss. The obvious leg fracture is a source, and the pelvic fracture can lead to significant blood loss into his retroperitoneum. The initial hematocrit of 30% should not create a sense of security, as it generally takes 1 to 4 hours for the hematocrit to accurately reflect red blood cell loss, depending on the rapidity of the bleeding and the aggressiveness of the fluid replacement.

30–2, B. Learning objective: *After initial attempts of crystalloid infusion, the use of blood is appropriate.* Begin transfusion of packed red blood cells immediately. If typed and cross-matched blood is unavailable, use un-cross-matched O-negative blood. If the patient requires more than 4 units of packed red blood cells in the first 1 to 2 hours of resuscitation, assess his platelet count and coagulation status and replace factors as necessary.

30–3. A. Learning objective: *Know the differential diagnosis of postoperative bleeding. Recognize that DIC is most often NOT the cause of postoperative bleeding.* A number of possible causes of the blood loss exist. A differential includes postoperative bleeding due to inadequate hemostasis, low body temperature, specific coagulation factor deficiency, DIC, and medication-related factor dysfunction (such as heparin or warfarin [Coumadin] administration).

30–3, B. Learning objective: *Understand how to rule out various causes of bleeding.* Low body temperature is not likely to be the cause of the bleeding because the patient is not significantly hypothermic. The normal INR and aPTT exclude DIC and most specific clotting factor deficiencies. Although aspirin ingestion or von Willebrand's disease are possible, they are far less likely than bleeding from a missed injury or inadequate hemostasis (e.g., a knot coming off a bleeding vessel).

30–3, C. Learning objective: *Provide initial care that arrests the patient's bleeding and maintains hemodynamic stability.* This patient should be taken directly to the operating room for exploration of his operative sites. Fluid resuscitation with blood and crystalloid should be initiated. At this time, transfusion of specific clotting factors is not appropriate because the patient's coagulation profile is normal.

30–4, A. Learning objective: *Know how to recognize DIC when it is present.* This patient has classic DIC. He is hyperthermic, and thus hypothermia is excluded as a diagnosis. His coagulation studies are abnormal; therefore, DIC cannot be ruled out. Given his fever, elevated WBC, and hypotension, he is exhibiting septic shock (a hypercoagulable state). His infected necrotic leg is providing the clotting stimulus. His low fibrinogen is indicative of severe DIC.

30–4, B. Learning objective: *Provide supportive care, correct the hypercoagulable state and remove the clotting stimulus.* Care should be directed at providing supportive care, regaining hemodynamic stability, and correcting the coagulation defect. Fluid resuscitation with crystalloid, blood, and clotting factors should be initiated to reverse the hypotension and correct the hypercoagulable state. The infectious basis for DIC should be addressed with both antibiotics and surgical removal of the infected leg (the clotting stimulus).

30–5, A. Learning objective: *Recognize clinical features of life-threatening splenic trauma.* One should always suspect a splenic injury in any trauma patient who presents with abdominal pain or distention, left upper quadrant tenderness, palpable left upper quadrant mass (Ballance's sign), hypotension, tachycardia, acute blood loss, anemia, left lower rib fractures, or referred left shoulder pain (Kehr's sign). Hemodynamic instability or a falling hematocrit with evidence of free intra-abdominal fluid on ultrasound or diagnostic peritoneal lavage mandates emergency exploratory laparotomy.

30–5, B. Learning objective: *Understand appropriate indications for nonoperative management of splenic trauma.* Penetrating splenic injuries have a high association with other intrathoracic or intra-abdominal injuries and are always explored. Nonoperative management of blunt splenic injuries requires less than a grade IV splenic injury as diagnosed by abdominal CT scan, absence of peritonitis on abdominal examination, a neurologically intact patient whose abdominal examination can be followed reliably, hemodynamic stability, and the absence of concomitant intra-abdominal injuries.

30–5, C. Learning objective: *Identify clinical changes in nonoperative management of splenic trauma that mandate exploratory laparotomy.* Any patient who develops peritonitis or hemodynamic instability or who requires more than 2 units of blood transfusion due to the splenic injury should be explored expediently.

30–6, A. Learning objective: *Recognize clinical signs of thrombocytopenia.* Patients with a platelet count <50,000/mm^3 usually notice easy bruisability, ecchymoses, or petechiae. Once the platelets reach 10,000/mm^3, spontaneous mucosal bleeding can occur, manifesting as epistaxis, bleeding gums, abnormal vaginal bleeding, hematuria, gastrointestinal bleeding, and, rarely, intracranial hemorrhage.

30–6, B. Learning objective: *Know the appropriate tests to diagnose ITP.* Laboratory findings in ITP include a moderate to severe thrombocytopenia with a platelet count always <100,000/mm^3, prolonged bleeding time but normal prothrombin and activated partial thromboplastin times, and normal or increased numbers of megakaryocytes in a bone marrow aspirate. Platelets may be absent from a peripheral blood smear. An iron deficiency anemia suggests chronic bleeding.

30–6, C. Learning objective: *Understand that medical management in ITP precedes surgical management.* Initial therapy for symptomatic ITP consists of steroids gradually tapered over 6 to 8 weeks (usually starting with prednisone 60 mg daily), intravenous gamma globulin, and, occasionally, plasmapheresis. This regimen increases the platelet count in 75% of individuals, thereby averting the risk of major hemorrhage, but only 15% to 20% are cured. Splenectomy should be performed in the following situations: when thrombocytopenia does not respond to aggressive medical therapy; when thrombocytopenia recurs with steroid taper or discontinuation; when side effects from the medical treatment prove unacceptable; or when intracranial hemorrhage occurs. Splenectomy produces a sustained remission in 80% of patients.

▶ **INFECTIOUS DISEASE**

31–1, A. Learning objective: *The diagnosis of Fournier's gangrene requires a high degree of suspicion.* The chief concern would be a necrotizing infection of the perineal area (Fournier's gangrene), because this would be a life-threatening infection.

31–1, B. Learning objective: *Recognize the signs of Fournier's gangrene.* Carefully inspect the wound and check for pain, tenderness, and crepitus. If these signs are present, surgical exploration is most likely necessary.

31–2, A. Learning objective: *Remember that necrotizing infection is possible even in the immediate postoperative period.* The differential diagnosis would also include wound infection and atelectasis.

31–2, B. Learning objective: *Physical exam is mandatory in the work-up of postoperative fevers.* The patient should be examined and the wound must be inspected. Further studies may then be warranted.

31–3, A. Learning objective: *Have a high degree of suspicion for necrotizing fasciitis in diabetic patients.* Because this is a life-threatening process, this should be your chief concern.

31–3, B. Learning objective: *Recognize the need for prompt antibiotic therapy.* You should initiate broad coverage for both gram-positive and gram-negative organisms, including clostridial species.

31–4, A. Learning objective: *Recognize sepsis in the postoperative period.* The differential diagnosis should include sepsis from surgical complication such as abscess, wound infection, anastomotic leak, urinary tract infection, pneumonia, and catheter infection.

31–4, B. Learning objective: *Know the important management steps of sepsis.* Treatment should include fluid resuscitation, transfer to an ICU, broad-spectrum antibiotics, and investigation of the source.

> ► **NEPHROLOGY**

32–1, A. Learning objective: *Identify the primary acid-base disorder.* The pH is below 7.37, so an acidosis is present. The HCO_3^- is low, suggesting that the primary disorder is a metabolic acidosis.

32–1, B. Learning objective: *Identify the appropriate respiratory compensation to a primary metabolic acidosis.* The pH is 7.35 and the expected Pco_2 for this situation would be $Pco_2 = 1.5 \times HCO_3^- + 8 (\pm 2)$ or, more simply, the expected Pco_2 would be near the last two digits of the pH. This is indeed the case, so in this metabolic acidosis there has been the expected respiratory compensation.

32–1, C. Learning objective: *Identify mixed acid-base disorders.* We have calculated the expected respiratory compensation and found that it was the appropriate compensation, so no primary respiratory acidosis or respiratory alkalosis is present. The anion gap is 22 [140 – (98 + 20) = 22] . This indicates that we are dealing with a high anion gap metabolic acidosis. The excess or delta anion gap is 22 – 12 = 10. Adding 10 to the serum $HCO_3^- = 30$. This value of 30 is higher than the normal bicarbonate value of 24 mmol/L, indicating that a metabolic alkalosis is also present.

32–1, D. Learning objective: *Recognize clinical scenarios that result in acid-base disturbances.* This patient was admitted with vomiting and has lost H^+ and Cl^- in the vomitus. This resulted in a metabolic alkalosis. However, on the second hospital day, the patient deteriorated and became hypotensive, perhaps due to a perforated viscus. With hypotension and inadequate peripheral circulation, he developed a lactic acidosis that was superimposed on the preexisting metabolic alkalosis.

32–2, A. Learning objective: *Identify the primary acid-base disorder.* The pH is above 7.40, indicating an alkalosis and the Pco_2 is low, indicating that this is a primary respiratory alkalosis.

32–2, B. Learning objective: *Identify the appropriate metabolic compensation to a primary respiratory alkalosis.* At first glance, it would appear that the HCO_3^- is low as a metabolic compensation for acute respiratory alkalosis, but actually the HCO_3^- is inappropriately low. A 20 mm Hg decrease in Pco_2 from normal would decrease the HCO_3^- by 4 mEq/L. So, the decrease in HCO_3^- is beyond the normal compensation.

32–2, C. Learning objective: *Identify mixed acid-base disorders.* We calculate the anion gap as being $133 - (96 + 14) = 23$. This suggests that a second primary disorder is present, a high anion gap metabolic acidosis. Next, the excess or delta anion gap is determined to be $23 - 12 = 11$. Adding this excess anion gap to the serum HCO_3^- reveals $11 + 14 = 25$, which is essentially normal. This indicates that no further primary disorders are present.

32–2, D. Learning objective: *Recognize clinical scenarios that result in acid-base disturbances.* The patient was admitted with chest trauma and was noted to be quite tachypneic, resulting in a respiratory alkalosis. A chest radiograph subsequently showed a broken rib and pneumothorax, explaining the tachypnea. This was treated with chest tube placement. Additionally, he was noted to have hyperglycemia and a high anion gap metabolic acidosis most consistent with diabetic ketoacidosis. Indeed, he had ketones in his urine. The normal blood pressure ruled against lactic acidosis.

32–3, A. Learning objective: *Recognize the most common causes of ARF in hospitalized patients.* The patient has developed ARF possibly due to a reduction in renal perfusion. This may have occurred as a result of intravascular volume depletion, peripheral vasodilation due to the fever, or an impairment in the cardiac output. It is also possible that an intrinsic injury to the renal tubular cells has occurred. A recently started medication may have triggered an allergic interstitial nephritis or tubular necrosis. The hypotension may have led to an ischemic insult resulting in tubular necrosis. A postrenal cause should be considered if the bladder catheter is not functioning properly due to blood clots or mucus.

32–3, B. Learning objective: *Initiate a work-up of ARF.* A physical exam should be performed to determine the intravascular volume status, paying close attention to the blood pressure, skin turgor and temperature, and jugular venous pressures. A careful review of medications should be performed, noting any medication that may be temporally related to the onset of ARF. A spot urine should be sent for sodium and creatinine along with a serum sodium and serum creatinine to calculate an FE_{Na}. A urinalysis should be sent to screen for urinary cells or casts. A reduction in cardiac output may be suggested by the discovery of lung rales, an S_3 heart sound, or tachycardia.

32–3, C. Learning objective: *Initiate a proper treatment for ARF based on the initial findings.* If the intravascular volume status was reduced based on the physical exam, low U_{Na}, and $FE_{Na} < 1\%$, a fluid challenge should be initiated followed by an increase in the hourly fluid intake. If there are physical findings of congestive heart failure, a low U_{Na} and low FE_{Na}, the congestive heart failure should be treated to improve renal perfusion. If the U_{Na} and FE_{Na} are elevated, suggesting intrinsic tubular damage, any offending medication should be stopped, and inputs and outputs should be carefully balanced. If oliguria develops, a potassium restriction should be instituted.

32–4, A. Learning objective: *Recognize the causes of hyponatremia.* This patient has small cell lung cancer that is associated with SIADH. The inappropriately concentrated urine is consistent with this diagnosis.

32–4, B. Learning objective: *Recognize the symptoms of acute hyponatremia and know how to correct the sodium concentration.* This patient developed neurologic symptoms consistent with hyponatremia over a short period and requires acute management with hypertonic saline. First, calculate the sodium deficit to raise the sodium level to a safe value of 120 mEq/L:

$$\text{Sodium deficit} = (0.5 \times 80) \times (120 - 100) = 800 \text{ mEq}$$

This requires (800 mEq/ 513 mEq/L) of 3% saline, or 1560 mL. The time required to correct the sodium concentration by 0.5 mEq/L/hr is (120 - 100)/0.5 = 40 hours. So the rate at which the 3% saline should be given is 1560/40 = 39 mL/hr.

32–5, A. Learning objective: *Recognize the causes of hyperkalemia.* This patient has multiple reasons for hyperkalemia. Chronic renal failure, metabolic acidosis, as well as his medications, the angiotensin-converting enzyme inhibitor and β-blocker, all play a role.

32–5, B. Learning objective: *Know how to treat severe hyperkalemia.* The patient has not only symptoms from his hyperkalemia but also ECG changes of hyperkalemia. Therefore, the cardiac membrane can be stabilized by IV calcium gluconate. Afterward, potassium is shifted back into cells with the use of IV glucose and insulin or inhaled α-agonists (bicarbonate does not work well in chronic renal failure). Finally, sodium polystyrene sulfonate should be given orally or by enema.

32–5, C. Learning objective: *Recognize the treatment differences between mild and severe hyperkalemia.* If no ECG changes are seen, treatment need only include the sodium resin exchange (a repeat potassium level might also be useful). Loop diuretics may be helpful.

32–6, A. Learning objective: *Recognize the causes of hypercalcemia.* This patient has the laboratory values and clinical history of someone who has ingested a great amount of milk or calcium carbonate. The history of peptic ulcer disease suggests that he may have self-administered calcium carbonate, and his hypercalcemia, metabolic alkalosis, and renal insufficiency confirm this.

32–6, B. Learning objective: *Be able to treat a patient with hypercalcemia.* In this patient without neurologic symptoms and at the current calcium concentration, IV hydration with or without furosemide is adequate. Renal function usually returns to baseline after cessation of milk or calcium carbonate intake.

32–7, A. Learning objective: *Volume deficits should be corrected quickly and before induction of anesthesia.* First, insert a large-bore IV, nasogastric tube, and Foley catheter. Based only on the history of no fluid intake for 12 hours, the volume of vomitus and stomach contents likely, and the third-space losses found in bowel obstruction, the patient must be depleted at least 2 or 3 L. Begin with a 1000-mL bolus and continue rapid IV fluids until urine output and vital signs are normal. Replete fluids prior to beginning the operation.

32–8, A. Learning objective: *The best measure of fluid status may be the physiologic response to a fluid bolus.* This patient has an indeterminate fluid status. She is over admission weight, but at least several liters of third-space losses are expected from the peritonitis. The patient's vital signs are only slightly abnormal. Invasive measures of vascular volume appear within normal range but may be falsely elevated by the positive end-expiratory pressure breathing. Persistent metabolic acidosis and oliguria point to inadequate perfusion. Her lung function is tenuous and may deteriorate if too much fluid is given. The physician should give a fluid bolus of 500 to 1000 mL and base further fluid management on the response of vitals, urine output, pulmonary wedge pressures and Po_2, and cardiac output.

▶ SURGICAL NUTRITION

33–1, A. Learning objective: *Estimated caloric needs are a good starting place; however, the calculated caloric needs may more accurately reflect the true needs.* This patient has an estimated need of 2220 to 2590 kcal/day based on the estimated nutritional requirements for trauma patients (see Table 33–2). The calculated caloric need that takes into account the height as well at the weight more accurately reflects the lean body mass. For instance, a 74-kg person who is 5 ft, 2 in tall has a lower calorie requirement by the calculated caloric needs than our patient who is 6 ft, 2 in because much of the weight most likely is not lean muscle mass. It also takes into account the severity of the injury, the degree of surgical stress, and the effects that sepsis have on metabolism. For instance, the range of caloric needs for our patient is 2490 to 4074 kcal/day, depending on the number that is assigned to the injury factor. Severe trauma or sepsis can profoundly affect caloric needs, and nutritional support should be modified to account for this or the patient will begin to catabolize proteins and lose muscle mass, which can adversely affect recovery from injury or surgery.

33–1, B. Learning objective: *The amount of protein should be adjusted to balance the number of kilocalories given.* Patients do best when on a balanced nutritional formula that contains carbohydrates, fats, and proteins. The usual requirement for protein is 60 g in an adult man, but this can go much higher with severe stressors such as injury or major surgery. Based on the trauma, this patient's need is 59 to 148 g. With total resting starvation the amount of time between ceasing all protein intake and exhausting the supplies of protein in the body is 40 to 60 days. Certainly, chronic underfeeding of both calories and proteins (protein malnutrition) leads to loss of lean muscle mass. Standard enteral formulas are supplied in balanced formulations, and you usually need to do little more than calculate the caloric requirements and the proper amount of proteins will be delivered. There is a little variability in the amount of protein relative to calories that you can deliver in TPN; however, ranges are set by the pharmacy to avoid overloading with protein, which can be detrimental. You should periodically check indices of nutrition to be sure that you are giving adequate nutrition. It is important to be aware and use specialized formulas for patients with underlying medical problems such as renal insufficiency or liver failure whose recovery and health may be adversely affected by protein overload.

33–1, C. Learning objective: *Factors specific to the clinical situation need to be accounted for when deciding on a route of nutritional access.* The preferred route for nutritional supplementation is enteric. It is cheaper, better able to replete nutritional deficit, and less prone to swings in electrolyte balance, glucose metabolism, and acid-base status. This patient has major intra-abdominal injuries as well as a lumbar spine injury associated with a complete cord transection. These contribute to some degree of postoperative ileus. Young healthy trauma victims may have the reserve to wait for these to resolve, and a nasoenteric feeding tube can be placed in anticipation of starting enteral feeding as soon as the clinical situation allows. If the anticipated period without nutrition is longer than 6 to 8 days, TPN should be started until the GI tract can be used. In patients who do not have the physiologic reserve to withstand even a short period without nutrition, TPN should be started immediately to avoid getting too far behind in their nutrition.

33–2, A. Learning objective: *An enteral route of feeding is always preferable if it is feasible.* This patient should have an open jejunostomy tube or a radiographically placed gastrostomy tube. The placement of a percutaneous endoscopic gastrostomy (PEG) tube in cases of oropharynx and esophageal malignancy has been associated with gastric tube site tumor implants. The published complication rate for gastric tubes placed either surgically or radiographically is equal. Some esophageal surgeons prefer not to have a gastric feeding tube because they think it potentially compromises the gastric tube used to replace the segment of removed esophagus; however, the tubes are frequently placed prior to consultation with the surgeon. The patient is likely to be on enteral feeds for a prolonged period even if he could swallow before his neoadjuvant therapy is started because many patients develop severe esophagitis that lasts throughout therapy. The goal of supplemental nutrition for him is to replace the losses he has already had and to maintain optimal nutrition throughout therapy.

33–2, B. Learning objective: *Objective measures of nutritional status at the beginning of nutritional supplementation should be determined.* Patients who have a serum albumin of less than 3.3 or who have lost more than 10% of their body weight are severely malnourished. Measuring objective nutritional parameters at the start and during the period of supplementation helps determine whether the nutritional goals are being met. He is going to have a planned long period where he will potentially have no intake except the gastric tube feeding. He should be given trace elements and vitamins as well as long as they do not interfere with the effectiveness of the chemotherapy.

33–2, C. Learning objective: *Complete repletion of weight loss is not required to have a clinically significant improvement in nutritional status.* The patient has not attained his premorbid weight; however, when tested, his albumin level had returned to normal limits. His nutritional status was no longer considered a factor when counseling him about his operative risks. Because he had lost a substantial weight, he would be a patient who was still considered to have depleted some of his physiologic reserve and should receive supplemental nutrition either enterally or parenterally as soon as possible in the postoperative course.

▶ **SURGICAL ONCOLOGY**

34–1, A. Learning objective: *Suspect melanoma with this history.* Any significant history of sun exposure should alert you to the possibility of a sun-related neoplasm. The diagnosis is pathologic, so a biopsy must be done. Because this lesion is on a part of the body that may be hidden by clothing, a full-thickness excisional biopsy should be done.

34–1, B. Learning objective: *Know the likely spread of melanoma.* The most likely spread of melanoma is lymphatic. Be sure to perform a complete lymph node evaluation, noting any nodal beds with firm, palpable nodes. Also, search the remaining skin to see if any other lesions warrant biopsy.

34–1, C. Learning objective: _Recognize that melanoma may drain to unexpected lymphatic beds._ A lymphoscintigram should be performed to identify any lymphatic beds that drain the site of the primary lesion. This is especially important in patients presenting with lesions of the head, trunk, neck ,or shoulder, because as many as 47% of these do not drain into an expected lymph node bed.

34–1, D. Learning objective: _Know the surgical treatment of melanoma._ This is a thin lesion. In patients with no evidence of lymphatic spread, the primary lesion should be excised with at least 1-cm margins. For lesions deeper than 1 mm, a 2-cm margin is indicated. Re-examination of regional lymph node beds is necessary at frequent intervals, and lymph node dissection is performed if any nodes are suspicious.

34–2, A. Learning objective: _A mass of this size is a sarcoma until proven otherwise._ A tissue diagnosis is required. Plan to obtain a biopsy.

34–2, B. Learning objective: _Understand that the biopsy technique is important._ The size of the tissue sample is important, because cellular architecture is important in grading the tumor. Another consideration is the orientation of the biopsy incision, because this needs to be completely excised at the time of definitive treatment.

34–2, C. Learning objective: _The three most important staging criteria are histologic grade, tumor size, and extent of spread._ After biopsy, the patient should undergo sizing of the primary tumor by MR imaging. The choice of additional staging depends on the grade of the tumor and the site of presentation. An extremity tumor tends to spread to the lungs, so a low-grade tumor may be evaluated by chest radiograph and a high-grade tumor may be evaluated by chest CT. A visceral tumor tends to spread to the liver, so abdominal CT scanning or MR imaging is required, regardless of the grade.

34–2, D. Learning objective: _Know that the primary treatment of sarcomas is surgery._ Surgery is required to control the primary tumor site. Excision of the tumor with 2- to 3-cm margins is preferable, but consideration of the functional losses to the limb is important. There is no advantage to amputation versus adequate surgical excision. Radiation therapy with either external-beam therapy or brachytherapy is necessary following surgical excision. Pulmonary sites of metastasis are surgically excised if possible.

► **TRAUMA**

35–1, A. Learning objective: _Know how to prioritize trauma assessment._ First, a patent _A_irway should be assured. Absent breath sounds and crepitus are adequate indications for a left chest tube, which should improve his *B*reathing. *C*irculatory assessment reveals obvious shock, and he should have at least two large-bore IVs and probably a large femoral vein catheter, and a 2-L bolus of warm Ringer's lactate. If the vital signs don't normalize, packed red blood cells are given. Neurologic *D*isability should be assessed initially and when the vital signs normalize. Thereafter, even if his airway is patent, if his Glasgow Coma Scale score remains <9, it is safer to proceed with paralysis and endotracheal intubation. Following a simultaneous parallel track, the cause of the shock is investigated with control of any external bleeding and with chest radiograph, pelvis radiograph, and ultrasound. Subsequent care is based on the results of the secondary survey and these tests.

35–1, B. Learning objective: *Know the commonly missed blunt injury syndromes.* The answer should include an aortic tear, diaphragmatic disruption, carotid dissection/thrombosis, pancreatic injury, and intestinal injury.

35–2, A. Learning objective: *Identify which patients with penetrating injury need immediate operation.* The physician should check chest tube output, perform a FAST (ultrasound) exam, and take the patient to the operating room. Pericardial tamponade must be considered in all patients with penetrating chest injury. Detecting Beck's triad (systolic hypotension, distended neck veins, and muffled heart sounds) may be difficult in the trauma room; the diagnosis is usually now made by ultrasound. If Beck's triad is found, the patient should be taken immediately to the operating room for median sternotomy and repair of the cardiac injury. Pericardiocentesis may help temporize but is rarely used. The one valid indication for emergency department thoracotomy may be the loss of vital signs in a patient with stab wound to the heart. Immediate release of the pericardial blood may be life-saving. Though chest tube placement causes expansion of the lung and tamponade of most pulmonary bleeding, bleeding from systemic vessels may persist. Patients with >200 mL/hr of chest tube output should be considered for thoracotomy. Stable patients with abdominal stab wounds and no peritoneal signs may be observed for development of signs of injury. However, patients with abdominal stab wounds and shock should be taken directly to the operating room for laparotomy for control of hemorrhage.

35–3, A. Learning objective: *Recognize and evaluate blunt abdominal trauma in the hemodynamically stable patient.* Further testing to rule out intra-abdominal injury should be performed on all patients with abdominal pain or tenderness. The diagnostic modalities available to the trauma surgeon include DPL, CTA, ultrasonography, and DL. Each has its own inherent advantages and disadvantages. In this setting, CTA has become the diagnostic test of choice to evaluate stable patients after blunt abdominal trauma. It can identify specific solid-organ injury (allowing nonoperative management) and provide assessment of renal perfusion, retroperitoneal structures, and the pelvis.

35–3, B. Learning objective: *Recognize the fact that physical examination is not always reliable in the trauma patient.* The presence of central nervous system injury (either closed head injury or spinal cord injury), substance abuse (drugs or alcohol), or distracting injuries (long bone and/or pelvic fractures) can render the physical examination unreliable in the blunt trauma victim. In addition, the need for sedation, intubation, respiratory support, or operative intervention for extra-abdominal injuries (head injury, orthopedic fractures) limits the utility of the physical examination. As a result, the trauma surgeon must rely on those modalities mentioned in 35–3, A.

35–3, C. Learning objective: *Recognize and diagnose the possibility of intra-abdominal hemorrhage in the unstable patient.* DPL should be performed for rapid screening of intra-abdominal hemorrhage in the unstable patient. A positive tap or aspirate indicates the need for urgent celiotomy. Ultrasonography can also provide rapid information regarding the presence or absence of intra-abdominal fluid in the resuscitation room. Remember, however, that ultrasonography is operator dependent.

35–4, A. Learning objective: *Recognize and definitively evaluate abdominal stab wounds.* The main point to recognize is the location of the wound. Stab wounds to the anterior abdominal wall can be evaluated by several methods: observation, local wound exploration, DL, and, less commonly, DPL. Each method is progressively more invasive. With a stable patient, an acceptable course of action involves admission to the ward with serial abdominal examinations by the same examiner. Local wound exploration can be done in the resuscitation room, and, if negative, allows the patient to be discharged. DL requires general anesthesia but provides definitive information regarding peritoneal penetration. DPL is not used as commonly for initial evaluation of stab wounds secondary to conflicting criteria concerning positive results.

35–4, B. Learning objective: *Recognize the need for urgent laparotomy in patients with penetrating abdominal trauma.* In unstable patients or in the mentally and neurologically intact patient with unequivocal signs and symptoms of abdominal injury, further diagnostic measures are unnecessary and urgent laparotomy should be performed.

35–5, A. Learning objective: *Understand the steps in triage and management of thermal injury patients.* Given the extent of burn and the high likelihood of smoke inhalation, this patient is likely to develop massive airway edema and early endotracheal intubation is indicated. Carbon monoxide inhalation is likely and a carboxyhemoglobin should be sent and 100% oxygen instituted. Fluid requirement should be calculated using the Parkland formula of 4 mL/kg per percentage of body burn, giving one-half over the first 8 hours postburn. Fluid therapy should begin at the calculated rate but should be modified depending on vital signs and urine output. Pain medication and tetanus prophylaxis should be given. The patient should be kept warm and the burned tissue should be covered with clean, dry towels. This patient should be treated in a regional burn center.

35–6, A. Learning objective: *Know the priorities of treatment of chest injuries.* The first priority is the assessment of the ABCDs. His *A*irway is patent. Assessment of *B*reathing reveals decreased breath sounds in the left chest and significant tachypnea. A left tube thoracostomy should be performed immediately to alleviate a possible tension pneumothorax or hemothorax. An evaluation of *C*irculation reveals tachycardia and relative hypotension. Two peripheral large-bore IVs also should be inserted to allow fluid resuscitation. Assessment of his neurological status (*D*isability) reveals no abnormal findings. *E*xposure is essential to rule out the presence of additional injuries. A *F*oley and a *G*astric (nasogastric) catheter are extremely important for diagnosis and monitoring. Finally, the performance of FAST is invaluable to rapidly examine the pericardium and abdominal cavity. A secondary survey with a thorough examination of all systems should follow. Physical examination of the chest and abdomen merits special attention.

35–6, B. Learning objective: *Become familiar with the possible injuries that would need to be addressed.* Injury to the thoracic wall with possible laceration of intercostal vessels can cause significant hemorrhage that may necessitate a surgical procedure. The possibility of laceration of the underlying lung is also present. Although most bleeding from the lung parenchyma is self-limited, injury to the pulmonary hilum may result in massive blood loss. Injury to the heart must also be considered. Injury to the left hemidiaphragm with associated intra-abdominal injuries should also be considered. Intra-abdominal organs most likely to be injured include the spleen, stomach, and left colon.

35–6, C. Learning objective: *Be able to prioritize the care of a patient with a chest injury.* Treatment is mainly determined from the hemodynamic status of the patient and the findings during the primary survey. If the patient becomes normotensive after the insertion of the left chest tube with resolution of his tachypnea and tachycardia, the decision for operation will be based on findings in the abdominal examination and chest tube output. The presence of peritonitis and excessive persistent bleeding from the chest tube are indications for surgical intervention. In the absence of an indication for surgical exploration, laparoscopic or thoracoscopic evaluation of the left hemidiaphragm is advisable.

35–7, A. Learning objective: *Recognize life-threatening chest injuries.* This patient appears to have an isolated chest injury. Multiple rib fractures and flail chest with underlying pulmonary contusion are likely. Pneumothorax and hemothorax are commonly associated with this condition and should be treated with tube thoracostomy without undue delay. Although blunt cardiac rupture is rare, blunt cardiac injury should be suspected. Blunt diaphragmatic rupture is rarely an isolated injury in blunt thoracic trauma. Finally, injury to the thoracic aorta should be carefully ruled out.

35–7, B. Learning objective: *Be able to diagnose and treat a flail chest.* Observation of the paradoxical movement of the thoracic wall and the presence of multiple rib fractures on the chest radiograph should raise the suspicion of flail chest. Close monitoring of arterial saturation and arterial blood gases is essential. Many patients that initially appear to have relatively normal breathing may progressively develop respiratory insufficiency. Selective early intubation is critical. The role of pain control and particularly of epidural analgesia cannot be overemphasized.

35–8, A. Learning objective: *Given the trauma mechanism and loss of consciousness, a closed head injury is likely.* With the patient's hypotension and tachycardia, significant blood loss is present. Thus, a full trauma evaluation is necessary to identify possible injury with bleeding in the thoracic cavity, peritoneal cavity, and retroperitoneal space. Bleeding intracranially and into extremity compartments does not result in hypovolemia. Significant external blood loss through lacerations, open fractures, and epistaxis can occur, but other sources must be excluded when mechanisms are severe. Blurred vision and numb cheeks suggest that orbit and/or zygomaticomaxillary fractures are present. Epistaxis can occur with each of them due to either nasal mucosal lacerations secondary to maxillary fractures or blood draining from the maxillary sinus due to orbit, zygoma, or maxillary bone fractures.

35–8, B. Learning objective: *A full trauma survey is necessary.* With respect to the face, laceration location and unstable bone segments must be identified. Blurred vision and epistaxis are associated with orbital-zygoma fractures. The orbit, zygoma, and maxillary bones are palpated to identify unstable segments and bony step-offs. For orbital floor fractures, examination may show enophthalmos and extraocular muscle entrapment. Displaced zygoma fractures show a retruded malar eminence. These findings can be present in any combination. Cheek numbness occurs with infraorbital nerve injury, which is also associated with orbital floor and zygoma fractures.

35–8, C. Learning objective: *The extent of facial injury is determined by physical exam findings and CT imaging of the craniomaxillofacial skeleton.* This patient also needs a full neurologic evaluation, including head CT scan, to identify intracranial bleeding and injury.

35–8, D. Learning objective: *Life-threatening injuries are treated first, then facial fractures are addressed.* If displaced, orbit, maxillary, and zygoma fractures require operative reduction and fixation. There are many exposure approaches to the facial skeleton, and a plan is determined to achieve adequate exposure for fixation of each of the fractures. Commonly, eyelid, brow, and intraoral incisions are used for orbital floor blow-out and zygomatic complex fracture repair.

35–9, A. Learning objective: *With the patient not able to close the mouth, a malocclusion exists.* Thus, mandible and/or maxillary fracture(s) are present. Given his trauma mechanism and an intraoral laceration, a mandible fracture is most likely.

35–9, B. Learning objective: *Determine whether the mandible or maxilla is stable by looking for movement with direct pressure.* Infraorbital nerve defects are associated with maxillary/orbit fractures, and mental nerve sensory deficits are associated with mandible fractures. Location of the intraoral laceration is usually directly over the fracture when the laceration is along the alveolus. Intraoral lip lacerations are due to the soft tissue hitting teeth and do not always correlate with facial bone fractures.

35–9, C. Learning objective: *The extent of injury is determined by physical exam findings and CT imaging of the craniomaxillofacial skeleton.* Physical examination alone is not sufficient to diagnose all injuries.

35–9, D. Learning objective: *Mandible fractures are reduced with arch bar placement with interdental wiring and mandibular-maxillary fixation.* The fractures are then exposed and plated, and the incision is closed with resorbable suture. The MMF is released to ensure that the mandibular condyles are properly seated. MMF is then reinstituted, depending on the fracture pattern and the plating technique used. This patient has the classic findings of a mandibular fracture. An intraoral laceration is commonly at the fracture site when in the body or symphyseal region. A maxillary fracture can also be present and should be excluded with the CT scan that will be done to localize all fractures. Physical exam should also address the function of the mental and marginal mandibular nerves, which can be contused. He will need operative reduction with internal fixation.

35–10, A. Learning objective: *Understand the treatment priorities in managing a patient with fractures.* Colles' fractures are common injuries. The typical deformity can best be described by the mnemonic RADIUS, as follows:

*R*adial displacement
*A*nterior angulation
*D*orsal displacement
*I*mpaction
*U*lnar styloid fracture (possibly associated)
*S*hortening

Acute carpal tunnel syndrome can occur with severe deformities. The initial treatment is to close reduce the fracture, either with intravenous sedation or a hematoma block. After reduction of the fracture, definitive treatment options include plaster immobilization, percutaneous pinning, external fixation, or open reduction and internal fixation.

35–11, A. Learning objective: *Understand the treatment options for treating hip fractures.* Hip fractures are common in elderly patients, especially women with osteoporosis. There are two common types of fractures: femoral neck (subcapital) fractures and intertrochanteric hip fractures. Blood supply to the femoral head can be disrupted in displaced subcapital fractures, leading to avascular necrosis. There is also a higher incidence of non-union in femoral neck fractures. All hip fractures need surgical intervention. Most elderly patients have medical comorbidities that need addressing prior to surgery. Intertrochanteric hip fractures are treated with surgical stabilization of the fracture with sliding plates and screw constructs or sometimes intramedullary nails. Treatment options include pinning versus hip replacement for femoral neck fractures, as in this case. The most important determinants of treatment are based on both patient and injury factors. Important patient factors include physiologic age, prior ambulatory status, and overall medical comorbidities. Important fracture factors include the amount of displacement, comminution, and overall bone quality.

35–12, A. Learning objective: *Understand the treatment priorities in treating traumatic fractures.* After the ABCDs and life-threatening injuries have been addressed, attention should be

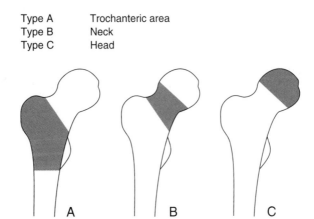

Type A	Trochanteric area
Type B	Neck
Type C	Head

Case 35–11. (From Rüedi TP, Murphy WM [eds]: AO Principles of Fracture Management. Davos, Switzerland, AO Publishing, 2000, p 52.)

turned to this injury, which is limb-threatening. Fractures associated with lacerations are assumed to be open fractures even though the bone may not be protruding through the skin at the time of exam. This patient requires an arteriogram to determine the presence and site of vascular injury to guide the repair, irrigation, and débridement of contaminated and devitalized soft tissue and stabilization of the fracture. At most centers the patient would be taken directly to the operating room (OR), where all these steps would be accomplished. Recurrent trips to the OR for débridement, cleaning, and ultimate soft tissue coverage will be required. This is an open fracture with significant soft tissue compromise as well a vascular injury. The patient should be informed that prolonged and poor healing are likely, and possibly even amputation may result.

35–13, A. Learning objective: *Know the importance of treating shock in head injuries.* The initial priorities of patients with head injury are the same as those without. *A*irway, *B*reathing, and *C*irculation. A comatose patient requires tracheal intubation to ensure an adequate airway. Immediate attention to airway and breathing preserve oxygen supply to the brain. Cerebral perfusion is best maintained by rapid restoration of systolic blood pressure, even if this requires thoracotomy or laparotomy to control life-threatening hemorrhage prior to evaluation of the head.

35–13, B. Learning objective: *Choose the correct diagnostic test for severe head injury.* After vital signs are restored, a rapid neurologic assessment should be performed and the patient taken immediately for head CT scan. A neurosurgeon should be immediately consulted. If the CT scan reveals a mass lesion, immediate craniotomy may be indicated for decompression.

35–13, C. Learning objective: *Be able to provide optimal intensive care to a patient with head injury.* The patient is taken to the ICU for continued resuscitation and cerebral protection maneuvers. Optimum blood pressure is maintained by fluid resuscitation to a normovolemic state. Ventilator therapy is adjusted to ensure an oxygen saturation at 99% to 100% and a Pco_2 around 35. The head of the bed is elevated. Electrolyte, glucose, and coagulation abnormalities are corrected.

35–13, D. Learning objective: *Know the indications for ICP monitoring.* Yes, unless there are contraindications, the neurosurgeon will place a monitor in this patient. ICP monitoring is indicated for all patients with a Glasgow Coma Scale score of 3 to 8 and an abnormal head CT scan (see Table 35–13).

35–13, E. Learning objective: *Respond to increased ICP with appropriate measures.* ICP elevations are treated with intermittent hyperventilation or mannitol infusion. Persistent elevations in ICP should be evaluated by a repeat CT scan to exclude new or blossoming focal lesions. The goal is to consistently maintain a CPP of a least 70 mm Hg. If the patient is adequately fluid resuscitated, blood pressure may be elevated with vasopressors to maintain a CPP of greater than 70.

35–14, A. Learning objective: *Recognize that severely injured patients should be initially evaluated in a rapid and systematic fashion so as to diagnose and treat immediately life-threatening problems.* This patient has sustained significant blunt trauma to the torso after a fall, and although her bloody urine is a dramatic finding, it should not distract the clinician from a rapid assessment of other vital organ systems. A rapid "primary survey" of the patient should first be performed to address problems most likely to cause immediate death or disability; this consists of the five ABCDEs: *A*irway, *B*reathing, *C*irculatory status, neurologic (or *D*isability) function, and full *E*xposure to allow complete viewing of all body surface areas. A compromised airway takes precedence over any other abnormalities and should be immediately secured via endotracheal intubation when possible. Oxygen delivery to the tissues should be maximized by assisting the patient with breathing and addressing thoracic injuries such as tension pneumothorax, flail chest with pulmonary contusion, and sucking chest wound. The circulatory status of the patient must next be evaluated, looking for causes of inadequate intravascular volume such as hemorrhage, neurogenic shock from spinal cord injury, or inadequate cardiac output from heart injury or tamponade. Signs of inadequate perfusion may be subtle, such as delayed capillary refill and confusion, or dramatic, such as hypotension and tachycardia. Adequate intravenous access is mandatory with volume replacement with crystalloid or blood products. Neurologic function as demonstrated by pupil size and reactivity and by Glasgow Coma Scale score should next be determined, since patients with alterations in these components are at high risk for traumatic brain injury. Finally, the patient should be fully exposed by removal of all articles of clothing to allow a complete head-to-toe examination.

35–14, B. Learning objective: *Understand that the history and initial physical examination can assist you in focusing on a specific portion of the urologic system and thus increase your diagnostic yield with respect to tests and procedures.* This patient's gross hematuria establishes the fact that the urologic system has been injured, but which part? Given the history of a fall from a height and the patient's pain and tenderness in the left flank, one may reasonably suspect that the left kidney is involved. Of course, a ruptured bladder may be another etiology of gross hematuria, but our patient's physical examination does not support the diagnosis of pelvic fracture. Thus, diagnostic efforts at delineating urologic injury in this case should be directed toward the upper urologic system. Because this patient is in shock, an emergency exploratory celiotomy is indicated once other sources of hypovolemia have been ruled out (e.g., tension pneumothorax, pelvic fracture, long-bone fracture, spinal cord injury).

35–14, C. Learning objective: *Be aware that other nonurologic organ systems may be injured and may require specific therapy.* Blunt injury to the left kidney is accompanied by splenic laceration with intraperitoneal bleeding, often requiring surgical exploration for control of hemorrhage via splenic repair or splenectomy. Also, it is not uncommon for blunt injuries in this region to result in multiple rib fractures, which may compromise breathing and oxygenation by virtue of the associated pain and possible pneumothorax. Blunt injuries to the right kidney are frequently associated with blunt hepatic lacerations and hematomas, which may bleed massively and require operative intervention even if the injured kidney itself does not. In addition to the solid organs mentioned, penetrating injuries to the kidneys from bullets are even more frequently associated with wounds to the hollow viscera, including the colon, small intestine, duodenum, and stomach. It is for this reason that gunshot wounds to the abdomen with suspicion of intra-abdominal or retroperitoneal violation are almost always immediately explored in the operating room.

35–15, A. Learning objective: *Know that blunt or penetrating trauma to the lower abdomen, pelvis, and perineum is associated with specific injuries of the lower urologic system.* Again, the history and physical examination provide important clues to the most probably locations of injury. This patient's suprapubic pain, combined with the radiographic evidence of a fractured anterior pelvis, places him at high risk for both traumatic urethral and bladder disruptions. Gross hematuria in this case would be an additional clue that the lower urinary tract may have been significantly injured. Subsequent diagnostic maneuvers must be chosen that focus on these specific areas of the urologic system.

35–15, B. Learning objective: *Recognize that a scrotal hematoma is a marker for urethral disruption in the male.* Urethral disruptions may occur at the base of the bladder as a result of severe direct pelvic trauma or over the length of the anterior urethra secondary to fractures of the pubic rami or straddle-type injuries. Signs that should alert you to the possible presence of a urethral injury are perineal or scrotal hematoma or subcutaneous urine, the inability to void urine spontaneously, the presence of gross blood at the urethral meatus, and a high-riding or nonpalpable prostate on digital rectal examination. All of these findings should be sought out in patients with pelvic and perineal injuries during the initial physical examination, and, if present, mandate retrograde contrast urethrography to visualize the urethra and determine its integrity.

35–15, C. Learning objective: *Recognize the contraindications for catheterization of the male urethra after trauma.* No patient suspected of harboring a urethral injury should undergo urethral catheterization until the injury is ruled out. By performing an RUG, the integrity of the urethra can be documented. A normal urethrogram allows safe insertion of the Foley catheter into the bladder without fear of further disrupting a partially torn urethra or misplacing the catheter tip in the perineal soft tissues below the bladder. Should the urethrogram reveal an injury, bladder decompression is best achieved through a percutaneously placed suprapubic cystostomy tube until the injury can be fully evaluated and repaired by a urologic surgeon.

35–16, A. Learning objective: *Know that microscopic hematuria may occur after injury to any portion of the urologic system.* Blood visible only on microscopic examination or "dipstick" testing may originate in the kidneys, ureters, bladder, or urethra. In addition, traumatic bladder catheterizations may produce varying amounts of hematuria in patients with no prior urologic injury as well. The history and physical examination help you narrow your differential diagnosis considerably and thus avoid ordering unnecessary and expensive tests and diagnostic procedures. Also be aware that a first-voided urine specimen is the most likely to contain blood and should be collected preferentially for analysis when hematuria is a concern.

35–16, B. Learning objective: *Understand that kidney injuries can be imaged by various techniques, although not all patients suspected of having renal trauma require specific imaging studies.* This patient's history of blunt trauma to the flanks puts her at higher risk for kidney injury, yet her normal vital signs makes it unlikely that she will require more than just observation and reassurance once the kidneys are imaged and an injury, if present, is diagnosed. In fact, many investigators believe that patients presenting with microscopic hematuria and no evidence of shock rarely require specific imaging studies at all, given their extremely low likelihood of harboring significant urologic injuries. In the stable patient with gross hematuria and physical signs or symptoms of renal injury (flank pain, ecchymosis or tenderness), a CT scan is the imaging study of choice because of its high sensitivity and specificity for upper urologic tract injuries. If a CT scan is not available, an IVP is an acceptable alternative, although it is not as sensitive or specific and can be more difficult to interpret due to overlying intestinal gas.

35–17, A. Learning objective: *The hematoma can be caused by injury to underlying soft tissue, a fracture of the underlying bone, or injury to a vein (nonpulsatile hematoma).* A radiograph of the area determines whether a fracture of the humerus is present. If there is not a fracture, the most likely injury causing the hematoma is bleeding from soft tissue or a vein that is tamponaded.

35–17, B. Learning objective: *Other than the radiograph of the humerus, no diagnostic tests are indicated.* With a normal pulse palpable at the wrist *and* a normal BBI, the likelihood of a significant arterial injury requiring operative repair is extremely low.

35–17, C. Learning objective: *This patient does not need an emergency operation.* If the hematoma is not expanding and is not excessively large, venous bleeding has stopped secondary to local tamponade and normal mechanisms of coagulation. The wound can be gently irrigated and dressed, an injection of tetanus toxoid given, and the patient discharged home with early follow-up.

35–18, A. Learning objective: *A severe blunt injury at the level of the left knee joint that is associated with a cool, pulseless left foot has most likely caused thrombosis or transection of the popliteal artery.* Because both pedal pulses are absent, the injury involves the popliteal artery or both the anterior and posterior tibial arteries. The latter scenario is less likely because of the level of the dislocation.

35–18, B. Learning objective: *The patient does not need any diagnostic tests because there is clearly loss of arterial inflow to the leg and foot from an arterial injury at the level of the dislocation.* There is an urgent need to restore arterial inflow to the ischemic leg and foot, and the patient should be moved to the operating room immediately. For the novice surgeon, a percutaneous surgeon-performed femoral arteriogram with a radiograph delayed 3 to 4 seconds after injection of the contrast agent would confirm that the occlusion or transection is at the level of the knee joint, but this is really not necessary.

35–18, C. Learning objective: *Understand the treatment options.* After preparation of the skin and draping of the area around the knee joint, a 4- to 5-inch-long medial incision overlying the course of the distal superficial femoral artery and the popliteal artery is made. After proximal and distal control around the injured segment of the popliteal artery is obtained, the segment is excised. An autogenous reversed saphenous vein graft removed from the opposite thigh is inserted as an interposition graft to restore arterial inflow to the leg and foot. The suture lines of the graft and distal arterial flow are assessed by an intraoperative popliteal-shank vessel arteriogram. Pressures in the anterior and posterior muscle compartments are measured to see if fasciotomies are needed.

> ▶ **VASCULAR DISEASE**

36–1, A. Learning objective: *Elderly patients with symptoms of back pain need immediate medical attention and should be monitored very closely.* Time is important, and thus the evaluation should be quick but thorough. One must obtain a detailed history of present symptoms (i.e., onset, duration, severity) and relevant past medical history and perform a thorough physical exam, concentrating on abdominal findings (pulsatile mass or tender aneurysm) and lower extremity pulses. Repeat vital signs and close monitoring are extremely important. In addition, electrocardiogram leads, intravenous access, and a Foley catheter should be placed.

36–1, B. Learning objective: *Back pain has many etiologies, including trauma, lumbar disc disease, muscle spasms, kidney stones, and retroperitoneal masses.* In an elderly patient with history of heart and vascular disease, the most important etiology to rule out is aortic aneurysm. Once this is ruled out, other etiologies can be considered and evaluated.

36–1, C. Learning objective: *Understand the work-up of an aortic aneurysm in a stable patient.* In a stable patient who has a symptomatic abdominal aortic aneurysm, after completing the evaluation and notifying the operating room, appropriate lab tests include CBC, prothrombin time, partial thromboplastin time, BUN, creatinine, urinalysis, chest radiograph, and electrocardiogram. Stable patients can be imaged by obtaining an abdominal ultrasound or CT scan of the abdomen and pelvis with IV contrast agent, assuming normal renal function. The CT scan is better and helps (1) evaluate for a leak, (2) exclude inflammatory aneurysms, (3) evaluate iliac arteries, (4) describe the proximal extent of the aneurysm in relation to the renal arteries, and (5) evaluate for venous anomalies. The important point is that ordering tests and imaging should not delay the patient's arrival in the operating room.

36–1, D. Learning objective: *Understand the need for urgent operation.* Symptomatic aortic aneurysms are treated in the operating room immediately. This can be done through either a retroperitoneal or transperitoneal approach. Depending on the patient's anatomy, aortic clamping is either suprarenal or infrarenal. Aneurysm repair entails opening the aneurysm sac after obtaining proximal and distal control and replacing the aorta with a prosthetic graft. In certain centers with vast experience, select symptomatic aortic aneurysms can be treated with endovascular modalities.

36–1, E. Learning objective: *Understand the differences in acuity between a stable and unstable patient.* A hypotensive patient with back pain and a pulsatile mass needs immediate exploration in the operating room. No time should be wasted obtaining lab results or imaging. After notifying the operating room and placing important access lines, the patient should be brought immediately to the operating room for initial resuscitation and operative intervention. Operative mortality is higher than 50% in these cases.

36–2, A. Learning objective: *Patients with asymptomatic carotid bruits are commonly referred to vascular centers.* Important facts to be obtained in the history include any fixed or transient neurologic deficits (motor, speech, vertigo), heart disease history, smoking history, present medications, and any history of amaurosis fugax. Of course, a complete and thorough physical exam are also needed.

36–2, B. Learning objective: *Understand the work-up of a carotid bruit.* In addition to routine blood work and an electrocardiogram, the patient should have a high-quality carotid duplex/ultrasound to evaluate the flow characteristics and percent stenosis in each artery. Angiograms are reserved for recurrent lesions or those in which carotid stenting is a consideration.

36–2, C. Learning objective: *Treatment of carotid artery disease is based on the percent stenosis and the clinical presentation of each patient.* Indications for carotid endarterectomy are (1) asymptomatic, internal carotid artery stenosis greater than 70%, (2) TIA with greater than 50% internal carotid stenosis, and (3) cerebrovascular accident with substantial neurologic recovery and greater than 50% stenosis.

36–3, A. Learning objective: *Know the common postoperative complications of cardiac endarterectomy.* Any patient who has a carotid endarterectomy must be monitored closely for hypertension, hypotension, and neurologic changes. Any acute changes in blood pressure must be medically treated to ensure a stable mean arterial pressure. New neurologic symptoms must be examined and immediately recognized. Once confirmed, the patient should be systemically heparinized and plans to return to the operating room should be in place.

36–3, B. Learning objective: *The patient needs immediate anticoagulation and reoperation.* Aside from heparin, no other orders are required. If time allows, a quick bedside carotid duplex can be performed to document the extent of carotid thrombosis. This is not a requirement and should not delay the return to the operating room.

36–3, C. Learning objective: *The patient should return to the operating room for re-exploration of the carotid artery.* The prior carotid artery repair should be opened and thrombus should be removed. The carotid artery surface should be inspected and the distal end point should be carefully evaluated. Most carotid thromboses in the early postoperative period are due to technical complications.

36–4, A. Learning objective: *Understand the common etiologies of leg pain.* Isolated leg pain with swelling has multiple etiologies including trauma, infection, heart failure, and venous occlusions. Full evaluation includes complete history of the event, risk factor assessment, previous hematologic history, and thorough physical exam looking for Homans' sign and phlegmasia cerulea dolens.

36–4, B. Learning objective: *Understand the initial work-up of leg pain.* Important tests to order are a hypercoagulable panel as described in the chapter and a lower extremity venous duplex ultrasound.

36–4, C. Learning objective: *Be able to strategize patients by risk factors.* Risk factors for venous thrombosis are patient specific.

The common risk factors include age older than 40 years, immobilization, malignancy, obesity, pregnancy, abdominal distention, and hypercoagulable states.

36–4, D. Learning objective: *Know the treatment options for DVT.* Acute DVTs of the lower extremity should be treated with the appropriate anticoagulation regimen whether it be unfractionated heparin, LMWH, or warfarin (Coumadin). Close monitoring is needed for abnormal bleeding and other complications of anticoagulation treatment.

36–5, A. Learning objective: *Recognize that peripheral arterial occlusive disease is a differential diagnosis in patients presenting with foot pain and nonhealing ulcers.* The evaluation should start with a thorough history and physical exam, with particular attention paid to risk factors for atherosclerotic disease and physical stigmata of atherosclerosis. Characteristics of the foot pain and factors that alleviate or worsen the pain should also be investigated. Ischemic rest pain usually manifests as a severe, burning pain located at the metatarsal heads. The patient may report some degree of pain relief with dangling of the foot. The foot ulcers should be thoroughly examined for evidence of infection.

36–5, B. Learning objective: *An ABI should be performed at the bedside.* If arterial occlusive disease is the etiology, this patient's ABI should be less than 0.5 unless his arteries are noncompressible due to diabetes mellitus. Baseline renal function test should be obtained, especially since this patient would likely require a radiologic test such as an angiogram prior to revascularization. A baseline complete blood count should also be obtained. If his creatinine level is normal, aortography with distal run-offs is the diagnostic test of choice to guide revascularization.

36–5, C. Learning objective: *The patient should be admitted for surgical intervention.* An antibiotic should be started if there is evidence of infection. Preangiogram and postangiogram hydration is important to prevent contrast-induced renal failure. His treatment option depends on the angiographic findings. With rest pain and nonhealing ulcers, this patient likely has multilevel disease and more than likely would require infrapopliteal bypass, with autogenous vein being the conduit of choice.

36–6, A. Learning objective: *The patient is in urgent need of dialysis; therefore, a central venous catheter should be placed.* A tunneled, cuffed central venous catheter should be placed via an internal jugular vein. (The right internal jugular usually provides easier catheter placement.) Subclavian veins should not be cannulated because of the high incidence of late stenosis and thrombosis. His renal failure is potentially reversible, but several weeks of dialysis may be needed before renal function returns. An uncuffed catheter is not likely to function that long but might be used for a few days if the patient is not stable enough to go to the operating room for placement of a tunneled, cuffed catheter. Only if renal function does not return after 6 to 8 weeks should an autologous fistula be created. A graft should never be placed if a fistula is possible. Forearm veins should not be used for venipunctures (blood draws, infusions) but preserved for possible future access procedures.

36–7, A. Learning objective: *The patient is in urgent need of dialysis; therefore a central venous catheter should be placed.* *A tunneled, cuffed central venous catheter should be placed via an internal jugular vein, and an autologous fistula should be created at the wrist. All other things being equal, the nondominant arm is preferred so as to allow the patient use of his dominant arm during dialysis.* His renal failure is not reversible; therefore, a tunneled, cuffed catheter is chosen to allow time for an autologous fistula, the preferred type of long-term access, to mature. As noted in 36–6, A, an uncuffed catheter might be used temporarily until the patient is stable enough to undergo the more extensive operative procedures.

36–8, A. Learning objective: *Autologous fistulas are the optimal type of long-term access but require 6 to 8 weeks to mature before they are usable.* *An autologous fistula should be created at the wrist in the patient's nondominant hand.* This type of fistula should ideally be created 2 to 3 months before it will be needed. The rate at which renal function deteriorates, however, is not the same for all patients; the nephrologists must make an educated guess as to when hemodialysis will need to be started. Fistulas generally enlarge and improve with time. Even if dialysis is not needed as soon as predicted, the patient will be well served by having a fistula created several months in advance. A central venous catheter would be needed only if the patient's condition deteriorated and she required hemodialysis before her fistula was useable.

36–9, A. Learning objective: *An autologous fistula is not possible.* *No access procedure should be performed for this patient at this time.* All prosthetic arteriovenous grafts deteriorate over time. Unlike autologous fistulas, they should not be created too long before dialysis is needed. They will be ready for use after 10 to 14 days. Central venous catheters are usually not needed and certainly would not be placed in this patient at this time because immediate dialysis is not indicated.

PRACTICE **EXAMINATION**

1. A 58-year-old alcoholic man has had several admissions for acute and chronic pancreatitis. He presents with progressive inability to eat, vomiting, abdominal discomfort, and a large palpable mass in the center of his epigastric region. What would be a reasonable first approach to diagnosis?

   A. No diagnosis is necessary because the disease process is benign. Simply reassure the patient.

   B. Emergency exploratory laparotomy

   C. CT scan or ultrasound

   D. Serum CEA and CA19-9

2. History and physical exam have not narrowed the differential diagnosis down for a 25-year-old man with a mass in his retroperitoneum. CT scan is only marginally helpful, and FNA was nondiagnostic. What is your next step?

   A. Perform exploratory laparoscopy with biopsies for tissue diagnosis.

   B. Treat presumptively for lymphoma, because that is the most common cause of nondiagnostic FNAs.

   C. Order an MRI and lymphangiogram.

   D. Observe the patient until the mass is large enough to be defined by CT scan.

3. A 72-year-old man with longstanding hypertension presents with a large pulsatile mass in his mid abdomen. He is not in pain but has noted that occasionally his toes develop blue spots that are tender to touch. Which of the following is *not* appropriate in the work-up of this mass?

   A. Ultrasound of the abdomen

   B. FNA of the mass

   C. CT scan of the abdomen with IV contrast

   D. Arterial angiography

4. A 56-year-old man presents with a 1-day history of abdominal distention, crampy abdominal pain, and obstipation. A diagnosis of small bowel obstruction is made on a KUB film. What are the three most likely etiologies of the obstruction?

   A. Crohn's disease, volvulus, adhesions

   B. Diverticulitis, hernias, radiation enteritis

   C. Adhesions, hernias, tumors

   D. Gallstone ileus, Crohn's disease, foreign body

   E. Adhesions, hernias, volvulus

5. A 78-year-old man comes to the emergency department with fever, abdominal distention, and pain. Which of the following findings help distinguish ileus from bowel obstruction?

   A. Rushes and tinkles on abdominal auscultation

   B. Air-fluid levels on KUB

   C. Fever

   D. Vomiting

   E. All of the above

6. A 32-year-old woman describes a 1-week history of progressively worsening lower abdominal distention and vague discomfort. She had an appendectomy as a child. Examination reveals localized lower abdominal distention that is rather dull to percussion. Which one of the following is the least likely cause for her problem?

   A. Closed-loop small bowel obstruction

   B. Cystadenoma of the ovary

   C. Ascites due to cirrhosis

   D. Retroperitoneal liposarcoma

   E. Pregnancy

7. A 21-year-old woman presents to the urgent care department with a 12-hour history of abdominal pain. She complains of pain in her right flank that radiates to her right groin. She states that her urine has looked "pink." She is afebrile and states that she has had similar pain on two prior occasions. Based on this history alone, the next steps would best include

   A. Reassurance and anticipatory care

   B. Treatment of her pain, urinalysis, and CT scan of her abdomen with IV contrast agent

   C. Treatment of her pain, full chemistry panel, amylase, lipase, urinalysis, liver function tests, serum pregnancy test, CT scan of her abdomen and pelvis, ultrasound of her right upper quadrant, and mesenteric angiogram

   D. Urgent exploratory laparotomy

8. Particular care should be taken when evaluating patients with abdominal pain and the following other condition(s)

   A. Extreme age

   B. History of spinal cord injury

   C. Chronic steroid use

   D. Undergoing chemotherapy

   E. All of the above

9. Tachycardia is a frequent associated symptom of abdominal pain. Which of the following is *not* a cause of tachycardia?

   A. Severe pain

   B. Anxiety

   C. Normal intravascular fluid volume

   D. Fever

   E. Cardiac dysrhythmia

10. Of the following, which would be an indication to *not* consider operative therapy?

    A. Abdominal pain associated with hypotension

    B. Complete bowel obstruction

    C. Evidence of bowel perforation on radiographic studies

    D. Comorbidities that would make surgical therapy more risky than the disease process itself

    E. Not knowing the etiology of the abdominal pain

11. Which of the following accurately characterizes a fibroadenoma?

    A. Irregular borders on ultrasound, with internal calcifications

    B. More commonly seen in older perimenopausal or postmenopausal women

    C. Is considered a precancerous lesion

    D. Is firm with smooth borders on physical exam

12. A 20-year-old patient presents with a painful breast mass. You aspirate the mass and remove 15 mL of clear yellow fluid and the mass completely resolves. Which of the following is true about cysts?

    A. Cysts cannot be seen on mammogram or ultrasound.

    B. Cysts are not associated with an increased cancer risk.

    C. Cysts are uncommon causes of a breast mass in women who have never breast-fed.

    D. Cysts that return should not be reevaluated.

13. Needle biopsies

    A. Are rarely helpful in the evaluation of breast masses

    B. May be used to replace surgical biopsy

    C. Should not be used when there is a high clinical suspicion for malignancy

    D. Can yield false-negative results due to sampling error

14. A 20-year-old man presents with 3 days of fevers, chills, nausea, vomiting, and diarrhea. Symptoms began with nausea, and he has protracted vomiting with some flecks of blood. He does feel light-headed on standing and almost passed out this morning. The diarrhea is green and loose and occurs at least every other hour. He denies any other significant past history and states that he does not remember anyone else eating the same food that he ate. On arrival, his blood pressure lying down was 109/40 mm Hg, heart rate was 114 beats/min, respiratory rate 24 breaths/min, and temperature is 101.5°F. Stool is green and guaiac positive. Emesis is bilious and has flecks of blood. The most likely etiology of this patient's acute illness is

   A. Gastric ulcer
   B. Ulcerative colitis
   C. Viral gastroenteritis
   D. *Staphylococcus aureus*
   E. *Giardia*

15. The proper plan of management of patient in question 14 includes all of the following *except*

   A. Intravenous hydration
   B. Checking stools for fecal leukocytes
   C. Lomotil to control diarrhea
   D. Complete blood count and SMA 7
   E. Stool cultures

16. A 60-year-old man presents in the office with a history of recent change in bowel habit to loose stools for 6 months associated with history of rectal bleeding for 4 months. He had lost 10 lb in the last 6 weeks. His family history was significant for father dying of colon cancer at 40 years of age. His hemoglobin was 9.1 with hematocrit of 25. He was hemodynamically stable. The most appropriate initial step in making a diagnosis will be to arrange for

   A. Barium enema
   B. Stool analysis for ova and parasites
   C. Stool for culture and sensitivity
   D. Colonoscopy with biopsy
   E. Blood transfusion

17. The most sensitive radiographic exam to evaluate for free intraperitoneal air is

   A. Abdominal CT
   B. "Three-way" of the abdomen

C. Upper and lower GI series

D. Upright chest radiograph

18. Which cause of free intraperitoneal air always requires surgical intervention?

   A. Perforated duodenal ulcer

   B. Perforated sigmoid diverticulitis

   C. Stab wound to the abdomen

   D. 3 days post–laparoscopic cholecystectomy

19. A 75-year-old man recently was discharged from the hospital following a myocardial infarction. He returns to the emergency department complaining of upper abdominal pain. He has mid-epigastric tenderness to palpation but no guarding or rebound tenderness. His bowel sounds are normal. An upright chest radiograph demonstrates a small amount of free intraperitoneal air beneath the right hemidiaphragm. How would you manage this patient?

   A. Tell him not to worry, because he does not have signs of peritonitis.

   B. Prepare him immediately for exploratory laparotomy.

   C. Make him DNR and admit him to the hospital for comfort care.

   D. Institute IV fluid resuscitation and nasogastric suction and admit him for observation and serial abdominal exams.

20. The most common cause of significant acute blood loss in a 15-year-old boy is

   A. Gastric varices

   B. Peptic ulcer disease

   C. Hemorrhoids

   D. Juvenile polyps

21. Patients with cirrhosis and portal hypertension often bleed from

   A. Gastroesophageal varices

   B. Mallory-Weiss tear

   C. Peptic ulcer disease

   D. Congestive gastropathy

   E. All of the above

22. A 60-year-old woman has melena and anemia. Early treatment priorities include
    A. Operative intervention
    B. Correction of anemia and colonoscopy
    C. Angiography
    D. Bleeding scan

23. Mortality related to massive hemoptysis is secondary to
    A. Myocardial infarction secondary to blood loss
    B. Exsanguination
    C. Inability to ventilate
    D. Cancer spread

24. Important treatment steps include all of the following *except*
    A. Emergent surgery
    B. Type and cross match
    C. Chest radiograph
    D. Bronchoscopy

25. Causes of hemoptysis include all of the following *except*
    A. Tuberculosis
    B. Swan-Ganz catheter
    C. Lung abscess
    D. Myocardial infarction

26. A 65-year-old man with COPD and BPH presents to the emergency department with a painful mass in his right groin that he noticed 12 hours earlier. The mass is located above the inguinal ligament and along its medial aspect and cannot be reduced. His abdomen is mildly distended and his temperature is 100.5°F. What is the next most appropriate step?
    A. Ultrasound of groin
    B. Aspirate the mass for Gram stain and culture
    C. Immediate surgical exploration
    D. CT scan of abdomen
    E. Admit for observation

27. A 15-year-old boy presents with acute scrotal swelling and pain. Which of the following findings would suggest testicular torsion?
    A. Anteriorly located epididymis
    B. Posteriorly located epididymis

   C. Low-lying, vertically oriented testicle

   D. A blue dot sign

   E. Alleviation of the pain with elevation of the scrotum

28. Which of the following is (are) typically nonpainful?

   A. Varicocele

   B. Hydrocele

   C. Undescended testicle

   D. Testicular tumor

   E. All of the above

29. A 70-year-old man presents with a 6-week history of increasing jaundice, anorexia, weight loss, and clay-colored stools. He reports no abdominal pain. On physical examination, there is a deep scleral icterus, temporal wasting, and a palpable right upper quadrant abdominal mass. Laboratory studies indicate a total bilirubin of 12.3 mg/dL, conjugated bilirubin of 11.1 mg/dL, alkaline phosphatase of 698 IU/L, ALT of 49 IU/L, and albumin of 2.9 g/dL. What is the most likely diagnosis?

   A. Choledocholithiasis

   B. Cholecystitis

   C. Pancreatic or biliary cancer

   D. Acute viral hepatitis

30. All of the following conditions are associated with unconjugated hyperbilirubinemia, *except*

   A. Neonatal jaundice

   B. Gilbert's syndrome

   C. Hereditary spherocytosis

   D. Rotor's syndrome

31. A 38-year-old woman underwent laparoscopic cholecystectomy for symptomatic cholelithiasis 8 months earlier. She now presents with recurrent episodes of right upper quadrant pain and jaundice. Ultrasound examination reveals a dilated common bile duct of 1.1 cm. The next procedure of choice is

   A. Liver biopsy

   B. Laparotomy with common bile duct exploration and stone extraction

   C. Percutaneous transhepatic cholangiography

   D. Endoscopic retrograde cholangiopancreatography (ERCP) with stone extraction

32. Which of the following is *not* a cause of leg pain?
    A. Deep venous thrombosis
    B. Compression of the neurospinal canal
    C. Infection
    D. Peripheral vascular disease
    E. Hyperkalemia and hypercalcemia

33. Buerger's disease is highly related to
    A. Cholesterol level
    B. Blood pressure
    C. Female sex
    D. Tobacco use
    E. Inactivity

34. A 22-year-old man presents to your clinic with a 3-day history of a tender lump in his neck. Last week he had the flu and now feels fine. On exam he has a 2-cm, slightly tender mass anterior to the left sternocleidomastoid muscle. All of the following are true *except*
    A. Complete blood count, Monospot, and chest radiograph would be the initial studies.
    B. Benign etiologies are more likely than malignancy.
    C. A period of short observation can be undertaken.
    D. Immediate excisional biopsy should be done.

35. Factors that warrant biopsy in lymphadenopathy include
    A. Smoking or tobacco use
    B. Age >50 years
    C. Lymph nodes >1.5 cm
    D. Associated constitutional symptoms
    E. All of the above

36. A 48-year-old woman presents with a complaint of a left axillary node. On exam she has a firm 1.5-cm node in the axilla. Additional nodes are found in the right axilla and cervical and inguinal regions. Important parts of the work-up include
    A. Presence of breast masses
    B. Associated constitutional symptoms
    C. HIV risk factors
    D. Chest radiograph
    E. All of the above

37. Hypoglycemia should be excluded as a cause of stupor in a diabetic patient by

    A. Drawing a panel of blood tests for the lab, including glucose, and giving graded glucose supplementation, depending on the serum level of glucose

    B. Ordering a fasting glucose tolerance test to be performed the next morning

    C. Giving potassium as needed to restore the serum level to normal

    D. Either infusing an intravenous glucose solution or performing an immediate bedside glucose test and acting immediately on the results

38. In a febrile adult recovering from meningioma resection, with suspected meningitis as a cause of lethargy, a lumbar puncture should be performed

    A. As the first step in the evaluation

    B. After the CBC, electrolytes, and drug screen have excluded other causes

    C. After the intraventricular drain has been irrigated

    D. After an examination has excluded papilledema or a CT has excluded increased intracranial pressure as a cause of lethargy

39. Which of the following are indicated in the management of delirium tremens (alcohol withdrawal)?

    A. Aggressive intravenous fluid replacement

    B. Sedation with benzodiazepines

    C. Multivitamins, thiamine, and folate

    D. All of the above

40. What is the most common cause of small bowel obstruction in North America?

    A. Hernia

    B. Postoperative adhesions

    C. Ulcerative colitis

    D. Small bowel malignancy

41. What is the most common electrolyte abnormality seen after prolonged vomiting?

    A. Hypermagnesemia

    B. Hypophosphatemia

    C. Metabolic acidosis

    D. Hypokalemia

42. What class of therapeutic agent is *not* commonly associated with nausea and vomiting in the postoperative patient?

    A. Proton pump inhibitors

    B. Narcotics

    C. Oral antibiotics

    D. General anesthetic agents

43. Neck masses can be caused by which of the following?

    A. Lymphadenopathy

    B. Thyroid mass

    C. Salivary gland tumor

    D. All of the above

44. Fine-needle aspiration would be appropriate for all of the following neck masses *except*

    A. Lymphadenopathy

    B. Salivary masses

    C. Hemangioma

    D. Thyroid mass

45. The most common etiology of midline neck masses is

    A. Lymphadenopathy

    B. Congenital

    C. Salivary

    D. Thyroid

46. Medications usually cause nipple discharge by

    A. Restoring serotonin levels

    B. Causing gynecomastia

    C. Increasing serum prolactin levels

    D. Mimicking pregnancy

47. Which of the following is a true statement?

    A. Bloody nipple discharge is always red.

    B. Discharge from multiple ducts is associated with a higher rate of malignancy.

    C. Ductography alone can sometimes distinguish between benign and malignant causes of nipple discharge.

    D. Paget's disease of the breast presents with erosions of the areola.

48. Intraductal papillomas are

    A. Found only in women
    B. Malignant and should be completely excised
    C. Are occasionally associated with malignant transformation
    D. Decreased by breast-feeding

49. A 72-year-old man in the intensive care unit who had undergone a left hepatic lobectomy has been diagnosed with a severe coagulopathy and given aggressive resuscitation with blood products and crystalloid fluid. Postresuscitation laboratory studies reveal the following: hematocrit 28%, aPTT 36 seconds, PT 15 seconds, platelet count 98,000/mm³ and fibrinogen 73 mg/dL. Which of the following would be most indicated to help maintain hemostatic mechanisms?

    A. Fresh frozen plasma
    B. Whole blood
    C. Protamine
    D. Cryoprecipitate
    E. Platelets

50. A 78-year-old woman diagnosed with a pancreatic head mass is being evaluated for a pancreaticoduodenectomy (Whipple procedure). She has a history of type 2 diabetes mellitus, a 90 pack-year smoking history, and reported heavy alcohol use for many years. She now smokes only one pack per week and quit drinking alcohol 1 year ago. She has no significant family history and denies any bleeding tendencies. On physical examination you find a thin woman with mildly icteric sclera and several spider angiomata on her chest wall. Aside from coarse breath sounds, her exam is otherwise unremarkable. Which of the following laboratory studies should be included as part of her preoperative work-up?

    A. Fibrinogen level
    B. Prothrombin time
    C. Bleeding time
    D. Factor IX level
    E. aPTT inhibitor study

51. A 54-year-old man is 3 hours out from an abdominal aortic aneurysm repair. During your postoperative rounds you find him to be tachycardic with a heart rate of 122 beats/min. His other vital signs reveal a blood pressure of 92/48 mm Hg, respiratory rate of 36 breaths/min, oxygen saturation of 91% on 6 L/min of O_2 per nasal cannula. His central venous pressure is 2 mm Hg, and his urine output for the past hour has been 12 mL.

Over the past 40 minutes his operative drains have put out more than 600 mL of blood. His CBC sent STAT 15 minutes earlier demonstrated a hematocrit of 31.2%, white blood cell count of 16,300/mm³, and platelets of 112,000/mm³. His INR and aPTT sent at the same time were 1.4 and 44 seconds, respectively. You suspect he has an acute bleed from his anastomosis. Which of the following was least useful in making this determination?

A. Urine output

B. Heart rate

C. Drain output

D. CBC

E. CVP

52. At night the nurse calls you to report that a patient who had had a colon resection earlier that morning has a fever of 102°F. The appropriate first management step is

A. Order acetaminophen and ice packs.

B. Order blood cultures and a chest radiograph.

C. Examine the patient.

D. Obtain a stat CT of the abdomen.

53. A patient who is postoperative day 4 after a stomach resection has a temperature of 101.5°F. All of the following are appropriate management steps *except*

A. Obtain a urinalysis and culture.

B. Examine all IV sites.

C. Order a chest radiograph.

D. Open the surgical incision.

54. On the first postoperative night the nurse calls you to inform you that a patient who had just undergone a mastectomy has a fever of 101.5°F. You examine the patient and find no causes of the fever. The most likely cause of the temperature is

A. Urinary tract infection

B. Atelectasis

C. Pneumonia

D. Wound infection

55. The primary defect in hypovolemic shock is

A. Decreased intravascular volume

B. Tachycardia

C. Low hemoglobin

D. Increased stroke volume

E. Increased extraction

56. The first step in treating hypovolemic shock is

   A. Transfusion

   B. Crystalloid infusion

   C. Normal saline infusion

   D. Ringer's lactate infusion

   E. Ensuring adequate airway

57. In septic shock, the defects include all the following *except*

   A. Decreased maximal O_2 extraction

   B. Decreased O_2 extraction

   C. Hypovolemia

   D. Decreased contractility

   E. Increased afterload

58. A 75-year-old man with diabetes is 2 days out from a right hemicolectomy for adenocarcinoma. His respiratory rate is 35 breaths/min, heart rate is 132 beats/min, and blood pressure is 150/90 mm Hg. He complains that he "can't catch his breath." *Immediate* actions include all of the following *except*

   A. Supplementary oxygen by face mask

   B. Transfer to the intensive care unit

   C. Placement of a central venous catheter

   D. Measurement of atrial oxygen (ABG or pulse oximetry)

   E. Preparation for intubation

59. A 50-year-old woman with recently diagnosed ovarian cancer presents to your clinic with shortness of breath and pleuritic chest pain. Her respiratory rate is 22 breaths/min and her Sao_2 is 93%. After administering supplementary oxygen, appropriate tests include all BUT the following

   A. Arterial blood gas

   B. Electrocardiogram

   C. Chest radiograph

   D. $\dot{V}/\dot{Q}$ scan

   E. Bedside spirometry

60. A 29-year-old man admitted on the medicine service for endocarditis secondary to IV drug abuse suddenly develops acute SOB. His respiratory rate is 34 breaths/min and the Sao_2 is 85%, and he is sitting upright complaining that he "cannot breathe." What should be *immediately* done for this patient?

    A. Transthoracic echocardiogram
    B. Electrocardiogram
    C. Supplementary oxygen administration
    D. Arterial blood gas
    E. Anticoagulation with heparin

61. You receive a call from the pediatric ICU nurse that the urine output of your 2-year-old (10-kg) patient who is several hours postappendectomy for severe perforated appendicitis was 5 mL for the last hour. What is the best course?

    A. Carefully clinically assess the patient's fluid status on morning rounds, and if the patient is dehydrated, bolus judiciously with 100 mL of normal saline.
    B. Ask the nurse to send blood and serum electrolytes and begin a 24-hour creatinine clearance test. You will see the patient immediately after the electrolytes are back.
    C. Ask the nurse to begin an IV bolus of 200 mL (20 mL/kg) and to irrigate the Foley bladder catheter while you are coming to evaluate the patient.
    D. Ask the nurse to give 5 mg of furosemide (Lasix).

62. An example of a contaminated wound in surgery is

    A. Elective laparoscopic cholecystectomy
    B. Inguinal hernia
    C. Splenectomy
    D. Perforated appendicitis

63. A patient has a warm and tender incision 6 days after colon surgery. The most appropriate step is

    A. Administer intravenous antibiotic.
    B. Return the patient to the operating room.
    C. Open the wound at the bedside.
    D. Swab the wound with povidone-iodine (Betadine).

64. A patient comes to the emergency department with a hedge trimmer cut to the forearm that occurred 8 hours earlier. There is only skin involvement. Appropriate treatment includes all of the following *except*

A. Wound closure with nylon

B. Irrigation of defect

C. Tetanus shot

D. Débridement of foreign material

65. A 35-year-old man presents with a 4-month history of a painful right groin swelling. It is easily reducible, and he has no symptoms of nausea or vomiting. He is otherwise healthy and has never had surgery before. What would you recommend?

A. Observation and reassurance

B. Open primary repair without mesh

C. Open repair with synthetic mesh

D. Bilateral laparoscopic repair

66. A 62-year-old woman had open cholecystectomy 10 years ago. She has complained for several months of a bulge at her incision site. This has been nontender and readily reducible, but it is unsightly. Over the last few days the bulge has increased in tenderness and she is unable to reduce it. She is nauseated, tachycardic, and running a low-grade fever. What would you recommend?

A. Observation and reassurance

B. Make a greater effort to reduce the hernia with increased pressure (using sedation or pain medicine if needed)

C. Schedule an elective laparoscopic hernia repair for next week

D. Arrange an urgent operation to explore the hernia

67. Which of the following is *not* a contraindication to breast-conserving therapy?

A. Diffuse indeterminate or malignant-appearing calcifications

B. Multifocal DCIS in addition to an invasive cancer

C. An invasive ductal carcinoma measuring 3 cm

D. Prior radiation therapy to the involved breast

68. Which of the following patients has the highest risk stratification for breast cancer?

A. A 30-year-old patient with fibrocystic disease, and a third cousin who has unilateral postmenopausal breast cancer

B. A 65-year-old nulliparous woman who smokes a pack per day and has a sister who contracted breast cancer at 35 years of age with a history of LCIS in the contralateral breast

C. A 20-year-old woman, whose mother died of breast cancer when she was 12 years old, with a painful breast mass and bilateral nipple discharge

D. A 70-year-old woman whose aunt was recently diagnosed with DCIS at 92 years of age

69. Which of the following is *not* a risk factor associated with recurrence of breast cancer after treatment?

A. Breast-conservation therapy

B. Estrogen- and progesterone-receptor–negative tumor

C. Her 2-neu–positive tumor

D. Lymph-vascular invasion

70. A 60-year-old male smoker presents with complaints of right shoulder pain, tingling paresthesias of the right upper extremity, and blurred vision. Physical exam reveals asymmetrical pupils with a right-sided ptosis, clavicular adenopathy, and right upper extremity sensory loss. What lung cancer syndrome is this?

A. Superior vena cava syndrome

B. Horner's syndrome

C. Pancoast's syndrome

D. Cerebellar ataxia syndrome

71. A 53-year-old woman presented 6 weeks ago with fever, productive cough, and a right lower lobe infiltrate. Antibiotic therapy initially improved her symptoms. She returns now complaining of continued cough, fever, and new abdominal pain. Laboratory tests are remarkable for an elevated AST and a mild anemia. Further work-up reveals a non–small cell lung cancer. An abdominal CT reveals hepatic and adrenal lesions. What is her most likely clinical stage at diagnosis?

A. IIA

B. IIB

C. IIIB

D. IV

72. A 45-year-old male smoker presents to you for possible resection of a pulmonary nodule. While taking the history, the patient admits to a 15-kg weight gain in the last 3 months and persistent fatigue. Physical exam reveals a moon-faced, obese male with ecchymoses over his forearms and striae across his abdomen. What is the most likely type of lung cancer that he has?

A. Small cell carcinoma

B. Adenocarcinoma

C. Squamous cell carcinoma

D. Large cell carcinoma

73. A 65-year-old man returns to your clinic for follow-up 4 weeks after discharge from a hospitalization for a COPD exacerbation. The patient has finished a tapering course of steroids and a 2-week course of antibiotics. He reports that he feels well and his sputum production and exercise tolerance have returned to his baseline. He received the pneumococcal vaccine 2 years ago at the time of his COPD diagnosis. What preventive therapy do you recommend at this time?

    A. Pneumococcal vaccine

    B. Pseudomonal vaccine

    C. Influenza vaccine

    D. *Haemophilus influenzae* type B vaccine

74. A 38-year-old man with a smoking history presents to your office with a 6-month history of slowly progressive dyspnea on exertion. Physical exam reveals a barrel-chested man with a prolonged expiratory phase and scattered wheezes on chest auscultation. Chest radiograph and PFTs are consistent with a diagnosis of COPD. What test do you order next?

    A. α_1-Antitrypsin concentration

    B. High-resolution CT of the chest

    C. Polysomnography

    D. Carbon monoxide diffusing capacity (DLCO)

75. A 70-year-old man with a history of severe COPD comes to you with complaints of night-time insomnia and anxiety. His current medications include albuterol, ipratropium (Atrovent), prednisone, and theophylline, and they have been stable for several weeks. Physical exam reveals a resting pulse of 90 beats/min and a fine tremor in his outstretched hands. What test do you order next?

    A. Thyroid function tests

    B. Fingerstick blood glucose

    C. Theophylline level

    D. Electrocardiogram

76. A 26-year-old woman presents to the emergency department with an "asthma attack." She reports 1 day of worsening shortness of breath, wheezing, and cough. On physical exam, she is tachypneic with a respiratory rate of 26 breaths/min and tachycardic with a heart rate of 115 beats/min. She appears moderately distressed and has some accessory muscle use with respiration. Chest auscultation elicits diffuse wheezing without rhonchi. A reasonable first step would be

    A. Ask her about any triggers that may have started this "attack."

    B. Have her perform a peak flow test now.

    C. Order 125 mg of IV methylprednisolone (Solu-Medrol) to be given now.

    D. Ask for assistance and prepare for urgent intubation.

77. A 69-year-old asthmatic woman comes to you for preoperative evaluation. She wishes to have an elective artificial hip replacement. She states that her arthritic hip and not her asthma limits her activities. She has not had an asthma exacerbation for more than a year and she reports that her PEFR has remained at 450 L/min (85% of predicted) during that time. Her medications include an albuterol metered-dose inhaler that she has not used this month and an inhaled steroid preparation that she uses daily. On physical exam, she appears well and in no distress. Chest exam is normal, and auscultation elicits wheezing only on forced expiration. What is the most appropriate preoperative recommendation?

    A. No pulmonary function tests before surgery

    B. Spirometry before surgery

    C. No elective surgery should be done

    D. Spirometry and ABG before surgery

    E. Spirometry before and after surgery and bronchodilator therapy before surgery

78. A 42-year-old woman is referred to your pulmonary office for preoperative evaluation for an elective ventral hernia repair. The patient's history is remarkable for a long history of moderate, persistent asthma. She has had four or five admissions for asthma and one intubation in the last 10 years. She recognizes several triggers of her asthma symptoms including cold air, cats, and seasonal pollens. She tells you that the last couple of weeks have been particularly bad for her asthma because she has had daily symptoms and has used extra albuterol to control her symptoms. Other than the albuterol, her medications include an inhaled steroid preparation and salmeterol. During the springtime, she also takes an antihistamine medication and a nasal steroid for her seasonal allergies. Her physical exam is remarkable for a heart rate of 102 beats/min and for diffuse wheezing with a prolonged expiratory phase on chest auscultation. A chest radiograph obtained at the time of her visit shows hyperinflated lung fields but no infiltrates. What do you recommend to your surgical colleagues and to the patient?

    A. Proceed with her surgery after obtaining pulmonary function tests to assess the adequacy of her FEV_1.

B. Proceed with surgery and be extra vigilant in having the patient perform postoperative pulmonary toilet.

C. Do not consider this elective surgery at all; the patient's asthma is too severe for her to have an uncomplicated course.

D. Postpone this elective surgery and intensify the patient's medical regimen to better control her symptoms at this time.

79. An 18-year-old woman presents to the emergency department with a 1-day history of shortness of breath. She notices that she now has difficulty walking from her bedroom to the bathroom without feeling faint and panting for breath. She is an exchange student who recently flew to the United States from England to begin school. She is otherwise healthy and her only medications are oral contraceptive pills. On physical exam, her heart rate is 110 beats/min, her blood pressure is 95/42 mm Hg, and her respiratory rate is 24 breaths/min. On pulse oximetry her oxygen saturation is 92% on 4 L of O_2 via nasal cannula. Other than her tachypnea and tachycardia, her physical exam is unremarkable. Her chest radiograph shows no apparent disease and her ABG reveals a pH of 7.46, Pco_2 of 32, and a Po_2 of 64 on 4 L of O_2 via nasal cannula. What is the appropriate next step?

A. Order a CT angiogram of the chest to rule out PE.

B. Order ventilation/perfusion scintigraphy to rule out PE.

C. Bolus with IV heparin based on the patient's weight and then titrate a heparin drip to keep the PTT between 60 and 80 seconds.

D. Order an echocardiogram to evaluate for right ventricular strain.

80. The patient in question 79 is eventually taken to the CT scanner for a CT angiogram of her chest. This test reveals a heavy clot burden in bilateral pulmonary artery distributions but no signs of thrombus in the veins of her legs. An echocardiogram reveals right ventricular dilation with markedly elevated estimated pulmonary artery pressures. Despite these findings, the patient remains comfortable and alert with oxygen therapy, with tachycardia and mild hypotension as the only signs of her massive pulmonary embolus. What step would you take next?

A. Administer systemic thrombolytic therapy after admitting the patient to an ICU.

B. Start heparin anticoagulation and admit the patient to the ICU.

C. Start heparin anticoagulation, begin overlap therapy with warfarin, and admit the patient to the ICU.

D. Call the cardiothoracic surgeon for an urgent evaluation for embolectomy.

81. You are called to see a 66-year-old man with a recently diagnosed colon cancer. The patient is hospitalized for a lower GI bleed thought to be attributable to his colon cancer. The patient is feeling better today after receiving 2 units of packed red blood cells for his GI bleed, but he noticed that his right leg is swollen compared to his left. He also notes pain in his calf with ambulation. He would like a pain medication for his calf discomfort. His vital signs are stable and without abnormality and his oxygen saturation is 99% on room air. You order an ultrasound of his right leg, and the results confirm your suspicion that he has a DVT in that leg. What do you do next?

   A. Start aspirin therapy for partial anticoagulation and monitor his hematocrit closely.

   B. Start a heparin drip without an initial bolus to minimize the patient's risk of further GI bleeding as you treat his DVT.

   C. Give a heparin bolus based on the patient's weight and then titrate a heparin drip to a PTT of 60 to 80 seconds while closely monitoring his hematocrit.

   D. Call Interventional Radiology and have the patient evaluated for an inferior vena cava filter device.

82. You are called to see a healthy 60-year-old man admitted today from home in anticipation of his radical prostatectomy for prostate cancer. The patient reports that he has had a 3-day history of productive cough, fever, and malaise. He attributes it to a cold that he caught from his wife. He would like some cough syrup and a sleeping pill. You review his vital sign log and examine him. He has a low-grade temperature but otherwise has normal vital signs. He appears flushed and mildly diaphoretic but otherwise well. He coughs through your attempt to auscultate his chest, but you think you hear rales in his right lower lung field. A chest radiograph confirms your suspicion and reveals an infiltrate in his right base. What is appropriate therapy for this patient?

   A. Intravenous beta-lactam and a macrolide

   B. A macrolide only

   C. A macrolide, cough suppressant, and antipyretic

   D. An antipseudomonal IV antibiotic and an antipneumococcal fluoroquinolone

83. You are called to see a 46-year-old woman for oxygen desaturation. She has been hospitalized for 8 days after undergoing an emergent open cholecystectomy for gangrenous cholecystitis. Her postoperative course has been

complicated by respiratory failure requiring mechanical ventilation. You evaluate the patient and note that she has a low-grade temperature today and that her oxygen saturations have fallen to 92% from 100% while her ventilator is set to deliver an Fio_2 of 40%. Her chest exam has coarse rhonchi throughout. Her suction canister attached to her endotracheal tube contains purulent secretions. You review her lab results and chest radiograph and note that she has a persistent leukocytosis and bilateral basilar infiltrates that have progressed since her morning chest radiograph. You diagnose a nosocomial pneumonia. What is appropriate antibiotic therapy in this patient?

A. An antipneumococcal fluoroquinolone and a macrolide

B. Two IV antibiotics that each have activity against *Pseudomonas*

C. A beta-lactam and an aminoglycoside

D. A broad-spectrum antibiotic, such as piperacillin/tazobactam, that covers gram-negative, gram-positive, and anaerobic bacteria

84. A 62-year-old male smoker presents to you with a 3-month history of productive cough, malaise, and weight loss. He has been unable to work for the last week because of his symptoms. He has received two courses of antibiotic therapy for a right middle lobe infiltrate. With each course of antibiotics, his symptoms have improved, only to recur with discontinuation of the antibiotics. His last course was completed a little over 1 week ago. The patient is otherwise healthy and takes only an aspirin because "another doctor told me it was good for me." He is frustrated by his illness and seeks more therapy so he can return to his job at a nursing home. His physical exam reveals a thin man in no apparent distress. Vital signs, including his temperature, are normal. Lung exam is notable for rhonchi over the right anterior chest. Chest radiograph reveals obliteration of the right heart border by a right middle lobe infiltrate. What should your next step be?

A. Prescribe a third course of antibiotics with an antibiotic that will cover the patient's probable pseudomonal infection.

B. Obtain a sputum Gram stain and culture and begin antibiotics based on the preliminary findings on the Gram stain.

C. Refer the patient to an Interventional Radiologist for CT-guided percutaneous aspiration of secretions from the right middle lobe infiltrate and begin antibiotics based on the culture results of those secretions.

D. Refer the patient to a pulmonologist for bronchoscopy with lavage and bronchoscopic biopsy of any suspicious lesions.

85. You are called to see a 27-year-old woman who has been admitted to the ICU for monitoring after having postpartum hemorrhage earlier in the day. During her resuscitation the patient received 10 units of packed red blood cells, 4 units of fresh frozen plasma, a six-pack of platelets, and 5 L of crystalloid. With this resuscitation and with emergent embolization of her pelvic vasculature, the patient has had a stable hematocrit and hemodynamic status for the last 6 hours. She now complains of shortness of breath, especially when trying to lie flat to sleep, and her nurse has noted that the patient has an oxygen saturation of 88% on room air. You examine the patient and note tachypnea, tachycardia, and rales throughout her posterior chest. You order a chest radiograph and it shows diffuse fluffy infiltrates. You diagnose volume overload with pulmonary edema from the patient's massive resuscitation. What is your first step in treatment?

   A. Order 40 mg of IV furosemide (Lasix) and attempt a brisk diuresis.

   B. Order oxygen therapy with nasal cannula or a face mask to keep the patient's oxygen saturation above 90%.

   C. Order a BiPAP device to be placed on the patient to deliver positive-pressure breaths and help redistribute the fluid that has accumulated in the alveoli back into the lymphatic drainage of the lung.

   D. Order a CT angiogram of the chest because a DIC picture can worsen bleeding but also cause a paradoxical PE that may explain this patient's symptoms.

86. You are called to see the patient in question 85 for obtundation. You find the patient unresponsive. A quick look at her vital signs reveals that she has a respiratory rate of 6 breaths/min and an oxygen saturation of 86% on 4 L of O_2 via nasal cannula. You urgently call for the respiratory therapist and take a moment to speak with the patient's nurse. He reports that the patient had improved with the oxygen therapy to an oxygen saturation of 98% and was able to lie flat. However, the patient complained of residual pelvic pain and had received a dose of 4 mg of IV morphine and 1 mg of IV lorazepam about 30 minutes ago. The nurse has already sent an arterial blood gas, and the results return as you place a bag mask over the patient's face to assist her respiration. The pH is 7.22, the Pco_2 is 58, and the Po_2 is 56. What do you do next?

   A. Ask the nurse for a dose of naloxone (Narcan) to be given intravenously.

   B. Ask the nurse for a dose of flumazenil to be given intravenously.

   C. Apply the bag mask to the patient's face with a tight seal and begin ventilating the patient.

D. Ask the respiratory therapist to apply a BiPAP mask to the patient to assist with her ventilation until the sedative and narcotic medications wear off.

87. You are an anesthesiologist and have just completed a long case in the OR. The case was that of a 78-year-old man who underwent an emergent repair of a ruptured abdominal aortic aneurysm under general anesthesia. The patient was in the OR for several hours and required large-volume resuscitation with blood products and crystalloid during the procedure. The general surgery attending physician asks you to extubate the patient prior to his departure from the OR. Your response is

A. To comply with the attending surgeon and extubate the patient in the operating room

B. To tell the surgeon you are worried about the patient and would prefer to do the extubation on arrival to the ICU

C. To express concern to the surgeon and ask that the patient be monitored and evaluated fully in the ICU prior to extubation

D. To tell the surgeon that the patient is at high risk for prolonged respiratory failure and will be ventilator dependent and require eventual tracheostomy

88. A 45-year-old man is evaluated for a neck mass and is found to have medullary carcinoma of the thyroid. He has a history of poorly controlled hypertension. Prior to surgery, what other disease must be looked for?

A. Renal artery stenosis

B. Hyperaldosteronism

C. Pheochromocytoma

D. Cushing's disease

89. The initial localization study for a suspected gastrinoma is

A. MRI

B. Scintigraphy

C. CT scan

D. Angiography with selective venous sampling

90. The incidence of thyroid cancer in a patient with a large goiter is

A. Much greater than that in the population at large

B. Equal to that in the population at large

C. Less than that in the population at large

D. Unknown

91. Which of the following statements is *not* true when operating for appendicitis?

    A. Free pus throughout the peritoneal cavity should be treated with external drainage.

    B. A normal appendix should be routinely removed when operating for presumed appendicitis.

    C. Antibiotics should be given after the decision has been made to take the patient for surgical exploration.

    D. Open and laparoscopic appendectomies are equally acceptable approaches.

92. Which answer best describes the etiology of periumbilical pain in appendicitis?

    A. The appendix often extends toward the umbilicus, and local inflammation irritates that area.

    B. The infection travels retrograde along the small bowel and refers pain to the umbilicus.

    C. Distention of the appendix causes somatic pain along nerves referred to the umbilicus.

    D. Periumbilical pain occurs only in cases in which perforation has already occurred.

93. Which group of signs and symptoms would be most suggestive of appendicitis?

    A. Suprapubic pain, febrile, shaking chills, pain with urination

    B. Suprapubic pain, diarrhea, febrile, similar pain several months ago

    C. Periumbilical abdominal pain that later migrates to right lower quadrant, low-grade temperature, anorexia, two episodes of vomiting

    D. Abdominal pain in right lower quadrant, no fever, diarrhea that preceded the abdominal pain, white blood cell count of 14/mm^3

94. A 27-year-old woman presents with pain on defecation lasting for 1 hour. She also has noted some bright red blood on the tissue. The most likely diagnosis is

    A. Bleeding internal hemorrhoids

    B. Proctitis

    C. Thrombosed external hemorrhoids

    D. Proctalgia fugax

    E. Anal fissure

95. A 42-year-old man presents with pain in the anal area and a circumferential, irreducible mass. He is afebrile. The most likely diagnosis is

    A. Rectal abscess

    B. Condyloma acuminata

    C. Anal carcinoma

    D. Prolapsed thrombosed hemorrhoids

    E. Hypertrophied anal papillae

96. A 35-year-old man presents to the emergency department with rectal pain and fever. The pain is aggravated by coughing. External examination is negative. The most likely diagnosis is

    A. Proctalgia fugax

    B. Intrasphincteric abscess

    C. Hidradenitis suppurativa

    D. Thrombosed internal hemorrhoids

    E. Infected anal fissure

97. Bile consists of all of the following *except*

    A. Cholesterol

    B. Lecithin

    C. Melanin

    D. Bile salts

98. Which of the following clinical syndromes does *not* result from occlusion of the biliary tree?

    A. Gallstone pancreatitis

    B. Biliary colic

    C. Ascending cholangitis

    D. Acute hepatitis

99. Charcot's triad is made up of all of the following *except*

    A. Clay-colored stools

    B. Jaundice

    C. Fever

    D. Right upper quadrant pain

100. Which of the following is the most useful imaging study in the initial evaluation of biliary disease?

    A. Magnetic resonance cholangiopancreatography (MRCP)

    B. Endoscopic retrograde cholangiopancreatography (ERCP)

C. Right upper quadrant ultrasound

D. Transhepatic cholangiography (THC)

101. Which of the following may make a HIDA scan unreliable?

    A. Recent ingestion of fat

    B. Hyperbilirubinemia

    C. Hepatic dysfunction

    D. All of the above

102. Which of the following statements is true?

    A. Any patients with documented gallstones needs a chole-cystectomy.

    B. Ascending cholangitis requires urgent drainage of the bile duct.

    C. All acute cholecystitis is caused by gallstones.

    D. Once the gallbladder is removed, the patient will be forever cured of gallstones.

103. Which of the following metabolic derangements are most likely to accompany a bowel obstruction with protracted vomiting?

    A. Hypernatremic metabolic acidosis

    B. Hypovolemic hyperchloremic metabolic alkalosis

    C. Hypochloremic hypokalemic metabolic alkalosis

    D. Hypochloremic hyperkalemic metabolic acidosis

104. An abdominal radiograph demonstrating distended colon from the cecum to the descending colon without small bowel gas is indicative of

    A. Ileus

    B. Colonic obstruction with a competent ileocecal valve

    C. Complete small bowel obstruction

    D. Partial small bowel obstruction

105. Rapidly worsening pain, reflexive vomiting, progressive tenderness, and minimal abdominal distention are signs and symptoms that are most consistent with which of the following types of bowel obstruction?

    A. Proximal small bowel obstruction

    B. Distal small bowel obstruction

    C. Closed-loop obstruction

    D. Large bowel obstruction

106. All of the following statements about sigmoid diverticular disease are true, *except*

    A. Diverticulosis is an asymptomatic state in which diverticula are discovered incidentally.

    B. Diverticular disease is associated with inflammation.

    C. Sigmoid diverticula usually involve all three layers of the bowel wall.

    D. Diverticular disease can be simple or complicated.

    E. Sigmoid diverticula can be associated with diverticulosis in other parts of the colon.

107. All of the following statements about diverticular disease are true, *except*

    A. Diverticulitis involves perforation of a diverticula.

    B. A connection between the colon and the bladder is the most common fistula that results from diverticular disease.

    C. Diverticular bleeding always requires surgical intervention.

    D. Contrast enema, ultrasound exam, and abdominal CT all have a role in the evaluation of diverticular disease.

    E. Endoscopy is generally contraindicated in patients with acute diverticulitis.

108. With regard to Zenker's diverticulum, which of the following abnormalities would *not* be observed?

    A. Bird-beak deformity of the distal esophagus with mega-esophagus

    B. Abnormal relaxation of the upper esophageal sphincter with deglutition

    C. Frequent regurgitation of undigested food

    D. Aspiration pneumonia

109. A 50-year-old woman presents with a history of chest pain, dysphagia of both solids and liquids and odynophagia, and weight loss of 20 lb. Cine-esophagram shows multiple simultaneous contractions of the esophagus leading down to a smooth narrowing at the gastroesophageal junction. The contractions are high amplitude and are associated with a non-relaxing lower esophageal sphincter. Treatment options include all of the following *except*

    A. Bougie dilation

    B. Nissen fundoplication

    C. Botulinum toxin injection

    D. Heller myotomy

110. A 37-year-old woman with longstanding heartburn that is minimally responsive to proton pump inhibitors is referred by her primary care physician for surgical treatment of GERD. Of the following tests, which is *not* required prior to antireflux surgery?

    A. 24-hour pH monitoring
    B. Manometry
    C. Upper endoscopy with biopsy to rule out Barrett's esophagus
    D. Botulinum toxin injection

111. A 50-year-old otherwise healthy woman was seen by her primary care physician for her annual physical exam. She was found to have an incidental finding of gastric air bubble in the thorax. An upper GI series confirms the diagnosis of a paraesophageal hiatal hernia (type II). She is completely asymptomatic. The appropriate treatment is

    A. None; she should wait until she has symptoms
    B. A hiatal hernia repair with Nissen fundoplication
    C. A transhiatal esophagectomy
    D. Bougie dilation

112. A 39-year-old woman having no adverse symptoms is found to have a 10-cm mass in the right upper quadrant of the abdomen. Routine blood studies and physical exam are otherwise unrevealing. CT scan of the abdomen reveals a 10-cm irregular mass overlying the hepatic flexure of the colon and abutting but not invading the liver. Biopsy shows a spindle cell neoplasm. Treatment is

    A. Preoperative chemotherapy
    B. Surgical resection and postoperative radiation
    C. Surgical resection and submission of tumor for *c-kit* mutation testing
    D. ERCP and placement of bile duct stent
    E. Total proctocolectomy

113. A 55-year-old man complains that swallowed food hangs up at his xiphoid process and is associated with mild pain. He has lost 15 lb. Stool is positive for occult blood. Appropriate diagnostic tests include

    A. Upper gastrointestinal endoscopy
    B. Biopsy of visible lesions and distal esophageal mucosa
    C. Endoscopic ultrasound of distal esophagus
    D. Abdominal CT scan
    E. All of the above

114. An 80-year-old man presents with signs of peritoneal inflammation and a tender left lower quadrant abdominal mass. He reports progressive diarrhea over several weeks, mild to moderate crampy abdominal pain, weakness, and rapid exacerbation of severe, steady abdominal pain 6 hours before admission, plus he has had chills. His skin is clammy and he is pale and quite thin. The *least* likely diagnosis is

A. Sigmoid diverticulitis
B. Perforation of a carcinoma of the sigmoid colon
C. Large lymphoma of the distal small bowel
D. Gastrointestinal stromal tumor
E. Carcinoma of the body and tail of the pancreas

115. All of the following statements about IBD are true, *except*

A. Crohn's disease can affect any part of the GI tract from the mouth to the anus.
B. Whereas Crohn's disease is a transmural process, mucosal ulcerative colitis usually involves only the colonic mucosa.
C. Strictures are common in both forms of IBD.
D. Surgery can be curative for mucosal ulcerative colitis.
E. Pseudopolyps are common in mucosal ulcerative colitis.

116. Indications for surgery in Crohn's disease include

A. Intestinal obstruction
B. Toxic megacolon
C. Free perforation
D. Interloop abscess
E. All of the above

117. The differential diagnosis of mucosal ulcerative colitis includes

A. Diverticulitis
B. Ischemic or infectious colitis
C. Crohn's disease
D. Lymphoma
E. All of the above

118. Which of the following is *not* true of hepatic abscesses?

A. Bacterial abscesses are usually caused by enteric organisms.
B. All hepatic abscesses must be drained.

C. The incidence of bacterial hepatic abscesses has decreased over the last few decades.

D. Amebic abscesses can be diagnosed by serologic testing or abdominal CT scans.

E. Hepatic abscesses can be associated with appendicitis.

119. All of the following statements about hepatocellular carcinoma (HCC) are true, *except*

   A. HCC is more common in Asians than in Americans or Europeans.

   B. HCC is strongly associated with hepatitis B virus infection.

   C. Ultrasound is an accurate means of diagnosing HCC.

   D. Abdominal pain is the most common symptom of HCC.

   E. Transplantation can cure some HCC patients.

120. Which of the following statements about liver disease is *not* true?

   A. Patients with liver disease have an increased risk of complications following surgery.

   B. The primary management of patients with variceal bleeding is early surgical intervention.

   C. Hepatic hemangiomas are usually asymptomatic.

   D. Metastatic neoplasms of the liver are much more common than primary tumors.

121. All of the following statements about adenocarcinoma of the pancreas are correct, *except*

   A. Only about 20% of patients have disease confined to the pancreas at the time of diagnosis.

   B. The best staging tool is a thin-cut helical CT scan through the pancreas and surrounding tissue.

   C. Percutaneous biopsy of a suspected pancreatic cancer is helpful and should be done before proceeding with operative resection.

   D. Long-term survival of patients undergoing "curative resection" of pancreatic cancer has steadily improved over the last two decades.

   E. The most common complication of pancreatic resection is pancreatic anastomotic leak.

122. Pancreatitis

   A. Has been described as a retroperitoneal "burn"

   B. Is most frequently due to gallbladder disease or alcohol abuse

   C. Can be severe enough to cause SIRS, sepsis or death

   D. Can cause obstruction of the bile duct, stones in the pancreatic duct, pancreatic ductal obstruction, or "pseudocysts"

   E. All of the above

123. Surgical indications in patients with ulcer disease include

   A. Inability to stop bleeding following endoscopic therapy

   B. Free perforation

   C. Gastric outlet obstruction

   D. Recurrent ulceration following ulcer surgery

   E. All of the above

124. The current treatment of Zollinger-Ellison syndrome is

   A. Total gastrectomy

   B. High-dose H_2 blockade

   C. Antibiotic therapy

   D. Aggressive surgical resection of the probable gastrinoma after evaluation with imaging studies and/or portal venous sampling

   E. Life-long administration of proton pump inhibitors

125. What is *not* true of the "dumping syndrome"?

   A. It can occur after either pyloroplasty or gastric resection.

   B. Most patients require surgery for relief of their symptoms.

   C. It is associated with rapid transit of food into the small intestine.

   D. Symptoms include tachycardia, sweating, abdominal pain, and dizziness.

   E. A Roux-en-Y gastroenterostomy is currently the preferred surgical correction procedure.

126. Which of the following patients does *not* have a standard indication for transfusion of packed red blood cells?

   A. A neonate with pulmonary failure who has a hemoglobin of 9 g/dL

   B. A 65-year-old man with a hemoglobin of 8 g/dL in the midst of an acute myocardial infarction

   C. A 60-year-old asymptomatic woman with a hemoglobin of 9 g/dL

   D. A 55-year-old man with a history of coronary disease, a hemoglobin of 8 g/dL, and persistent oliguria despite being euvolemic

127. Which of the following patients does *not* have an indication for transfusion of platelets?

    A. A 62-year-old man with a platelet count of 60,000/mm^3 about to undergo brain surgery

    B. A 70-year-old woman admitted for cellulitis who has a platelet count of 25,000/mm^3 as an incidental finding

    C. A 35-year-old trauma victim who has diffuse, small vessel bleeding, a falling hematocrit, and a platelet count of 60,000/mm^3

    D. A patient with severe pneumonia who develops a platelet count of 4000/mm^3

128. Which of the following statements is true?

    A. A "PLA" can be derived from as many as six donors.

    B. Cryoprecipitate is rich in factor VII.

    C. There is enough plasma in packed red blood cells to maintain normal coagulation in cases of major bleeding.

    D. Angina can be a symptom of anemia.

129. DIC results from the presentation of a clotting stimulus to the intravascular space in a patient with which of the following conditions?

    A. Hypothermia

    B. A hypercoagulable state

    C. Hemophilia

    D. Aspirin use

    E. Von Willebrand's disease

130. When treating a patient with ongoing bleeding, which of the following should be corrected?

    A. Hypothermia

    B. Volume depletion

    C. Underlying infection

    D. Depressed levels of clotting factors

    E. All of the above

131. Depletion of which of the following factors would result in a hypercoagulable state?

    A. Fibrinogen

    B. Thrombin

    C. Calcium

    D. Protein C

    E. Tissue factor

132. Which of the following has been shown to reverse DIC?

    A. Antithrombin

    B. Heparin

    C. Aminocaproic acid (Amicar)

    D. Tissue plasminogen activator

    E. None of the above

133. Splenectomy is most commonly indicated for which one of the following congenital hemolytic anemias?

    A. Thalassemia major

    B. Hereditary elliptocytosis

    C. Sickle cell anemia

    D. Pyruvate kinase deficiency

    E. Hereditary spherocytosis

134. Which of the following statements regarding splenic rupture is true?

    A. The spleen is the most commonly injured organ in penetrating abdominal trauma.

    B. The spleen is the most commonly injured organ in blunt abdominal trauma.

    C. Spontaneous splenic rupture rarely involves an underlying infectious or hematologic disorder.

    D. Grade IV splenic injuries can usually be managed nonoperatively.

    E. Nonoperative management of splenic injury is effective in 80% of cases.

135. Regarding splenectomy in the treatment of ITP,

    A. Splenectomy always results in disease remission.

    B. Open splenectomy is preferred over laparoscopic splenectomy.

    C. Symptomatic splenomegaly is a common indication.

    D. Splenectomy should be performed only after steroid therapy fails.

    E. Splenectomy is contraindicated.

136. Necrotizing infections have the following components *except*

    A. Rapid spread of infection

    B. Multiple organisms

    C. Good response to antibiotics

    D. Tenderness to palpation

137. Standard treatment of necrotizing infection includes all of the following *except*
    A. Hyperbaric oxygenation
    B. Surgical débridement
    C. Broad-spectrum antibiotics
    D. Second-look surgery

138. An example of appropriate antibiotic therapy could be all of the following *except*
    A. Piperacillin/tazobactam
    B. Cephalexin
    C. Penicillin and clindamycin
    D. Imipenem/cilastatin

139. Sepsis can cause which of the following?
    A. Renal dysfunction
    B. Respiratory failure
    C. Hypotension
    D. All of the above

140. Treatment of sepsis includes all of the following *except*
    A. Emergency exploratory laparotomy
    B. Treatment of hypotension
    C. Broad-spectrum antibiotic
    D. Pan-culture of blood, urine, sputum

141. Significant signs of sepsis include
    A. Hypotension
    B. Hypothermia
    C. Organ dysfunction
    D. All of the above

142. A 63-year-old diabetic man is in the 7th day after a small bowel resection. He is requiring nasogastric suctioning. He is noted to have worsening hyperglycemia and tachypnea. A chest radiograph reveals pneumonia. Laboratory studies show Na^+ of 130 mmol/L, Cl^- of 85 mmol/L, HCO_3^- of 15 mmol/L, glucose of 452 mg/dL, pH 7.50, and Pco_2 of 20 mm Hg. The most likely acid-base disturbance is
    A. Respiratory alkalosis with a metabolic compensation
    B. Metabolic acidosis with a respiratory compensation

    C. Three superimposed primary acid-base disorders: respiratory alkalosis, metabolic acidosis, and metabolic alkalosis

    D. Respiratory acidosis and metabolic acidosis

143. A 52-year-old man develops acute renal failure 7 days after an abdominal aortic aneurysm is repaired. The urinalysis and urine indices suggest acute tubular necrosis. A serum potassium measurement returns at 8 mEq/L and an ECG shows prolonged PR interval, QRS widening, and peak T waves. Increased cardiac ectopy is noted on the monitor. The initial treatment of this potential life-threatening complication of hyperkalemia is

    A. Reduced potassium intake and administration of a diuretic

    B. Calcium gluconate 10 mL of a 10% solution

    C. Oral sodium polystyrene sulfonate (Kayexalate)

    D. Sodium bicarbonate

144. A 68-year-old woman is admitted with cholelithiasis. Her laboratory values show a creatinine value of 2.4 mg/dL. The initial evaluation reveals a benign urinalysis, U_{Na} <20 mEq/L, and FE_{Na} <1%. The most likely explanation for the renal insufficiency is

    A. An infection-related glomerulonephritis

    B. Obstructive uropathy

    C. Acute tubular necrosis

    D. Prerenal azotemia

145. A sodium deficit on routine laboratory screening may be caused by which of the following?

    A. Normal total body sodium in a setting of excess total body fluid

    B. Decreased total body sodium in a setting of normal total body fluids

    C. Laboratory error

    D. All of the above

146. Symptoms of hypocalcemia include all the following *except*

    A. Tetany

    B. A negative Chvostek's sign (no facial twitch after tapping the patient near the facial nerve)

    C. A positive Trousseau's sign (carpal spasm with prolonged application of a blood pressure cuff)

    D. Abdominal cramping

    E. Irritability

147. Treatment of a patient with suspected hyperkalemia may include all of the following *except*

    A. ECG and cardiac monitoring
    B. Administration of calcium gluconate
    C. Administration of glucagon
    D. Administration of bicarbonate
    E. Administration of sodium polystyrene sulfonate (Kayexalate)

148. A 59-year-old man presents to the emergency department with a several-day history of vomiting. He has not been able to keep any food or liquid down for 3 days. Which of the following bedside exams gives reasonable confirmation of severe dehydration?

    A. Decreased urine output
    B. Diminished mental status
    C. Decreased skin turgor
    D. Tachycardia
    E. All of the above

149. A 72-year-old man is 2 days out from elective repair of sigmoid diverticulitis. Despite his receiving intravenous fluids in the postoperative period, you suspect that he is still under-fluid-resuscitated. What is a reasonable initial work-up to assess his fluid status?

    A. Swan-Ganz catheter placement and initiation of dopamine
    B. Serum and urine osmolality measurements
    C. Placement of a urinary catheter and a fluid challenge
    D. Cardiac echo

150. An 18-year-old man drove his car off a cliff. He presents to the trauma center with multiple injuries including bilateral femur fractures, a distended abdomen, and closed head injury. His heart rate is 150 beats/min, his respirations are 40 breaths/min and shallow, and his initial blood pressure is 80/40 mm Hg. What is his estimated fluid loss class?

    A. Class I (15% of blood volume, <750 mL)
    B. Class II (15–30% of blood volume, 750–1500 mL)
    C. Class III (30–40% of blood volume, 1500–2000 mL)
    D. Class IV (>40% of blood volume, >2000 mL)
    E. Cannot assess because the patient is unconscious

151. With regard to line sepsis,

    A. Sudden development of hyperglycemia or increased insulin requirements is an early sign of line sepsis.

B. Most catheter infections can be treated with antibiotics without replacing the line.

C. The most common complication of parenteral nutrition is pneumothorax.

D. *Escherichia coli* is the most commonly isolated bacteria in TPN-associated line sepsis.

152. Which of the following patients is most appropriate for perioperative TPN?

A. A 20-year-old patient admitted for a stab wound to the left upper quadrant that sustains an isolated diaphragmatic injury

B. An elderly man with a bleeding gastric cancer with an albumin of 2.6 preoperatively

C. A 65-year-old woman with esophageal cancer with a pre-operative albumin of 3.7

D. A 40-year-old woman admitted for bilateral mastectomy

153. All of the following are important indicators of nutritional deficiency *except*

A. Serum albumin

B. Temporal muscle wasting

C. Poor skin turgor

D. Increased serum glucose

154. Which of the following is *not* a recommended technique to decrease the spread of cancer during an operation?

A. Early ligation of vascular pedicles of the tumor

B. Wide excision, avoiding cutting into the tumor

C. Squeezing out any remaining venous blood from the tumor after ligation of the feeding artery

D. Protection of the wound edges with gauze or plastic sheets

155. Lymphoscintigraphy should be considered in patients with an extremity melanoma of

A. Thin depth (<0.76 mm) and negative lymph node exam

B. Intermediate depth (0.76–4.0 mm) and negative lymph node exam

C. Thick depth (>4.0 mm) and bulky palpable nodes

D. Any depth

156. All of the following are risk factors for the development of melanoma *except*

    A. Celtic heritage
    B. Use of moisturizing creams
    C. Dysplastic nevus syndrome
    D. Family history of melanoma

157. Which of the following is *not* a poor prognostic sign in staging soft tissue sarcomas?

    A. Age
    B. Tumor size
    C. Histologic grade
    D. Lymph node spread

158. Which of the following is *not* an acceptable biopsy technique for a mass suspicious for sarcoma?

    A. Incisional biopsy of a 10-cm mass of the thigh with an incision lengthwise down the leg
    B. Excisional biopsy of a 2-cm buttock lesion with 2-cm margins
    C. FNA of a 3-cm lesion on the back of the hand
    D. Core tissue biopsy of a 20-cm mass on the back of the shoulder

159. A 25-year-old woman is the driver of an automobile involved in a high-speed motor vehicle accident. She complains of abdominal pain but does not have peritoneal signs. Her vitals signs are stable and normal. Which one of the following would *not* be considered as part of the initial work-up of this patient?

    A. CT scan of the abdomen
    B. Ultrasonography
    C. Diagnostic peritoneal lavage
    D. Arteriography

160. Which of the following associated injuries in the multiply injured trauma patient is likely to account for the greatest blood loss?

    A. Facial fractures
    B. Humerus fracture
    C. Femur fracture
    D. Sacroiliac/pelvic fracture

161. Which of the following cell counts constitutes a positive diagnostic peritoneal lavage for blunt abdominal trauma?

    A. >1000 RBC/mm^3
    B. $>10,000$ RBC/mm^3

    C. >100,000 RBC/mm^3

    D. >100 WBC/mm^3

162. Which of the following increases the likelihood of a patient's dying from a major burn injury?

    A. Age >70 years

    B. Age <1 year

    C. Smoke inhalation

    D. Preexisting cardiac and renal disease

    E. All of the above

163. Calculate, using the Parkland formula, the initial hourly fluid requirements for a 70-kg man who arrives at your emergency department 3 hours after sustaining a 50% full-thickness body burn.

    A. 100 mL/hr

    B. 175 mL/hr

    C. 270 mL/hr

    D. 1400 mL/hr

164. Electrical burns are characterized by all of the following *except*

    A. More extensive deep injury than is obvious from the superficial appearance

    B. The possibility of myonecrosis, rhabdomyolysis, and resultant renal failure

    C. Frequent necrosis of the bony areas transmitting the current

    D. The possibility of development of compartment syndrome

165. Which of the following is an indication of thoracic aortic injury?

    A. Free air under the diaphragm

    B. Right pleural effusion

    C. Left pneumothorax

    D. Loss of aortopulmonary window

    E. Left lung contusion

166. What is the gold standard for diagnosis of an aortic injury?

    A. Plain chest radiograph

    B. CT of the chest

    C. Aortography

    D. Transesophageal echocardiogram

    E. Transthoracic echocardiogram

167. Which of the following statements concerning cardiac injuries is *not* true?

    A. They are among the most lethal injuries.

    B. In penetrating injuries, patients with stab wounds have better survival rates.

    C. Emergency department thoracotomy yields better results in patients with penetrating cardiac trauma.

    D. All patients with suspected cardiac injury should be evaluated with a CT scan to exclude associated thoracic injuries.

    E. Subxiphoid pericardial window can be used in the diagnosis of cardiac injuries.

168. A 27-year-old man is brought to the hospital after suffering a single gunshot wound to the left chest. He is hypotensive and tachycardic and has decreased breath sounds in the right hemithorax. A right chest tube is inserted and yields 1800 mL of blood. What should be the next step in his management?

    A. Perform an emergent right thoracotomy.

    B. Transfuse 2 units of blood and obtain a CT of the chest to further evaluate the extent of his injuries.

    C. Autotransfuse the blood evacuated from the right chest and observe closely for continuing hemorrhage.

    D. Obtain an emergency angiogram because the large amount of blood loss is suggestive of a vascular injury.

    E. Perform pericardiocentesis to exclude cardiac injury.

169. What is Beck's triad; in what percentage of patients with cardiac tamponade is it seen?

    A. Bradycardia, hypotension, pulsus paradoxus; 15%

    B. Pulsus paradoxus, hypertension, bradycardia; 15%

    C. Tachycardia, hypotension, Kussmaul's sign; 20%

    D. Muffled heart sounds, hypotension, jugular venous distention; 10%

    E. Muffled heart sounds, hypertension, tachycardia; 15%

170. Which of the following is *not* an indication to perform an emergency department thoracotomy?

    A. Cardiopulmonary arrest

    B. Profound shock

    C. Cardiopulmonary arrest due to blunt trauma

    D. Exsanguinating injuries

    E. Pericardial tamponade

171. Which of the following is *not* a clinical sign or symptom of cardiac tamponade?

    A. Beck's triad

    B. Restlessness

    C. Shock

    D. Strong peripheral pulses

    E. Weak peripheral pulses

172. Which of the following is true concerning tension pneumothorax?

    A. It is an immediately life-threatening injury and requires an emergency department thoracotomy.

    B. It can be treated with needle thoracostomy alone.

    C. Presentation can be similar to cardiac tamponade.

    D. Hemodynamic consequences are a result of respiratory failure.

    E. It is only seen following penetrating chest injuries.

173. Which of the following is *not* an indication for tube thoracostomy?

    A. Hemothorax

    B. Lung contusion

    C. Pneumothorax

    D. Tension pneumothorax

    E. Patients with multiple rib fractures requiring air transfer

174. Tube thoracostomy

    A. Requires sterile technique and should not be performed outside the operating room

    B. Should be performed under general anesthesia

    C. Is the sole treatment required in a large number of patients with thoracic trauma

    D. Using special trocars is faster and safer

    E. Should be placed as low as possible to provide better evacuation of hemothorax

175. Flail chest can be life-threatening because

    A. It causes significant pain that results in respiratory compromise

    B. Of the underlying lung parenchymal injury

    C. It requires intubation and prolonged mechanical ventilation

    D. It is associated with tension pneumothorax

    E. The flail segment follows independently the chest wall motion

176. Concerning thoracic injuries, which of the following is *not* true?

    A. Diaphragmatic injuries can be easily diagnosed with helical CT scan of the chest.

    B. Traumatic esophageal injuries are rare.

    C. Hemodynamically stable patients with transmediastinal gunshot wounds should be evaluated systematically to exclude cardiac, great vessel, or esophageal injuries.

    D. Emergency department thoracotomy is more successful in patients with penetrating thoracic trauma.

    E. Tube thoracostomy output of 1500 mL is an indication for thoracotomy.

177. Which facial bone fracture is associated with cheek numbness?

    A. Frontal bone

    B. Nasal

    C. Maxillary arch

    D. Mandibular

    E. Orbit

178. Le Fort II fracture segments contain which of the following bones?

    A. Mandible, nasal

    B. Maxilla, temporal arch

    C. Maxilla, zygoma

    D. Maxilla, nasal, zygoma

    E. Maxilla, nasal

179. What is the significance of epiphyseal fractures?

    A. They occur through thick cortical bone.

    B. They are often associated with extensive bleeding.

    C. They commonly are intra-articular and have segments with articular cartilage.

    D. They require extensive energy transfer compared to other fractures.

180. What is the worst type of Salter-Harris physeal fracture in children?

    A. Type I—transphyseal separation

    B. Type II—through the metaphysis and physis

    C. Type V—crush injury of the physis

    D. All types carry a poor prognosis for anatomic healing.

181. Which of the following require(s) emergency management?

   A. Fracture of the tibia with an overlying 1-cm laceration

   B. Dislocation of the hip following motor vehicle collision

   C. Dislocation of the ankle without vascular compromise

   D. All of the above

182. Which of the following is true concerning brain injury?

   A. Epidural hematomas often result from arterial bleeding associated with skull fracture.

   B. Subdural hematomas often result from venous bleeding and usually are associated with brain parenchymal injury.

   C. Diffuse axonal injury may not manifest on initial CT but may be associated with brain edema, increased cerebral pressure, and decreased brain perfusion.

   D. All of the above

183. Which of the following may be used to exclude cervical spine injury in an injured patient?

   A. An examination demonstrating no neurologic abnormality

   B. A normal lateral cervical spine film

   C. A normal three-view cervical spine film with C1 through C6 clearly visualized

   D. Absence of neck pain or tenderness in an alert, not-intoxicated patient with no distracting injuries

184. A 34-year-old man sustains two stab wounds, the first to the right flank and the second to the mid-anterior abdomen. He complains of abdominal pain and presents to the emergency department with a blood pressure of 85/50 mm Hg. You rapidly insert two large-bore intravenous catheters and begin infusing warm isotonic crystalloid while a nurse inserts a Foley catheter into the bladder—the urine returns bright red. A supine chest radiograph is normal. How do you best proceed with this patient?

   A. Obtain a CT scan with intravenous contrast of the lower abdomen and pelvis to better delineate the extent of his injuries.

   B. Obtain a retrograde contrast cystogram via the Foley catheter to rule out a bladder laceration as the cause of the hematuria.

   C. Obtain an immediate surgical consultation for a possible emergency exploratory celiotomy.

   D. Order an intravenous pyelogram to determine the extent of his possible right kidney and ureter injury.

E. Arrange for emergency renal angiography to study the kidneys and any possible renal vascular injury.

185. A 50-year-old woman is brought to your emergency department after crashing her automobile into a freeway bridge abutment. She complains of headache and pain in her left knee and leg. She is alert and denies back, abdominal, flank, or hip pain. Her pelvis is nontender to your repeated examinations. A routine urinalysis reveals 20 to 30 red blood cells per high-power field, although her urine appears to be grossly normal. How would you approach this patient's hematuria?

A. Obtain a CT scan with intravenous contrast of the lower abdomen and pelvis to better delineate the extent of her injuries.

B. Obtain a retrograde contrast cystogram via the Foley catheter to rule out a bladder laceration as the cause of the hematuria.

C. Obtain an immediate urologic consultation for a possible emergency exploratory celiotomy.

D. Order an intravenous pyelogram to determine the extent of a possible kidney or ureter injury.

E. Observe the patient without ordering any specific urologic imaging studies.

186. An 18-year-old male is thrown from his bicycle under a moving vehicle. In the emergency department, he has stable vital signs but complains of severe pain over his right lateral rib cage, in the suprapubic area, and over the right hip. Examination is significant for point tenderness over the right lateral rib cage and a small scrotal hematoma. A chest radiograph obtained shortly after arrival is normal. The pelvic radiograph demonstrates displaced fractures of the right superior and inferior pubic rami. What is this patient's most likely urologic injury and how would you diagnose it?

A. Right renal contusion; obtain a CT scan of the abdomen with intravenous contrast agent.

B. Bladder rupture; insert a Foley catheter and perform retrograde contrast cystogram.

C. Any injury is possible; obtain a catheterized urine specimen for microanalysis to determine the degree of hematuria and guide you in further selection of appropriate diagnostic tests.

D. Urethral disruption; obtain a retrograde contrast urethrogram.

E. Right ureteral injury; obtain an IVP to fully delineate the ureters and check for extravasation.

187. A 28-year-old man with a gunshot wound anterior to the left sternocleidomastoid muscle arrives in the emergency department with a large cervical pulsatile hematoma and difficulty in breathing and speaking. What is the most appropriate management?

    A. Call for a chest radiograph.

    B. Incise the hematoma with a scalpel.

    C. Arrange for a CT scan of the neck.

    D. Call for a thoracic surgery consult.

    E. Establish an airway.

188. A 5-year-old girl with a supracondylar fracture of the left humerus complains of pain in the forearm and hand and has no radial/ulnar pulses at the left wrist. What is the most appropriate management?

    A. Put the unreduced fracture in a loose sling.

    B. Inject the site of the fracture with local anesthesia.

    C. Call for an orthopedic surgeon to realign the fracture.

    D. Perform a forearm fasciotomy.

    E. Give an injection of morphine sulfate.

189. A 20-year-old man who was the driver in a head-on motor vehicle crash has a hematoma in his superior mediastinum on the admission chest radiograph, but no other obvious injuries. A thoracic aortogram documents the presence of extravasation of contrast from the aorta just beyond the origin of the left subclavian artery. What is the most appropriate management?

    A. Obtain a thoracic CT to confirm the injury.

    B. Call the operating room and a thoracic surgeon.

    C. Repeat the chest radiograph.

    D. Call the hospital chaplain.

    E. Put the patient in the head-down position.

190. Leriche's syndrome is associated with all of the following *except*

    A. Aortoiliac disease

    B. Impotence

    C. Aortic aneurysms

    D. Hip/buttock claudication

    E. Seen in men only

191. Yearly risk of rupture for an aneurysm greater than 7 cm is

    A. 5%

B. 80%

C. 30%

D. 15%

E. 60%

192. Which of the following is *not* true regarding endovascular treatment of abdominal aortic aneurysms?

    A. It is still experimental.

    B. It requires appropriate patient anatomy.

    C. It can be performed safely in most patients.

    D. It has less blood loss than open surgery.

193. Complications of aortic surgery include all of the following *except*

    A. Myocardial infarction

    B. Acute renal failure

    C. Hemorrhage

    D. Atheroembolism

    E. Colonic ischemia secondary to superior mesenteric ligation

194. Proper treatment for an asymptomatic carotid dissection is

    A. Carotid endarterectomy

    B. Carotid angioplasty

    C. Anticoagulation

    D. Observation

    E. Carotid artery stenting

195. The diagnostic test of choice to evaluate a carotid bruit is

    A. CT scan of the head and neck

    B. Carotid duplex scan

    C. Carotid angiogram

    D. MRI/MRA

    E. Oculoplethysmography

196. Which of the following is *not* an indication for carotid endarterectomy?

    A. Asymptomatic internal carotid lesion <50%

    B. TIA with >50% internal carotid stenosis

    C. Stroke with neurologic recovery and >50% stenosis

    D. Asymptomatic internal carotid lesion >70%

    E. Amaurosis fugax from ulcerated plaque

197. Risk factors for deep venous thrombosis (DVT) include all of the following *except*
    A. Immobilization
    B. Malignancy
    C. Protein C and S deficiency
    D. Factor V Leiden mutation
    E. Decreased homocysteine levels

198. Appropriate anticoagulation regimen for a pregnant patient with a DVT is
    A. Aspirin
    B. Coumadin
    C. Heparin therapy
    D. Compression stockings
    E. Clopidogrel (Plavix)

199. Risk factors for peripheral vascular disease include all of the following *except*
    A. Hypertension
    B. Active lifestyle
    C. Smoking
    D. Diabetes
    E. Hypercholesterolemia

200. Claudicants usually have an ankle:brachial index (ABI) in the range of
    A. >0.85
    B. 0.6–0.8
    C. <0.2
    D. 0.2–0.4

201. Intermittent claudication symptoms are first treated by
    A. Smoking cessation and exercise
    B. Medical therapy
    C. Angioplasty
    D. Bypass surgery
    E. Lowering cholesterol

202. Placement of dialysis catheter via the subclavian vein should be avoided whenever possible because
    A. Cannulation of these vessels by large-bore catheters frequently leads to stenosis and thrombosis, rendering the ipsilateral arm unsuitable for further access attempts.

B. Excessively high flow rates through these large central veins can cause hypotension.

C. The brachial plexus is frequently injured during the insertion of these large-bore catheters.

D. Recirculation is more likely to occur with this site compared to catheters placed in the internal jugular veins.

E. Successful dialysis requires arteriovenous, not venovenous, flow.

203. Which of the following access systems will improve with time?

    A. An uncuffed central venous catheter

    B. A cuffed central venous catheter

    C. An autologous arteriovenous fistula

    D. A polytetrafluoroethylene (PTFE) graft

    E. A modified bovine arterial arteriovenous heterograft

204. Which of the following access systems is the safest to use in an acutely ill patient who is severely uremic, suffering from congestive heart failure, pericardial effusion, and coagulopathy?

    A. An uncuffed central venous catheter

    B. A cuffed central venous catheter

    C. An autologous arteriovenous fistula

    D. A polytetrafluoroethylene (PTFE) graft

    E. A modified bovine arterial arteriovenous heterograft

205. Successful hemodialysis of an adult requires blood flow of at least

    A. 50 mL/min

    B. 100 mL/min

    C. 250 mL/min

    D. 500 mL/min

    E. 1 L/min

PRACTICE **EXAMINATION** ANSWERS

1.	C	36.	E	71.	D	106.	C	141.	D	176.	A
2.	A	37.	D	72.	A	107.	C	142.	C	177.	E
3.	B	38.	D	73.	C	108.	A	143.	B	178.	E
4.	C	39.	D	74.	A	109.	B	144.	D	179.	C
5.	A	40.	B	75.	C	110.	D	145.	D	180.	C
6.	C	41.	D	76.	B	111.	B	146.	B	181.	D
7.	B	42.	A	77.	A	112.	C	147.	C	182.	D
8.	E	43.	D	78.	D	113.	E	148.	E	183.	D
9.	C	44.	C	79.	C	114.	E	149.	C	184.	C
10.	D	45.	B	80.	A	115.	C	150.	D	185.	E
11.	D	46.	C	81.	D	116.	E	151.	A	186.	D
12.	B	47.	B	82.	C	117.	E	152.	B	187.	E
13.	D	48.	C	83.	D	118.	B	153.	D	188.	C
14.	E	49.	D	84.	D	119.	D	154.	C	189.	B
15.	A	50.	B	85.	B	120.	B	155.	B	190.	C
16.	D	51.	D	86.	C	121.	C	156.	B	191.	C
17.	A	52.	C	87.	C	122.	E	157.	A	192.	A
18.	C	53.	D	88.	C	123.	E	158.	C	193.	E
19.	D	54.	B	89.	B	124.	D	159.	D	194.	C
20.	D	55.	A	90.	B	125.	B	160.	D	195.	B
21.	E	56.	E	91.	A	126.	C	161.	C	196.	A
22.	B	57.	E	92.	C	127.	B	162.	E	197.	E
23.	C	58.	C	93.	C	128.	D	163.	D	198.	C
24.	A	59.	E	94.	E	129.	B	164.	C	199.	B
25.	D	60.	C	95.	D	130.	E	165.	D	200.	B
26.	C	61.	C	96.	B	131.	D	166.	C	201.	A
27.	A	62.	D	97.	C	132.	E	167.	D	202.	A
28.	E	63.	C	98.	D	133.	E	168.	A	203.	C
29.	C	64.	A	99.	A	134.	B	169.	D	204.	A
30.	D	65.	C	100.	C	135.	D	170.	C	205.	C
31.	D	66.	D	101.	D	136.	C	171.	D		
32.	E	67.	C	102.	B	137.	A	172.	C		
33.	D	68.	B	103.	C	138.	B	173.	B		
34.	D	69.	A	104.	B	139.	D	174.	C		
35.	E	70.	C	105.	C	140.	A	175.	B		

Appendix 1: Useful Formulae*

1. Determination of serum osmolality (mOsm)

$$\text{Serum osmolality} = 2[\text{Na}] + \frac{[\text{glucose}]}{[18]} + \frac{[\text{BUN}]}{[2.8]}$$

Na   Serum sodium concentration (in mEq/L)
Glucose   Serum glucose concentration (in mg/dl)
BUN   Blood urea nitrogen concentration (in mg/dl)
Normal range   280–295 mOsm

2. Determination of free water deficit (in L) in settings of hypernatremia

$$\text{Water deficit} = \frac{[\text{Na (observed)} - \text{Na (desired)}]\,[0.6]\,[\text{Wt}]}{[\text{Na (desired)}]}$$

Na (observed)   Serum sodium concentration (in mEq/L)
Na (desired)   Assume 140 mEq/L
0.6   Volume of distribution of sodium
Wt   Weight (in kg)

3. Determination of actual serum sodium in settings of hyperglycemia

$$\text{Na (corrected)} = \frac{[\text{glucose (observed)} - \text{glucose (normal)}]\,[1.4]}{[\text{glucose (normal)}] + \text{Na (observed)}}$$

Na (corrected)   Actual serum concentration of sodium (in mEq/L)
Na (observed)   Serum sodium concentration (in mEq/L)
Glucose (observed)   Serum glucose concentration (in mg/dl)
Glucose (normal)   Assume 200 mg/dl
1.4   Correction factor, which considers the shift of water that follows glucose into the interstitial space

---

*From Adams GA, Bresnick SD: On Call Surgery, 2nd ed. Philadelphia, WB Saunders, 2001.

4. Determination of sodium deficit in settings of hyponatremia

$$\text{Na deficit} = [\text{Na (desired)} - \text{Na (observed)}]\,[0.6]\,[\text{Wt}]$$

Na (desired)	Assume 135 mEq/L
Na (observed)	Serum sodium concentration (in mEq/L)
0.6	Volume of distribution of sodium
Wt	Weight (in kg)

5. Determination of bicarbonate (HCO_3) deficit (in mEq/L)

$$HCO_3 \text{ deficit} = [\text{Wt}]\,[0.4]\,[HCO_3 \text{ (desired)} - HCO_3 \text{ (actual)}]$$

HCO_3 (desired)	Assume 15–20 mEq/L
HCO_3 (observed)	Serum concentration of bicarbonate (in mEq/L)
Wt	Weight (in kg)
0.4	Correction factor, which considers intracellular buffering of bicarbonate
Goal of therapy	Serum pH >7.2

6. Determination of bicarbonate (HCO_3) deficit (in mEq/L) by using base deficit

$$HCO_3 \text{ deficit} = \frac{[\text{Base deficit}]\,[\text{Wt in kg}]\,[0.4]}{2}$$

7. Determination of anion gap (in mEq/L)

$$\text{Anion gap} = (\text{Na} + \text{K}) - (\text{Cl} + HCO_3)$$

Na	Serum sodium concentration (in mEq)
K	Serum potassium concentration (in mEq)
Cl	Serum chloride concentration (in mEq)
HCO_3	Serum bicarbonate ion concentration (in mEq)

8. Henderson-Hasselbalch equation

$$pH = 6.1 + \log\left(\frac{HCO_3}{0.03 \times P_{CO_2}}\right)$$

6.1	pH of the bicarbonate buffer system
HCO_3	Serum bicarbonate ion concentration (in mEq)
0.03	Solubility constant of CO_2 in arterial blood
P_{CO_2}	Partial pressure of CO_2 in serum (in mm Hg)

9. Nitrogen balance (in g/day, may be a positive or a negative value)

$$N_2 \text{ balance} = \frac{24\text{-hour protein intake}}{6.25} - [(24\text{-hour UUN}) + (4)]$$

24-hour UUN	Urinary urea nitrogen excretion (in g/day)
4	Obligatory loss (in g/day)

6.25   The number of grams of protein that yield 1 g N_2

Goal of therapy   +3 to 6 g/day balance

10. Calculation of fractional excretion of Na (FE_{NA})

$$\frac{U_{Na} \times P_{Cr}}{P_{Na} \times U_{Cr}}$$

U_{Na} Urinary sodium concentration (in mEq)
P_{Cr} Plasma creatinine concentration (in mg)
P_{Na} Plasma sodium concentration (in mEq)
U_{Cr} Urinary creatinine concentration (in mg)

As all units cancel, results are reported as %. May be performed on spot urine and plasma samples. A value <1% is indicative of pre-renal causes of renal failure, a value >1% is indicative of renal causes of failure.

CARDIAC PHYSIOLOGY

1. Determination of cardiac output (CO)

$$CO = [HR] [SV]$$

CO   Cardiac output (in L/min)
HR   Heart rate (in beats/min)
SV   Stroke volume (in L/beat)

Normal CO = 3.5–8.5 L/min
Cardiac index (CI) = CO/patient surface area

2. Determination of blood pressure (BP)

$$BP = [CO] [SVR]$$

BP   Blood pressure (in mm Hg)
CO   Cardiac output (in L/min)
SVR   Systemic vascular resistance $\left(\frac{\text{in dyne-sec}}{cm^5} \right)$

3. Determination of mean arterial blood pressure (MAP)

$$MAP = \frac{DBP + [SBP - DBP]}{[3]}$$

MAP   Mean arterial pressure (in mm Hg)
DBP   Diastolic blood pressure (in mm Hg)
SBP   Systolic blood pressure (in mm Hg)

4. Determination of systemic vascular resistance (SVR)

$$SVR = \frac{[MAP - CVP]\,[80]}{[CO]}$$

SVR   Systemic vascular resistance $\left(\dfrac{\text{in dyne-sec}}{cm^5}\right)$

MAP   Mean arterial pressure (in mm Hg)
CVP   Central venous pressure (in mm Hg)
CO   Cardiac output (in L/min)

5. Conversion of pressure in millimeters of mercury (mm Hg) to pressure in centimeters of water (cm H$_2$O)

$$mm\ Hg = \frac{cm\ H_2O}{1.36}$$

6. Calculation of cerebral perfusion pressure (CPP)

$$CPP = MAP - ICP$$

CPP   Cerebral perfusion pressure (in mm Hg)
MAP   Mean arterial pressure (in mm Hg)
ICP   Intracranial pressure (in mm Hg)

CPPs should run ≥65 mm Hg for adequate cerebral perfusion.

RESPIRATORY PHYSIOLOGY

1. The Fick law for transfer of gases

$$V_{gas} = \frac{(A)}{0.5}\,(k)\,(P_1 - P_2)$$

V_{gas} Rate of gas transfer across a membrane
A   Tissue area
0.5   Thickness of the pulmonary membrane (in μm)
k Solubility coefficient of the gas
$P_1 - P_2$ Partial pressure gradient of the gas across the membrane (in mm Hg)

CO_2 diffuses 20 times faster than O_2 due to differences in their solubility coefficients.

2. Calculation of the alveolar oxygen partial pressure (PAo$_2$)

$$PAo_2 = (713)\,(Fio_2) - \frac{Paco_2}{0.8}$$

PAo$_2$ Alveolar oxygen partial pressure (in mm Hg)
713   Sea level barometric pressure (760 mm Hg) minus the
            partial pressure of water vapor (PH$_2$O, 47 mm Hg)
Fio$_2$ Fractional concentration of inspired oxygen
Paco$_2$ Partial pressure of CO_2 (in mm Hg, from arterial blood
            gas data)
0.8   Respiratory quotient

3. Calculation of the alveolar-arterial oxygen gradient (P[A-a]o$_2$)

$$P[A-a]o_2 = PAo_2 - Pao_2$$

P[A-a]o$_2$ Alveolar-arterial oxygen gradient (in mm Hg)
PAo$_2$ Alveolar oxygen partial pressure (in mm Hg)
Pao$_2$ Arterial oxygen partial pressure (in mm Hg, from
               arterial blood gas data)

Normal P[A-a]o$_2$ is 12 mm Hg in young adults and increases to 20 mm Hg by the age of 70 years. In failure of ventilation, the P[A-a]o$_2$ will increase.

RENAL PHYSIOLOGY

1. Creatinine clearance (CrCl)

$$CrCl = \frac{(140 - age)\,(wt)}{(72)\,(Cr)}$$

CrCl   Creatinine clearance (in ml/min)
Age   Patient's age (in years)
Wt   Patient's weight (in kg)
Cr   Serum creatinine concentration (in mg/dl)
Normal   90–150 ml/min
  CrCl

Appendix 2: Formulary*

This formulary includes medications which are commonly encountered while on call. Dosages listed are for adults, and generic names are listed. Antibiotic dosages are listed in Appendix C. Always be mindful of the renal and hepatic function of the patient before administration of medications, and be aware that many patients require individualization of medications. Also, be aware that many medications require individualization of dose. For further information, consult the pharmacy or the medication insert instructions.

Acetaminophen

Proprietary name(s)	Tylenol and others
Therapeutic class	Analgesic and antipyretic
Indications	Pain and fever
Actions	Diminishes pain response and has direct action on hypothalamus temperature regulation centers
Metabolism	Hepatic
Excretion	Renal
Side effects	Uncommon; rash, drug fever, mucosal ulcerations, leukopenia, pancytopenia, and hepatic toxicity
Dose	325–1000 mg PO/PR every 4–6 hr as needed, to 4000 mg/24 hr.
Notes	Little to no anti-inflammatory action. Does not affect the aggregation of platelets. Does not interact with anticoagulants. Antidote for overdose is N-acetylcysteine.

Albuterol

Proprietary name(s)	Proventil and Ventolin
Therapeutic class	β_2-Adrenergic agonist

*From Adams GA, Bresnick SD: On Call Surgery, 2nd ed. Philadelphia, WB Saunders, 2001.

Indications	Bronchospasm due to asthma, bronchitis, or chronic obstructive pulmonary disease (COPD)
Actions	β_2-Adrenergic agonist
Metabolism	Hepatic; less than 20% of the inhaled dose is absorbed systemically.
Excretion	Renal
Side effects	Headache, tachycardia, lightheadedness, dizziness, tremor, palpitations, and nausea
Dose	2.5–5 mg in 3 ml normal saline (NS) by nebulizer every 4 hr as needed. Severe acute bronchospasm may require doses every 3–5 min initially.
Notes	May alternate with metaproterenol.

Allopurinol

Proprietary name(s)	Zyloprim
Therapeutic class	Xanthine oxidase inhibitor
Indications	Symptomatic gout, uric acid nephropathy, and lysis of tumor
Actions	Inhibits formation of uric acid
Metabolism	Metabolite oxipurinol is also active
Excretion	Renal
Side effects	Rash, fever, gastrointestinal (GI) upset, cataracts, renal toxicity, and hepatotoxicity
Dose	100–300 mg PO every day after meals. Severe cases may require doses up to 800 mg/day.
Notes	Reduce the dose in renal or hepatic insufficiency. Acute gout episodes may follow initiation of therapy. Aminophylline, mercaptopurine, and azathioprine levels may be increased by allopurinol. Nonsteroidal anti-inflammatory drugs (NSAIDs) are the first-line therapy for acute gout.

Aluminum hydroxide

Proprietary name(s)	Amphojel and ALternaGEL
Therapeutic class	Antacid
Indications	Epigastric pain due to peptic ulcer disease or gastritis. Prophylaxis for stress ulcers. Reduction of urinary phosphate in patients with phosphate-containing renal stones.

Actions	Buffers gastric acid; binds to phosphate in the GI tract
Side effects	Constipation, anorexia, nausea, hypophosphatemia, and aluminum toxicity in patients with renal failure
Dose	For acute symptoms, 30–60 ml PO every 1–2 hr as needed.
	For maintenance therapy, 30–60 ml PO every 1–3 hr when symptomatic and before bedtime as needed.
Notes	May bind to and reduce the absorption of tetracycline, thyroxine, and other medications.

Aluminum hydroxide/Magnesium hydroxide

Proprietary name(s)	Maalox and Mylanta
Therapeutic class	Antacid
Indications	Pain due to peptic ulcer disease, reflux esophagitis, and prophylaxis of stress ulcers
Actions	Buffers gastric acidity
Side effects	Diarrhea, hypermagnesemia, or aluminum toxicity in patients with renal failure
Dose	For acute symptoms, 30–60 ml PO every 1–2 hr as needed.
	For maintenance therapy, 30–60 ml PO every 1–3 hr when symptomatic and before bedtime as needed.
Notes	Aluminum salts cause constipation. Magnesium salts cause diarrhea. The mixture of the salts tends to balance the effects.
	May bind to and reduce the absorption of tetracycline, thyroxine, and other medications.

Amikacin (See antibiotic listing in Appendix 3)

Aminocaproic acid

Proprietary name(s)	Amicar
Therapeutic class	Plasminogen activator inhibitor
Indications	Hemorrhage due to fibrinolysis
Actions	Inhibits plasminogen activator; also has antiplasmin activity
Metabolism	65% of drug is excreted unchanged
Excretion	Renal

Side effects
: Increased risk of deep venous thrombosis (DVT), cerebral embolism, and pulmonary embolism. Nausea, abdominal cramps, dizziness, rash, and headaches.

Dose
: Loading dose of 4–5 g IV over 1 hr, followed by maintenance infusion of 1–1.25 g/hr to achieve plasma levels of 0.13 mg/ml or until clinical bleeding stops.
Maximum dose, 30 g/24 hr.
Loading dose may be given PO.

Notes
: Rule out disseminated intravascular coagulation (DIC) before administration.

Aminophylline

Therapeutic class
: Bronchodilator

Indications
: Bronchospasm due to asthma

Actions
: Methylxanthine; inhibits phosphodiesterase activity, resulting in smooth muscle relaxation and bronchodilation. Also activates respiratory centers.

Metabolism
: Hepatic (90%)

Excretion
: Renal

Side effects
: Tachycardia, increased ventricular ectopy, nausea, vomiting, headaches, seizures, insomnia, and nightmares

Dose
: Loading dose of 6 mg/kg IV, followed by maintenance infusion of 0.5–0.7 mg/kg/hr. Use 0.5 loading dose if the patient is already taking theophylline.

Notes
: May follow plasma level, but patient side effects generally limit therapeutic usefulness. Decrease the dose in patients with congestive heart failure (CHF) and liver disease and in elderly patients.
Aminophylline clearance is decreased by erythromycin, cimetidine, propranolol, allopurinol, and a number of other medications.

Amoxicillin (See antibiotic listing in Appendix 3)

Amphotericin B

Proprietary name(s)
: Fungizone

Therapeutic class
: Polyene antifungal

Indications	Systemic fungal infections
Actions	Disruption of fungal cell membrane
Excretion	Renal
Side effects	Fever, chills, nausea, vomiting, diarrhea, hypotension, nephrotoxicity, hypokalemia, hypomagnesemia, and thrombophlebitis
Dose	Initial test dose: 0.1 mg/kg in 100 ml 50% dextrose in water IV over 2 hr.
	If tolerated, further doses of 10 mg may be given on the first day.
	Daily dose then may be increased by 0.25 mg/kg/day until the desired dose of 0.5–1.0 mg/kg/day is achieved. Administer IV over 4–6 hr.
	It is more important to administer a complete total course than it is to achieve the desirable daily dose. If the patient does not tolerate that high a concentration, simply lower the daily dose and extend the length of therapy.
Notes	Patients vary with respect to how well they tolerate amphotericin B therapy. Premedicate before each dose with antipyretics, antihistamines, antiemetics, and corticosteroids to reduce side effects. Follow serial potassium and magnesium levels during therapy and watch for renal insufficiency.
	Liposome-conjugated amphotericin B (Abelcet) may be given in doses of 5 mg/kg/day.

Ampicillin (See antibiotic listing in Appendix 3)

Aspirin (acetylsalicylic acid)

Therapeutic class	Analgesic, antipyretic, and anti-inflammatory
Indications	Pain due to inflammation, fever, and anti-platelet aggregation agent in coronary syndromes
Actions	Acts peripherally by interfering with the production of prostaglandins, thus reducing pain and inflammation
	Acts centrally to reduce pain perception and reduce temperature by increasing heat loss

Side effects	Gastric erosion and bleeding, tinnitus, fever, thirst, and diaphoresis
	Severe allergic reactions can occur, including asthma-like symptoms.
Dose	For mild pain or fever, 325–650 mg PO every 4–6 hr.
	For chest pain due to pericarditis, 650 mg PO 4 times per day.
	For angina and antiplatelet effects, 30–325 mg PO every day or every other day.
	For treatment of rheumatoid arthritis, 2.6–5.2 g/day in divided doses.

Aztreonam (See antibiotic listing in Appendix 3)

Beclomethasone

Proprietary name(s)	Beclovent and Vanceril
Therapeutic class	Inhaled corticosteroid
Indications	Bronchial asthma and long-term therapy
Actions	Topical anti-inflammatory
Excretion	Fecal
Side effects	Oral and pharyngeal candidiasis, laryngeal myopathy
Dose	2 inhalations 2–4 times per day. May be more effective if administered 3–5 min after a bronchodilator dose.
Notes	Not indicated for acute bronchospasm.

Bisacodyl

Proprietary name(s)	Dulcolax
Therapeutic class	Laxative
Indications	Constipation
Action	Stimulates peristalsis
Metabolism	Poorly absorbed
Side effects	Abdominal cramping, nausea, rectal burning or bleeding
Dose	10–15 mg PO every night as needed.
	10-mg suppository PR every night as needed.
Notes	Avoid in pregnancy or after a myocardial infarction (MI). May worsen orthostatic hypotension, weakness, and incoordination in elderly patients.

Avoid in acute abdomen and intestinal
  obstruction or with recent intestinal
  anastomoses.
Onset of action is 6–10 hr after PO
  dose, 15–60 min after a PR dose.

Bumetanide

Proprietary name(s)	Bumex
Therapeutic class	Loop diuretic; rapid onset, short duration of action
Indications	Edema associated with CHF, cirrhosis, renal disease, or nephrotic syndrome
Actions	Inhibits the reabsorption of Na^+ and Cl^- in the ascending limb of the loop of Henle. Increases potassium excretion.
Excretion	Renal (80%)
Side effects	Electrolyte depletion, rash, hyperuricemia, and reversible deafness
Dose	0.5–2.0 mg PO/IV per day in a single dose. May repeat every 20 min, if necessary, to a maximum of 3 mg.
Notes	1 mg bumetanide is equivalent to 40 mg furosemide.

Calcium gluconate

Therapeutic class	Calcium supplement
Indications	Symptomatic hypocalcemia and hyperkalemia. Adjunct therapy in cardiopulmonary resuscitation (CPR)
Actions	Replacement. Decreases cardiac automaticity and raises cardiac cell resting potential.
Side effects	Administration to patients concurrently on digoxin therapy may precipitate ventricular dysrhythmias due to combined effects of digoxin and Ca^{2+}.
Dose	For control of hypocalcemia, 1–15 g PO every day. For more rapid response, 5–10 ml of 10% solution IV.
Notes	500 mg of calcium gluconate = 2.3 mmol ionized Ca^{2+}. 10% solution contains 0.45 mmol ionized Ca^{2+}/ml.

Captopril

Proprietary name(s)	Capoten
Therapeutic class	Angiotensin-converting enzyme (ACE) inhibitor
Indications	Hypertension, CHF, and prophylaxis against diabetic nephropathy
Actions	Inhibits the enzyme responsible for pulmonary conversion of angiotensin I to angiotensin II
Excretion	Renal (59%)
Side effects	Hypotension, impaired taste, cough, rash, angioedema, neutropenia, proteinuria, and renal insufficiency
Dose	Begin with a test dose of 6.25 mg PO and monitor blood pressure (BP) for 4 hr.
	For hypertension, titrate to 25–50 mg PO 2–3 times per day.
	For CHF, titrate to 25–50 mg PO 3 times per day.
Notes	May cause hyperkalemia if used in patients receiving potassium-sparing diuretics or receiving potassium supplementation.

Cefazolin (See antibiotic listing in Appendix 3)

Cefotaxime (See antibiotic listing in Appendix 3)

Cefoxitin (See antibiotic listing in Appendix 3)

Ceftazidime (See antibiotic listing in Appendix 3)

Ceftriaxone (See antibiotic listing in Appendix 3)

Cefuroxime (See antibiotic listing in Appendix 3)

Celecoxib

Proprietary name(s)	Celebrex
Therapeutic class	Selective COX-2 inhibitor
Indications	Osteoarthritis, rheumatoid arthritis, familial adenomatous polyposis
Actions	Inhibition of prostaglandin production via inhibition of cyclooxygenase-2
Metabolism	Cytochrome P450 2C9
Excretion	Hepatic metabolism
Side effects	Rare; hepatic dysfunction, fluid retention, edema, GI bleeding
Dose	For arthritis pain relief, 100–200 mg PO two times per day.

Notes | For familial adenomatous polyposis, 400 mg PO two times per day.
Not recommended in patients who have aspirin allergy. Not recommended in patients with sulfa allergy. Less GI upset reported than wih nonselective NSAIDs.

Chloral hydrate

Therapeutic class | Alcohol hypnotic
Indications | Insomnia
Actions | Hypnotic
Side effects | Gastric irritation, rash, paradoxical agitation
Dose | 0.5–1.0 g PO/PR every night as needed.
Notes | Avoid in patients with liver or kidney disease.

Chlordiazepoxide

Proprietary name(s) | Librium and others
Therapeutic class | Benzodiazepine
Indications | Anxiety and alcohol withdrawal
Actions | Benzodiazepine sedative and anxiolytic agent
Metabolism | Hepatic
Excretion | Renal
Side effects | Central nervous system (CNS) depression, drowsiness, ataxia, confusion, and pruritic rash
Dose | For anxiety, 5–25 mg PO 3–4 times per day.
For alcohol withdrawal, 50–100 mg intramuscularly (IM)/IV every 2–6 hr as needed, maximum dose of 500 mg in the first 24 hr.
Notes | Dose must be individualized.
Unpredictable absorption after IM injection.
Antidote is flumazenil.

Chlorpromazine

Proprietary name(s) | Thorazine
Therapeutic class | Phenothiazine antipsychotic and antiemetic
Indications | Agitation, nausea, vomiting, and hiccoughs

Actions	Antagonist of dopamine, histamine, muscarine, and α_1-adrenergic responses
Side effects	CNS depression, hypotension, extrapyramidal effects, and jaundice
Dose	For mild agitation, 25–75 mg PO every day.
	For more severe cases, 150 mg PO every day or 25–50 mg IM with repeated doses every 3–4 hr, as needed.
	For hiccoughs, nausea, and vomiting, 10–15 mg PO/IM every 6–8 hr.
Notes	For acute agitation, haloperidol may be a more appropriate choice as it has less effect on BP.

Chlorpropamide

Proprietary name(s)	Diabinese and others
Therapeutic class	Oral hypoglycemic agent
Indications	Non–insulin-dependent diabetes mellitus (NIDDM)
Actions	Sulfonylurea. Stimulates insulin secretion, and increases the effects of insulin on the liver to increase gluconeogenesis and on the muscle to increase glucose use.
Metabolism	Renal excretion
Side effects	Hypoglycemia, rash, blood dyscrasias, jaundice, hyponatremia, and edema
Dose	100–500 mg PO every day in 1 or 2 doses.
Notes	Has a long duration of action (20–60 hr). Hypoglycemic reactions may be prolonged in elderly patients and in those patients with renal impairment.
	Drug associations causing hypoglycemia: NSAIDs, salicylates, sulfonamides, chloramphenicol, cimetidine, ranitidine, probenecid, warfarin, monoamine oxidase (MAO) inhibitors, β-blockers, and metformin.
	Drug associations causing hyperglycemia: Thiazides, diuretics, corticosteroids, phenothiazines, thyroid hormone replacement agents, oral contraceptive agents, phenytoin,

sympathomimetics, calcium channel blockers, and isoniazid.

Cimetidine

Proprietary name(s)	Tagamet
Therapeutic class	Histamine$_2$ antagonist
Indications	Peptic ulcer disease and gastroesophageal reflux
Actions	Inhibits histamine-induced secretion of gastric acid
Metabolism	Hepatic
Excretion	Renal
Side effects	Gynecomastia, impotence, confusion, diarrhea, leukopenia, thrombocytopenia, and increased serum creatinine
Dose	For peptic ulcer, 300 mg PO or IV every 6–8 hr, or 800 mg PO every night. For reflux, 400 mg PO 2 times per day.
Notes	Reduces microsomal enzyme metabolism of medications, including oral anticoagulants, phenytoin, and theophylline.

Ciprofloxacin (See antibiotic listing in Appendix 3)

Clindamycin (See antibiotic listing in Appendix 3)

Clopidogrel

Proprietary name(s)	Plavix
Therapeutic class	ADP-binding agent, inhibits platelet aggregation
Indications	Atherosclerotic disease
Actions	Inhibition of ADP-dependent platelet aggregation
Metabolism	Hepatic
Excretion	50% urine, 46% stool
Side effects	Rare, GI bleeding, neutropenia, rash
Dose	75 mg PO each day.
Notes	Risks of bleeding are similar to aspirin.

Codeine

Therapeutic class	Narcotic analgesic
Indications	Pain, cough, and diarrhea
Actions	Narcotic analgesic, depresses the medullary cough center, and decreases propulsive contractions of the small bowel

Metabolism	Hepatic
Excretion	Renal (90%)
Side effects	Dysphoria, agitation, pruritus, constipation, lightheadedness, and sedation
Dose	For analgesia, 30–60 mg PO/subcutaneously (SC)/IM every 4–6 hr, as needed.
	For cough or diarrhea, 8–30 mg PO/SC/IM every 4 hr, as needed.
Notes	Useful for mild to moderate pain. May be habit forming.

Clotrimazole

Proprietary name(s)	Lotrimin and Mycelex
Therapeutic class	Antifungal
Indications	Esophageal, vaginal, and intertrigonal candidiasis
Actions	Damages fungal cell membranes
Side effects	Local irritation
Dose	For esophageal candidiasis, 10-mg troche PO 4 times per day.
	For vaginal candidiasis, 100 mg intravaginally every night × 7 nights.
	For intertrigonal candidiasis, 1% cream or solution applied 2 times per day.

Diazepam

Proprietary name(s)	Valium and others
Therapeutic class	Benzodiazepine
Indications	Anxiety, seizures, and alcohol withdrawal
Actions	Benzodiazepine sedative and anxiolytic agent
Metabolism	Hepatic (to active metabolites)
Excretion	Renal
Side effects	Sedation, hypotension, respiratory depression, and paradoxical agitation
Dose	For anxiety, 2–10 mg PO/IM/IV 2–4 times per day.
	For status epilepticus, 2 mg/min IV until the seizure ceases or to a total dose of 20 mg.
	For alcohol withdrawal, 5–10 mg IV at a rate of 2–5 mg/min every 30–60 min until the patient is sedated, then maintain on 10–20 mg PO 4 times per day.

| Notes | Dose must be individualized.
Unpredictable absorption after IM injection.
Rectal and endotracheal tube (ET) administration possible in emergency situations.
Antidote is flumazenil. |

Digoxin

Proprietary name(s)	Lanoxin
Therapeutic class	Digitalis glycoside
Indications	Supraventricular tachycardia and CHF
Actions	Slows atrioventricular (AV) conduction, increases the force of cardiac contraction, and is Na^+/K^+-ATPase inhibitor
Metabolism	Hepatic (<10%)
Excretion	Renal (80%)
Side effects	Dysrhythmias, nausea, vomiting, and neuropsychiatric disturbances
Dose	Load with 0.125–0.5 mg IV every 6 hr to a total dose of 1 mg, or load with 0.125–0.5 mg PO every 6 hr to a total dose of 1.5 mg, then maintain on 0.125–0.25 mg PO/IV every day. Some supraventricular tachycardias may require higher doses.
Notes	Reduce dose in elderly patients and in those patients with renal impairment. May cause arrhythmias in settings of hypokalemia or hypercalcemia.

Diltiazem

Proprietary name(s)	Cardizem
Therapeutic class	Calcium channel blocker
Indications	Angina pectoris, coronary spasm, and hypertension
Actions	Calcium channel blocker and vasodilator
Metabolism	Hepatic
Excretion	Renal and biliary
Side effects	First-degree AV block, bradycardia, flushing, dizziness, headache, peripheral edema, nausea, rash, and asthenia
Dose	Initial dose, 30 mg PO 3–4 times per day, with titration to 180–360 mg/day administered in divided doses.

Notes

Maximum antihypertensive effect is seen at 14 days.
Sustained-release forms are available.

Diphenhydramine

Proprietary name(s)
Therapeutic class
Indications
Actions
Metabolism
Excretion
Side effects

Dose

Notes

Benadryl
Antihistamine
Allergic reactions
Antihistamine and anticholinergic
Hepatic
Renal
Drowsiness, dizziness, dry mouth, and urinary retention
25–50 mg PO/IV/IM every 6–8 hr as needed.
Anticholinergic effects may be additive to those noted with other medications such as tricyclic antidepressants.

Docusate

Proprietary name(s)
Therapeutic class
Indications
Actions

Side effects
Dose
Notes

Colace and Dialose
Laxative
Prevention of constipation
Stool softener and lowers surface tension
Nausea and bitter taste
100 mg PO 3 times per day.
Effects not immediate, may not be noticeable for 1–2 days.

Enalapril

Proprietary name(s)
Therapeutic class
Indications
Actions

Metabolism

Excretion
Side effects

Dose

Vasotec
ACE inhibitor
Hypertension and CHF
Inhibits the enzyme responsible for conversion of angiotensin I to angiotensin II
Hepatic (to active metabolite, enalaprilat)
Renal
Hypotension, headache, nausea, and diarrhea
Begin with a test dose of 2.5 mg PO and monitor BP for 4 hr.

For hypertension, titrate to 2.5–40
mg PO every day.
For CHF, titrate to 10–25 mg PO 2
times per day.

Notes   May cause hyperkalemia if used in
patients receiving potassium-sparing
diuretics or receiving potassium
supplementation.

Erythromycin (See antibiotic listing in Appendix 3)

Ethacrynic acid

Proprietary name(s)	Edecrin
Therapeutic class	Loop diuretic
Indications	CHF and edema
Actions	Inhibition of the reabsorption of Na$^+$ and Cl$^-$ in the ascending limb of the loop of Henle
Side effects	Electrolyte depletion, hyperuricemia, hyperglycemia, anorexia, nausea, vomiting, diarrhea, and sensorineural hearing loss
Dose	50 mg IV × 1 or 2 doses.
Notes	May have more side effects than other loop diuretics. Onset is rapid, within 30 min of a PO dose or within 5 min of an IV dose.

Famotidine

Proprietary name(s)	Pepcid
Therapeutic class	Histamine$_2$ antagonist
Indications	Peptic ulcer disease and gastroesophageal reflux
Actions	Inhibits histamine-induced secretion of gastric acid
Metabolism	Hepatic (to inactive metabolite)
Excretion	Renal (70%)
Side effects	Headache, dizziness, constipation, diarrhea, GI upset, and rash
Dose	For acute disease, 40 mg PO every day or 20 mg IV 2 times per day. For maintenance, 20 mg PO every night.
Notes	Less effect on microsomal enzymes or androgen blocking than cimetidine.

Ferrous sulfate

Therapeutic class	Iron supplement
Indications	Iron deficiency
Actions	Replaces iron stores
Side effects	Constipation, nausea, diarrhea, and abdominal cramping
Dose	325 mg PO 3 times per day.
Notes	300 mg ferrous sulfate = 60 mg elemental iron.
	Stool may turn black.
	GI absorption enhanced on an empty stomach with concomitant vitamin C administration (200 mg vitamin C/30 mg iron).
	Iron stores will not be completely replaced for up to 4–6 mo of therapy after normalization of the hematocrit.

Fluconazole

Proprietary name(s)	Diflucan
Therapeutic class	Antifungal
Indications	Oropharyngeal, esophageal, and systemic candidiasis; cryptococcal meningitis
Actions	Inhibition of cell membranes of yeasts and fungi
Excretion	Renal
Side effects	Nausea, vomiting, headache, rash, abdominal pain, diarrhea, and hepatic necrosis
Dose	For oral or esophageal disease, initial dose of 200 mg PO followed by 100 mg PO every day.
	For systemic candidiasis and cryptococcal meningitis, 200–400 mg PO every day.
	Reduce the dose in those patients with renal impairment.
Notes	Many drug interactions due to the microsomal enzyme inhibition, including sulfonylureas, phenytoin, warfarin, and cyclophosphamide.

Flumazenil

Proprietary name(s)	Romazicon
Therapeutic class	Benzodiazepine antagonist

Indications	Reversal of benzodiazepine-induced sedation
Actions	Benzodiazepine receptor antagonist
Metabolism	Hepatic
Excretion	Renal
Side effects	Seizures, headache, vasodilation, nausea, vomiting, agitation, dizziness, abnormal vision, and paresthesias
Dose	For reversal of sedation, 0.2 mg IV over 15 sec. Repeat as necessary in increments of 0.2 mg every 60 sec, to a maximum dose of 1 mg. For treatment of benzodiazepine overdose, 0.2 mg IV over 30 sec. An additional 0.3 mg IV may be administered after 30 sec, if necessary. Further doses of 0.5 mg may be given IV every 30 sec as needed to a maximum of 3 mg.
Notes	Avoid in patients with evidence of cyclic antidepressant overdose. Does not reverse benzodiazepine-induced respiratory depression. Monitor for return of benzodiazepine-related symptoms of sedation and respiratory depression.

Furosemide

Proprietary name(s)	Lasix
Therapeutic class	Loop diuretic
Indications	CHF, edema, hyperkalemia, and hypercalcemia
Actions	Inhibition of the reabsorption of Na^+ and Cl^- in the ascending limb of the loop of Henle
Metabolism	Hepatic
Excretion	Renal
Side effects	Electrolyte depletion, hyperuricemia, hyperglycemia, and reversible deafness
Dose	For acute pulmonary edema, 20–40 mg PO/IV with repeat doses every 60–90 min as needed, to a maximum of 600 mg/day.

Notes

Higher doses may be required in
patients with severe disease or renal
failure.
Loop diuretics are well absorbed orally
with rapid onset of action.

Gentamicin (See antibiotic listing in Appendix 3)

Haloperidol

Proprietary name(s)	Haldol
Therapeutic class	Antipsychotic
Indications	Psychotic disorders and acute agitation
Actions	Antipsychotic neuroleptic butyrophenone
Side effects	Extrapyramidal reactions, postural hypotension, sedation, galactorrhea, jaundice, blurred vision, bronchospasm, and neuroleptic malignant syndrome
Dose	0.5–2.0 mg PO 3 times per day. For acute psychotic crises, 2–10 mg IM every 1 hr as needed.
Notes	Extrapyramidal side effects are more pronounced, but hypotension is less frequent than with phenothiazines.

Heparin sodium

Therapeutic class	Anticoagulant
Indications	Prophylaxis and treatment of DVT, pulmonary embolism, embolic cerebrovascular accident (CVA). Adjunct in treatment of unstable angina, and thrombolytic therapy.
Actions	Acts in conjunction with antithrombin III, which neutralizes several activated clotting factors. Antithrombin effect.
Metabolism	Hepatic
Excretion	Renal
Side effects	Hemorrhage and thrombocytopenia
Dose	For DVT or pulmonary embolus, load IV with 5000–10,000 U followed by continuous infusion of 1000–2000 U/hr IV. Low-dose SC: 5000 U every 8–12 hr. High-dose SC: 10,000–12,500 U every 8–12 hr. Titrate to desired partial thromboplastin time (PTT) (generally 1.5–2 × control).

| Notes | Monitor PTT closely. Also prolongs prothrombin time (PT). Overheparinization is treated with protamine sulfate. Usual dose is 1 mg protamine/100 U heparin given slowly IV. |

Hydralazine

Proprietary name(s)	Apresoline
Therapeutic class	Arterial vasodilator
Indications	Hypertension
Actions	Arterial vasodilator
Metabolism	Hepatic
Side effects	Tachycardia, headache, blood dyscrasias, nausea, vomiting, diarrhea, systemic lupus erythematosus (SLE) reaction at higher doses (>200 mg/day)
Dose	10–25 mg PO every 6 hr. 20–40 mg IV/IM every 3–6 hr as needed.
Notes	Very limited effect on veins, so minimal postural hypotension. Monitor carefully in patients with coronary artery disease.

Hydrochlorothiazide

Proprietary name(s)	Esidrix and HydroDIURIL
Therapeutic class	Thiazide diuretic
Indications	Hypertension, CHF, and edema
Actions	Blocks Na^+ and Cl^- reabsorption in the cortical diluting segment of the loop of Henle
Excretion	Renal
Side effects	Electrolyte depletion, hyperuricemia, hyperglycemia, hypercalcemia, pancreatitis, jaundice, nausea, vomiting, and diarrhea
Dose	12.5–50 mg PO every day.
Notes	Adequate potassium replacement necessary with long-term therapy.

Hydrocortisone

| Therapeutic class | Corticosteroid |
| Indications | Severe bronchospasm, anaphylaxis, hypercalcemia, and adrenal insufficiency |

Actions — Anti-inflammatory

Side effects — Na^+ retention, hyperglycemia, and K^+ loss. Behavioral disturbances.

Dose — 250 mg IV followed by 100 mg IV every 6 hr.

Notes — Contraindicated in settings of systemic fungal infections.

Hydroxyzine

Proprietary name(s) — Atarax and Vistaril

Therapeutic class — Antihistamine and antiemetic

Indications — Anxiety, pruritus, nausea, and vomiting

Actions — Suppression of activity in subcortical CNS sites

Metabolism — Hepatic

Side effects — Drowsiness, dry mouth, and tremor

Dose — For anxiety, 50–100 mg PO/IM 4 times per day.
For pruritus or nausea, 25–100 mg PO/IM 3–4 times per day.

Notes — May potentiate the sedation effects of other CNS depressants.

Ibuprofen

Proprietary name(s) — Motrin and others

Therapeutic class — NSAID

Indications — Inflammation due to arthritis, soft-tissue injuries, and analgesia

Actions — Propionic acid derivative. Interferes with the production of prostaglandins.

Metabolism — Hepatic

Excretion — Renal

Side effects — Nausea, diarrhea, gastric pain, gastric erosions, dizziness, headache, tinnitus, and vision changes. May compromise renal function in patients with renal impairment.
Contraindicated in the syndrome of aspirin sensitivity, nasal polyps, and bronchospasm.

Dose — For analgesia, 200 mg PO 3–4 times per day.
For anti-inflammatory effects, 200–400 mg PO 3–4 times per day.
Maximum dose: 3200 mg/day.

Notes — Available in many over-the-counter preparations.

Should be used with caution in patients receiving anticoagulant medications.

Imipenem (See antibiotic listing in Appendix 3)

Indomethacin

Proprietary name(s)	Indocin
Therapeutic class	NSAID
Indications	Inflammation due to arthritis, acute gout, soft-tissue injury, and pericarditis
Actions	Indole acetic acid derivative. Interferes with the production of prostaglandins.
Metabolism	Hepatic
Excretion	Renal
Side effects	Headache, dizziness and lightheadedness, and epigastric pain. May compromise renal function in patients with renal impairment. Contraindicated in the syndrome of aspirin sensitivity, nasal polyps, and bronchospasm.
Dose	25–50 mg PO 3 times per day. Maximum daily dose: 150–200 mg/day.
Notes	May increase the risk of bleeding in patients receiving anticoagulants. Take with food to minimize GI upset.

Insulin

Therapeutic class	Hypoglycemic
Indications	Diabetes mellitus
Actions	Enhances hepatic glycogen storage, enhances entry of glucose and potassium into cells, and inhibits the breakdown of protein and fat
Side effects	Hypoglycemia, local skin reactions, and lipohypertrophy
Dose	Must be individualized
Notes	Less immunogenicity is seen with recombinant human insulin than with insulins from animal sources.

Isosorbide dinitrate

Proprietary name(s)	Isordil and Sorbitrate
Therapeutic class	Vasodilator
Indications	Angina pectoris and CHF
Actions	Venous, coronary, and arterial vasodilator

Side effects	Headache, hypotension, and flushing
Dose	5–30 mg PO 4 times per day.
Notes	Nitrate tolerance may develop with prolonged continuous administration.

Ketoconazole

Proprietary name(s)	Nizoral
Therapeutic class	Imidazole antifungal
Indications	Esophageal candidiasis, pulmonary histoplasmosis
Actions	Inhibition of yeast and fungal cell growth
Metabolism	Hepatic
Excretion	Biliary (>80%)
Side effects	Nausea, anorexia, vomiting, rash, pruritus, gynecomastia, and impotence. Inhibits microsomal enzymes, so may interfere with the metabolism of warfarin, cyclophosphamide, and other medications.
Dose	200–400 mg PO every day.
Notes	Absorption is impaired in patients receiving medications that reduce gastric acidity.

Labetalol

Proprietary name(s)	Normodyne and Trandate
Therapeutic class	α_1- and β-blocker
Indications	Hypertensive emergencies
Actions	α_1-Blocking action is predominant in acute use but is accompanied by nonspecific β-blockade
Metabolism	Hepatic
Excretion	Renal
Side effects	Postural hypotension, bronchospasm, jaundice, bradycardia, and negative inotropic effect. Avoid in patients with asthma or with severe bradycardia.
Dose	20 mg IV every 10–15 min. Increase the dose incrementally (e.g., 20 mg, 20 mg, 40 mg, 40 mg . . .) every 10 min until the desired supine BP is achieved. Alternatively, a continuous drip may be started at 2 mg/min with titration to desired BP response, with a maximum daily dose of 2400 mg.

Notes   Contraindicated in patients in whom β-blockade is undesirable.

Levodopa-carbidopa

Proprietary name(s)	Sinemet
Therapeutic class	Dopamine agonist
Indications	Parkinson's disease
Actions	Levodopa is converted to dopamine in the basal ganglia. Carbidopa inhibits the peripheral destruction of levodopa.
Side effects	Anorexia, nausea, vomiting, abdominal pain, dysrhythmias, behavioral changes, orthostatic hypotension, and involuntary motions
Dose	Begin with 1 tablet (100 mg/10 mg) PO 2 times per day. Increase the dose until the desired response is obtained, with a maximum daily dose of 8 tablets (800 mg/80 mg).
Notes	Side effects are common.

Lidocaine

Proprietary name(s)	Xylocaine
Therapeutic class	Class IB antiarrhythmic
Indications	Ventricular arrhythmias, prophylaxis, and treatment
Actions	Lengthens the effective refractory period in the ventricular conduction system. Decreases ventricular automaticity.
Metabolism	Hepatic
Excretion	Renal
Side effects	Nausea, vomiting, hypotension, confusion, seizures, perioral paresthesias, drowsiness, and dizziness
Dose	Load with 1 mg/kg IV over 2–3 min. Further doses of 50 mg IV may be given at 5–10-min intervals to a total dose of 300 mg. Maintain with 1–4 mg/min continuous IV infusion. For prophylaxis, a loading dose of 200 mg given in 50-mg increments every 5 min, followed by maintenance IV infusion of 3 mg/min.

Notes   Lower maintenance doses are required in elderly patients or in those with CHF, hepatic failure, or hypotension.

Lorazepam

Proprietary name(s)   Ativan
Therapeutic class   Benzodiazepine
Indications   Insomnia and anxiety
Actions   Benzodiazepine sedative-hypnotic
Metabolism   Hepatic
Excretion   Renal
Side effects   Sedation and respiratory depression
Dose   For sleep, 0.5–1.0 mg PO/IM every night. For anxiety, 1 mg PO/IM 2 times per day. Maximum dose: 4 mg/dose.
Notes   Peak effect in 1–6 hr. Antidote is flumazenil.

Mannitol

Proprietary name(s)   Osmitrol
Therapeutic class   Osmotic diuretic
Indications   Peripheral edema, cerebral edema, and hemolytic transfusion reactions
Actions   Osmotic diuresis
Excretion   Renal
Side effects   Volume overload, hyperosmolality, hyponatremia, nausea, and headache
Dose   Test dose of 12.5 g over 3–5 min. Effects should be noted within 2 hr. 25–100 g IV over 15–30 min every 2–3 hr as needed.
Notes   Requires functioning kidneys to work, contraindicated in renal failure. Monitor electrolytes.

Meperidine

Proprietary name(s)   Demerol
Therapeutic class   Narcotic analgesic
Indications   Moderate to severe pain
Actions   Narcotic analgesic
Metabolism   Hepatic
Excretion   Renal
Side effects   Respiratory depression, hypotension, nausea, vomiting, constipation, agitation, and rash

Dose	50–150 mg SC/IM/PO every 4 hr.
Notes	60–80 mg meperidine (SC/IM/PO) is equivalent to 10 mg morphine (SC/IV). Often administered with concomitant antinausea medication.
	Antidote is naloxone.
	May be habit forming.

Mesalamine

Proprietary name(s)	Asacol, Pentasa
Therapeutic class	Delayed-release sulfasalazine, anti-inflammatory
Indications	Inflammatory bowel disease
Actions	Luminal anti-inflammatory, inhibition of prostaglandin synthesis
Metabolism	Acetylated by gut mucosa
Excretion	72% stool (not absorbed), 28% kidney
Side effects	Mild; headache, GI upset, diarrhea, asthenia
Dose	400–800 mg PO 3 times per day.
Notes	May cause aberrations in liver function tests.

Metaproterenol

Proprietary name(s)	Alupent
Therapeutic class	β_2-Adrenergic agonist
Indications	Bronchospasm due to asthma, bronchitis, or COPD
Actions	β_2-Adrenergic agonist
Metabolism	Hepatic. 3% of aerosol dose is systemically absorbed.
Side effects	Headache, tachycardia, hypertension, lightheadedness, dizziness, tremor, palpitations, nausea, and vomiting
Dose	0.2–0.3 mg in 3 ml NS by nebulizer every 4 hr as needed.
	Severe acute bronchospasm may require doses every 3–5 min initially.
Notes	May alternate with albuterol.

Metformin

Proprietary name(s)	Glucophage
Therapeutic class	Antihyperglycemic agent
Indications	NIDDM as monotherapy or in conjunction with sulfonylureas

Actions	Decreases hepatic glucose production, decreases intestinal absorption of glucose, and increases peripheral glucose uptake and utilization
Excretion	Renal
Side effects	Lactic acidosis, diarrhea, nausea, vomiting, abdominal bloating, flatulence, and anorexia
Dose	Dose must be individualized. Start with 500 mg PO 2 times per day and increase to desired blood glucose effect, to a maximum daily dose of 2500 mg. Decrease dose in renal failure.
Notes	Hypoglycemic reactions are not seen as with sulfonylureas.

Metolazone

Proprietary name(s)	Zaroxolyn
Therapeutic class	Quinazoline diuretic
Indications	Hypertension, CHF, edema, and some types of renal failure
Actions	Blocks Na^+ and Cl^+ reabsorption in the cortical diluting segment of the loop of Henle
Excretion	Renal
Side effects	Electrolyte depletion, hyperuricemia, hyperglycemia, and hypomagnesemia. Do not use in anuric patients.
Dose	2.5–10 mg PO every day.
Notes	Similar properties to thiazide diuretics but longer acting than hydrochlorothiazide. Monitor electrolytes. Additive effects when administered with furosemide.

Metronidazole (See antibiotic listing in Appendix 3)

Midazolam

Proprietary name(s)	Versed
Therapeutic class	Benzodiazepine
Indications	Sedation before surgery or diagnostic procedure
Actions	Benzodiazepine sedative-hypnotic
Side effects	Sedation, paradoxical agitation, respiratory depression

Dose	Induction dose, 0.20–0.35 mg/kg IV as needed over 20–30 sec. Reduce dose in elderly patients and in those already receiving other sedative medications.
Notes	Inject slowly to avoid complications of respiratory depression and hypotension. Should be used with appropriate monitoring for respiratory complications. Antidote is flumazenil.

Misoprostol

Proprietary name(s)	Cytotec
Therapeutic class	Synthetic prostaglandin E_1 analogue
Indications	Prophylaxis of NSAID-related gastric ulcers
Actions	Inhibits gastric acid secretion and protects mucosal cells
Excretion	Renal (80%)
Side effects	Diarrhea, abdominal pain, nausea, headache, flatulence, and dyspepsia
Dose	0.1–0.2 mg PO 4 times per day with food.
Notes	Do not administer to pregnant women.

Morphine sulfate

Therapeutic class	Narcotic analgesic
Indications	Moderate to severe pain and pulmonary edema
Actions	Narcotic analgesic and splanchnic venodilation
Metabolism	Hepatic
Excretion	Renal (90%) and biliary (7–10%)
Side effects	Respiratory depression, hypotension, sedation, nausea, vomiting, and constipation
Dose	For pulmonary edema or chest pain due to coronary ischemia, 2–4 mg IV every 5–10 min to a maximum dose of 10–12 mg. For pain, 2–15 mg IV/IM/SC every 4 hr as needed.
Notes	10 mg morphine (IM/SC) is equivalent to 60–80 mg meperidine (IM/SC/PO). Often administered with concomitant antinausea medication. May be habit forming. Antidote is naloxone.

Naloxone hydrochloride

Proprietary name(s)	Narcan
Therapeutic class	Narcotic antagonist
Indications	Reversal of narcotic-induced effects
Actions	Narcotic receptor antagonist
Metabolism	Hepatic
Excretion	Renal
Side effects	Nausea, vomiting, and may precipitate withdrawal in narcotic abusers
Dose	0.2–2.0 mg IV/IM, SC every 5 min to a maximum dose of 10 mg.
Notes	Effects are shorter than most narcotics. Monitor for return of narcotic-induced symptoms, and repeat naloxone dose as necessary. May be administered via ET in emergency situations.

Naproxen

Proprietary name(s)	Naprosyn
Therapeutic class	NSAID
Indications	Inflammation due to arthritis, soft-tissue injury, and pericarditis
Actions	Propionic acid derivative; interferes with production of prostaglandins
Metabolism	Hepatic
Excretion	Renal
Side effects	Headache, dizziness and lightheadedness, and epigastric pain May compromise renal function in patients with renal impairment. Contraindicated in the syndrome of aspirin sensitivity, nasal polyps, and bronchospasm.
Dose	250 mg PO 2 times per day. Maximum dose: 1250 mg/day.
Notes	Should be used with caution in patients receiving anticoagulant medications.

Nifedipine

Proprietary name(s)	Adalat and Procardia
Therapeutic class	Calcium channel blocker
Indications	Angina pectoris, coronary spasm, and hypertension
Actions	Calcium channel blocker and vasodilator
Metabolism	Hepatic
Excretion	Renal (80%)

Side effects	Hypotension, flushing, dizziness, headache, and peripheral edema
Dose	10–30 mg PO 3 times per day. Maximum dose: 180 mg/day.
Notes	The edema due to nifedipine is due to vasodilation and does not respond to diuretics. Hypotension is often difficult to treat with fluids alone and may require vasopressor agent administration. Nifedipine has a greater effect than verapamil and diltiazem on peripheral vasculature.

Nitroglycerin

Therapeutic class	Vasodilator
Indications	Angina pectoris and CHF
Actions	Venous, coronary, and arterial vasodilation
Metabolism	Hepatic
Excretion	Renal
Side effects	Headache, hypotension, and flushing
Dose	Sublingual (SL) 0.15–0.6 mg every 3–5 min. Lingual aerosol 1–2 sprays onto or under the tongue every 3–5 min to a maximum dose of 3 sprays/15 min. Transdermal patch 0.2 mg/hr, increasing to 0.4 mg/hr. Patch should be left on for 10–12 hr and then removed for 12–14 hr to avoid tolerance. Transdermal paste 0.5–4 inches every 4–8 hr. Rotate sites. Oral (sustained-release) 2–9 mg PO 2–3 times per day. IV 0–3 μg/kg/min. Titrate to desired BP.
Notes	Nitrate tolerance may develop with prolonged continuous administration. Dose must be individualized.

Nystatin

Proprietary name(s)	Mycostatin
Therapeutic class	Antifungal
Indications	Oral and esophageal candidiasis
Actions	Disruption of fungal cell membranes
Excretion	Fecal for a PO dose
Side effects	Minimal; nausea and vomiting

Dose   400,000–600,000 U PO swish and
swallow 4 times per day.

Notes   Not absorbed orally.

Omeprazole

Proprietary name(s)   Prilosec

Therapeutic class H^+/K^+-ATPase inhibitor

Indications   Active peptic ulcer disease,
gastroesophageal reflux, severe erosive
esophagitis, gastric acid hypersecretion

Actions   Gastric acid pump inhibitor

Excretion   Renal (77%), remainder biliary

Side effects   Headache, diarrhea, abdominal pain,
nausea, vomiting, rash, dizziness

Dose   For ulcer, reflux, and esophagitis,
20 mg PO every day.
For hypersecretion syndromes, start
with 60 mg PO every day, increase to
120 mg 3 times per day as required
to achieve desired results.

Notes   Not recommended for long-term
maintenance therapy.

Oxazepam

Proprietary name(s)   Serax

Therapeutic class   Benzodiazepine

Indications   Insomnia and anxiety

Actions   Benzodiazepine sedative-hypnotic

Side effects   Sedation, respiratory depression, and
confusion

Dose   For sleep, 10–30 mg PO every night as
needed.
For anxiety, 30–100 mg PO every day in
divided doses.

Notes   Peak effect in 1–4 hr. Relatively short
duration.
Antidote is flumazenil.

Penicillin (See antibiotic listing in Appendix 3)

Pentamidine isethionate

Proprietary name(s)   Pentam

Therapeutic class   Anti-PCP agent

Indications   *Pneumocystis carinii* pneumonia (PCP)

Actions   Unknown

Excretion   Renal

| Side effects | Hypotension, renal failure, cardiac arrhythmias, hypoglycemia, and pancreatitis |
| Dose | 4 mg/kg/day in 50–250 ml 5% dextrose in water IV over 2 hr. Reduce dose in renal-impaired patients. |

Phenazopyridine

Proprietary name(s)	Pyridium
Therapeutic class	Urinary analgesic
Indications	Cystitis and urethritis
Actions	Analgesic effect on inflamed urinary tract mucosa
Excretion	Renal
Side effects	Orange discoloration of secretions including urine, tears, and semen; nausea, headache, rash, and pruritus
Dose	200 mg PO 3 times per day after meals, as needed.
Notes	No antibacterial effects. May stain contact lenses.

Phenytoin

Proprietary name(s)	Dilantin
Therapeutic class	Anticonvulsant
Indications	Seizure disorders, prophylaxis, and treatment
Actions	Anticonvulsant and reduces Na^+ transport across cerebral cell membranes
Metabolism	At therapeutic doses, phenytoin is metabolized by the liver in zero-order kinetics (a fixed amount of drug is metabolized per unit time). Relatively small changes in the dose can cause major changes in serum concentrations in the long term. Serum levels are greatly affected by medications altering microsomal enzyme activity.
Excretion	Renal
Side effects	Hypotension, cardiac dysrhythmias, ataxia, nystagmus, dysarthria, hepatotoxicity, gingival hypertrophy, hirsutism, megaloblastic anemia, lymphadenopathy, fever, and rash

Dose	For status epilepticus, 18 mg/kg IV in NS loading dose at a rate of 25–50 mg/min, followed by a maintenance dose of 300 mg PO/IV every day.
Notes	Dose must be individualized. Follow serum levels.
	IM administration is erratically absorbed.
	Abrupt withdrawal may precipitate seizure activity.

Phytonadione (vitamin K_1)

Proprietary name(s)	AquaMEPHYTON
Therapeutic class	Vitamin replacement
Indications	Replacement in vitamin K deficiency and reversal of warfarin effects
Actions	Vitamin K is essential for hepatic synthesis of clotting factors II, VII, IX, and X
Side effects	Hematoma formation with SC/IM administration
Dose	For reversal of overcoumarinization: 2.5–5.0 mg PO/SC/IM.
	For vitamin supplementation in total parenteral nutrition (TPN): 2.5 mg IM weekly.
Notes	Avoid IV administration because of hypotension and anaphylaxis.
	Severe hemorrhage due to warfarin therapy is best treated with fresh frozen plasma. The effects of vitamin K take several days to overcome with continuous warfarin therapy.

Piperacillin (See antibiotic listing in Appendix 3)

Potassium

Proprietary name(s)	Slow K, Micro-K, and Kay Ciel
Therapeutic class	Potassium supplement
Indications	Hypokalemia
Actions	Potassium supplement
Side effects	Nausea, vomiting, diarrhea, abdominal discomfort, and hyperkalemia
Dose	For prevention, 24–40 mEq/day.
	For treatment, 60–120 mEq/day.
Notes	Danger of hyperkalemia in patients with renal impairment, patients receiving

potassium-sparing diuretics, and
those on ACE inhibitors.

Procainamide

Proprietary name(s)	Procanbid
Therapeutic class	Class IA antiarrhythmic
Indications	Atrial and ventricular arrhythmias
Actions	Reduces the maximum rate of depolarization in atrial and ventricular conducting tissues
Metabolism	Hepatic
Excretion	Renal
Side effects	Hypotension, anorexia, nausea, vomiting, heart block, proarrhythmia, rash, fever, SLE-like syndrome, and arthralgias
Dose	Load with 1 g PO followed by 250–500 mg PO every 3 hr. Delayed-release formulations may be given every 12 hr. For life-threatening tachydysrhythmias, 100 mg IV over 2 min, repeating the dose until the arrhythmia abates or to a maximum dose of 1 g. Follow with a maintenance infusion of 2–4 mg/min.
Notes	Actions are similar to quinidine except no atropinic effect. Cross-allergic with procaine.

Prochlorperazine

Proprietary name(s)	Compazine
Therapeutic class	Phenothiazine
Indications	Agitation, nausea, and vomiting
Actions	Antagonist of dopamine, histamine, muscarine, and α_1-adrenergic responses
Metabolism	Hepatic, with enterohepatic recirculation
Excretion	Renal
Side effects	Drowsiness, dizziness, amenorrhea, blurred vision, skin reactions, hypotension, extrapyramidal effects, jaundice, tardive dyskinesia, and neuroleptic malignant syndrome
Dose	For nausea, 5–10 mg PO/IM every 6–8 hr, as needed, or 2.5–10 mg IV every 6–8 hr, as needed.

Notes — Extrapyramidal symptoms may be treated with diphenhydramine.

Promethazine

Proprietary name(s)	Phenergan
Therapeutic class	Phenothiazine
Indications	Sedation, antianxiety, nausea, and vomiting
Actions	Antihistamine and anticholinergic
Metabolism	Hepatic
Excretion	Renal and fecal
Side effects	Extrapyramidal symptoms, drowsiness, dizziness, constipation, dry mouth, and urinary retention
Dose	25–50 mg PO/PR/IM every 4–6 hr, as needed.
	12.5–25 mg IV every 4–6 hr, as needed.
Notes	Anticholinergic effects are additive with those of other medications such as tricyclic antidepressants.

Propranolol

Proprietary name(s)	Inderal
Therapeutic class	Nonspecific β-blocker
Indications	Angina pectoris, post-MI treatment of supraventricular tachycardia (SVT), hypertension, and thyrotoxicosis
Actions	Nonspecific β-blockade
Metabolism	Hepatic
Excretion	Renal (<1%)
Side effects	Hypotension, bradycardia, bronchospasm, CHF, nausea, vomiting, fatigue, nightmares, and may mask symptoms of hypoglycemia
Dose	10–80 mg PO 2–4 times per day. Begin with a low dose and adjust to desired effect.
Notes	Abrupt withdrawal may precipitate symptoms of angina in patients with coronary artery disease.
	Dose must be individualized.

Protamine sulfate

Therapeutic class	Heparin antagonist
Indications	Reversal of heparin-induced anticoagulation
Actions	Binds to and inactivates heparin

Side effects	Hypotension, bradycardia, and flushing
Dose	1 mg/100 mg heparin. Administer by slow IV push, no more than 50 mg in a 10-min period.
Notes	Overdosage may paradoxically worsen hemorrhage as protamine also possesses anticoagulant properties. Effects may be transient.

Quinine sulfate

Therapeutic class	Antimalarial
Indications	Nocturnal leg cramps
Actions	Increases muscular refractory period, decreases motor endplate excitability, and affects the distribution of calcium within the muscle fiber
Side effects	Nausea, visual disturbances, hemolytic anemia, and thrombocytopenia
Dose	300 mg PO every night as needed.
Notes	Side effects are unusual at this dose, which is $1/10$ that used to treat malaria.

Ranitidine

Proprietary name(s)	Zantac
Therapeutic class	Histamine$_2$ antagonist
Indications	Peptic ulcer disease and gastroesophageal reflux
Actions	Inhibits histamine-induced secretion of gastric acid
Metabolism	Hepatic
Excretion	Renal (30% of PO dose, 70% of IV dose)
Side effects	Jaundice, gynecomastia, headache, confusion, and leukopenia
Dose	For acute symptoms, 50 mg IV every 8 hr or 150 mg PO 2 times per day or 300 mg PO every night. For maintenance therapy, 150 mg PO every night.
Notes	Generally well tolerated. Does not have the same effect as cimetidine on microsomal enzymes or androgen blocking.

Retinol (vitamin A)

Proprietary name(s)	Aquasol A
Therapeutic class	Vitamin replacement
Indications	Replacement in vitamin A deficiency

Actions	Vitamin A is essential in the production of rhodopsin in the eye and preserves the integrity of epithelial cells
Metabolism	Fat-soluble vitamin, stored in liver and excreted in feces
Side effects	Due to overdose. Fatigue, malaise, lethargy, abdominal discomfort, anorexia, nausea, irritability, headache, and skin changes.
Dose	100,000–500,000 U every day × 3 days PO/IM, followed by 50,000 U PO/IM every day × 2 mo.
Notes	May facilitate wound healing in steroid-dependent patients.

Rofecoxib

Proprietary name(s)	Vioxx
Therapeutic class	Selective COX-2 inhibitor
Indications	Osteoarthritis, treatment of acute pain in adults
Actions	Inhibition of prostaglandin production via inhibition of cyclooxygenase-2
Metabolism	Cytosolic enzymes
Excretion	Hepatic metabolism
Side effects	Rare; hepatic dysfunction, fluid retention, edema, GI bleeding
Dose	12.5–50 mg PO per day.
Notes	Not recommended in patients who have aspirin allergy. Less GI upset reported than with nonselective NSAIDs.

Sodium polystyrene sulfonate

Proprietary name(s)	Kayexalate
Therapeutic class	Cation exchange resin
Indications	Hyperkalemia
Actions	Nonabsorbable cation exchange resin
Side effects	Nausea, vomiting, gastric irritation, and sodium retention
Dose	15–30 g in 50–100 ml NS, or 20% sorbitol PO every 3–4 hr, or 50 g in 200 ml 20% sorbitol or 20% dextrose in water PR by retention enema for 30–60 min.
Notes	20 mEq Na^+ is exchanged for 20 mEq K^+ for each 15 g resin given PO. Mg^{2+} and Ca^{2+} may also be exchanged. Actual results are highly variable.

Spironolactone

Proprietary name(s)	Aldactone
Therapeutic class	Aldosterone antagonist and diuretic
Indications	Ascites, edema, hypertension, and hyperaldosteronism
Actions	Aldosterone antagonist
Metabolism	Hepatic (into many active metabolites)
Excretion	Renal > biliary
Side effects	Hyponatremia, gynecomastia, confusion, and headache
Dose	50–100 mg PO per day (may be divided into 4 doses per day as desired). Higher doses may be required in states of hyperaldosteronism.
Notes	Most effective in states of hyperaldosteronism; however, equipotent to thiazide diuretics in the treatment of hypertension.

Sucralfate

Proprietary name(s)	Carafate
Therapeutic class	Sulfated disaccharide
Indications	Peptic ulcer disease, prophylaxis, and treatment
Actions	Formation of an ulcer-adherent complex that acts as a barrier to damage from gastric acid, bile salts, and pepsin; minimal antacid properties
Excretion	Fecal, not absorbed
Side effects	Side effects are rare: constipation, nausea, gastric discomfort, pruritus, rash, dizziness, headache, insomnia, and vertigo
Dose	1 g PO 4 times per day.
Notes	May reduce the absorption and effects of many medications including cimetidine, ciprofloxacin, digoxin, ketoconazole, norfloxacin, phenytoin, ranitidine, tetracycline, and theophylline. Sucralfate binds and sequesters aluminum. Use with caution in renally impaired patients.

Sumatriptan succinate

Proprietary name(s)	Imitrex
Indications	Intermittent treatment of migraine
Actions	Selective 5-hydroxytryptamine-like receptor agonist

Side effects	Causes vasoconstriction, particularly of the dilated carotid circulation in migraine disorder
	May cause coronary artery spasm. Contraindicated in patients with coronary artery disease, concomitant use of ergot alkaloid medication, concomitant use of MAO inhibitors, uncontrolled hypertension, or hemiplegic migraine disorder.
	Flushing, dizziness, feelings of heat, pressure, malaise, fatigue, drowsiness, nausea, and vomiting
Dose	6 mg SC or 100 mg PO.
	If initial dose is partially or completely successful, may repeat doses with an additional 6 mg SC or 100 mg PO.
	Do not exceed a maximum daily PO dose of 300 mg.
	Do not repeat if initial dose has no effect.
Notes	Peak effect in 15 min with SC dose, in 0.5–5 hr with PO dose. A nasal spray formulation is also available.

Tetracycline (See antibiotic listing in Appendix 3)

Thiamine (vitamin B_1)

Therapeutic class	Vitamin replacement
Indications	Thiamine deficiency and prophylaxis of Wernicke's encephalopathy
Actions	Water-soluble vitamin B_1 replacement
Side effects	IV administration associated with hypotension or anaphylactic shock
Dose	100 mg PO/IM/IV every day × 3 days. If given IV, administer over 5 min.
Notes	Well absorbed orally. Consider the PO route, even in emergencies.

Tobramycin (See antibiotic listing in Appendix 3)

Vancomycin (See antibiotic listing in Appendix 3)

Verapamil

| Proprietary name(s) | Isoptin and Calan |
| Therapeutic class | Calcium channel blocker |

Indications	Angina pectoris, treatment of SVTs, hypertension, and left ventricular diastolic dysfunction
Actions	Calcium channel blockade and depresses AV conduction
Metabolism	Hepatic
Excretion	Renal (70%) and fecal
Side effects	CHF, bradycardia, hypotension, headache, dizziness, and constipation
Dose	For angina and hypertension, 80–120 mg PO 3 times per day. For SVT, 5–10 mg IV; IV administration should occur only in monitored patients.
Notes	Calcium gluconate 1–2 g IV may reverse the negative inotropic and hypotensive effects, but not the AV block.

Warfarin

Proprietary name(s)	Coumadin
Therapeutic class	Oral anticoagulant
Indications	Prophylaxis and treatment of DVT, pulmonary embolism, and embolic CVA
Actions	Inhibits vitamin K–dependent clotting factors
Metabolism	Hepatic and microsomal
Excretion	Renal
Side effects	Hemorrhage, nausea, vomiting, skin necrosis, fever, and rash
Dose	10 mg PO every day × 2 days, then estimate maintenance dose at 5–7.5 mg every day PO based on PT.
Notes	Dosage must be individualized to maintain PT in the desired range. Many medications interact to increase or decrease the effects of warfarin. Always look up the interactions with warfarin of any newly prescribed medication. Fresh frozen plasma is the treatment of choice to reverse warfarin-associated hemorrhage. Vitamin K is used if further warfarin therapy is not desired.

Appendix 3:
Antibiotic Standard Doses and Susceptibility Guidelines*

*From Adams GA, Bresnick SD: On Call Surgery, 2nd ed. Philadelphia, WB Saunders, 2001.

TABLE 3–1

Antibiotic Standard Doses and Indications for Patients with Normal Renal Function

Drug	Dosage Range (g/day) IV/IM*	Usual Dosage (g/dosing interval) IV/IM*	Special Comments and Usage
Amikacin	15 mg/kg	7.5 mg/kg every 12 hr	Good coverage for Gram-negative rods Useful for organisms resistant to gentamicin and tobramycin Consider use in patients with Gram-negative infections with contraindication to aminoglycoside use
Amoxicillin	1–6	0.5–1.0 every 8 hr	Good for group B streptococcus, *Streptococcus viridans*, *S. pneumoniae*, and staphylococcus
Ampicillin	2–12	1 every 6 hr	Drug of choice for enterococcus, group B streptococcus, *Listeria*, and actinomycete Useful for treatment of sepsis in combination with an aminoglycoside and either metronidazole or clindamycin
Aztreonam	1–8	0.5–2 every 8 hr	Good Gram-negative coverage Consider use in patients with Gram-negative infections with renal insufficiency or contraindication to aminoglycoside use
Cefazolin	3–6	1 every 8 hr	Most common preoperative antibiotic Good *Staphylococcus aureus* and *Staphylococcus epidermidis* coverage Moderate streptococcus groups A and B coverage Does not cover enterococcus
Cefotaxime	3–8	1–2 every 6–8 hr	Moderate coverage of streptococcus and staphylococcus, but does not cover enterococcus Useful in meningitis due to Gram-negative rods resistant to ampicillin
Cefoxitin	3–6	1–2 every 6–8 hr	Some staphylococcus and streptococcus coverage, and moderate anaerobic Gram-positive (*Clostridium*) and anaerobic Gram-negative coverage (*Bacteroides fragilis*) with a single agent
Ceftazidime	3–6	1 every 8 hr	Good *Pseudomonas* coverage Consider use when Gram-negative infection and aminoglycosides inappropriate

continued

Table 3–1. Antibiotic Standard Doses and Indications for Patients with Normal Renal Function *continued*

Drug	Dosage Range (g/day) IV/IM*	Usual Dosage (g/dosing interval) IV/IM*	Special Comments and Usage
Ceftriaxone	1–4	1–2 every 12–24 hr	Longer half-life than other cephalosporins Moderate staphylococcus and streptococcus coverage
Cefuroxime	2–4.5	0.5–1 every 8 hr	Useful in meningitis due to Gram-negative rods resistant to ampicillin Mixed lung infections in penicillin-allergic patients *Haemophilus influenzae* resistant to ampicillin
Ciprofloxacin	0.4–0.8	200–400 mg every 12 hr	Good coverage for streptococcus and staphylococcus except MRSA and enterococcus Broad-spectrum agent for urinary tract infections and as adjunct for complicated skin infection; also, good bone penetration 500 mg PO every 12 hr has equal bioavailability as 400 mg IV every 12 hr
Clindamycin	0.6–2	0.6 every 8 hr	Good coverage for anaerobes "above the diaphragm" *B. fragilis* dosing
Erythromycin	1–4	0.5 every 6 hr	Drug of choice for *Legionella, Chlamydia, Mycoplasma* Moderate *S. aureus* and streptococcus groups A and B coverage Does not cover *S. epidermidis* or enterococcus
Gentamicin	3–5 mg/kg	1–1.5 mg/kg every 8 hr	Serious aerobic Gram-negative rod infections Follow gentamicin levels and creatinine
Imipenem	1–2	0.5 every 6 hr	Good staphylococcus coverage, except MRSA Good anaerobic and aerobic enteric coverage Consider "big-gun agent"
Metronidazole	1–2	0.5 every 8 hr	Good Gram-negative enteric coverage Good for anaerobes "below the diaphragm" Well absorbed orally Good for pseudomembranous colitis caused by *Clostridium difficile*

Penicillin	2–20 mu	1–4 mu every 4–6 hr	Drug of choice for streptococcal infections Good for oral infections, human bites, and anaerobic infections "above the diaphragm"
Piperacillin	6–12	1.5–2 every 4 hr	Use for *Pseudomonas* infections Moderate Gram-negative enteric coverage
Tetracycline	1–2	0.5 every 6 hr	Avoid use in children or pregnant patients, because bone and tooth development are affected
Tobramycin	3–5 mg/kg	1.5 mg/kg every 8 hr	More effective than gentamicin for *Pseudomonas* infection
Vancomycin	1–2	1 every 12 hr	Drug of choice for MRSA Useful in multidrug-resistant Gram-positive infections

*Unless otherwise specified.
MRSA = methicillin-resistant *Staphylococcus aureus*; mu = million units.

TABLE 3-2

Antibiotic Susceptibility Guidelines (Sensitivities Must Be Checked)

Drug	Pneumococci	Staphylococcus aureus (penicillin resistant)	Haemophilus influenzae	H. influenzae (ampicillin resistant)	Escherichia coli (community acquired)	Klebsiella	Pseudomonas	Coliforms	Above Diaphragm Excluding Bacillus fragilis	B. fragilis
									(Aerobes)	*(Anaerobes)*
Amikacin	–	?	–	–	+	+	+	+	–	–
Ampicillin/amoxicillin	+	–	‡	–	‡	–	–	±	+	–
Cefazolin	+	+	–	–	+	+	–	±	+	–
Cefotaxime	+	?	+	+	+	+	–	+	?	–
Cefoxitin	+	+	–	–	+	+	–	±	+	+
Ceftazidime	?	?	+	+	+	+	+	+	?	–
Ceftriaxone	+	?	+	+	+	+	–	+	–	–
Cefuroxime	+	+	+	+	+	+	–	±	+	–
Chloramphenicol	+	+	+	+	+	+	–	+	+	+
Ciprofloxacin	–	+	+	+	+	+	+	±	–	–
Clindamycin	+	+	–	–	–	–	–	–	+	+
Cloxacillin	+	‡	–	–	–	–	–	–	–	–
Co-trimoxazole	±	±	+	+	+	–	–	–	–	–
Erythromycin	+	+	?	?	–	–	–	–	?	?

	1	2	3	4	5	6	7	8	9	10
Gentamicin	−	?	−	+	+	+	+	−	−	−
Imipenem	+	+	+	+	+	+	+	+	+	+
Metronidazole	−	−	++	−	−	−	−	++	++	++
Penicillin	++	−	+	+	−	−	−	++	−	−
Piperacillin	+	−	+	+	+	+	+	+	+	+
Tetracycline	±	?	−	±	±	±	±	±	±	±
Tobramycin	−	−	−	+	++	+	+	+	+	+
Vancomycin	+	+	−	−	−	−	−	−	−	−

Courtesy of St. Paul's Formulary, St. Paul's Hospital, Vancouver, British Columbia, Canada.
++ = drug of choice; + = effective; − = not effective; ± = depends on sensitivities; ? = clinical efficacy not proven.

Index

Note: Page numbers followed by f indicate figures; those followed by t indicate tables.

754

Index

Index